HEALTH PROMOTION FOR NURSES

A PRACTICAL GUIDE

THE PEDAGOGY

Health Promotion for Nurses: A Practical Guide drives comprehension through various strategies that meet the learning needs of students, while also generating enthusiasm about the topic. This interactive approach addresses different learning styles, making this the ideal text to ensure mastery of key concepts. The pedagogical aids that appear in most chapters include the following:

Learning Objectives

These objectives provide instructors and students with a snapshot of the key information they will encounter in each chapter. They serve as a checklist to help guide and focus study. Objectives can also be found on the companion website at http://go.jblearning.com/healthpromotion.

Key Terms

Found in a list at the beginning of each chapter, these terms will create an expanded vocabulary. The "www" icon directs students to the companion website http://go.jblearning.com/healthpromotion to see these terms in an interactive glossary and use flashcards and word puzzles to nail the definitions.

LEARNING OBJECTIVES

Upon completion of this chapter, you will be able to:

1. Define theory and concept.
2. Discuss the relationship between theory and concept.
3. Differentiate between a grand theory and a midrange theory.
4. Describe a model and its relationship to theory and concepts.
5. Define a schematic model.
6. Discuss the role of theories in health promotion and disease prevention.
7. Explain the development of the health belief model.
8. Reiterate the beliefs needed to

KEY TERMS   www.

Bio-psycho-social-spiritual model

Clark wellness model

Concept

Conceptual model

Expanded health belief model

Grand theories

Health belief model

Health education mod

Health promotion mod

Hypothesis

Midrange theories

Model

1. Define theory and concept.
2. Discuss the relationship between theory and concept.
3. Differentiate between a grand theory and a midrange theory.
4. Describe a model and its relationship to theory and concepts.
5. Define a schematic model.
6. Discuss the role of theories in health promotion and disease prevention.

Ask Yourself

The Ask Yourself feature encourages active learning and promotes critical thinking skills in learners. Students can analyze the situation they are presented with and solve problems so they can learn how the information in the text applies to everyday practice online at http://go.jblearning.com/healthpromotion.

> ### ASK YOURSELF
>
> You are planning to study a population of clients who have high cholesterol levels, with the goal of developing a prevention program. You have decided to use the health belief model as your framework. What areas might you explore?

Hot Topics

Encourage students to research current trends and topics in the field of health promotion.

outweigh all of the arguments in favor of performing the

HOT TOPICS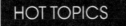

Here are some topics to explore:
- Bandura's self-efficacy theory
- Value-expectancy theories
- HR3200 (healthcare bill)
- Health insurance and health promotion
- Theory of planned behavior
- Theory of reasoned action

THE PEDAGOGY

Health Promotion Challenges

Each chapter includes health promotion challenges to introduce new content to students and encourage them to reflect on key concepts.

environment, culture, gender, and other social factors have on the decision-making and implementation process.

HEALTH PROMOTION CHALLENGE

Most smokers are well aware of the risks of smoking. Even smokers who contemplate quitting take no actions toward it because they find the side effects of quitting to be too great a challenge. What strategies can be employed to help a smoker in the contemplation stage of quitting move to preparation and action?

Case Studies

Case studies encourage active learning and promote critical thinking skills in learners. Students can analyze the situation they are presented with and solve problems so they can learn how the information in the text applies to everyday practice online at http://go.jblearning.com/healthpromotion.

CASE STUDY

Charles, a 28-year-old man, started smoking an occasional cigarette while in high school. After he graduated, he attended a community college where his friends also smoked. His own parents had smoked for years, and he grew up in a household exposed to secondhand smoke. Currently, Charles has two jobs: During the daytime he works at a local mall as a cell phone salesman, and in the evenings and on weekends he is a musician, playing keyboards with a local band, which requires traveling to gigs and late hours. The late hours he works as a musician, the atmosphere of the venues he often plays (bars, clubs, and restaurants), and the fact that many of his friends and acquaintances smoke makes it difficult for him to avoid smokers.

Although Charles does not consider himself a real smoker, as he smokes less than a pack per day, he always thought he could just quit at anytime. Last year, however, his live-in girlfriend (a nonsmoker), asked him to quit. He found that quitting was not as easy as he expected, and while he stopped smoking in their apartment, he continued smoking cigarettes when he was around others who smoke, mostly during or after gigs. Charles says that he probably would have continued this way indefinitely, but his father was diagnosed with Stage IV lung cancer only a few weeks ago. "My mother is devastated," he says. "It's a real wake-up call. She's quitting because of it, and she wants me to quit, too. And I know she's right—if I don't quit, this could happen to me." Nevertheless, despite ...king now, Charles says his behavior ...ven knowing that it's the last thing I

CASE STUDY

Charles, a 28-year-old man, started smoking an occasional cigarette while in high school. After he graduated, he attended a community college where his friends also smoked. His own parents had smoked for years, and he grew up in a household exposed to secondhand smoke. Currently, Charles has two jobs: During the daytime he works at a local mall as a cell phone salesman, and in the evenings and on weekends he is a musician, playing keyboards with a local band, which requires traveling to gigs and late hours. The late hours he works

Summary   69

REVIEW QUESTIONS   [www.]

1. A value expectancy theory
   a. Incorporates the idea that one has the desire to get well and a belief that a specific health action would prevent illness.
   b. Is a theory that helps define health for an individual.
   c. Explains a belief by an individual that there are too many barriers to successfully achieving disease prevention.
2. The PRECEDE-PROCEED framework
   a. Was developed by Pender.
   b. Includes the defining concept of self-efficacy.
   c. Includes assessments of environment, ecology, and education of a community/individual.
3. The health promotion model includes the following assumption:
   a. Perceived benefits and barriers to achievement of health behaviors regulate health seeking activities.
   b. Individuals seek to actively regulate their own behavior.
   c. Health and health risks have multiple determinants.
4. Self-efficacy theory is
   a. A belief or conviction by the individual that he or she is able to successfully execute the behavior needed for producing the desired outcome.
   b. A systematic planning process with the primary goal of empowering individuals and communities to understand and engage in efforts to improve the quality of their lives.
   c. A theory that incorporates the assumptions that one has the desire to avoid illness or get well and a belief that a specific health action by that person would prevent illness.
5. The expanded health belief model includes
   a. The self-efficacy concept.
   b. Epidemiologic assessment.
   c. The proposition that when positive emotions or affect are associated with a behavior, the probability of commitment and action is increased.
6. A theory
   a. Links practice to theory.
   b. Is a set of interrelated ideas that represent a way to describe a phenomenon.
   c. Is a systematic collection of concepts and propositions.
   d. Is all of the above.
7. The relationship between a concept and a theory is
   a. Concepts are constructed from multiple theories.
   b. Theories are extensively tested before they generate concepts.
   c. Concepts put together will make a theory.
   d. Concepts are more abstract than theories.

Review Questions

Utilize these multiple-choice questions to review key topics and apply information in the text to everyday practice. Students can test their knowledge online at http://go.jblearning.com/healthpromotion.

REVIEW QUESTIONS   [w]

1. A value expectancy theory
   a. Incorporates the idea that one has the desire to get well and a belief that a specific health action would prevent illness.
   b. Is a theory that helps define health for an individual.
   c. Explains a belief by an individual that there are too many barriers to successfully achieving disease prevention.
2. The PRECEDE-PROCEED framework

Exercises

Each chapter includes exercises that students can work on individually or in a group after reading through the material. The "www" icon directs students to the companion website http://go.jblearning.com/healthpromotion to delve deeper into concepts by completing these exercises online.

EXERCISES

1. Find research in your area of interest that uses the expanded health belief model work. Discuss the incorporation of the model's key concepts and definitions

2. Apply the PRECEDE-PROCEED framework to a community health problem ested in. Outline the various activities and assessments you would complete problem and devise a plan of action and evaluation based on your supposed

3. Search the literature for information on self-efficacy theory. Prepare a short studies that you found to be particularly interesting.

4. Find two studies that used the health promotion model for their framework. assumptions and propositions the studies were based on.

HEALTH PROMOTION FOR NURSES

A PRACTICAL GUIDE

Carolyn Chambers Clark, EdD, RN, ARNP, FAAN
Director of Wellness, Self-Care and Relationship Resources
Nursing and Health Services
Walden University
Minneapolis, Minnesota

Karen K. Paraska, PhD, MSN, CRNP
Assistant Professor
Duquesne University
Pittsburgh, Pennsylvania

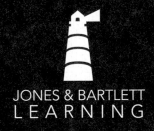

JONES & BARTLETT
LEARNING

World Headquarters
Jones & Bartlett Learning
5 Wall Street
Burlington, MA 01803
978-443-5000
info@jblearning.com
www.jblearning.com

Jones & Bartlett Learning books and products are available through most bookstores and online booksellers. To contact Jones & Bartlett Learning directly, call 800-832-0034, fax 978-443-8000, or visit our website, www.jblearning.com.

Additional credits appear on page 719, which constitutes a continuation of the copyright page.

Production Credits
Publisher: Kevin Sullivan
Acquisitions Editor: Amanda Harvey
Editorial Assistant: Sara Bempkins
Developmental Editor: Elizabeth Platt
Associate Production Editor: Cindie Bryan
Senior Marketing Manager: Elena McAnespie

V.P., Manufacturing and Inventory Control: Therese Connell
Composition: Publishers' Design and Production Services, Inc.
Cover Design: Kristin E. Parker
Rights & Photo Research Assistant: Joseph Veiga
Cover Image: © Myper/ShutterStock, Inc.
Printing and Binding: Courier Companies
Cover Printing: Courier Companies

To order this product, use ISBN: 1-978-1-4496-8667-3

Library of Congress Cataloging-in-Publication Data
Clark, Carolyn Chambers.
  Health promotion for nurses : a practical guide / Carolyn Chambers Clark and Karen Paraska. — 1st ed.
      p. ; cm.
  Includes bibliographical references and index.
  ISBN 978-0-7637-8163-7 (pbk.) — ISBN 0-7637-8163-0 (pbk.)
  I. Paraska, Karen. II. Title.
  [DNLM: 1.   Health Promotion. 2.   Nursing Care. 3.   Nurse's Role.   WY 100.1]
  610.73—dc23
                                                                                          2012012920

6048

Printed in the United States of America
16   15   14   13   12   10 9 8 7 6 5 4 3 2 1

DEDICATION

To all the nurses past, present, and future, who promote health and wellness.

—Carolyn Chambers Clark

CONTENTS

Part 1: Health Promotion and Theory   1

Part 2: Health Promotion In Action 143

Part 3: Health Promotion and Evidence-Based Practice   307

Part 4: Appendix 477

INTRODUCTION

Health Promotion for Nurses: A Practical Guide is meant for you, the basic nursing student. This book is important because health promotion and illness prevention are major avenues for reducing healthcare costs and early death. For this reason, we have included many activities to help you start thinking about health promotion opportunities and practicing ways to act on them. As you are a role model for health promotion, we also present ways to help you on your journey to health and wellness.

Part 1 introduces you to health and health promotion. It differentiates concepts, models and theories and outlines the nurse's role in health promotion.

Part 2 provides definitions, measures, and nursing interventions for physical, mental, and family health. It also takes a broader look at the issue of health promotion with an in-depth discussion of healthcare policy and how it affects health promotion in the United States.

Parts 3 and 4 are more advanced and include specific interventions.

Because they are evidence-based, they could also be used by RNs, graduate nursing students and nurse practitioners.

Part 3 includes information about evidence-based health promotion, including how to develop evidence-based health promotion research questions; how to use natural and noninvasive approaches to promote health; and how to develop, facilitate, measure and evaluate health promotion programs, with a focus on community. Part 3 also identifies the four main causes of death in the United States: insufficient exercise, poor nutrition, smoking, and drinking. Because the number of consumers with chronic conditions related to these four issues is growing at an astonishing rate, we present ways to help you learn how to assist clients with self-management and prevention activities.

Although the medical healthcare system is based on treating acute disease, nursing is in the forefront of developing interventions for the much larger population of clients who suffer from chronic conditions and in teaching self-management procedures, which have become a high priority for chronic conditions.

Part 4 contains an appendix of health promotion interventions for 32 chronic conditions. Each intervention is evidence-based and focuses on self-management and complementary approaches to health and wellness.

Taken as a whole, *Health Promotion for Nurses, A Practical Guide* offers a valuable and unique approach to health promotion and wellness. The book provides not only in-depth coverage of theory and research, but also provides specific information for the clinical application of preventive and health promotion actions.

CONTRIBUTORS

Pamela P. DiNapoli, PhD, RN
Associate Professor of Nursing
University of New Hampshire, Department of Nursing
Durham, New Hampshire

Judith Gammonley, EdD, ARNP, BC
Morton Plant Mease BayCare Health System

Cecile A. Lengacher, PhD, RN, FAAN
Professor and Director of the BS-PhD Program
University of South Florida, College of Nursing
Tampa, Florida

Carolyn T. Martin, PhD, RN, CFNP
Graduate Coordinator
California State University, Stanislaus, Department of Nursing
Turlock, California

Susanne M. Tracy, PhD, RN
Assistant Professor of Nursing
University of New Hampshire, Department of Nursing
Durham, New Hampshire

REVIEWERS

Joyce Azzaline, DHSc, APRN-BC
Associate Professor of Nursing
Trinity Christian College
Palos Heights, Illinois

Jeri L. Brandt, PhD, RN
Professor of Nursing
Nebraska Wesleyan University
Lincoln, Nebraska

Betty Dornbrook, MSN, ANP-C
Associate Professor
Madonna University
Livonia, Michigan

Debra A. Hunt, PhD, ARNP-BC
Assistant Professor
University of Central Florida
College of Nursing
Orlando Florida

Barbara James, DSN, RN, CNE
Dean & Professor
Southern Adventist University School of Nursing
Collegedale, Tennessee

Debora E. Kirsch, RN, MS, CNS, PhDc
Director of Undergraduate Nursing Studies
Clinical Assistant Professor of Nursing
SUNY Upstate Medical University
Syracuse, New York

Mary J. Kulp, MSN, RN
Associate Professor
Jefferson Community and Technical College
Carrollton Campus
Louisville, Kentucky

Margaret Lunney, PhD, RN
Doctoral Faculty, CUNY Graduate Center
Professor and Graduate Nursing Programs Coordinator
College of Staten Island
Department of Nursing
Staten Island, New York

Patricia S. Martin, MSN, RN
Assistant Professor
RN-BSN Program Coordinator
University of Louisville
School of Nursing
Louisville, Kentucky

Paula L. McNiel, DNP, RN
Assistant Professor
College of Nursing
University of Wisconsin, Oshkosh
Oshkosh, Wisconsin

Vanessa Miller, PhD
Department of Psychology
Texas Christian University
Fort Worth, Texas

Elizabeth R. Pratt, MSN, RNC
Assistant Professor of Nursing
Southern Arkansas University
Magnolia, Arkansas

Charlene Thomas, PhD, RN
Assistant Professor
Aurora University
Aurora, Illinois

Diane Whitehead, EdD, RN, ANEF
Director Doctorate Nursing Practice
Program/Professor
Nova Southeastern University
Fort Lauderdale, Florida

PART 1

Health Promotion and Theory

Upon completion of this chapter, you will be able to:

1. Discuss the concepts of patient versus client.

2. Analyze the historical evolution of the multidimensional aspects of health.

3. Contrast the concepts of health and wellness.

4. Compare the dimensions of health on the health–illness continuum.

5. Contrast the various definitions of health promotion.

6. Identify the six key aspects of health and analyze the factors that are determinants of health.

7. Define ethnomedical ethnic systems and explain how cultural factors may affect health promotion.

8. Differentiate the three levels of disease prevention: primary, secondary, and tertiary.

9. Discuss key aspects of Leavell and Clark's conceptual map of prevention.

Adaptive dimension

Client

Clinical dimension

Determinants of health

Dimensions of health

Disease prevention

Eudaimonistic dimension

Health

Health versus wellness

Health promotion

Healthy People 2020

High-level wellness

Primary prevention

Quality of life

Role-performance dimension

Secondary prevention

Tertiary prevention

Wellness

CHAPTER 1

Health and Health Promotion

http://go.jblearning.com/healthpromotion

For a full suite of assignments and learning activities, use the access code located in the front of your book to visit the exclusive website: http://go.jblearning.com/healthpromotion If you do not have an access code, you can obtain one at the site.

Introduction

Despite being the central focus (and goal) of health promotion, health and its definitions are not simple matters. Health can mean different things to different people.

Health promotion often demands a significant, if not total, effort from each person in order to evolve. For that reason, throughout this book, we use the word **client** to indicate a more equal level of power in the relationship. As one client said,

> As a patient, I am clearly at the mercy of someone else who holds the cards. They decide things for me, not with me. They do things to me and I rarely have a real choice. It is often a subordinate relationship. The word "client" implies that I am a consumer with free will and the ability to make choices. (Baird, 2011, p. 1)

Given this power, a client's definition of what's healthy may conflict with the nurse's ideas about how to promote health. So, it is important to start with a few basic points about our central concept.

An Evolving Definition of Health

Florence Nightingale (FIGURE 1-1) described modern concepts of health and health promotion in her publication, *Notes on Nursing*. She published her book in 1860, but the interventions she described were decades ahead of their time.

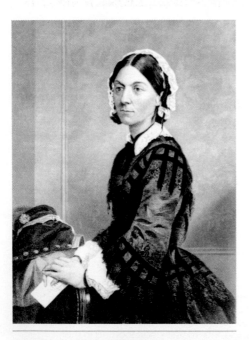

Nightingale developed her definitions of health during the Crimean War while working in unsanitary conditions. From these experiences, she developed a novel concept. She recognized that disease stemmed from factors that could be addressed *before illness developed* by paying attention to physiologic or environmental processes that laid the groundwork for the disease. She described how factors such as hunger, basic sanitation, overcrowding, poor nutrition, and lack of clean drinking water affect health. She argued that nurses must be concerned with each of these if we wish to support the reparative process that the body undertakes naturally (Nightingale, 1860).

In Nightingale's time, and up until World War II, infectious diseases caused most deaths worldwide. They defined **health** as the absence of infection in an individual. Prior to the war, international consensus defined health simply as the absence of disease or illness World Health Organization [WHO] (1958, p. 1).

FIGURE 1-1   Florence Nightingale
Source: National Library of Medicine

As knowledge grew, the term, *health*, became multidimensional. In recognition of this reality, in 1946, the World Health Organization (WHO) began its constitution by emphasizing the concept of wholeness and positive qualities of health with the following definition: "Health is a state of complete physical, mental, and social well-being and not merely the absence of disease and infirmity" (WHO, 1948, p. 1). This definition implies that there is an intrinsic relationship between the body and the welfare of the self.

In the more than 60 years since WHO's constitution was written, definitions of health have broadened to include spiritual and emotional aspects. In 1986, WHO (p. 1) expanded upon its original definition (see BOX 1-1) to note that "[h]ealth is a positive concept emphasizing social and personal resources, as well as physical capacities." In 2006, WHO added two new concepts to its health lexicon: that of wellness, which was defined in terms of optimal physical, psychological, spiritual, and economic health as well as the ability to fulfill social roles, and global health, which acknowledged for the first time the global impacts of certain health issues (Smith, Tang, & Nutbeam, 2006).

BOX 1-1 The World Health Organization's Evolving Definitions of Health and Wellness

» **WHO, 1946:** "*Health* is a state of complete physical, mental, and social well-being and not merely the absence of disease or infirmity."

» **WHO, 1986:** "*Health* is . . . a resource for everyday life, not the objective of living. Health is a positive concept emphasizing social and personal resources, as well as physical capacities."

» **SMITH, TANG, & NUTBEAM, 2006:** "*Wellness* is the optimal state of health of individuals and groups . . . [including] the realization of the fullest potential of an individual physically, psychologically, socially, spiritually and economically, and the fulfillment of one's role expectations in the family, community, place of worship, workplace and other settings."

» **SMITH, TANG, & NUTBEAM, 2006:** "*Global health* refers to the transnational impacts of globalization upon health determinants and health problems which are the beyond the control of individual nations."

REFERENCES

Smith, B. J., Tang, K. C., & Nutbeam, D. (2006). "WHO health promotion glossary: New terms." *Health Promotion International, 21*(4), 340–345.

World Health Organization. (1946). *Preamble to the Constitution of the World Health Organization.* Signed at the International Health Conference, New York, July 22, 1946.

World Health Organization. (1986). *Ottawa Charter for Health Promotion.* First International Conference on Health Promotion, Ottawa, Canada, November 21, 1986—WHO/HPR/HEP/95.1.

For our purposes, we will use Murray and colleagues' (2009) definition of health:

> Health is a state of well-being in which the person uses adaptive responses physically, mentally, emotionally, spiritually, and socially in response to external and internal stimuli or stressors. The purpose of health is to maintain relative stability and comfort and to achieve personal objectives that emphasize characteristics of strength, resilience, resources, and capabilities rather than on pathology. (p. 2)

Health is a state of well-being. Health is the place we are at at any given moment in relation to our physical, emotional, social, spiritual, and intellectual self. Health is believed to exist throughout life, interspersed with periods of injury, illness, or disease. Optimal health is a dynamic balance of physical, emotional, social, spiritual, and intellectual health. Health can be measured with thermometers, blood pressure machines, and blood tests, but **wellness** is the client's assessment of his or her physical, emotional, social, spiritual, environmental, and intellectual status. It is possible to be dying and still feel well if death is accepted and peace is prevalent.

Dunn (1961) coined the term **high-level wellness**. Key concepts include maximizing one's potential, having direction and purpose in life, meeting the challenges of the environment, looking beyond the needs of self to the needs of society, and doing it all with joy or a zest for life. In this framework, the nurse is a facilitator who teaches clients how to self-assess, decide on wellness goals, plan on actions to meet those goals, and self-evaluate success.

The evolution of the definitions of health and wellness reflects a growing understanding that while being healthy is primarily associated with the absence of disease, health and wellness are not absolute conditions, nor are they usually perceived that way.

Here is an example: According to results from the Canadian Community Health Survey–Healthy Aging, 76% of Canadians in mid-life (45 to 64 years old) and 56% of seniors reported that they experienced "good health" in 2009 (Ramage-Morin, Shields, & Martel, 2010). This is based on a definition of health composed of positive self-perceived general and mental health and wellness, functional ability, and independence in activities of daily living. Good health, according to this definition, was reported even by persons who had chronic conditions such as high blood pressure, arthritis, and back problems, all of which were common among people aged 45 or older.

Most individuals want to be healthy, however they define that state. Even when optimal health is not a reasonable possibility (in persons with chronic diseases or disabling conditions, for example), a wish to be healthier is common. At its foundation, **health promotion** is a method that seeks to help individuals, families, and communities reach this goal. We will further define health promotion later in this chapter.

Multiple Dimensions of Health

As noted earlier, health is multidimensional—so health can be promoted along a number of different routes. Before delving into a more complex definition of health promotion, it is worth discussing what these dimensions might be.

Smith (1983) provided a description of health that may be useful. This description involves underlying concepts of actualization and stability. In this description of health, each dimension is defined by extremes on the health–illness continuum.

1. *Clinical dimension:* In this dimension, the absence of disease signs and symptoms indicate health. Illness would be at the extreme opposite with obvious identifiable evidence of disease through specific signs and symptoms. Health extreme: absence of signs or symptoms of disease. Illness extreme: presence of signs or symptoms of disease.
2. *Role-performance dimension:* This dimension defines health as the ability of a person to perform social roles, including those involving work and family, based on societal expectations. Illness is when the person is unable to perform his or her role at this level of expectation. Health extreme: performance of social roles with maximum output. Illness extreme: failure to perform one's social roles.
3. *Adaptive dimension:* This is defined by the ability to adapt positively to social, mental, and physiological change for health, while illness means failure to adapt. Health extreme: flexible adaptation to the environment. Illness extreme: alienation and maladaptation to the environment.
4. *Eudaimonistic dimension:* This dimension is derived from a Greek term that means exuberant well-being. One end of the dimension includes positive interaction among the physical, social, psychological, and spiritual aspects of the environment, while the other includes a lack of involvement or apathy/wasting away due to illness. Health extreme: exuberant well-being. Illness extreme: devitalized with increasing debility.

When you seek to promote health in an individual, a family, or a community, any (or all) of these ***dimensions of health*** can become a focal point for health promotion efforts. Your role is to identify where, in each of these dimensions, the client can move toward wellness and to actively work to promote improvement along each axis (FIGURE 1-2). It is not enough to simply address the clinical dimension in a client who has a disease, given that many factors contributing to the disease occur along other dimensions.

Consider the following hypothetical example: Suppose you are asked to work with a 40-year-old man, married 15 years with two young children, who is suffering from chronic lower back pain related to a car accident that took place 18 months prior. He has been using opiate pain medications since the accident, but he complains that they are not always effective anymore. He has been offered higher doses by his doctor, but he worries about becoming

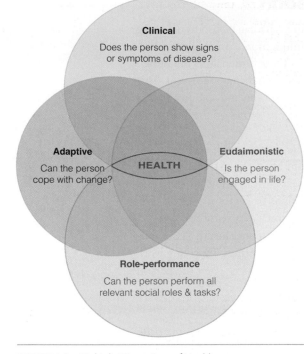

FIGURE 1-2   Multiple Dimensions of Health

addicted to opioids and fears that keeping such drugs in the house will make him vulnerable to thieves if anyone should find out he has them. As a result, he is often in significant pain. The pain affects the man's ability to work, play with and care for his children, and participate in sports and many other activities he used to enjoy. He tries to work through the pain but often is not successful, and his mood varies in accordance with his success. At times, he is irritable, depressed, and prone to lashing out at his wife and kids, and his relationship with his family has been adversely affected as a result. He comments that at 40, he did not expect to be a decrepit old man already.

This hypothetical client offers a number of opportunities for successful interventions. First, let us look at the clinical dimension. Pain management through opioid medications (e.g., oxycodone) is attractive because pain relief is thorough and, for short, acute bouts of pain, the likelihood of drug tolerance or dependence is limited. While they are an option for acute episodes of severe pain, opioids do not work better than NSAIDs for long-term, chronic pain conditions, yet they have a stronger likelihood of addiction and misuse when used for more than a few months (Jamison, Serraillier, & Michna, 2011; White, Arnold, Norvell, Ecker, & Fehlings, 2011). While concerns about addiction, the development of drug tolerance, and withdrawal symptoms upon discontinuation are probably the most significant drawbacks, of opioid use there are other clear-cut physiologic side effects, apart from addiction, that make opioids less attractive for treating chronic pain long-term (Furlan, Sandoval, Mailis-Gagnon, & Tunks, 2006; Gore, Sadosky, Leslie, Tai, & Emery, 2012; Von Korff, Kolodny, Deyo, & Chou, 2011). Constipation, dizziness, drowsiness, and nausea are among the most common side effects, and delayed gastric emptying, immune suppression, and muscle rigidity are known to occur in long-term opioid treatment. Opioids also tend to work less effectively on pain related to the central nervous system (brain and spinal cord) (Benyamin et al., 2008).

These clinical facts, taken together, support the client's wish to find an alternative to opioid pain medications. But even more important are the factors related to other dimensions of health. The client's physical condition impairs his ability to function in his roles as an employee, a husband, and a father—and, as revealed by his concern about theft, as a family protector. While pain may be causing some of his mood swings, it is likely that his poor health in the role-performance dimension is also affecting his mood. The stress he experiences as a result of his inability to meet the expectations of his roles may in turn be adding to his physical pain.

He is also doing poorly in terms of his adaptive and eudaimonistic dimensions. His sole strategy for coping is to work through the pain by ignoring his body's signals regarding its needs in order to meet the need to fulfill his roles. This decision puts his personal well-being in direct conflict with his role-performance needs and results in poor outcomes on *both* fronts. The outbursts of anger are a clear indication that he is unable to manage the stress of juggling these conflicts, and he is also is unable to find alternative solutions.

This is where a nurse trained in health promotion can offer some assistance. The nurse can address the clinical issue—back pain—by providing information about safe and effective nonmedical approaches and allowing the client to choose which method of safe pain relief might be best for him. You can ask the client if he would like to learn progressive relaxation or listen to a relaxation tape that can help relax his muscles and reduce pain. The nurse can also refer the client to a massage therapist or to physical or occupational therapy that will retrain him to use his body in ways that support his back's normal functioning. Other options include offering alternate forms of pain relief, such as acupuncture, which has been shown to be effective in pain relief (Manheimer, White, Berman, Forys, & Ernst, 2005; Moritz et al., 2011; Trigkilidas, 2010). These actions will not only address the clinical issue, but also will address one of the client's emotional concerns by supporting his desire to keep opioid drugs out of his home. Unless the other three dimensions on the health–illness continuum are addressed, his *total* health may not improve. This client needs to learn adaptive strategies for managing his pain, rather than ignore it. The nurse can offer the client cognitive behavioral therapy, meditation, and other methods of mind–body management as appropriate measures to help the client learn better coping skills and explore new ways of fulfilling his roles (Thorn et al., 2011). (These measures are discussed elsewhere in this text.) In such cases, the nurse's role is to look beyond the simple clinical manifestations of physical illness and address the factors that are causing the client distress on all levels.

To obtain more information about personal and global well-being, explore the website at http://www.nationalaccountsofwellbeing.org/explore/indicators/zsocial

☐ Mental Health

Throughout much of history, concepts of health focused primarily on the health of the body. It has not been until fairly recently that mental health has been recognized as a key factor in the health of a person in terms of the connections between body, mind, and spirit. The Surgeon General's 1999 report on mental health explained these connections succinctly:

> Considering health and illness as points along a continuum helps one appreciate that neither state exists in pure isolation from the other. In another but related context, everyday language tends to encourage a misperception that "mental health" or "mental illness" is unrelated to "physical health" or "physical illness." In fact, the two are inseparable. (Office of the Surgeon General, 1999, p.1)

Mental health overlaps physical health in that many psychiatric and developmental disabilities are founded in physiologic issues, which can include genetic disorders, injuries to the brain and nervous system, neurochemical imbalances, early learned behaviors, and even nutritional deficits. The manifestations of mental health disturbances often affect the emotional and social realms and vice versa. For this reason, mental health issues have often been met with fear, misunderstanding, and contempt by society at large and even some healthcare professionals. While great strides have been made in understanding the origins of psychiatric and psychological disorders, mental health issues still carry significant stigma (Parton, 2011). This stigma, as well as the disorder itself, can represent both a significant burden to physical health and a barrier to health promotion.

While this stigma continues, hope is born in a study that looks at primary prevention of mental health problems in Australia. The researchers investigated changes in standardized academic performance across the 2-year implementation of a mental health initiative in 96 Australian elementary schools that focused on improving student social–emotional competencies. They used the KidsMatter program, and after controlling for socioeconomic differences, they found a significant positive relationship existed between quality of implementation and academic performance. The difference between students in high- and low-implementing schools was equivalent to a difference in academic performance of up to 6 months of schooling. The key practitioner message is that, given the known relationship between student academic achievement and mental health, many nations are mounting school-based mental health interventions (Dix, Slee, Lawson, & Keeves, 2012).

☐ Quality of Life

Another consideration that has developed in recent decades is concern for an individual's **quality of life**. Quality of life is almost wholly subjective, because it centers around the individual's own sense of well-being, which is itself hard to define (Andrews & Withey, 1976; Diener, 2000; Ryff & Keyes 1995; Wiseman, McLeod, & Zubrick, 2007):

There is no consensus around a single definition of well-being, but there is general agreement that at minimum, well-being includes the presence of positive emotions and moods (e.g., contentment, happiness), the absence of negative emotions (e.g., depression, anxiety), satisfaction with life, fulfillment and positive functioning. (Centers for Disease Control and Prevention [CDC], 2011)

Individuals with significant physical disabilities can, and often do, have high quality of life. In the presence of significant physical illness, maximizing quality of life is often part of the health goal, particularly if there is no method of reducing or alleviating physical symptoms. In contrast, some mental health issues can markedly reduce the quality of life in even a person with good physical health—and in extreme cases, mental health issues affect physical health negatively, which further reduces quality of life. Quality of life is therefore a central concern for people suffering from both mental and physical illness. Taking a wellness approach and asking clients to define what they mean by quality of life could be a first step in clarifying the confusion.

HEALTH PROMOTION CHALLENGE

If you were to develop a tool to help clients define their quality of life, what would you include and how would you test it out?

What Is Health Promotion?

Health promotion has evolved over the past 30 years; as a result, it has as many definitions as the concept of health itself does. Each one generally entails the concept of improving the health of individuals, families, and communities.

In its 1986 *Ottawa Charter for Health Promotion* (p. 425), WHO defined health promotion as "the process of enabling people to increase control over, and to improve, their health." This definition was groundbreaking in that it directly states that individuals should be actively engaged in supporting their own health. However, the charter offers no suggestions as to how the health promotion process works. A more detailed definition of health promotion proposed by Maville and Huerta (2002) reflects the multiple themes and issues found in the literature:

Health promotion is any endeavor directed at enhancing the quality of health and well-being of individuals, families, groups, communities, and/or nations through strategies involving supportive environments, coordination of resources, and respect for personal choice and values. Related concepts, including health education, health protection, and disease prevention are part of the broader concept of health promotion. The definition that an individual or organization adopts depends upon political, societal, and philosophical viewpoints (p. 3).

These points are consistent with what the World Health Organization incorporates into its definition of health, including positive attributes that consider not only the person's physical aspects, but also their social and personal resources (WHO, 1986).

Still other definitions exist, and some have nuances that merit attention. For example, consider each of the following alternate definitions of health promotion:

1. Health promotion is behavior motivated by the desire to increase well-being and actualize human health potential, whereby disease prevention or health protection is behavior motivated by a desire to actively avoid illness (primary prevention), detect it early (secondary prevention), or maintain functioning within constraints of an illness (tertiary prevention) (Pender, Murdaugh, & Parsons, 2006).

2. Health promotion is the art and science of helping people discover the synergies between their core passions and optimal health, enhancing their motivation to strive for optimal health, and supporting them in changing their lifestyle to move toward a state of optimal health. Optimal health is a dynamic balance of physical, emotional, social, spiritual, and intellectual health. Lifestyle change can be facilitated through a combination of learning experiences that enhance awareness, increase motivation, and build skills and, most important, through the creation of opportunities that open access to environments that make positive health practices the easiest choice (O'Donnell, 2009, p. iv).

3. Health promotion is the process of advocating health in order to enhance the probability of personal (individual, family, and communities), private (professional and business), and public (federal, state, and local government) support of positive health (Dwore & Kreuter, 1980, p. 103).

In the first alternate definition, health promotion focuses on disease prevention and improving well-being in an individual client, with the emphasis on the client's own behavior. In the second, the focus is on lifestyle and optimal health, again for individuals, but with an emphasis on the provider's role in the process. The third expands its focus beyond the individual and defines health promotion from the point of view of advocacy.

What is interesting about all of the definitions discussed here is that they each have different ideas about where health promotion takes place and who is responsible for promoting health. We see definitions that focus on the individual and on society at large, and we also see a perspective that emphasizes personal initiative on the part of a client set in contrast to the role of the nurse or healthcare provider. Are any of these perspectives correct? Or are they all aspects of health promotion? We would argue that health promotion as a discipline encompasses them all.

In practice, health promotion includes any or all of the following:

- Providing a combination of educational and environmental supports for actions and conditions of living conducive to health
- Using various methods to induce lifestyle change through a combination of efforts to enhance awareness, change behavior, and create environments that support good health and have the greatest impact in producing lasting changes
- Helping people discover the synergies between their core passions and optimal health by facilitating lifestyle change through a combination of experiences that enhance awareness, increase motivation, and build skills by creating open access to environments that make positive health practices the easiest choice

Health Promotion: Perspectives and Concepts

The main concepts that separate health promotion from most other types of healthcare philosophy include:

1. A holistic view of health
2. A focus on participatory approaches
3. A focus on the determinants of health—the social, behavioral, economic, and environmental conditions that are the root causes of health and illness
4. Building on existing strengths and assets, not just addressing health problems and deficits
5. Using multiple, complementary strategies to promote health at the individual, family, and community levels

The previous list includes the term **determinants of health**. This term is important to comprehend not only to aid in understanding the definition of health promotion, but also when reviewing *Healthy People 2020* documents, which will be outlined in another chapter. Determinants of health is a very broad term that refers to a range of factors, including social, economic, and environmental factors that contribute to determining the health status of an individual, a family, or communities. These factors, outlined by Nutbeam (1998), include the following:

1. Income and social status
2. Social support networks
3. Education (including both literacy and health literacy)
4. Employment and working conditions
5. Physical environments
6. Social environments

7. Biology and genetic endowment
8. Health service
9. Cultural concepts of health

Other determinants of health may be identified as well; this list is not intended to be all-encompassing, but represents most of the basic factors that determine health.

HOT TOPICS

Here are some topics to explore:
- Quality of life research
- Holistic health
- Healthy People 2020
- Health insurance
- Health disparities

From the practical point of view, health promotion can be defined as any activity undertaken for the purpose of achieving a higher level of health and well-being. Health promotion activities are directed toward developing client resources that maintain or enhance well-being, not just avoiding or preventing disease. Health promotion includes both prevention and wellness activities and may be focused on physical, emotional, social, intellectual, spiritual, or environmental aspects of health.

Physical aspects of health include:
- Fitness
- Nutrition
- Self-care
- Substance abuse (note that substance abuse may also have emotional, social, and spiritual ramifications as well)

Emotional aspects of health include:
- Coping skills during an emotional crisis
- Stress management
- Quality of life
- Self-esteem and self-efficacy

Social aspects of health include:
- Community involvement
- Family relationships
- Friendships
- Geographical factors (rural vs. urban)
- Socioeconomic status and income

Intellectual aspects of health promotion include:
- Education
- Health literacy (note that well-educated people may still know little about health)
- Achievement
- Career development
- Access to technology

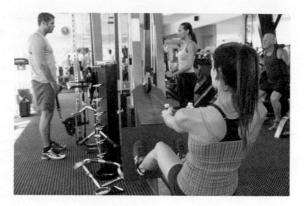

Spiritual aspects of health promotion include:
- Love
- Hope
- Charity
- Life purpose

Environmental aspects of health promotion include:
- Living in a nontoxic environment
- Working in a nontoxic environment
- Attending school in a nontoxic environment
- Availability of local resources to promote health (e.g., healthcare providers, pharmacies, facilities for exercise, wellness programs)

☐ Cultural Ideas about Health

There is another determinant of health that bears discussion: the cultural dimension of how health is defined. Individuals may have different perspectives on what health means within a culture, but, social groups that derive from different cultures of origin also sometimes have widely differing ideas of what constitutes health, both for the individual and for the society. When working with a client from a particular ethnic or cultural group, it is important that the nurse gain some understanding of the client's ethnomedical system (this is the client's cultural perspective on health)—both with respect to what constitutes health and how health is maintained. Medical anthropologist Mark Edburg explains why this matters:

> [We] can define an ethnomedical system as an applied cultural knowledge system related to health that sets out the kinds of health problems that can exist, their cause, and . . . appropriate treatments. . . . Of key importance when thinking about the cultural aspect of ethnomedical systems is that, across cultures, there are different answers to [medical] questions, from the range of potential health problems, to causes, to treatments, as well as the closely related question of what kinds of individuals are qualified to provide treatment. This means that if you are working in health promotion, prevention, or intervention efforts across cultures, you may define a health problem as, say, the flu, and understand it to be caused by a particular virus; while the people with whom you are working may define it differently—as, for example, a set of symptoms that are the result of improper social relations (e.g., behavior motivated by jealousy). Remember, human beings are biocultural. For this reason, in talking about

ethnomedical systems, some theorists have found it useful to make a distinction between a disease (an abnormal biomedical state caused by pathogens or physical anomalies) and an illness (a culturally defined state of not being well, with many culturally defined causes, including biomedical) . . . Diseases and illnesses may or may not refer to the same phenomenon. (Edburg, 2012, p. 39)

The impact of differences in ethnomedical concepts upon health promotion is illustrated by a study (Holdsworth, Gartner, Landais, Maire, & Delpeuch, 2004) in which women from Senegal—where having a large body is regarded as a sign of prosperity and fertility—were shown body silhouettes of various body types and asked to ascribe personality traits to those bodies. The outcomes of the study showed that the women considered the silhouettes showing an obese body type as having

a range of positive personal attributes—warm, happy, popular, friendly, proud, sociable, easy going, and having a strong personality. Body size profiles leaning towards the overweight were also seen as having the highest social status, a good job, enough money, a contented husband, children, proud family in-laws, and a higher likelihood of getting married. (Edburg, 2012, p. 18)

Knowing this, you can imagine that a nurse working with a female client from this cultural background might have difficulty convincing that client to undertake a weight management program—even if the client had developed weight-related physical diseases or conditions such as diabetes, hypertension, joint pain, breathing difficulties, and so forth. Regardless of what the client's biomedical circumstances might be, the cultural support for maintaining high body mass outweighs the incentive to lose weight.

Health promotion efforts in this case may involve raising the client's awareness of how her own cultural assumptions may impede her physical health, but understand that challenging deeply held cultural norms may not be a beneficial strategy unless the client appears open to it—for instance, a recent immigrant from Senegal may hold onto such norms as a way of maintaining contact with the familiar ideas of home, but a second-generation immigrant or younger woman might be more receptive to the idea that weight reduction would benefit her.

Another strategy may involve shifting emphasis from weight loss to improving physical fitness. That is, the nurse may have better results if instead of putting her Senegalese client on a weight loss program, she instead presents the client with an expectation of improved physiologic condition leading to relief of unpleasant symptoms related to poor fitness (e.g., joint pain, breathing issues). Make it clear to the client that part of the trade-off would be loss of some of the weight that the client prizes. Highlighting the benefits of this trade-off and keeping the client focused on the positive results ("Are you feeling less pain now in your joints?" "How has your blood pressure been lately?") can help alleviate some of the emotional distress the client may feel at undertaking a program that contradicts cultural imperatives.

Learn enough about the client's cultural perspectives to make effective suggestions without resorting to stereotyping. There are several ways to do this:

- Reading anthropological literature on the cultural history of the ethnic group in question (useful if you regularly serve individuals from this community, but not likely a good use of time if this ethnic group represents a small subset of clients)
- Reviewing the health literature for studies relating to interventions in the ethnic group of interest
- Interviewing the client and family members about cultural beliefs and expectations regarding health. (This might be your best bet because not all members of a cultural group adhere to all beliefs or expectations. Such action would also help build rapport with the client.)
- Developing a community-based research study to identify cultural beliefs about health (again, useful if the ethnic group of interest is widely represented among clients).

Keep in mind, though, that however well versed you might become in traditions and ethnomedical perspectives of a particular ethnic group, clients need to be regarded as individuals first, and representatives of their cultural tradition second. Individuals can and often do have ideas that conflict with their own cultural norms, and these should be respected and honored.

It is also important to recognize that ethnic origin and cultural background are not necessarily the same thing. International adoptions are very common,

CULTURAL RESEARCH STUDY

A review of: Health Disparities in Lifestyle Choices Among Hypertensive Korean Americans, Non-Hispanic Whites, and Blacks

This study gathered data from 100 hypertensive Korean Americans (KAs) about medications, diet, and exercise/physical activity and compared this data to matched individuals from the National Health and Nutrition Examination Survey (NHANES III) who were non-Hispanic Whites and Blacks. The results of the study indicated that the KAs were significantly less likely to reduce salt in their diets and follow advice for weight loss to reduce cholesterol levels. The KAs had lower body mass index, were older, and were more educated than the other two groups. They attended a KA clinic because of the respect they received and the use of the Korean language. The implications of this study included a suggestion of the need for KA healthcare providers to place more emphasis on health-promoting lifestyles with their patients. In addition, it was suggested that healthcare providers needed to treat all patients with respect and be sensitive to language needs.

Source: Kim, M. J., Ahn, Y. H., Chon, C., Bowen, P. & Khan, S. (2005). Health Disparities in Lifestyle Choices among Hypertensive Korean Americans, Non-Hispanic Whites, and Blacks. *Biological Research for Nursing, 7*(1), 67–74.

and you may encounter individuals who are ethnically from one population but who have grown up in a household with significantly different cultural norms from those of the ethnic group of origin. Make no assumptions about ethnomedical systems based on a client's ethnicity. Instead, ask what health and health care mean so that an intervention is tailored to the client's perspective, rather than a stereotype.

Disease Prevention

It is virtually impossible to discuss health promotion without taking into account one key component: disease prevention. **Disease prevention** is defined as taking steps to avoid illness and the agents of illness. These steps include measures to identify risk factors for illness, since avoiding illness is difficult when the factors that contribute to illness are not known. Risk assessment is particularly important for preventing noninfectious diseases like diabetes or cancer, but it is also key to preventing infections that have specific, controllable transmission vectors, such as sexually transmitted diseases, where risk rises in direct relation to an individual's use of safe sex practices and number of sexual partners. Much of the research around risk assessment for disease prevention has been done by the United States Preventive Services Task Force.

In 1965, Leavell and Clark outlined three different forms of prevention: primary, secondary, and tertiary (FIGURE 1-3). We will discuss each in turn.

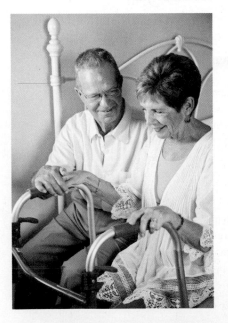

Primary Prevention

Primary prevention can only occur before someone contracts a disease or condition. Primary prevention aims to prevent the disease from occurring, thereby reducing both the incidence and prevalence of a disease. Prevalence (the proportion of a population that has the condition at a given time) depends on both the incidence (the rate of a new problem arising during a period of time) and the duration of the condition.

Primary prevention activities aimed at an individual's health are a set of actions that prevent a specific targeted condition. Prevention precedes the disease or condition. The activities decrease or even prevent the probability of occurrence of an injury, physical or mental illness, or a health-threatening situation in an individual or family, or an event or illness in a population. Some examples of primary prevention would include teaching new parents

Primary prevention:
avoiding exposure to a disease-causing agent.

Example: primary prevention
of skin cancer includes:
- wearing sunblock
- seeking shade
- limiting sun exposure
  during peak hours

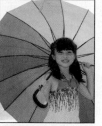

Secondary prevention:
taking steps to limit risk and detect disease after
exposure occurs.

Example: secondary prevention of skin cancer
includes:
- routinely checking skin for suspicious changes
- avoiding further sun exposure and sunburn

Tertiary prevention:
reducing effects of disease once symptoms are
apparent.

Example: tertiary prevention of skin cancer
includes:
- removing any suspect moles or lesions
- obtaining a biopsy specimen for analysis
- seeking immediate treatment if cancerous
  cells are detected

FIGURE 1-3   Three Types of Prevention

how to care for a newborn infant; the health problems being prevented are
both health issues in the newborn from improper care as well as stress-related
mental health problems in the parents. Another example would be working
with a client concerned about weight gain to develop better diet and exercise
habits (to prevent a variety of weight-related illnesses). Primary prevention is
not undertaken only by people with no health issues—very few people would
qualify! Primary prevention also includes encouraging a client with osteoporosis to use adequate daytime lighting, wear nonslip footwear, and have available
a bedside bell, flashlight, walker, cane, and/or assistance when necessary. Such
actions are known to prevent falls, which are the leading cause of debilitating

RESEARCH BOX: Sedatives, Mood-Altering Drugs Related to Falls Among Elderly

» BACKGROUND: There is increasing recognition that the use of certain medications contributes to falls in seniors. Our objective was to update a previously completed meta-analysis looking at the association of medication use and falling to include relevant drug classes and new studies that have been completed since a previous meta-analysis.

» METHODS: Studies were identified through a systematic search of English-language articles published from 1996 to 2007. We identified studies that were completed on patients older than 60 years, looking at the association between medication use and falling. Bayesian methods allowed us to combine the results of a previous meta-analysis with new information to estimate updated Bayesian odds ratios (ORs) and 95% credible intervals (95% CrIs)

» RESULTS: Of 11,118 identified articles, 22 met the inclusion criteria. Meta-analyses were completed on 9 unique drug classes, including 79 081 participants, with the following Bayesian unadjusted OR estimates: antihypertensive agents, OR, 1.24 (95% CrI, 1.01-1.50); diuretics, OR, 1.07 (95% CrI, 1.01-1.14); β-blockers, OR, 1.01 (95% CrI, 0.86-1.17); sedatives and hypnotics, OR, 1.47 (95% CrI, 1.35-1.62); neuroleptics and antipsychotics, OR, 1.59 (95% CrI, 1.37-1.83); antidepressants, OR, 1.68 (95% CrI, 1.47-1.91); benzodiazepines, OR, 1.57 (95% CrI, 1.43-1.72); narcotics, OR, 0.96 (95% CrI, 0.78-1.18); and nonsteroidal anti-inflammatory drugs, OR, 1.21 (95% CrI, 1.01-1.44). The updated Bayesian adjusted OR estimates for diuretics, neuroleptics and antipsychotics, antidepressants, and benzodiazepines were 0.99 (95% CrI, 0.78-1.25), 1.39 (95% CrI, 0.94-2.00), 1.36 (95% CrI, 1.13-1.76), and 1.41 (95% CrI, 1.20-1.71), respectively. Stratification of studies had little effect on Bayesian OR estimates, with only small differences in the stratified ORs observed across population (for β-blockers and neuroleptics and antipsychotics) and study type (for sedatives and hypnotics, benzodiazepines, and narcotics). An increased likelihood of falling was estimated for the use of sedatives and hypnotics, neuroleptics and antipsychotics, antidepressants, benzodiazepines, and nonsteroidal anti-inflammatory drugs in studies considered to have "good" medication and falls ascertainment.

» CONCLUSION: The use of sedatives and hypnotics, antidepressants, and benzodiazepines demonstrated a significant association with falls in elderly individuals. Falls among elderly people are significantly associated with several classes of drugs, including sedatives often prescribed as sleep aids and medications used to treat mood disorders, according to a study led by a University of British Columbia expert in pharmaceutical outcomes research.

The study, published Nov. 23, 2009, in the *Archives of Internal Medicine*, provides the latest quantitative evidence of the impact of certain classes of medication on falling among seniors. Falling and fall-related complications such as hip fractures are the fifth leading cause of death in the developed world, the study noted.

Source: Woolcott, J. C., Richardson, K. J., Wiens, M. O., Patel, B., Marin, J., Khan, M. K., & Marra, C. A. Meta-analysis of the Impact of 9 Medication Classes on Falls in Elderly Persons. *Archives of Internal Medicine, 169*(21), 1952–1960.

hip fractures in individuals with osteoporosis (Donat & Ozcan, 2007; Ruben-stein, 2006; Stevens & Olson, 2000).

Primary prevention on a broader scale works toward combating harmful forces that operate on the individuals of the community by strengthening the capacity of people to withstand these forces (Murray et al., 2009). The purpose of community-level primary prevention programs is to decrease the vulnerability of the individual or population to disease or dysfunction. This can include health education about specific risk factors for a disease, promoting practices such as the use of helmets or other safety equipment, or providing protection from infection through dissemination of vaccines.

ASK YOURSELF   [www]

Community health is a topic that is important to all of us. Imagine you have decided to become more active in your community and would like to channel your energies in the direction where you can have some major impact. How would you determine what direction you should take? Who might you talk to? What organizations might you contact?

Leavell and Clark (1965) developed a conceptual map for community-based primary prevention. It included:

Health Promotion

1. Health education
2. Good standard of nutrition adjusted to developmental phases of life
3. Attention to personality development
4. Provision of adequate housing, recreation, and agreeable working conditions
5. Marriage counseling and sex education
6. Genetic counseling
7. Periodic selective examination

Specific Protections

1. Use of specific immunizations
2. Attention to personal hygiene
3. Use of environmental sanitation
4. Protection against occupational hazards
5. Protection from accidents
6. Use of specific nutrients
7. Protection from carcinogens

HEALTH PROMOTION CHALLENGE

Read the information in the RESEARCH BOX and develop a primary prevention nursing intervention for falls based on the study findings.

Secondary Prevention

Secondary prevention is the identification and treatment of asymptomatic persons who have developed risk factors or who have a disease that is in a preclinical state (that is, not yet clinically apparent). The goal of secondary prevention is to find and treat disease early, because many diseases can be cured more easily with early diagnosis. Secondary prevention consists of measures taken after exposure to the disease-causing factor has occurred, but before the person notices that anything is wrong. For example, secondary prevention of colon cancer would involve getting a colonoscopy to look for precancerous polyps. In contrast, primary prevention for colon cancer would involve eating a high-fiber diet that limits red meat and alcohol (that is, taking steps to lower risk of developing polyps and neoplastic changes in the first place).

Secondary prevention activities include screening techniques (e.g., mammograms, blood glucose testing, and similar routine tests) intended to offer an early diagnosis and prompt treatment of the existing health problem, disease, or harmful situation. Such measures are undertaken with the goal of shortening the disease's duration and severity of consequences so that the individual can return to his or her maximum potential health or normal functioning as quickly as possible.

Secondary prevention can also include actions taken to resolve a known factor in the home or the environment that contributes to increased risk of disease for a community. For example, efforts to reduce air pollution in urban areas may be considered secondary prevention for diseases such as asthma and chronic obstructive pulmonary disease (COPD), both of which are related to the overall levels of air pollution in urban environments (Kelly & Fussell, 2011).

Tertiary Prevention

Tertiary prevention targets the person who already has symptoms of the disease. Since it is no longer possible to prevent the disease itself from developing, the goals of tertiary prevention are:

- Prevent or limit damage and pain from the disease
- Slow down progression of the disease
- Prevent the disease from causing complications
- Give better care to people with the disease
- Assist people with the disease to be able to do what they used to do

An example of tertiary prevention includes teaching people with COPD to gain control over their breathing and breathe more efficiently; this can be achieved by using their breath to play a computer game that teaches them to inhale more slowly and exhale more completely (Collins, Langbein, & Fehr, 2008).

It is important to recognize that tertiary prevention is not curing a disease or restoring a person to perfect health—it is undertaken, mostly, in the setting of an irreversible health problem. The goal of tertiary prevention is to prevent progression of a disease or any of its complications, therefore minimizing the disease effects and disability. Tertiary prevention activities may also involve maintenance activities or assessment for preventing complications. For example, physical therapy and occupational therapy for a patient who has experienced a cerebrovascular accident would be considered a tertiary prevention intervention. The therapy will prevent contractures on the patient's affected side and assist the patient in relearning some activities that are key to independent daily living, such as eating, dressing, or writing without assistance. In addition, the patient would be taught ways to maintain an appropriate blood pressure to limit the risk of another incident.

Final Thoughts: Evidence-Based Practice and Dealing with Data Overload

Health promotion does not consist of any one set of activities, techniques, or methods. As nursing practice is continually changing, with new therapies and tools being developed daily, so also are health promotion techniques. Nursing professionals advocate for evidence-based practice, but to create a health-promotion program supported by evidence, it is important to keep up with the latest research.

One of the best sources of the latest research is the government website, http://www.pubmed.gov. All you need do is type in one or two terms at the top search box and numerous studies will appear. At the very least, before accepting research findings as valid, be sure to check who is funding the study, that an adequate-sized and relevant population is used, and whether the outcomes are positive. Use only findings that are based on systematic study, not anecdotes or opinions.

The core foundation of health promotion is unchanging: Whatever the specifics of methods or evidence, the intent is always to assist clients—individuals, families, or communities—to obtain optimal health in all senses. Be it physical, mental, social, environmental, or spiritual, establishing a strong foundation for wellness is the cornerstone of health promotion practice.

Summary

Health may be defined from the viewpoint of caregivers and clients. Health and its determinants have been described since Florence Nightingale's *Notes on Nursing*. As infectious diseases were quelled, health started to attain a higher priority in society. Prior to World War II, emphasis was mainly on illness and disease. After the war, health concepts shifted to focus on maintaining not only the body, but the mind, the emotions, the family, and the community. Health began to be viewed as something the individual could affect through taking part in positive actions.

The World Health Organization (WHO) incorporated wholeness and positive qualities of health into its 1946 definition; by 1986, WHO had expanded its definition to include spiritual, psychological, and economic health as well as the ability to fulfill social roles. Later, concepts of wellness and global health were developed.

Smith (1983) described health within four dimensions, defined by extremes of the health–illness continuum: clinical dimension, role-performance dimension, adaptive dimension, and eudaimonistic dimension. In recent decades, mental illness and quality of life have become incorporated as inseparable to considerations of health. Your role is to help the client improve wellness in all dimensions.

Disease prevention is the avoidance of illness and agents of illness, plus identification of risks. Disease prevention may be categorized as primary, secondary, and tertiary prevention.

Primary prevention precedes disease and includes a set of actions that prevent a specific disease or condition. Secondary prevention is the identification and treatment of asymptomatic persons who have developed risk factors or are at a preclinical state. Tertiary prevention is the treatment and management of clinical and chronic disease, restoring the client to optimum function and maintenance of life skills. Leavell and Clark developed a conceptual map that outlines activities to be undertaken at each of the three levels of prevention.

Although health can be measured with clinical tools, wellness is self-assessed and self-evaluated. High-level wellness includes maximizing one's potential, having direction and purpose in life, meeting the challenges of the environment, looking beyond the needs of self to the needs of society, and doing it all with joy or a zest for life.

Health promotion has many definitions, most of which incorporate elements of well-being, quality of health, and avoidance of illness for individuals, families, and communities. Included under the concept of health promotion are health education, health protection, and disease prevention. Determinants of health may include a range of factors including social, economic, and environmental categories.

REVIEW QUESTIONS

www.

1. What is quality of life?
   a. General well-being as assessed by either that individual or by another person about that individual
   b. A set of actions that prevents a specific disease or condition
   c. Activities that promote well-being

2. Primary prevention is
   a. Treatment and management of the patient's clinical and chronic disease
   b. Identification and treatment of asymptomatic persons who have developed risk factors
   c. A set of actions that prevents a specific disease or condition

3. Tertiary prevention is
   a. Treatment and management of the patient's clinical and chronic disease
   b. Identification and treatment of asymptomatic persons who have developed risk factors
   c. A set of actions that prevents a specific disease or condition

4. Health promotion includes the following:
   a. Management of chronic disease
   b. Assessment and treatment of new-onset disease
   c. Health education and disease prevention

5. The eudaimonistic dimension of Smith's health definition is
   a. The positive interaction among the physical, social, psychological, and spiritual aspects of the environment
   b. The ability to adapt positively to social, mental, and physiological change for health versus illness
   c. The ability of the person to perform social roles, including work and family, based on societal expectations

6. The adaptive dimension of Smith's health definition is
   a. The positive interaction among the physical, social, psychological, and spiritual aspects of the environment
   b. The ability to adapt positively to social, mental, and physiological change for health versus illness
   c. The ability of the person to perform social roles, including work and family, based on societal expectations

7. Primary prevention includes
   a. Case-finding measures and mass screenings
   b. Provision of hospital and community facilities for retraining and education to maximize use of remaining capacities
   c. Use of environmental sanitation

8. Secondary prevention includes
   a. Genetic counseling
   b. Attention to personal hygiene
   c. Adequate treatment to arrest disease process and prevent further complications and sequelae

9. Determinants of health refers to
   a. A range of factors, including social, economic, and environmental
   b. Case-finding measures and mass screenings
   c. General well-being

10. Nutbeam's list of factors that are determinants of health includes
   a. Adequate treatment
   b. Social support networks
   c. Work therapy in hospitals

EXERCISES   [www.]

1. Explore the term *health*. Find dictionary definitions, discussions in textbooks, and links on the Internet. Read about nursing models and theories that discuss the concept of health.

2. Review the topic of disease prevention. Pick a special health-related issue or disease you are interested in and list the activities related to this issue or disease that could be categorized as primary prevention, secondary prevention, and tertiary prevention.

3. Go to the website http://www.nurses.info/nursing_theory_accepted_theories.htm Find a research instrument related to health or quality of life and briefly outline a study you might conduct using this instrument.

4. Find information about principles of health education. Apply these principles and devise a brief plan for patient education related to the issue or disease you identified in exercise No. 2.

5. Check out the following websites to learn more about primary, secondary, and tertiary prevention of skin and other cancers:

   http://www.cdc.gov/ChooseYourCover

   http://www.foundation.sdsu.edu/sunwisestampede/

   http://www.cancer.org

   http://www.cancer.gov

   http://www.preventcancer.org

   a. List at least two examples of skin or other types of cancer prevention at each of the prevention levels. Who would you target with each of the methods you described?
   b. Find out what your school or hospital setting is doing to protect people from the sun.
      • Have they built shade structures or planted trees?

- Do they encourage the use of hats and protective clothes when outside?
- Do they furnish sunscreen?

   c. The Centers for Disease Control and Prevention (CDC) is active in developing policies and programs on sun exposure and protection. For its latest information, go to http://www.cdc.gov/cancer/skin/basic_info/prevention.htm What can you do with this information to help prevent skin cancer?

6. California recently passed a law that says California schools must let children wear sun protective clothes at school. Share information on the following issues with one of your classmates:
   a. What are your thoughts on the law?
   b. What kind of barrier was the law trying to overcome?
   c. Does your state or school have a law or rule that prevents you from wearing hats or wearing sunscreens?

7. Overweight/obesity is linked with numerous illness conditions. Losing weight is an important goal for a significant number of adults and children. Check out the following weight-loss websites:

   http://www.healthcastle.com/easy-weightloss.shtml

   http://diet.health.com/2009/12/22/crash-diets/

- List two ways you could use this information with clients.
- List two ways you could use this information with yourself, your family, or friends.

Choose one wellness indicant as your goal for the next year; e.g., I will exercise for 1 hour a day by either riding a stationary bike or swimming, or I will reduce my stress by taking a yoga class and participating every week for 1 hour.

REFERENCES

Andrews, F. M., & Withey, S. B. (1976). *Social indicators of well-being*, (pp. 63–106). New York, NY: Plenum Press.

Baird, K. (2011). Inside the patient experience—Elizabeth's journey #10. Retrieved from http://baird-group.com/blog/inside-the-patient-experience-%E2%80%93-elizabeth%E2%80%99s-journey-10

Benyamin, R., Trescot, A. M., Datta, S., Buenaventura, R., Adlaka, R., Sehgal, N., . . . Vallejo R. (2008). Opioid complications and side effects. *Pain Physician, 11*(March; 2 Suppl), S105–S120.

Centers for Disease Control and Prevention [CDC]. (2011). *Health-related quality of life (HRQoL): Well-being concepts.* Retrieved from http://www.cdc.gov/hrqol/wellbeing.htm#three. Atlanta, GA: Centers for Disease Control and Prevention Health Related Quality of Life Surveillance Program.

Collins, E., Langbein, E., & Fehr, L. (2008). Can ventilation-feedback training against exercise tolerance in patients with chronic obstructive pulmonary disease. *American Journal of Respiratory and Critical Care Medicine, 177*(8), 844–852.

Diener, E. (2000). Subjective well being: The science of happiness and a proposal for a national index. *American Psychologist, 55*(1), 34–43.

Dix, K. L., Slee, P. T., Lawson, M. J., & Keeves, J. P. (2012). Implementation quality of whole-school mental health promotion and students' academic performance. *Child and Adolescent Mental Health, 17*(1), 45–51.

Donat, H., & Ozcan, A. (2007). Comparison of the effectiveness of two programmes on older adults at risk of falling: Unsupervised home exercise and supervised group exercise. *Clinical Rehabilitation, 21*(3), 272–283.

Dunn, H. (1961). *High level wellness.* Arlington, VA: Beatty Press.

Dwore, R. B. & Kreuter, M. W. (1980). Reinforcing the case for health promotion [Update]. *Family and Community Health, 2*(4), 103–119.

Edburg, M. (2012). *Essentials of health, culture, and diversity: Understanding people, reducing disparities.* Burlington, MA: Jones & Bartlett Learning.

Furlan, A. D., Sandoval, J. A., Mailis-Gagnon, A., & Tunks, E. (2006). Opioids for chronic noncancer pain: A meta-analysis of effectiveness and side effects. *Canadian Medical Association Journal, 174*(11), 1589–1594.

Gore, M., Sadosky, A. B., Leslie, D. L., Tai, K. S., & Emery, P. (2012). Therapy switching, augmentation, and discontinuation in patients with osteoarthritis and chronic low back pain. *Pain Practice* (January 9). Advance online publication. doi:10.1111/j.1533-2500.2011.00524.x

Holdsworth, M., Gartner, A., Landais, E., Maire, B., & Delpeuch, F. (2004). Perceptions of healthy and desirable body size in urban Senegalese women. *International Journal of Obesity, 28,* 1561–1568.

Jamison, R. N., Serraillier, J., & Michna, E. (2011). Assessment and treatment of abuse risk in opioid prescribing for chronic pain. *Pain Research and Treatment.* 2011:941808. Retrieved from www.ncbi.nlm.nih.gov/pmc/articles/PMC3200070/

Kelly, F. J., & Fussell, J. C. (2011). Air pollution and airway disease. *Clinical and Experimental Allergy, 41*(8), 1059–1071.

Leavell, H., & Clark, A. (1965). *Preventive medicine for doctors in the community.* New York, NY: McGraw-Hill.

Manheimer, E., White, A., Berman, B., Forys, K., & Ernst E. (2005). Meta-analysis: Acupuncture for low back pain. *Annals of Internal Medicine, 142*(8), 651–663.

Maville, J., & Huerta, C. (2002). *Health promotion in nursing.* Albany, NY: Delmar Publishers.

Moritz, S., Liu, M. F., Rickhi, B., Xu, T. J., Paccagnan, P., & Quan H. (2011). Reduced health resource use after acupuncture for low back pain. *Journal of Alternative and Complementary Medicine, 17*(11), 1015–1019.

Murray, R., Zentner, J., & Yakimo, R. (2009). *Health promotion strategies through the life span.* Upper Saddle River, NJ: Pearson Education.

Nightingale, F. (1860). *Notes on nursing, What it is and what it is not.* London, England: Gerald Duckworth & Co.

Nutbeam, P. (1998). Health promotion glossary. *Health Promotion International, 13*(4), 349–364.

O'Donnell, M. P. (2009). Definition of health promotion 2.0: Embracing passion, enhancing motivation, recognizing dynamic balance, and creating opportunities. *American Journal of Health Promotion, 24*(1), iv.

Office of the Surgeon General. (1999). *Mental health: A report of the surgeon general.* Washington, DC: U.S. Department of Health and Human Services: Retrieved from http://www.surgeongeneral.gov/library/mentalhealth/chapter1/sec1.html

Parton, D. (2011). Living with stigma is still the common experience for mental health service users. *Mental Health Today,* (July–August), 5.

Pender, N., Murdaugh, C., & Parsons, N. (2006). *Health promotion in nursing practice* (5th ed.). Upper Saddle River, NJ: Pearson Prentice Hall.

Ramage-Morin, P. L., Shields, M., & Martel, L. (2010). Health-promoting factors and good health among Canadians in mid- to late life. *Health Reports/Statistics Canada, 21*(3), 45–53.

Rubenstein, L. Z. (2006). Falls in older people: Epidemiology, risk factors and strategies for prevention. *Age and Ageing, 35*(2 Suppl.), ii37–ii41.

Ryff, C. D., & Keyes, C. L. M. (1995). The structure of psychological well-being revisited. *Journal of Personality and Social Psychology, 69*(4), 719–727.

Smith, J. (1983). *The idea of health: Implications for the nursing profession.* New York, NY: Teachers College Press.

Smith, B. J., Tang, K. C., & Nutbeam, D. (2006). WHO health promotion glossary: New terms. *Health Promotion International, 21*(4), 340–345.

Stevens, J. A., & Olson, S. (2000). Reducing falls and resulting hip fractures in older women. *Morbidity and Mortality Weekly Report, Recommendations and Reports, 49*(March 31, RR-2), 3–12.

Thorn, B. E., Day, M. A., Burns, J., Kuhajda, M. C., Gaskins, S. W., Sweeney, K., . . . Cabbil, C. (2011). Randomized trial of group cognitive behavioral therapy compared with a pain education control for low-literacy rural people with chronic pain. *Pain, 152*(12), 2710–2720.

Trigkilidas, D. (2010). Acupuncture therapy for chronic lower back pain: A systematic review. *Annals of the Royal College of Surgeons of England, 92*(7), 595–598.

Von Korff, M., Kolodny, A., Deyo, R. A., & Chou R. (2011). Long-term opioid therapy reconsidered. *Annals of Internal Medicine, 155*(5), 325–328.

White, A. P., Arnold, P. M., Norvell, D. C., Ecker, E., & Fehlings, M. G. (2011). Pharmacologic management of chronic low back pain: Synthesis of the evidence. *Spine (Phila Pa 1976), 36*(October 1; 21 Suppl), S131–S143.

Wiseman, J., McLeod, J., & Zubrick, S. R. (2007). Promoting mental health and well-being: Integrating individual, organisational and community-level indicators. *Health Promotion Journal of Australia, 18*(3), 198–207.

World Health Organization. (1946). *Preamble to the Constitution of the World Health Organization.* Signed at the International Health Conference, New York, July 22, 1946.

World Health Organization [WHO]. (1948). *Constitution of the World Health Organization.* Geneva, Switzerland: Author. Retrieved from http://apps.who.int/gb/bd/PDF/bd47/EN/constitution-en.pdf

World Health Organization [WHO]. (1958). *The first ten years of the World Health Organization.* Geneva, Switzerland: Author.

World Health Organization [WHO]. (1986). *Ottawa Charter for Health Promotion.* First International Conference on Health Promotion, Ottawa, Canada, November 21, 1986—WHO/HPR/HEP/95.1.

INTERNET RESOURCES

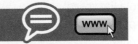

For a full suite of assignments and learning activities, use the access code located in the front of your book to visit this exclusive website: **http://go.jblearning.com/healthpromotion**. If you do not have an access code, you can obtain one at the site.

LEARNING OBJECTIVES

Upon completion of this chapter, you will be able to:

1. Define theory and concept.
2. Discuss the relationship between theory and concept.
3. Differentiate between a grand theory and a midrange theory.
4. Describe a model and its relationship to theory and concepts.
5. Define a schematic model.
6. Discuss the role of theories in health promotion and disease prevention.
7. Explain the development of the health belief model.
8. Reiterate the beliefs needed to promote health.
9. Define self-efficacy.
10. List three key variables of the expanded health belief model.
11. Provide three assumptions of the health promotion model.
12. Discuss the role theoretical propositions play in the health promotion model.
13. Explain the use of the PRECEDE-PROCEED framework.
14. Show the relationships between the propositions of the PRECEDE-PROCEED framework.
15. Discuss the various phases of the PRECEDE-PROCEED framework.

KEY TERMS

Bio-psycho-social-spiritual model

Clark wellness model

Concept

Conceptual model

Expanded health belief model

Grand theories

Health belief model

Health education model

Health promotion model

Hypothesis

Midrange theories

Model

Orem self-care model

PRECEDE-PROCEED framework

Schematic model

Self-determination theory

Self-efficacy

Stages of change theory

Theory

Theory of reasoned action

Value expectancy theory

Variables

CHAPTER 2

Concepts, Models, and Theories

- Introduction
- What Are Theories, Concepts, and Models?
- Nursing Theory
- Summary

http://go.jblearning.com/healthpromotion

For a full suite of assignments and learning activities, use the access code located in the front of your book to visit the exclusive website: http://go.jblearning.com/healthpromotion If you do not have an access code, you can obtain one at the site.

Introduction

In your nursing practice, you will use a set of ideas that explains what needs to be accomplished and how to best meet these goals. These ideas are expressed through concepts, theories, and models; we will begin by defining each of those terms before outlining key examples of each of these in health promotion.

Different sources define basic theoretical terminology in various ways, so this chapter will discuss the distinctions between these definitions. The goal of this chapter is to provide the theoretical foundation for health promotion concepts, theories, and models, and ways to apply them to research and practice.

What Are Theories, Concepts, and Models?

The word *theory* is misused and misunderstood. It is used colloquially to mean "an idea or explanation that someone has made up but has not proven." In nursing and other scientific fields, such an unsupported explanation for a phenomenon is called a hypothesis or a proposition, not a theory.

In scientific terminology, an idea that explains or describes a phenomenon (an observable fact or event), is called a **concept.** Some sources describe a set of interrelated ideas as a concept. Concepts can be concrete (that is, able to be described or measured directly, using the five senses) or abstract (described using mental or theoretical constructs that do not exist in physical reality).

An excellent example of an abstract concept is "health," which is complex and ever changing, and relates as much to the world of ideas and beliefs as it does to physical reality. Conversely, "table" is an example of a concrete concept; while tables can differ in size, shape, and materials, they are generally alike in function and overall appearance. An abstract idea is broader and less specific than a concrete idea. When discussing or developing concepts, be as specific as possible. Concepts are the building blocks of theory, because to develop a theory, you must test the validity of interrelated concepts. To test a concept, raise a question about the concept and then form a hypothesis or hunch about what the answer to that question might be. A **hypothesis** predicts the relationship of variables; the prediction is sometimes found to be true, false, or true, but not statistically significant. A **variable** is an attribute of the relationship between phenomena; for example, sunshine can be an attribute of depression. A hypothesis predicts how those variables interact with one another. When you test a hypothesis, you are trying to determine if the prediction is correct. If it is, then the study's outcome supports a story about how certain variables behave in relation to one another—and that story is the beginning of the theory. If the prediction is not correct, then you will need to develop a different theory, one that explains why the variables behave as they do, rather than as you expected.

For example, suppose you are working with a group of older adults in a nursing home. You observe that some of them like to spend a lot of time in the sun, while others prefer to stay indoors most of the time. You then observe that those who spend time in the sun seem happier and less depressed than those who do not. So you form a concept: exposure to sunlight improves mood in older adults. To test this concept, you develop a hypothesis that spending more time in the sun will make a positive change to their mood, and you ask the people who stay indoors to start going outside for a half hour to an hour each day to see if this occurs. After regular exposure to sunlight for a few weeks, you assess their mood. Do they seem happier, more cheerful? If the answer to that question is yes, then you have evidence that supports your hypothesis. If the answer to that question is no, then there are two possibilities: either something other than sunlight is making the difference in mood between the two groups, or the amount of sunlight exposure you have given the indoor group is not enough to make a difference. You could then go back and ask the indoor group to increase their time in the sun to see if that makes a change to their mood, and reassess again later.

But even if you get positive results to these tests, you still do not have a theory—yet. A concept supported by one piece of evidence isn't enough to make a theory. You need multiple tests, all of them successful, to show that your concept is valid, and you need to look further to identify other concepts that connect logically to your concept. You can either continue to do research into the effects of sunlight on older adults, or you can analyze research findings by others to see if their work also supports your hypothesis. This action will help you to determine if they have well-supported concepts that help to explain why your observations occur.

When you can connect a set of concepts that are well supported by evidence and observations, and hold up in the face of testing and challenges, *then* you have a theory. In this case, you have a theory about the benefits of sunlight for the mental health of older adults, as shown by not one, but numerous observations of the relationship between mood and light exposure.

As new observations are generated by continued research, they can be tested against the theory to see if they support it or not. If they do not, new theoretical constructs must be developed to explain how everything fits together. But even if they do, the development of the theory is not the end of the road; it becomes instead a starting point for generating new hypotheses about how the relationship you have observed came about, why and how it works, and how it may be used to improve the health and well-being of people other than those involved in the research.

A **theory**, then, is a way to organize a set of ideas or concepts, explain complex sets of research findings, and assist in developing and testing new hypotheses.

Identifying and Controlling for Variability: The Importance of Variables

If there are too many uncontrolled or unidentified variables affecting the relationship you are investigating, then the potential alternative explanations also weaken your theory.

☐ How Variables Affect Hypotheses: An Example

Your research question sought to explain the relationship between mood (variable *A*) and sunlight exposure (variable *B*). Your hypothesis proposes that variable *A* has a relationship with variable *B* that can be described this way: *B* acts upon *A* and alters it in a positive direction. Put another way, you are suggesting that if you add more of variable *B* (sunlight) to the people in your study population, you will see an improvement or positive increase in variable *A* (mood). Here, variable *B* is the independent variable because it is the variable you change, while variable *A* is the dependent variable because what you observe about that variable depends to what changes you apply.

There are other independent variables beyond sunlight exposure that could be affecting the dependent variable, and you need to take them into account before you can focus on the proposed relationship between *B* and *A*. Your study population consisted of older adults living in an assisted living facility. Right there, you have identified two specific attributes, or variables, that could affect the relationship you're concerned about: (1) the general age of the individuals under study (variable *C*), and (2) the circumstances in which the study participants live (variable *D*).

Age is a key health-related variable because the human body and mind change dramatically over time. You would not expect a group of 5-year-old children to behave, whether physically, mentally, emotionally, or spiritually, in the same ways as a group of 80-year-olds, simply because they are at different developmental and life stages. You would expect variation between these two groups simply because of differences in age—and that is why age is such an important variable in health promotion studies. One reason age is an important attribute in this population is that the skin's ability to absorb sunlight often decreases with age. It is important to make sure that all participants are within the same age/developmental stage of life, older adulthood. You might want to further refine this variable by grouping the subjects by decade, so that you would compare people aged 50–59, 60–69, 70–79, and 80+ to one another, instead of assuming that individuals ranging in age across 40 years were all alike.

The circumstances (or environment) in which the study group lives is an important variable, too. You might not expect people who live in different households, different communities, or different regions to behave in similar ways, but those who live in the same or similar settings—such as an assisted living facility—might be expected to have more in common with one another than those who do not. For example, you would expect all of the people living in this facility to eat similar foods, go to bed at the same time, and participate in similar activities. A certain amount of variation is possible among the residents of this facility. A 75-year-old man with rheumatoid arthritis and diabetes may differ in many respects from a 99-year-old woman whose health is good, but who lives in the facility because she lacks social support to help her care for herself on a day-to-day basis. But overall, by virtue of the fact that they share living circumstances, you could reasonably assume that these two people do not have major differences in lifestyle unless one has chronic insomnia and the other has relatives who sneak food into the facility.

Why is that important? Because of the apples-to-oranges rule. Simply put, when you are conducting a study to identify a relationship between two variables, you want to limit the number of other variables that could be affecting the relationship by ensuring that the subjects in your study are as similar as possible. In other words, you want to compare apples to apples and oranges to oranges, but you do *not* want to compare apples to oranges, because such major differences between subjects introduces another key variable that could alter the observed outcome of your comparison. If the 75-year-old man and 99-year-old woman did not live in the same environment, they could have very different lifestyles, so they would be less appropriate for comparison.

Considering these two individuals brings up another point. There are both men and women in this facility. Could the gender of the participants matter in how sunlight affects mood? Well, yes, it could; men and women have different neurological and psychological profiles, and women in general have a higher rate of depression than men. A study in Australia suggests this difference may diminish with age (Pachana, McLaughlin, Leung, Byrne, & Dobson, 2012), but it is unclear whether this applies to the U.S. population as well. So it would probably be best to assume that gender is a variable, E, that might affect the outcome of the study. You can eliminate its effects very simply by analyzing the study participants separately according to gender—comparing men to men and women to women—to see whether you find differences in the results based on gender. Taking such steps to make study participants more similar to one another is called controlling for variability. If you cannot select subjects that are all similar, you can use statistical analyses to find out whether their differences truly matter when it comes to the problem you are studying.

Here's another example of how that works. Let us say that this facility houses about 200 people, who come from all races and ethnic backgrounds—Asian Americans, African Americans, Latinos, Caucasians, Native Americans, people of mixed race, and so forth. Is race a variable to consider? Well, it could be. Different races absorb sunlight into skin at different rates because of the amount of melanin (protective skin pigment) in their skin cells. Very dark-skinned people are known, from vitamin D studies, to require as much as an hour in sunlight to generate the same amount of vitamin D synthesis as Caucasians—and vitamin D synthesis is a possible explanation for the proposed effect of sunlight upon mood. If your population of 200 is very diverse, with no more than two-thirds belonging to any one ethnic group, you may also want to come up with a way of categorizing your subjects by skin pigmentation as a way of controlling for variation in skin color (variable *F*) for your study.

On the other hand, if you have a population of 200 people, and 190 of them are White, then you would probably do better to lump everyone together without considering skin color because the number of participants whose skin color could be a mitigating factor is fairly small—less than 1% of the group—so skin color is unlikely to be a significant cause of variation in this group.

You could find other differences and distinctions in the study population that you could name as variables *G* through *Z* and beyond—but that would not be helpful to the purpose of the study. Ideally, you would want to identify only those key variables that had the potential to strongly affect the study outcome, categorize the participants so that the differences between and among them are diminished, and then perform your tests. The tests themselves would be set up to reduce the chance of variation; for example, you would ask all of your participants who were going out into the sunlight to do so for the same amount of time, at the same time of day, during the same season, to avoid variation in the amount and intensity of sunlight to which the participants are exposed.

☐ Statistics and Evidence: Not All Hypotheses Are Created Equal

A theory is only as strong as the evidence that supports it, and the evidence, in turn, is only as strong as the hypotheses and data collection that formed it. You can see from the previous example that developing hypotheses about phenomena may seem simple, but actually testing the hypothesis in order to develop or support a theory can be complicated.

Develop a solid understanding of statistics and statistical methods to identify for yourself what qualifies as solid (versus questionable) evidence. Whether conducting your own research or reviewing someone else's, always look at what variables the study or studies took into account, focusing on these two important questions: (1) how were key variables identified, and (2) what was done to reduce the effects of, or control for, these variables?

At minimum, study participants should be similar in age, gender, and ethnicity; other common variables that are often taken into account include education, socioeconomic status, and the presence or absence of specific diseases or physiologic conditions or states (for example, whether a woman has given birth or has passed through menopause). On the other hand, very large studies, which tend to include a broader cross-section of the population, should include some type of analysis differentiating groups along these lines as part of the study.

We discuss this later in the text, but one great resource is a collection of articles from the *New England Journal of Medicine*'s archives, published under the title *Medical Uses of Statistics* (Bailar & Hoaglin, 2009), which offers a clear explanation of many different aspects of study design and statistical methods.

When Is a Theory Not a Theory? When It Is Theory

Looking at variables when you are talking about theories is sort of like considering the molecular structure of an object: It tells you what that object is composed of, but it does not tell you what that object is. Examining the object itself—the specific theory—does not really give you a sense of its place in the universe.

For that, turn to generalized theory. Our earlier definition of a theory as a set of concepts that have been tested and are supported by evidence is a concrete concept. It should not be confused with the idea of general theory, which itself is an abstract concept based upon generalization about the nature of theories. As an abstract concept, theory can be defined a number of ways:

- Theory is systematically organized knowledge applicable in a relatively wide variety of circumstances devised to analyze, predict, or otherwise explain the nature of behavior of a specified set of phenomena that could be used as the basis for action (vanRyn & Heaney, 1992).
- Theory is a systematic collection of concepts and relationships, also known as propositions; they form a set of statements about how some part of the world works (Powers & Knapp, 1995).
- Theory is a set of interrelated propositions, including concepts that describe, explain, or predict a phenomenon (Glanz, Rimer, & Lewis, 1997).

From these definitions, you can conclude the following:

1. *Theory is complex.* Each definition emphasizes the presence of multiple ideas, concepts, or propositions.
2. *Theory is systematic.* The nature of theory as an organizing principle is underscored in each description.
3. *Theory describes relationships between components.* Simply listing ideas or concepts does not establish theory; development of a theoretical construct is a creative process that describes how the parts work together

to form a working whole—one that consistently fits with observed phenomena.

In the concrete sense, theories are used in any discipline to organize its body of knowledge in a scientific manner and to help establish an empirical (observation- or experience-based) background about a specific phenomenon. So the image or idea is a concept, and the connections between concepts describe a theory. The traditional definition of theory that has been used in education is actually the interweaving of at least two concepts per theory, to provide that image or example.

In the abstract sense, theory is what links practice to research. As a nurse, you will make decisions about how to work with a client depending on the theory that informs your practice. For example, if you are a proponent of Dossey's (2008) theory of integral nursing, you support the idea that there are four factors that define an individual's integral self (interior self, exterior self, self in relation to others, and self in relation to systems). As such, you would work in the context of that theory's core concepts, both by maintaining awareness and promoting care of the client's integral self.

You may also make use of one or more concrete theories to help make decisions about what activities to undertake in helping the client's specific problem. For example, if the client has an addiction problem, you may call upon the 12-step process originally developed by Alcoholics Anonymous (Krentzman et al., 2010), and adapted by other treatment methods, to guide the client toward better health. You may also make use of activities grounded in other theories that have proven helpful in treating addictions, such as the stages of change theory (described later in this chapter).

Why offer the client alternatives based in a variety of theories? This is important because integral nursing theory promotes addressing *all* aspects of the client's self in treatment.

INFORMATION BOX 2-1

» HTTP://www.nurses.info/nursing_theory.htm
This site has a compilation of worldwide information on nursing theories, models, research resources, and links to other nursing theory websites. It is a useful site for finding just that right theory or model.

Nursing Theory

Much of modern nursing theory was developed in the 1980s and 1990s and correlates with the increase in PhD and EdD programs in nursing. Most of nursing theory focuses on explaining phenomena related to clinical practice, but while specific theories can spring from observations made in the clinical setting, they cannot be applied to clinical practice until they have been tested via research.

Nursing theory has two traditional types: grand and middle range (midrange). **Grand theories** are all-inclusive, conceptual structures that describe and explain large segments of the human experience. Grand theories are very abstract and tend to form the core of a knowledge base. Some examples of grand theories are Dossey's (2008) theory of integral nursing (described previously), Roy's (1999; Roy & Andrews, 1991) adaptation theory, and Leininger and McFarland's (1996) cultural care and diversity and universality theory. Conversely, **midrange theories** are less abstract, more focused, and lead to a narrow explanation of a specific phenomenon. Many times, midrange theories are more attractive for a researcher because they are very specific and concrete, making them ideal to be used as a theoretical framework (see the next section) to guide a study. Midrange theories include resilience theory and the theory of uncertainty in illness.

What Is a Theoretical Framework?

If you are a researcher who wishes to test or develop a hypothesis or theory, you need to create a logical set of actions and analyses that will allow you to gather data from your research subjects, analyze the data to ascertain the relationships between and among these subjects, and draw meaningful conclusions about these relationships. These conclusions will become evidence in support of (or refuting of) your hypothesis or theory. The theoretical framework is a representation of all of the factors that determine what this set of actions and analyses can be. It consists of the following:

1. The question or problem you wish to investigate
2. Concepts that underlie the theory or hypothesis that you plan to test
3. Findings from prior research on your subject or on related subjects (scientific literature)
4. The set of variables you have identified as affecting your problem or question
5. The relationships between/among variables and concepts that you or other researchers have already identified
6. Assumptions and biases that you identify in yourself as a researcher, or that you are aware your data set might contain

The point of creating the theoretical framework is to clearly delineate exactly what you as the researcher are attempting to describe or measure, so that the limits or parameters of the research problem are laid out and made clear. The theoretical framework outlines or encompasses the problem you are seeking to address.

☐ The Theoretical Framework Structure: A Fictional Case

Suppose that 15 years ago, eminent scientist C. Georgiana Monquey, RN, PhD, discovered a previously unknown enzyme, found in bananas, that she has named platanoase. Dr. Monquey has done many years of research studies consisting of repeated series of in vitro experiments (that is, experiments done in test tubes and petri dishes) and in vivo experiments (experiments done on living creatures) in mice to determine what platanoase does in the human body. Her findings suggest that this enzyme appears to have a key role in activating killer T cells, the immune cells that eliminate viral infections.

Dr. Monquey now wants to find out if platanoase works in people the way it works in test tubes and lab mice. She proposes that if schoolchildren, who are notoriously susceptible to viruses, eat more bananas, they will have more platanoase available in their bodies, and that this will result in stronger immune protection against viruses. She intends to test this hypothesis by randomly feeding or withholding bananas from a group of school children at Yellowhat School and keeping track on how often members of either group of children get sick.

Dr. Monquey's theoretical framework is built upon the following factors:

1. The concept that many childhood illnesses are caused by viral infections
2. Research findings that show that platanoase affects killer T cell functioning in vitro and in vivo
3. The proposition (assumption) that a response seen in a test tube and in a mouse will also be seen in a human child
4. The concept of the ability to alter bodily system functioning via nutritional inputs
5. The proposition (theory) that there is a cause-and-effect relationship between what the children eat and how their immune system responds to viruses
6. The proposition (hypothesis) that eating a specific food (bananas) will result in a specific change to the immune response (improved resistance to viruses)

Some of Dr. Monquey's framework factors are clear-cut: It is well known that many childhood illnesses are caused by viral infections, for example. Her own work on how platanoase affects killer T cell function might be strong or weak, depending on how often she ran the experiments and how carefully she obtained and analyzed this data. For the sake of this example, let us imagine that her work in this area has held up to scrutiny and received wide acceptance. So we can include this scientific knowledge of the actions of platanoase as a more solid piece of this framework.

Less solid are the remaining four contributing factors. It is often the case that relationships found in vitro and in experiments on lab animals *do* translate to the same response in humans, but it is equally common that they do not, or that the response is present but weaker or stronger in humans. Dr. Monquey may need to present evidence supporting the idea that it is likely that the children will show the same response to platanoase as the mice did. Also, while there is some evidence that diet determines the capacity of bodily systems to function well, the idea that specific nutrient inputs have direct effects is open for debate. Yet, evidence gathered from randomized trials supports a valid association of a Mediterranean dietary pattern with CHD (Mente, deKoning, Shannon & Anand, 2009).

Dr. Monquey will need to argue the case based on research evidence she uncovers in the scientific literature if she wishes to use this idea in support of her study of platanoase. Dr. Monquey's research methods should take into account the fact that her theoretical framework contains a few debatable factors and potential variables that need to be addressed.

In the course of designing and implementing her study, she may find that there are variables she hasn't considered. For example, what if she randomly assigns some students to the no bananas group and others to the bananas group, only to discover that half of the no bananas group loves bananas and eats them at home when they are not at school participating in the study? If she's right that bananas have a powerful effect on immunity, the fact that non-banana-eating study participants are actually eating bananas could skew (alter) the study results. Or, what if one teacher, Mrs. Jones, is a germaphobe who makes her students wash their hands six times a day, while another, Mrs. Smith, is so disorganized, it is a miracle if any of her students wash their hands even once during the day? Frequent hand washing is known to help protect against virus transmission, so this factor might also skew the study results. If Dr. Monquey creates her framework by taking these variables into consideration, she may anticipate such biases and take steps to eliminate them.

☐ Theoretical Frameworks and Evidence-Based Practice

All of this matters because when you develop programs for health promotion of individuals, families, and communities they must be based partly upon the theories about how clients function, learn, and change, and partly upon the research findings and experiences of those who have been in practice before and alongside them. It is vital for you to assess the validity of existing methods of addressing and promoting health.

Evidence-based practice means doing exactly that—reviewing the evidence found in research and clinical experience and using it as the basis of deciding how to help clients. We will discuss the nature of healthcare evidence later in this text, but here, the important message is that theory is not the be-all and end-all of nursing and health promotion—theory and evidence-based practice must go hand in hand for you to be effective.

Health Promotion Theory

Theories are used in health promotion to understand, guide, and explain health promotion at the individual, family, and community level. Theories are used and applied in multiple ways in health promotion. The theories can help researchers in understanding with whom they may be working, in guiding the selection and development of the appropriate health-promotion strategy, and in explaining the factors promoting and inhibiting change in the sample being studied.

Health promotion theories come from a multitude of disciplines, primarily behavioral and social sciences, specifically from psychology, sociology, management, and political science. This diverse group reflects that health promotion is not only concerned with just a specific individual's health behavior, but also with the organization of society and the role of policy and organizational and community structures in promoting health. These approaches are theories in that they are continually being tested empirically.

What Is the Difference Between a Theory and a Model?

A model for a building lays out all of the structural components under construction. A **model** for health promotion similarly outlines the structural components of a health phenomenon. If theory's goal is to determine how and why phenomena occur, then the goal of modeling is to identify the structure or composition of the phenomenon under investigation.

Types of Models

Modeling can also be used to organize concepts that do not have formal relationships established—that is, that are not held within the structure of a theory. A **conceptual model** is a less formal way of organizing ideas or concepts than the theories themselves. Conceptual modeling of this kind might be considered a pretheory in that it is used to help develop the hypotheses that, once tested, can support the formulation of theories. Conceptual models deal with concepts that are placed together because of their relevance to a common theme.

Conceptual models are not readily observable in the empirical world. In our fictional example of Dr. Monquey's banana enzymes, her idea of testing the effects of platanoase on immunity by feeding it to children is based on the conceptual model of animal testing. Not until she tried out her ideas with a animals did she consider using a human sample because developing a research strategy without doing the preliminary step first might prove to be a waste of time and research dollars. Conceptual models are very important in helping to formulate a hypothesis for research, and they can help refine the direction in which research goes.

A **schematic model** is a visual representation that uses concepts as building blocks but models the relationships between them using a minimal number of words. All types of research use schematic models. A list of concepts using boxes, arrows, or symbols to define the linkages is an example. Schematic models are also referred to as conceptual maps or conceptual frameworks. In nursing, there are multiple theoretical approaches, so the terms conceptual models, conceptual frameworks, and schematic models are used interchangeably.

FIGURE 2-1 is an example of a schematic model of factors affecting successful weight loss. In this model, a number of factors that affect an individual's ability to lose weight are depicted as boxes, and their relationships with one another are shown by means of arrows. Does the model encompass all factors? Probably not—but it outlines the interaction of a number of important, interrelated factors so that it becomes easier to think about them and consider how they work in the real world. The model itself does not offer any practical tips

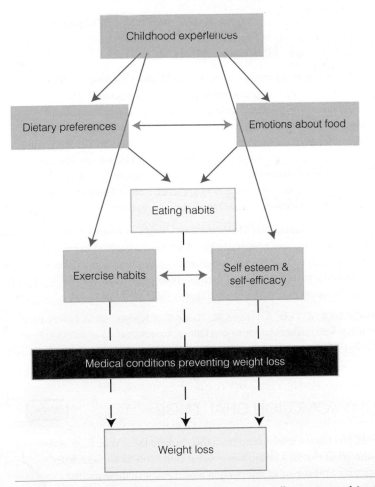

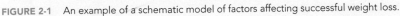

FIGURE 2-1   An example of a schematic model of factors affecting successful weight loss.

for how to work with a specific client, but it does provide suggestions as to what factors may need to be considered, discussed, and addressed.

RESEARCH BOX 2-1   Research Example: Health Promotion for Kidney Stones

» STUDY PURPOSE: Lack of fluid intake is an important factor in the development of kidney stones, but many factors can interfere with this health promotion action.

» POPULATION: Clients with kidney stones from an academic and a community practice were recruited for key informant interviews and focus groups.

» CONCEPTUAL FRAMEWORK: Groups were guided based on the framework of the health belief model. Content analysis was done on transcriptions using qualitative data analysis software.

» PROCEDURE: Key informant interviews were completed with 16 patients and with a total of 29 subjects in 5 focus groups. Content analysis revealed that all participants were highly motivawted to prevent stones.

» FINDINGS: An important strategy to increase fluid intake was insuring fluid availability by providing containers. Participants were more consistently confident in the ability to increase fluid, in contrast to ingesting medicine or changing the diet. While barriers to increasing fluid were multifactorial among individuals, the barriers aligned into three progressive stages that were associated with distinct patient characteristics. Stage 1 barriers included not knowing the benefits of fluid or not remembering to drink. Stage 2 barriers included disliking the taste of water, lack of thirst, and lack of availability. Stage 3 barriers included the need to void frequently and related workplace disruptions.

» CONCLUSIONS: Clients with kidney stones are highly motivated to prevent recurrence and were more amenable to fluid intake change than to another dietary or pharmaceutical intervention. Barriers preventing fluid intake success aligned into three progressive stages. Tailoring fluid intake and counseling based on patient stage may improve fluid intake behavior.

Source: McCauley, L. R., Dyer, A. J., Stern, K., Hicks, T., & Nguyen, M. M. (2012). Factors influencing fluid intake behavior among kidney stone formers. *Journal of Urology, 187*(4), 1282–1286.

HEALTH PROMOTION CHALLENGE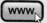

How could you use the information from this study to tailor your work with clients who are at risk for kidney stones? What could you do to make water more palatable? What kind of information would you give these clients?

Theories and Models Used in Nursing and Health Promotion

There are entire books devoted to nursing theory and models, so we cannot hope to provide a comprehensive description of the full body of nursing theory available. Instead, we will briefly touch upon those theories and models that are important components of health promotion practice, because familiarity with their concepts will help to support the discussions in later chapters. Note that the theories described here are midrange theories that focus on how human behavior can be changed and influenced—so an understanding of these theories has direct consequences for how you approach health promotion. Grand theories are beyond the scope of this chapter, and for the most part lack direct utility for health promotion practice.

Self-Determination Theory

Self-determination theory suggests that every person has three basic psychological needs that must be satisfied to foster well-being and health (Baumeister & Leary, 1995; Deci & Vansteenkiste, 2004). These are:

1. Competence, defined as a feeling of being effective in dealing with the environment or situation
2. Relatedness, defined as the wish to interact with, be connected to, or experience caring for and by others
3. Autonomy, defined as the universal urge to be the principal actors in our own life and act in ways that harmonize with our integrated self— that is, according to our values, morals, and cultural norms

Self-determination theory makes distinctions between different types of motivation and the consequences of actions that spring from them. Extrinsic motivation comes from external sources—for example, the desire for a good grade or payment can motivate individuals to do work they otherwise would have no interest in doing. The work itself is not the source of the reward or motivating factor. Intrinsic motivation, on the other hand, is motivation that comes from within. Intrinsic motivating factors include the pleasures felt upon doing something one enjoys as well as the natural, inherent drive to seek out challenges and new possibilities that are associated with cognitive and social development.

In this theory, motivation is a key determinant of behavior, so it is also a major factor in health promotion activities. You may want clients to engage in specific behaviors, but they may feel no motivation to do so—even if they understand why the behavior will benefit health. The promise of an extrinsic factor—"You'll be able to return to hiking and playing tennis after you complete 10 weeks of physical therapy."—may seem too remote or unreal in comparison to the challenge or obstacle presented by the desired behavior.

Deci and colleagues found that providing an emotionally meaningful reason for engaging in otherwise uninteresting behavior, along with support for a sense of autonomy and relatedness, can lead to internalization of the motivating factors and result in positive, integrated behaviors (Deci & Vansteenkiste, 2004; Jang, 2008). To help the client in the example to engage in health behaviors that are uninteresting or challenging, provide a more meaningful reason to undertake the challenge, such as, "I know how frustrating it is to be unable to hike or play tennis [expression of empathy]. But I'll help you every step of the way [support to build relatedness] through your 10 weeks of physical therapy. If you make a commitment to this therapy [autonomy], in the end, you'll have the freedom to do everything you enjoy [reward = autonomy and emotional satisfaction]."

The nature of self-determination predicts that the subject of health promotion activities *must be actively involved* for the activities to be effective. Each of the three factors of self-determination theory may be intertwined with the others. For example, giving positive feedback on a task increases intrinsic motivation to complete the task because it fulfills the need for competence, reinforcing to clients they're capable (Weiss, Amorose, & Wilko, 2009). Negative feedback has the opposite effect because it decreases the sense of competence (Berger, Steckelberg, Meyer, Kasper, & Mühlhauser, 2010).

In both instances, the feedback given has a similar effect on the client's sense of autonomy—a client who is given an experience of competence feels supported in his or her sense of autonomy, while a client who receives a message of incompetence will feel his or her autonomy is reduced. At the same time, providing positive feedback can fulfill the need for relatedness, while negative feedback leaves that need unfilled. When relatedness needs are not fulfilled, clients may have lower intrinsic motivation to engage in healthy behaviors. A simple, supportive act such as telling a client, "good job," will enhance relatedness, competence, and autonomy, which increases motivation—while negative behaviors such as scowling or pressuring the client will decrease each factor and reduce motivation. These responses have profound implications for health promotion; they suggest that it is important for nurses to be warm and caring, not cold and distant, if they hope to enhance healthy behaviors in clients.

According to self-determination theory, it is important that the three psychological needs be considered when developing motivational tools for a client. For example, offering extrinsic rewards (money, prizes, etc.) undermines behavior that is intrinsically motivated, because the client grows less interested in complying if the reward offered is not seen as equal in worth to the loss or reduction of autonomy. Other external factors like deadlines, which restrict and control, also decrease intrinsic motivation (Murayama, Matsumoto, Izuma, & Matsumoto, 2010). In contrast, situations that increase autonomy, as opposed to reducing it, support intrinsic motivation. Studies examining the effects of choice have found that increasing participant options and choices (increasing autonomy) increases intrinsic motivation to engage in the activities offered as options (Serneels et al., 2010).

The utility of the self-determination theory is demonstrated by the findings of a study published in the *Journal of the American Dietetic Association* that used a model founded upon this theory to study whether adolescents could be motivated to reduce obesity risk behaviors when offered opportunities to meet each of the three psychological needs. Middle-school students in low-income New York City schools were given a curriculum that stressed individual scientific inquiry and personal autonomy in decision making around food choices, exercise, and decisions about portion size. The outcome of the study was that those students who were offered the curriculum "showed substantial increases in positive outcome expectations about the behaviors, self-efficacy, goal intentions, competence, and autonomy" (Contento, Koch, Lee, & Calabrese-Barton, 2010, p. 1830).

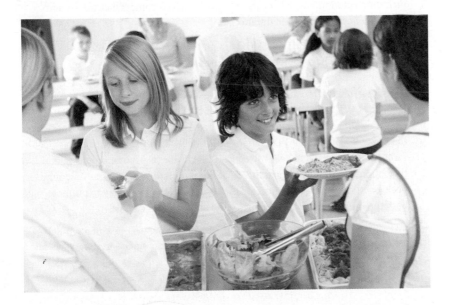

RESEARCH BOX 2-2 provides information about a computerized intervention to promote leisure-time physical activity and uses a self-determination theory model.

HEALTH PROMOTION CHALLENGE

Use self-determination theory to explain Charles's behavior.

RESEARCH BOX 2-2

» OBJECTIVES: To provide a methodological overview of a computerized intervention to promote leisure-time physical activity (PA) and to apply self-determination theory (SDT) to PA initiation to better understand the psychological mechanisms underlying PA frequency, intensity, and duration in previously sedentary individuals.

» DESIGN: Based on SDT, two computerized personal trainers were developed for use with sedentary young adults. One personal trainer was designed to be supportive, empathic, and structured while the other was designed to be more controlling, evaluative, and judgmental.

» METHOD: Participants were randomly assigned to work with either the need-supportive or controlling computerized personal trainer. They completed a series of seven weekly training sessions. In between training sessions, participants completed daily records of PA behaviors and experiences including autonomous self-regulation and perceived competence for PA and PA frequency, intensity, and duration.

» POTENTIAL CONTRIBUTIONS: The design of this intervention and its theoretical basis have important implications for advancing the field of exercise science specifically and health behavior change more broadly. Computerized interventions have the benefit of standardizing intervention content as well as reducing clinical contact burden for practitioners. Daily recording procedures reduce the likelihood of retrospection bias and allow for the modeling of (1) daily fluctuations in PA behavior and (2) the psychological mechanisms believed to be involved in PA behavior (e.g., autonomous self-regulation). Finally, as a broad theory of human motivation, SDT is uniquely positioned to offer explanations for the conditions that are likely to promote both the initiation and maintenance of health behavior change.

Source: Patrick, H., & Canevello, A. (2011). Methodological overview of a self-determination theory-based computerized intervention to promote leisure-time physical activity. *Psychology of Sport and Exercise, 12*(1), 13–19.

Social Cognitive Theory

Social cognitive theory is a learning theory based on the idea that we learn by watching what others do, and that human thought processes are central to understanding personality. This theory is most widely associated with the writings of Canadian psychologist Albert Bandura, who suggested that people who observed others behaving in a certain way adopted the behavior as their own. Bandura (1962, 1977) argued that promoting desired behaviors could best be done by modeling those behaviors to the individuals who needed to adopt them,

CASE STUDY

Charles, a 28-year-old man, started smoking an occasional cigarette while in high school. After he graduated, he attended a community college where his friends also smoked. His own parents had smoked for years, and he grew up in a household exposed to secondhand smoke. Currently, Charles has two jobs: During the daytime he works at a local mall as a cell phone salesman, and in the evenings and on weekends he is a musician, playing keyboards with a local band, which requires traveling to gigs and late hours. The late hours he works as a musician, the atmosphere of the venues he often plays (bars, clubs, and restaurants), and the fact that many of his friends and acquaintances smoke makes it difficult for him to avoid smokers.

Although Charles does not consider himself a real smoker, as he smokes less than a pack per day, he always thought he could just quit at anytime. Last year, however, his live-in girlfriend (a nonsmoker), asked him to quit. He found that quitting was not as easy as he expected, and while he stopped smoking in their apartment, he continued smoking cigarettes when he was around others who smoke, mostly during or after gigs. Charles says that he probably would have continued this way indefinitely, but his father was diagnosed with Stage IV lung cancer only a few weeks ago. "My mother is devastated," he says. "It's a real wake-up call. She's quitting because of it, and she wants me to quit, too. And I know she's right—if I don't quit, this could happen to me." Nevertheless, despite feeling a more urgent desire to quit smoking now, Charles says his behavior hasn't changed. "I will bum a cigarette even knowing that it's the last thing I should do, and I'll think about my Dad and feel guilty—but I'll still smoke it and even bum another one," he comments. "I just can't seem to stop."

and by encouraging the expectation of success by showing those persons that they, or individuals like them, were capable of mastering the new behaviors.

A key concept in social cognitive theory is that of **self-efficacy**. Bandura defined self-efficacy as "the belief in one's capabilities to organize and execute the courses of action required to manage prospective situations" (1992; 1995, p. 2). Self-efficacy beliefs function as important determinants of human motivation, affect, and action. Clients who believe they can perform a certain behavior are more apt to do so (Bandura, 2006). Client perception of capability may be different from actual capability. A goal for utilizing this theory in practice is to take action to increase self-efficacy in the client. Self-efficacy can be developed through a variety of methods. Information about past performances, accomplishments, vicarious experiences, social and verbal persuasion, physical or emotional arousal, and even imagery all can be offered in support of a client's self-efficacy (Bandura, 2006).

Benight and Bandura (2004) reviewed a number of studies that looked at the generalized role of perceived coping self-efficacy in individuals' ability to recover from different types of traumatic experiences. These experiences include natural disasters, technological catastrophes, terrorist attacks, military combat, and sexual and criminal assaults. In these analyses, perceived coping self-efficacy emerges as a key player in posttraumatic recovery. The fact that self-efficacy could be shown to contribute to posttraumatic recovery across a wide range of traumas supports the idea that promoting belief in a person's capability to exercise some measure of control over traumatic adversity is an important factor in healing from trauma.

Social cognitive theory is applied today in many different arenas. Mass media, public health, and education are just a very few. To ensure the success of a health promotion program, choose a model of the proper gender, age, and ethnicity so that participants can identify with a recognizable peer. Models can be those of an interpersonal imitation or media sources. Effective modeling teaches general rules and strategies for dealing with different situations (Bandura, 1988).

A study by Poddar and colleagues (Poddar, Hosig, Anderson, Nickols-Richardson, & Duncan, 2010) examined the use of a web-based nutrition education intervention to improve self-efficacy and self-regulation related to increased dairy intake in college students. They found that the intervention was effective in modifying some social cognitive theory constructs; strategies that positively impact outcome expectations and social support through online interventions require further development.

HEALTH PROMOTION CHALLENGE

Devise a way to use social cognitive theory to positively impact a group of clients. Share your ideas with at least two of your classmates and ask for feedback and suggestions.

Stages of Change Theory

Stages of change theory was originally developed in the context of smoking cessation, and later expanded to look at other efforts to change behavior. It draws upon other motivation theories to argue that any effort to change behavior passes through a set of specific stages before the behavior becomes permanent or ongoing (Prochaska & DiClemente, 1986). These stages are:

- Precontemplation—an individual has a behavioral problem in need of resolution (via behavioral change), but does not yet recognize the existence of that problem
- Contemplation—an individual recognizes the presence of a problem and is giving consideration to changing behavior
- Preparation—an individual recognizes a problem and makes an intention to change behavior within a set period of time

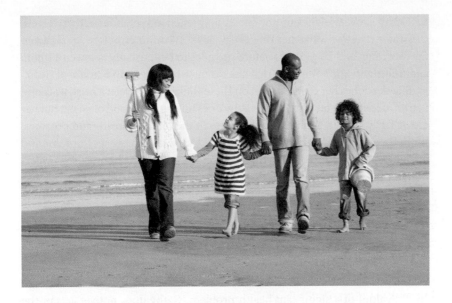

- Action—an individual actively and consistently undertakes the desired new behavior for at least 6 months
- Maintenance—an individual practices the behavior for longer 6 months or more

Clients do not necessarily progress from one stage to the next in a linear (or even forward-moving) fashion. A person who wants to exercise more, for instance, may stay in the contemplation stage for many years, occasionally make preparations to change and begin to take action, but lack the consistency that the action phase requires. This person may lapse back into contemplation for a time before moving, again, into preparation. Or, that same person, perhaps motivated by a health-related revelation (e.g., learning that he or she is has dangerously high blood pressure and is at risk of a stroke), may skip from precontemplation straight into action, bypassing the contemplation and preparation stages.

☐ Transitioning from Precontemplation: A Case Example

Jean, a nurse who is also a clinical diabetes educator, has a new client, Cathy, who has just been referred to her for diabetes education after being diagnosed with type 2 diabetes. Cathy's hemoglobin A_{1c} value is 8.3, showing that her average blood glucose levels are well above normal (a normal HbA_{1c} value is ~6.0), so the referring physician wants Cathy to learn to take her blood glucose in the morning and evening, eat a lower carbohydrate diet, lose some weight, and exercise more in an effort to bring her blood glucose levels down to a normal range.

Cathy is overweight but not obese, and when asked about activity levels, she states that she walks her dog every day—10 minutes before breakfast in the morning, and 20 minutes before she goes to bed, usually between 11 p.m. and midnight. She complains that she rarely gets more than 5 hours of sleep.

She describes her exercise level on these walks as "between a brisk walk and a stroll, depending on my mood." Cathy does not eat junk food or sugar, but her diet is fairly high in simple carbohydrates in the form of breads and potatoes.

In their initial meeting, Jean learns that Cathy has no overt symptoms and is having a hard time believing that her condition is real. Although she understands what diabetes means in terms of her long-term health, the need to use a blood glucose meter and take the actions her doctor recommends to address her blood sugar levels do not resonate with Cathy. "I don't feel sick," she tells Jean, "and I don't understand why he wants me to change what I'm doing. I get half an hour of exercise every day, and I don't really eat a lot of sugar—isn't that enough?"

Despite having a definitive diagnosis with evidence (in the form of a high HbA_{1c} value) of a significant health problem, Cathy does not yet accept the reality that a problem exists. She is in the precontemplation stage when it comes to changing her diet and exercise habits.

Jean's task will be to help Cathy reach acceptance that her situation is real and must be addressed right away, and to get her started on making lifestyle changes that will help her manage her blood glucose levels. This may not be an easy task given the lack of overt symptoms. One way Jean might help Cathy reach acceptance is by doing a simple test of Cathy's blood glucose values—and a demonstration. Their conversation might go as follows:

Jean: "OK, Cathy, let's do a little math. Can you tell me when you last ate something, and what you ate?"

Cathy: "Well, I had lunch about 2 hours ago. I had a peanut butter and jelly sandwich with a glass of milk and a handful of potato chips, and a small orange for dessert."

Jean: "That's not so bad in terms of nutrition, but I wonder if you know how many grams of carbohydrates that contains—here, let's look at this chart. Was the bread in your sandwich white or whole wheat?"

Cathy: "Whole wheat. I only eat white bread now and then."

Jean: "Good, good. Whole wheat is a better choice nutritionally. But even whole wheat bread is pretty high in carbohydrates—each slice has about 20 grams. The peanut butter isn't bad—only 3 grams for one tablespoon—but the jelly has 14 grams for a single tablespoon, which is a lot. Your orange probably had less than the jelly did—we'll say about 12 grams. The potato chips, hmm. . . let's assume you had about an ounce of chips. That would be maybe another 10 grams of carbohydrates. And your glass of milk adds another 12 grams. Altogether, your lunch included 91 total grams of carbohydrate."

Cathy: "Is . . . that a lot?"

Jean: "Well, that depends on what you eat at your other meals. Most adults who don't have diabetes need between 180 and 230 grams per day, and if you eat this much at every meal, you'd be taking in about 270 grams, which means you're going to exceed the max by almost 40 grams. And since you do have diabetes, you would probably find your blood sugar would be lower if you ate less than that 180-gram lower level. But that's not what I want to focus on right now. Can we test your blood sugar so we can see how that lunch has affected it? It's been 2 hours, so you should have digested most of it, and all of those carbs will have raised your blood glucose substantially. So it's a good time for us to take a look at what is going on in your blood."

Cathy: "Well, sure, I guess that's a smart thing to do. Will it hurt?"

Jean: "Just a little pinprick. Tell you what, I'll take mine too and we can compare them. I had lunch just about an hour and a half ago too."

Upon testing Cathy's blood glucose, they find it to be at 290 mg/dl, which is considerably higher than the 180 mg/dl maximum recommended for postmeal levels. Jean's blood glucose is 150 mg/dl.

Cathy: "Gosh. I'm 140 points higher than you are."

Jean: "Yes. That's part of what it means to have diabetes. You don't metabolize the glucose very well at this stage, so a lot of it stays in your bloodstream instead of going into your cells. Your body has to do something with it, so it's going to either store it as fat or pass it out through the urine—but that means potentially damaging your kidneys and causing all kinds of other problems down the line. Fortunately, there's an easy way to address it. C'mon, Cathy, let's get your blood sugar down right now!"

Cathy: "Huh? How?"

Jean: "We're going to walk it off."

Jean takes Cathy for a brisk, 20-minute walk around the office building, jogging up and down several flights of stairs and keeping a pace that has them both breathing harder, but still able to talk. When they return to Jean's office, Cathy's heart rate is noticeably higher and she's flushed, but energized. They take Cathy's blood glucose again, and Cathy is amazed to find that it has dropped by almost 50 mg/dl. It is still too high, but the message has been demonstrated very clearly—vigorous exercise is one key to bringing Cathy's diabetes under control. Jean can also start to talk to Cathy about ways to limit her carbohydrate intake. For instance, instead of peanut butter and jelly, Cathy can have turkey with lettuce and tomato—reducing her intake by about 15 to 18 grams of carbohydrate, and more if she buys a low-carb wheat bread rather than regular wheat bread. If she has a salad with lemon juice and olive oil in place of the potato chips, and water or unsweetened iced tea instead of milk, that brings her total intake down by another 15 to 18 grams—and she may even be eating *more* food, not less! She can still have her orange, but perhaps she will only eat half and save the rest for later, or choose a smaller mandarin orange, tangerine, or clementine instead, so she gets half as many grams of carbohydrate. Simply by changing her food choices to lower carbohydrate, lower glycemic options, Cathy can reduce her carbohydrate intake by 45% or more, which will help prevent blood sugar spikes. Increasing her exercise will also help her to maintain lower blood glucose. Jean talks to Cathy about the benefit of walking her dog for half an hour instead of 10 minutes before breakfast, and suggests she take the dog for its second walk about an hour after dinner, instead of before bedtime, so she can increase the impact these walks have on her blood glucose values. She might even consider adding another walk after lunch. Jean also suggests that she buy a pedometer and use it as a way of making sure her walks are briskly paced enough to bring her heart rate up, so she will burn off more glucose.

When Cathy understands that the changes Jean is asking her to make are not huge alterations to her lifestyle, she is more likely to contemplate making them—and having seen how her blood sugar responded directly to exercise, she is also more likely to accept that the changes are needed. In future meetings, Jean can reinforce the benefits of changing her behavior by addressing her sleep issues, which also will help her blood glucose levels.

☐ Using Stages of Change Effectively

While the stages of change theory does not address motivation, it does give concrete guidance as to how nurses can work to promote changes in behavior. Identifying where a client is in the process can be highly useful in determining how to proceed in promoting health. A client who engages in a risky behavior without knowledge of the potential consequences, for example, is unlikely to even be at a contemplation stage related to reducing or eliminating the risk by changing behavior. Explaining the risk is therefore a step the nurse can take toward bringing that client from precontemplation to contemplation. Offering a set of specific actions and sources of support for behavior change can help move the client from contemplation to preparation and subsequent action. Continued support can help the client make the final transition into maintenance. Reaching the maintenance stage does not mean that the behavior is set in stone; individuals who have reached that stage can, and often do, return to earlier stages. Even if regression occurs, returning to the maintenance stage is generally easier once the client has previously established the desired behavior.

The Centers for Disease Control and Prevention successfully incorporated the stages of change theory into a study of HIV/AIDS counseling at clinics treating individuals for sexually transmitted diseases during the 1990s (Coury-Doniger, Levenkron, Knox, Cowell, & Urban, 1999). A review by the World Health Organization (King, 1999) found that while this theory offered guidelines for interventions with diverse populations, it overlooked the role that environment, culture, gender, and other social factors have on the decision-making and implementation process.

HEALTH PROMOTION CHALLENGE

Most smokers are well aware of the risks of smoking. Even smokers who contemplate quitting take no actions toward it because they find the side effects of quitting to be too great a challenge. What strategies can be employed to help a smoker in the contemplation stage of quitting move to preparation and action?

Theory of Reasoned Action

The **theory of reasoned action**, developed by Martin Fishbein and expanded by Fishbein and Icek Ajzen (1975), is founded upon two basic assumptions: first, that human beings are rational and make systematic use of information available to them, and second, that people consider the implications of their actions before they decide to engage or not engage in certain behaviors. The theory proposes that individuals are more likely to decide to behave in certain ways (behavioral intention) if their attitudes and normative beliefs are pointing toward that behavior, but this decision is mitigated by perceived behavioral control, or the degree to which they feel capable of executing the behavior. Attitude is the degree to which a person feels positively or negatively about a behavior; one important aspect of attitude is the beliefs that the individual has about how valuable the behavior might be (behavioral beliefs). Normative beliefs are the individual's understanding of, and willingness to conform to, societal opinions or pressure surrounding the behavior in question. So, simply put, the theory of reasoned action suggests that a person who has a positive attitude, who feels social pressures or influences toward a behavior, and who has a greater degree of perceived behavioral control, is likely to set an intention to adopt the behavior.

There are certain problems with the theory. Its focus on the individual, as with the stages of change theory, does not allow for the influence of outside environmental or social factors on decision making and execution of behavioral change. It also does not address factors outside of the rational sphere—emotional, physiologic, and psychological factors that influence the individual away from the behavior that they may have made a conscious intention to adopt.

Health Belief Model

Turning from theories to models, one of the first models we will discuss is the **health belief model** (FIGURE 2-2). The health belief model is among the most widely used models for explaining change and maintenance of health

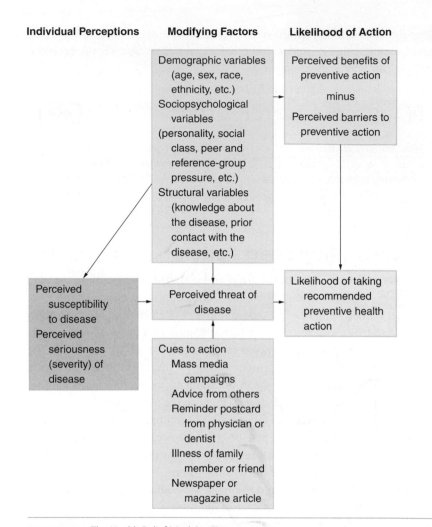

FIGURE 2-2   The Health Belief Model

Source: Strecher, V., & Rosenstock, I. (1977). The health belief model. *Health Behavior and Health Educa-*
tion, Theory, Research, and Practice (pp. 41–58). San Fransico, California: Jossey-Bass.

behavior, as well as for developing health behavior interventions (Strecher &
Rosenstock, 1997). The original health belief model was developed in the 1950s
by a group of social psychologists who were all part of the United States Public
Health Service (Hochbaum, 1958; Rosenstock, 1960; Rosenstock, 1966). The
purpose of the model was to aid in explaining the widespread failure of people
to participate in health promotion/prevention programs. The original concern
that led to the development of the model was the spread of infectious diseases,
specifically tuberculosis. At the time, the model was being tested to see if it
could successfully predict whether people would participate with preventive
measures, and if not, what interventions would encourage them to engage in
preventive behaviors.

ASK YOURSELF
www.

You are planning to study a population of clients who have high cholesterol levels, with the goal of developing a prevention program. You have decided to use the health belief model as your framework. What areas might you explore?

The model originated as a **value expectancy theory** that relied on the assumptions that an individual has the desire to avoid illness or to get well (value) and a belief that a specific health action by that person would prevent illness (expectancy). Therefore, the theory is based on an individual's idea and appraisal of perceived benefits compared to perceived barriers.

CULTURAL RESEARCH STUDY

A review of: Hispanic Chronic Disease Self-Management: A Randomized Community-Based Outcome Trial

This study, which was based on self-efficacy theory, applied the results of a successful English chronic disease self-management program to a Spanish-speaking population by using Spanish speakers and focus groups to validate the materials. Patient education courses were conducted in Spanish and included content related to healthy eating, exercise, problem solving, action planning, breathing problems, relaxation techniques, medications, and family relationships. At 4 months, the participants, compared with control subjects, had more improved health status and behaviors, more improved self-efficacy, and fewer emergency room visits. At 1 year, improvements were maintained.

Source: Lorig, K. R., Ritter, P. L., & Gonzáles, V. M. (2003). Hispanic chronic disease self-management: A randomized community-based outcome trial. *Nursing Research, 52*(6), 361–369.

Over the 40 years of the development of this model, numerous investigations have expanded and clarified the model and have extended its use to preventive actions as well as illness and sick-role behaviors (Becker & Maimam, 1980; Janz & Becker, 1984; Kirscht, 1974; Rosenstock, 1974). Rosenstock, Strecher, and Becker (1988) determined that, in general, individuals will take action to ward off, screen for, or control an ill-health condition if:

1. They regard themselves as susceptible to the condition (perceived susceptibility)
2. The condition will have potentially serious consequences (perceived severity)
3. A course of action available to them would be beneficial in reducing either their susceptibility or the severity of the condition (perceived benefits)

4. The anticipated barriers to or costs of taking the action are outweighed by its benefits (perceived barriers)

5. There are good reasons to believe that action is needed (cues to action)

Self-efficacy was eventually added to the model to increase explanatory power, and thus the term **expanded health belief model**. Self-efficacy, the belief or conviction that a person can successfully execute a behavior required to produce a desired outcome, is viewed as a key factor in determining the presence or absence of action. If self-efficacy is lacking, then a barrier is added to taking a recommended health action—even if all of the other five belief requirements are satisfied. To put it simply, "I can't do this" is a phrase that can outweigh all of the arguments in favor of performing the health-promoting act.

HOT TOPICS

Here are some topics to explore:
- Bandura's self-efficacy theory
- Value-expectancy theories
- HR3200 (healthcare bill)
- Health insurance and health promotion
- Theory of planned behavior
- Theory of reasoned action

The key variables of the expanded health belief model now include perceived susceptibility, perceived severity, perceived benefits, perceived barriers, self-efficacy, and cues to action (TABLE 2-1). In general, modifying factors include demographic, sociopsychological, and structural variables.

Bio-Psycho-Social-Spiritual Model

The **bio-psycho-social-spiritual model** is considered the most comprehensive for holistic health promotion. The model suggests that all disease has a psychosomatic component—that is to say, the client's state of mind, attitude, intellectual capacity, and belief systems all have influence on the disease course. The model emphasizes that the human spirit must be incorporated as a major healing force in reversing, stabilizing, and producing remission in diseases and illnesses. The spiritual aspect of this model incorporates individual values, meaning, and purpose in living (Dossey, 1999).

Hunter and Mann (2010) used a bio-psycho-social-spiritual framework to examine hot flushes and night sweats commonly experienced by mid-aged women during the menopause transition. These symptoms affect approximately 70% of women, but are regarded as particularly problematic for 15–20% largely due to physical discomfort, distress, social embarrassment, and sleep disturbance. The authors described a cognitive model of menopausal hot flushes that

Table 2-1 Key Concepts and Definitions of the Expanded Health Belief Model

Concept	Definition	Application
Perceived susceptibility	One's opinion of chance of getting a condition	Define population at risk
Perceived severity	One's opinion of how serious a condition is	Specify consequences of risk
Perceived benefits	One's opinion of the efficacy of the advised action	Define action to take
Perceived barriers	One's opinion of the tangible and psychological costs of the advised action	Identify barriers and help to reduce them
Cues to action	Strategies to activate one's readiness	Promote awareness
Self-efficacy	One's confidence in one's ability to take action	Demonstrate desired behavior
Modifying factors	One's demographic, sociopsychological, and structural variables	Education, age, and race

Source: Strecher and Rosenstock, 1997.

can explain symptom perception, cognitive appraisal, and behavioral reactions to symptoms. As part of Phase II intervention development, they described a cognitive behavioral treatment that links the bio-psycho-social-spiritual processes specified in the model to components of the intervention.

Clark Wellness Model

While the bio-psycho-social-spiritual model focuses on psychosomatic processes, the **Clark wellness model** (Clark, 1996) (FIGURE 2-3) exemplifies nurse–client interactions from a wellness perspective. It combines elements within systems theory. In this model, both nurse and client are complete systems that interact within themselves (that is, each has inputs, throughputs—activities within the system—and outputs), and interact with each other (intersystems) across interfaces to jointly plan and achieve goals and feelings of well-being. Your own wellness is an important facet of this theory, and you serve as a wellness role model for the client to emulate.

Trudeau and colleagues (Trudeau, Ainscough, Pujol, & Charity, 2010) used a wellness model to develop an online self-management program for arthritis pain sufferers. They reviewed both practitioners' and clients' views and published the differences they found. This information can help you gain insight into how to interact more effectively with clients. For example, suppose a nurse who is overweight is working with a client who has arthritis and is also overweight.

BIOLOGICAL, HISTORICAL,
SOCIAL, AND CULTURAL FACTORS ◄————————► WHOLE PERSON WELLNESS ◄————————► STRESSORS

Chance

Increases perceptions of the world and individual experiences as manageable and meaningful

Situational/
developmental crises/
changes/diseases/
disabilities

Seeks access to material goods, jobs, money, educational growth—
promoting and challenging environment

Childhood experiences

Interpersonal conflict

Uses problem solving creatively and imaginatively to solve life problems

Internal conflict

Cultural expectations

Presents self as coherent, consistent, integrated, stable, flexible, assertive

Uses self-care strategies to achieve optimum fitness and nutritional status

Daily hassles

Socioeconomic status and
role expectations

Is willing to examine contradictions to thinking and to readjust beliefs and
practices into an integrated and consistent whole

Community/world
change

Increases richness of social supports and ties; interrelatedness of energy
fields of individual with family and community

Genetic factors, such as immunological strength, charm,
beauty, plasticity of body systems

Physical and biochemi-
cal interactions

Maintains open communication channels with others

Gaps between goals
and means to meet
goals

Increases differentiation of self while increasingly able to work with and get
along with others

Participates and shows commitment to patterns (communication, action) of
behavior with self, significant people, objects, and environs; uses energy
efficiently in a goal-directed way.

Increases use of values to guide behavior toward coherence

Functions effectively in family and work or learner roles

Develops coping strategies that are flexible, reasonable, farsighted, and that
produce success

Source: This figure suggested by the work of Ahmed and Coehlho (*Toward a New Definition of Health*, New York, NY: Plenum, 1979);
Antonovasky (*Health, Stress and Coping*, San Francisco, CA: Jossey-Bass, 1979); and Dunn (*High Level Wellness*, Arlington, VA: R.W. Beatty, 1961.)

FIGURE 2-3 The Clark Wellness Model

Although their reasons for being overweight may differ, if the nurse puts pressure on the client to lose weight as a way of relieving his osteoarthritis symptoms, the client will not take the advice seriously—"After all," the client may think, "how can she expect me to do something she isn't doing herself?" But the nurse may have better success if she makes herself a role model instead. "I understand just how hard it is to lose weight," she could say. "I have a thyroid problem myself, and boy, I fight just to stay where I am, never mind losing weight. But I also know that if I don't persevere, I could end up with the same difficulties you have—pain, pain, and more pain. So it's worth it to keep trying even when progress is slow."

See RESEARCH BOX 2-3 for information about Trudeau and colleagues' study.

RESEARCH BOX 2-3

» OBJECTIVE: Self-management of pain is a critical component of arthritis care; but, limited mobility can restrict access to resources. Although the Internet has become a primary source of health information, few studies address what patients want and need from a self-management website.

» METHODS: Thirty-two people diagnosed with arthritis and 12 practitioners (1) participated in individual 1-hour interviews and (2) sorted and rated a list of 88 unique statements that were derived from the interviews. Qualitative data were analyzed using concept mapping procedures.

» RESULTS: The six-cluster map provided the best discrimination between statements. Follow-up analyses suggested that although clients with arthritis and practitioners generally agree on the categories of content on a self-management website about arthritis, they appear to disagree on the importance of each category. The conceptual map the researchers developed included: 1. Tools to manage pain, 2. Latest research findings on arthritis pain, 3. How to stop arthritis from getting worse, 4. Physical activity and diet needed to maintain strength to support joints, 5. Daily living things that could affect pain, and 6. How to e-mail questions to practitioners and obtain answers and support.

» CONCLUSIONS: These findings about client- and provider-desired content can be used by nurses to develop a curriculum for health education of clients with arthritis pain.

Source: Trudeau, K.J., Ainscough, J., Pujol, L.A., & Charity, S. (2010). What arthritis pain practitioners and patients want in an online self-management program. *Musculoskeletal Care 8*(4), 189–196.

Health Education Model

While the Clark wellness model focuses on the interaction between client and nurse, in the **health education model,** clients must have awareness, knowledge, skills, positive attitudes, appropriate or supportive cultural norms, requisite opportunities, and/or motivation to change to healthier behavior. These attributes are defined as follows:

- Awareness includes alerting a target group or individual to a danger or a positive factor
- Knowledge is awareness with understanding.

- Skills include the ability to problem solve, take advantage of an opportunity, or otherwise develop tools improve a health situation.
- An individual who believes that performing a certain behavior will lead to positive outcomes will tend to hold a favorable attitude toward that behavior. The converse is also true.
- Cultural norms and opportunity to participate in related health activities or services will expand or limit the effectiveness of any health education program.
- Motivation is an internalized construct of self-reinforcement—that is, a force within the individual's own thought processes that influences him or her to take action in a certain direction.

According to this model, motivation is necessary before an individual can take responsible actions. If motivation toward a healthy behavior is not present or is weak, the person's health beliefs and attitudes must be influenced or strengthened before a person becomes motivated to change a behavior in the direction of better health. If an individual is made aware, given relevant knowledge and skills, and has the opportunity to make necessary changes in attitude and participate in related health services, it is possible that motivation toward healthy behaviors will improve simply on the basis of having the needed tools. Motivation is also assumed to be a process that involves stages of change, which can be targeted with specific educational methods. Without motivation, the rest of the elements of health education will not be effective in changing health behaviors (Patterson & Campbell, 1995).

All these factors are interrelated; for example, awareness of the effect of diet on weight can stimulate curiosity and lead to an increase in knowledge or motivation to change the diet in order to lose weight, if attitude and cultural norms support weight loss.

RESEARCH BOX 2-4 describes a study that uses a health education model.

RESEARCH BOX 2-4

» BACKGROUND: Patient education is an important intervention for the management of heart failure, but in practice patient education varies considerably.

» AIM: To systematically review educational interventions that have been implemented for heart failure patients and assess their effectiveness.

» METHODS: Randomized controlled trials from 1998 to 2008 in CINAHL, MEDLINE, PsychInfo, EMBASE, and Cochrane were reviewed using the following search terms in combination with "heart failure" patient education, education, educational intervention, and self-care. There were 1,515 abstracts reviewed independently by 2 reviewers.

» RESULTS: A total of 2,686 patients were included in the 19 studies that met the inclusion criteria. Commonly, the initial educational intervention was a one-on-one didactic session conducted by nurses and supplemented with written materials and multimedia approaches. Seven studies referred to a theoretical model as a framework for their educational intervention. Studies used a variety of outcome measures to evaluate their effectiveness. Of the studies reviewed, 15 demonstrated a significant effect from their intervention in at least one of their outcome measures.

» CONCLUSION: Due to the heterogeneity of the studies included in this review, it was difficult to establish the most effective educational strategy as the educational interventions varied considerably in delivery methods and duration as well as the outcome measures that were used for the evaluation. A client-centered approach to education based on educational theory and evaluated appropriately may assist to develop an evidence base for client education.

Source: Boyde, M., Turner, C., Thompson, D. R., & Stewart, S. (2010). Educational interventions for patients with heart failure: A systematic review of randomized controlled trials. *Journal of Cardiovascular Nursing, 26*(4), E27–E35.

Orem Self-Care Model of Nursing

Unlike the health education model, which assumes clients will change once they have the knowledge to do so, or the Clark wellness model, which assumes the nurse is a role model for client behavior, Orem based her theory, the **Orem self-care model**, on the philosophy that all "patients wish to care for themselves" (Orem, 2001). According to this concept, individuals can recover more quickly and holistically if they are allowed to perform their own self-care to the best of their ability.

Self-care requisites are groups of needs or requirements that Orem placed in one of three categories:

1. Universal self-care requisites are those needs that all people have, including air, water, food, elimination, activity and rest, solitude, and social interaction, among others.

2. Developmental self-care requisites are needs that are either maturational (that is, needs dependent upon or important to life transitions from infancy to childhood to adolescence to adulthood) or situational (that is, needs that arise because of particular circumstances in life, such as transitioning through a divorce or coping with the death of a loved one).

3. Health deviation requisites include needs that arise as a result of a patient's condition (for example, the need for medication to treat an

illness, or the need for physical therapy to restore mobility after an accident).

When individuals are unable to meet their own self-care requisites, a self-care deficit occurs. From a health promotion standpoint, a deficit occurs when the individual lacks information or needs to be taught certain skills in order to perform self-care tasks. In contrast to the Clark wellness model, where client input is crucial, in the Orem model, the nurse determines these deficits and defines a support modality by rating dependencies for each of the self-care deficits from total compensation, to partial compensation, to educative/supportive.

Klainin and Ounnapiruk (2010) performed a meta-analysis of self-care behavior research on elders in Thailand. They used 20 studies undertaken from 1990 to 2008. Most studies were unpublished master's theses guided by Orem's self-care deficit theory. Data were collected in these studies by face-to-face interviews. Variables with the greatest effects on self-care encompassed self-concept, social support, and self-efficacy. Those with moderate effects included family relationships, overall health beliefs, internal locus of control, health status, and external locus of control.

Pender's Health Promotion Model

Unlike the other models, Pender's **health promotion model** is directed at increasing a client's level of well-being, with special focus on helping clients to associate positive feelings with health-promoting actions (Pender, Murdaugh, & Parsons, 2010).

The model is based on the following ideas:

1. Prior behavior and inherited and acquired characteristics influence beliefs, affect, and enactment of health-promoting behavior.
2. Persons commit to engaging in behaviors from which they anticipate deriving personally valued benefits.
3. Perceived barriers can constrain commitment to action, which can be a mediator of behavior as well as actual behavior.
4. Perceived competence (self-efficacy) to execute a given behavior increases the likelihood of commitment to action and actual performance of the behavior.
5. Greater perceived self-efficacy results in fewer perceived barriers to a specific health behavior.
6. Positive affect toward a behavior results in greater perceived self-efficacy, which can, in turn, result in increased positive affect.
7. When positive emotions or affect are associated with a behavior, the probability of commitment and action is increased.
8. Persons are more likely to commit to and engage in health-promoting behaviors when significant others model the behavior, expect the

behavior to occur, and provide assistance and support to enable the behavior.

9. Families, peers, and healthcare providers are important sources of interpersonal influence who can increase or decrease commitment to and engagement in health-promoting behavior.

10. Factors in the external environment can increase or decrease commitment to or participation in health-promoting behavior.

11. The greater the commitments to a specific plan of action, the more likely health-promoting behaviors are to be maintained over time.

12. Commitment to a plan of action is less likely to result in the desired behavior when competing demands over which persons have little control require immediate attention.

13. Commitment to a plan of action is less likely to result in the desired behavior when other actions are more attractive and thus preferred over the target behavior.

14. Clients or nurses can modify cognitions, affect, and the interpersonal and physical environment to create incentives for health actions.

A study used Pender's health promotion model to examine clients' diabetes self-management behaviors (Ho, Berggren, & Dahlborg-Lyckhage, 2010). Realizing that diabetes self-management is a challenge for both clients and nurses, and that empowerment plays a vital role in helping clients achieve successful self-management, Ho and colleagues adopted a metaethnographic approach. They synthesized the results of nine qualitative studies to identify what clients perceive as being important in an effective empowerment strategy for diabetes self-management. Four central metaphors that influenced empowerment were identified: trust in nurses' competence and awareness, striving for control, a desire to share experiences, and nurses' attitudes and ability to personalize. The lines-of-argument synthesis suggested the need for an evaluation system to appraise clients' diabetes knowledge, health beliefs, and negative emotions, as well as the outcome of interventions.

Based on Pender's health promotion model, this study emphasizes the fact that healthcare professionals need to understand and address modifiable behavior-specific variables. The study suggests that an effective empowerment strategy would be to use activity-related affect, as well as interpersonal and situational influences, as a means of facilitating and enhancing clients' health-promoting behaviors.

PRECEDE-PROCEED Framework

Another model used in health promotion is the **PRECEDE-PROCEED framework** (Green & Kreuter, 2005). PRECEDE stands for *p*redisposing, *r*einforcing, and *e*nabling *c*onstructs in *e*ducational/ecological *d*iagnosis and *e*valuation.

The acronym PROCEED stands for *p*olicy, *r*egulatory, and *o*rganizational *c*onstructs in *e*ducational and *e*nvironmental *d*evelopment. The purpose of health promotion within this model is not to do interventions for a person, but rather to empower him to do them himself.

The PRECEDE-PROCEED framework (FIGURE 2-4) acts as a systematic planning process that has the primary goal of empowering individuals and communities to understand and engage in efforts to improve their quality of life. The framework entails different phases that can easily be linked to different levels of theory for a health behavior change. The model was designed as a guide for planning and developing health education programs, by identifying the most appropriate intervention. The underlying assumption of the PRECEDE phase is that an educational diagnosis needs to be made prior to initiating an intervention plan. The second phase, PROCEED, was added to account for the contribution of environmental variables, or things that are outside of the individual, to health. The two propositions of the model are (1) health and health risks have multiple determinants, and (2) efforts to change the behavioral, physical, and social environment must be multidimensional and participatory.

The original planning process of the model included the following nine steps:

1. Social assessment/community assessment
2. Epidemiologic assessment
3. Behavioral/environmental assessment

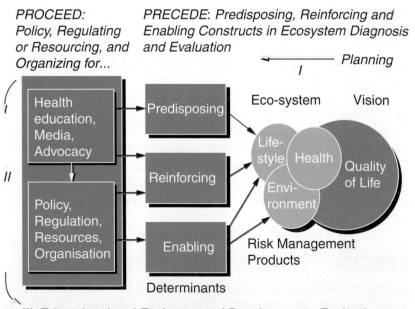

FIGURE 2-4   The PRECEDE-PROCEED framework

4. Educational and ecological assessment
5. Administration and policy assessment
6. Implementation of the planned intervention
7–9. Process and outcome evaluations

The model was condensed in 2004, merging the steps into the following six phases:

Phase one: Social assessment and situational analysis (formerly step 1)

Phase two: Epidemiological assessment and behavioral and environmental assessments (formerly steps 2 and 3)

Phase three: Educational and ecological assessment (formerly step 4)

Phases four, five, and six: Intervention, alignment, administrative and policy assessment, and evaluation (formerly steps 5–9)

Despite the efforts to compress it, the model is very time intensive, and enacting it drains human and financial resources. The authors of the model have a website of published papers with applications of the model, which can be found at http://www.lgreen.net/preccdc.htm

HEALTH PROMOTION CHALLENGE

Make a list of at least three ways you can influence clients to associate positive emotions with health promotion behavior. More advanced students can pick one of Pender's ideas upon which her model is based and develop a research design to test it.

Summary

Theories, Concepts, and Models

A theory is a set of interrelated ideas that represent an orderly way to describe a phenomenon. Theory links practice to research. A concept is a set of interrelated ideas that are the building blocks of a theory. A model focuses on a structure or composition of a phenomenon; it is a symbolic representation of concepts.

Theories need to be tested through research before being applied to clinical practice. There are two traditional types of theory: grand theories and midrange theories. Grand theories are all-inclusive, conceptual structures that describe and explain large segments of the human experience; they are very abstract and are used to establish a knowledge base. Midrange theories are more focused, less abstract, and have a narrower scope than grand theories. They can be used as a framework to guide a study. Midrange theories often referenced in health-promotion research studies include self-determination theory, social cognitive theory, stages of change theory, and the theory of reasoned action.

A conceptual model is less formal than a theory and is composed of concepts that have been placed together because of a common theme; they are more loosely structured than theories and may assist in the development of hypotheses in research. A schematic model is a visual representation that uses concepts as building blocks and minimizes the use of words. In nursing, the terms conceptual model, conceptual framework, and schematic model are often used interchangeably.

The health belief model was originally developed in the 1950s to aid in explaining the widespread failure of people to participate in health promotion/prevention programs. This model originated as a value expectancy theory, incorporating the assumptions that one has both the desire to avoid illness or get well (value) and a belief that a specific health action to oneself would prevent illness (expectancy). The expanded health belief model includes the addition of self-efficacy, a belief or conviction of expected success held by the client that health promotion behavior can be produced. The key concepts of the expanded health belief model are perceived susceptibility, perceived severity, perceived benefits, perceived barriers, cues to action, self-efficacy, and modifying factors.

The bio-psycho-social-spiritual model incorporates the understanding that mental constructs of varying types influence the progression of disease and healing. The Clark wellness model suggests that the nurse has an active role to play in promoting wellness; in contrast, the health education model suggests that the prime mover of health promotion is the client's level of understanding and acceptance of information, so that the nurse's role becomes more instructional and less interactive.

In the Orem self-care model, the nurse's role is to identify areas in which individuals lack needed requisites to perform self-care. The health promotion model developed by Pender contains seven assumptions that reflect nursing and behavioral science perspectives and 14 statements/propositions that provide a basis for investigative work on health behaviors. The PRECEDE-PROCEED framework developed by Green and Kreuter in 2005 is a systematic planning process with the primary goal of empowering individuals and communities to understand and engage in efforts to improve the quality of their lives. The process involves social, community, epidemiologic, behavioral, environmental, educational, ecologic, administration, and policy assessments, followed by implementation of the planned intervention and process and outcome evaluations. The two propositions of the model are that (1) health and health risks have multiple determinants, and (2) efforts to change the behavioral, physical, and social environment must be multidisciplinary and participatory.

REVIEW QUESTIONS

www

1. A value expectancy theory
   a. Incorporates the idea that one has the desire to get well and a belief that a specific health action would prevent illness.
   b. Is a theory that helps define health for an individual.
   c. Explains a belief by an individual that there are too many barriers to successfully achieving disease prevention.

2. The PRECEDE-PROCEED framework
   a. Was developed by Pender.
   b. Includes the defining concept of self-efficacy.
   c. Includes assessments of environment, ecology, and education of a community/individual.

3. The health promotion model includes the following assumption:
   a. Perceived benefits and barriers to achievement of health behaviors regulate health seeking activities.
   b. Individuals seek to actively regulate their own behavior.
   c. Health and health risks have multiple determinants.

4. Self-efficacy theory is
   a. A belief or conviction by the individual that he or she is able to successfully execute the behavior needed for producing the desired outcome.
   b. A systematic planning process with the primary goal of empowering individuals and communities to understand and engage in efforts to improve the quality of their lives.
   c. A theory that incorporates the assumptions that one has the desire to avoid illness or get well and a belief that a specific health action by that person would prevent illness.

5. The expanded health belief model includes
   a. The self-efficacy concept.
   b. Epidemiologic assessment.
   c. The proposition that when positive emotions or affect are associated with a behavior, the probability of commitment and action is increased.

6. A theory
   a. Links practice to theory.
   b. Is a set of interrelated ideas that represent a way to describe a phenomenon.
   c. Is a systematic collection of concepts and propositions.
   d. Is all of the above.

7. The relationship between a concept and a theory is
   a. Concepts are constructed from multiple theories.
   b. Theories are extensively tested before they generate concepts.
   c. Concepts put together will make a theory.
   d. Concepts are more abstract than theories.

8. A grand theory
   a. Is more concrete than a midrange theory.
   b. Explains large segments of the human experience.
   c. Contains no concepts.
   d. Has a narrower scope than a midrange theory.

9. A midrange theory
   a. Is more concrete than a grand theory.
   b. Explains large segments of the human experience.
   c. Contains no concepts.
   d. Has a wider scope than a grand theory.

10. A model
    a. Is used to illustrate the relationship between a proposition and a schematic model.
    b. Is the connection between theories and concepts with symbolic representations.
    c. Is used for illustration of disease frequency.
    d. Is used in primary prevention trials but not secondary prevention trials.

11. A conceptual model is also known as
    a. A conceptual framework.
    b. A schematic model.
    c. A proposition.
    d. A theory.

12. The purpose of a hypothesis is
    a. To explain the relationship between the model and the theory.
    b. To guide the direction of the study through prediction.
    c. To explain the utility of a concept.
    d. To help in selecting the theory to support.

EXERCISES

1. Find research in your area of interest that uses the expanded health belief model as its framework. Discuss the incorporation of the model's key concepts and definitions into the study.

2. Apply the PRECEDE-PROCEED framework to a community health problem you are interested in. Outline the various activities and assessments you would complete related to this problem and devise a plan of action and evaluation based on your supposed findings.

3. Search the literature for information on self-efficacy theory. Prepare a short summary of two studies that you found to be particularly interesting.

4. Find two studies that used the health promotion model for their framework. Identify the assumptions and propositions the studies were based on.

REFERENCES

Bailar, J. C., III, & Hoaglin, D. C. (Eds.). (2009). *Medical uses of statistics* (3rd ed.). Hoboken, NJ: Wiley.

Bandura, A. (1988). Organizational applications of social cognitive theory. *Australian Journal of Management, 13*, 275–302.

Bandura, A. (1962). *Social learning through imitation*. Lincoln: University of Nebraska Press.

Bandura, A. (1977). Self-efficacy: Toward a unifying theory of behavioral change. *Psychological Review, 84*, 191–215.

Bandura, A. (1992). Exercise of personal agency through the self-efficacy mechanisms. In R. Schwarzer (Ed.), *Self-efficacy: Thought control of action* (p. 2). Washington, DC: Hemisphere.

Bandura, A. (1995). *Self-efficacy in changing societies*. New York, NY: Cambridge University Press.

Bandura, A. (2006). *Psychological modeling*. Piscataway, NJ: Aldine.

Baumeister, R., & Leary, M. R. (1995). The need to belong: Desire for interpersonal attachments as a fundamental human motivation. *Psychological Bulletin, 117*, 497–529.

Becker, M., & Maimam, L. (1980). Strategies for enhancing patient compliance. *Journal of Community Health, 6*(2), 113–135.

Benight, C. C., & Bandura, A. (2004). Social cognitive theory of posttraumatic recovery: The role of perceived self-efficacy. *Behaviour Research and Therapy, 42*, 1129–1148.

Berger, B., Steckelberg, A., Meyer, G., Kasper, J., & Mühlhauser, I. (2010). Training of patient and consumer representatives in the basic competencies of evidence-based medicine: A feasibility study. *BMC Medical Education, 11*(10), 16.

Clark, C. C. (1996). Intersystems wellness nursing model. In *Wellness nursing: Concepts, theory, research and practice*. New York, NY: Springer Publishing Company.

Contento, I. R., Koch, P. A., Lee, H., & Calabrese-Barton, A. (2010). Adolescents demonstrate improvement in obesity risk behaviors after completion of choice, control & change, a curriculum addressing personal agency and autonomous motivation. *Journal of the American Dietetic Association, 110*(12), 1830–1839.

Coury-Doniger, P., Levenkron, J. C., Knox, K. L., Cowell, S., & Urban, M. A. (1999). Use of stage of change (SOC) to develop an STD/HIV behavioral intervention: Phase 1. A system to classify SOC for STD/HIV sexual risk behaviors—development and reliability in an STD clinic. *AIDS Patient Care & STDs, 13*(8), 493–502.

Deci, E. L., & Vansteenkiste, M. (2004). Self-determination theory and basic need satisfaction: Understanding human development in positive psychology. *Ricerche di Psicologia, 27*, 17–34.

Dossey, B. M. (1999). *Core curriculum for holistic nursing*. Gaithersburg, MD: Aspen.

Dossey, B. M. (2008). Theory of integral nursing. *Advances in Nursing Science, 31*(1), E52–E73.

Fishbein, M., & Ajzen, I. (1975). *Belief, attitude, intention and behavior: An introduction to theory and research*. Reading, MA: Addison-Wesley.

Glanz, K., Rimer, B. K, & Lewis, F. M. (Eds). (1997). *Health behavior and health education: Theory, research, and practice* (2nd ed.). San Francisco, CA: Jossey-Bass.

Green, L., & Kreuter, M. (Eds). (2005). Health promotion and a framework for planning. In *Health promotion planning* (pp. 1–28). Boston, MA: McGraw-Hill.

Ho, A. Y., Berggren, I., & Dahlborg-Lyckhage, E. (2010). Diabetes empowerment related to Pender's health promotion model: A meta-synthesis. *Nursing & Health Sciences, 12*(2), 259–267.

Hochbaum, G. (1958). *Public participation in medical screening programs: A sociopsychological study*. Washington, DC: U.S. Department of Health Education and Welfare.

Hunter, M. S., & Mann, E. (2010). A cognitive model of menopausal hot flushes and night sweats. *Journal of Psychosomatic Research, 69*(5), 491–501.

Jang, H. (2008). Supporting students' motivation, engagement, and learning during an uninteresting activity. *Journal of Educational Psychology, 100*(4), 798.

Janz, N., & Becker, M. (1984). The health belief model: A decade later. *Health Education Quarterly, 11*, 1–47.

King, R., for the Joint United Nations Programme on HIV/AIDS. (1999). Sexual behavioural change for HIV: Where have theories taken us? Geneva, Switzerland: UNAIDS.

Kirscht, J. (1974). The health belief model & illness behavior. *Health Education Monogram, 2*, 387–408.

Klainin, P., & Ounnapiruk, L. (2010). A meta-analysis of self-care behavior research on elders in Thailand: An update. *Nursing Science Quarterly, 23*(2), 156–163.

Krentzman, A. R., Robinson, E. A., Moore, B. C., Kelly, J. F., Laudet, A. B., White, W. L., . . . Strobbe, S. (2010). How Alcoholics Anonymous (AA) and Narcotics Anonymous (NA) work: Cross-disciplinary perspectives. *Alcohol Treatment Quarterly, 29*(1), 75–84.

Leininger, M., & McFarland, M. (1996). *Cultural care diversity & universality: A worldwide nursing theory* (2nd ed.). Sudbury, MA: Jones and Bartlett.

Mente, A., de Koning, L., Shannon, H. S., & Anand, S. S. (2009). A systematic review of the evidence supporting a causal link between dietary factors and coronary heart disease. *Archives of Internal Medicine, 169*(7), 659–669.

Murayama, K., Matsumoto, M., Izuma, K., & Matsumoto, K. (2010). Neural basis of the undermining effect of monetary reward on intrinsic motivation. *Proceedings of the National Academy of Sciences of the United States of America, 107*(49), 20911–20916.

Orem, D. (2001). *Nursing: Concepts of practice*. New York, NY: Mosby.

Pachana, N. A., McLaughlin, D., Leung, J., Byrne, G., & Dobson, A. (2012). Anxiety and depression in adults in their eighties: Do gender differences remain? *International Psychogeriatrics, 24*(1), 145–150.

Patterson, L., & Campbell, C. (1995). An extension service health education model. Mississippi State University. Retrieved from http://msucares.com/health/health/model2.html

Pender, N. J., Murdaugh, C. L., & Parsons, M. A. (2010). *Health promotion in nursing practice* (6th ed.). Upper Saddle River, NJ: Prentice-Hall.

Poddar, K. H., Hosig, K. W., Anderson, E. S., Nickols-Richardson, S. M., & Duncan, S. E. (2010). Web-based nutrition education intervention improves self-efficacy and self-regulation related to increased dairy intake in college students. *Journal of the American Dietetic Association, 110*(11), 1723–1727.

Powers, B., & Knapp, T. (1995). *A dictionary of nursing theory & research* (2nd ed.). Thousand Oaks, CA: Sage.

Prochaska, J. O., & DiClemente, C. C. (1986). Towards a comprehensive model of change. In U. Miller & N. Heather (Eds.), *Treating Addictive Behaviors* (pp. 3–27). New York, NY: Plenum Press.

Rosenstock, I. (1960). What research in maturation suggests for public health. *American Journal of Public Health, 50*, 295–301.

Rosenstock, I. (1966). Why people use health services. *The Millbank Memorial Fund Quarterly, 44*(3), 94–124.

Rosenstock, I. (1974). The health belief model & preventive health behavior. *Health Education Monographs, 2*, 354–386.

Rosenstock, I., Strecher, V., & Becker, M. (1988). Social learning theory and the health belief model. *Health Education Quarterly, 15*(2), 175–183.

Roy, C. (1999). *The Roy adaptation model*. Norwalk, CT: Appleton & Lange.

Roy, C., & Andrews, H. (1991). *The Roy adaptation model: The definitive statement.* Norwalk, CT: Appleton & Lang.

Serneels, P., Montalvo, J. G., Pettersson, G., Lievens, T., Butera, J. D., & Kidanu, A. (2010). Who wants to work in a rural health post? The role of intrinsic motivation, rural background and faith-based institutions in Ethiopia and Rwanda. *Bulletin of the World Health Organization, 88*(5), 342–349.

Strecher, V., & Rosenstock, I. (1997). The health belief model. In K. Glanz, I. Lewis, & B. Rimer (Eds.), *Health behavior and health education: Theory, research, & practice* (pp. 31–35). San Francisco, CA: Jossey-Bass.

Trudeau, K. J., Ainscough, J. L., Pujol, L. A., & Charity, S. (2010). What arthritis pain practitioners and patients want in an online self-management programme. *Musculoskeletal Care, 8*(4), 189–196.

vanRyn, M., & Heaney, C. (1992). What's the use of theory? *Health Education Quarterly, 19*(3), 315–330.

Weiss, M. R., Amorose, A. J., & Wilko, A. M. (2009). Coaching behaviors, motivational climate, and psychological outcomes among female adolescent athletes. *Pediatric Exercise Science, 21*(4), 475–492.

INTERNET RESOURCES

For a full suite of assignments and learning activities, use the access code located in the front of your book to visit this exclusive website: **http://go.jblearning.com/healthpromotion**. If you do not have an access code, you can obtain one at the site.

LEARNING OBJECTIVES

Upon completion of this chapter, you will be able to:

1. Discuss the concepts of active listening, empathy, and effective communication.
2. Identify barriers to effective communication.
3. Define differentiation.
4. Recognize what constitutes low versus high levels of differentiation.
5. Self-assess your level of differentiation.
6. Define boundaries and understand how boundaries determine appropriateness of behavior.
7. Understand triangles and how they can affect nurse–client relationships.
8. Describe effective communication practices and distinguish assertive from aggressive communication postures.
9. Develop practices for increasing self-awareness.
10. Pursue one personal wellness goal and chart progress.
11. Take action on one political or policy issue.

KEY TERMS

www.

Active listening

Affirmation

Aggressiveness

Assertiveness

Avoidance

Boundaries

Centering

Contracting

Differentiation

Empathy

Hidden agendas

Refuting irrational ideas

Self-talk

Shaping techniques

Triangulation

Value clarification

CHAPTER 3

The Nurse's Role in Health Promotion

- Introduction
- Effective Communication
- Personality Traits and Communication
- Communication Barriers
- Techniques for Enhancing Communication Skills
- Facilitating Movement Toward Health and Wellness
- Summary

http://go.jblearning.com/healthpromotion

For a full suite of assignments and learning activities, use the access code located in the front of your book to visit the exclusive website: http://go.jblearning.com/healthpromotion
If you do not have an access code, you can obtain one at the site.

Introduction

Definitions of health and health promotion, theories about how to undertake health promotion activities, and models for health promotion are all important foundation stones for the practice of health promotion. The final key element to successful health promotion practice is your ability to communicate with the client. As the person connecting a client to the health-promoting activities that seek to improve the client's overall health, your ability to assess needs, mediate problems, and motivate a client is crucial for success. Critical tasks include: (1) actively listening to the client; (2) communicating effectively with the client; and (3) educating the client.

Learning these tasks requires an understanding of how to identify social and familial communication patterns, not only in the client, but also in yourself. Listening, communicating, and educating are all bidirectional interactions that occur between you and the client. If you are not obtaining and processing input from the client, the client is unlikely to obtain and process the input from you.

In this chapter, we explain what constitutes effective communication between two people and describe how to mitigate obstacles to communication. We outline some social and familial factors that can limit or impede effective communication and offer strategies for getting around such obstacles. We will also address the internal factors that can prevent you from utilizing key communication methods so you can become aware of (and address) some of your own communication problem areas.

Effective Communication

Individuals, families, and communities turn to nurses to learn what steps to take to improve health. Doing so involves a process in which the person who has the required information (the nurse) communicates it to the client (an individual, family, or community). Sounds simple. It would be, were it not for the fact that communication is rarely simple. If you choose words or ideas that the client has trouble understanding, it is often difficult to tell where the communication breakdown lies. Some questions to ask yourself to unravel this puzzle are:

1. Am I assuming the client has a base knowledge that is lacking?
2. Are the ideas overly complicated or being communicated in an unclear or confusing fashion?
3. Is the client unable or unwilling to listen and learn in an active fashion?

In many instances, the problem may include elements of all of these issues.

Understanding how people communicate is a first step for you to take in learning how to teach clients more effective methods of listening, self-aware-ness, and self-expression, and how to identify barriers to communication. These techniques are all skills that you can develop and use to lay the ground-work for developing effective health promotion strategies.

What Is Communication?

Communication should be simple. You want to tell the client something or the client wants to tell you something. The process is complicated by the fact that information passed between two people is almost never composed of pure data free of encumbrances. Along with information, the person transmitting the information also gives a variety of messages, some conscious and inten-tional, some otherwise, that are received along with the information that the communication intends to pass along. These additional subtext messages may be transmitted by word choice, vocal tone, body language, or expression, and they may not always support the intended communication.

The recipient may also load the information *and* the messages with mean-ings not intended by the messenger. Most of us have played the game Tele-phone, where one person whispers a message to another, who then passes what he or she heard to a third person, and on down the line. The end result is usually greatly (and hilariously) different from the original message. This is the basic problem with communication: It is exceedingly rare for a recipient to obtain the *exact* information the messenger attempts to transmit without some sort of alteration occurring.

Communication Decisions

The act of message/information transmission is preceded by a variety of deci-sions—some made unconsciously—by the messenger. The most important of these decisions are:

1. *What information do I want or need to transmit to this person?* This decision includes smaller decisions about the amount of detail to be offered, whether there are points of information to be highlighted or suppressed, and it frequently involves an assessment of how urgent the transmission process is for both parties and what form the transmission process should take (e.g., "I need to tell Mr. Smith that his test came back negative, but it's not something he needs to do anything about—so I'll just send him an e-mail.")

2. *What words and tone will best accomplish the task of explaining this information?* In some cases, these decisions are made consciously (e.g., a speech, lecture, or prerehearsed conversation), while in others, choices are made unconsciously, in response to emotional impulses in the

moment. Or word choice might be made consciously, but tone is not, which can lead to conflicts between the information transmitted—for example, "I love you" stated in angry or bored tones transmits very different messages than the same words spoken in gentle or enthusiastic tones. Note that body language can have as strong an effect on transmission as tone, although the effect may not be as overt.

3. *How do I feel about transmitting information to this person?* A messenger who feels reluctance, unhappiness, guilt, anger, or other negative emotions related to the message being transmitted generally cannot hide these emotions unless a conscious attempt is made to recognize personal feelings and alter body language and expressions. If no such attempt is made, the *emotional subtext* (information about how the messenger is feeling) transmitted along with the verbal message may actually drown out or supersede the recipient's ability to receive the intended communication.

These decisions, and the subsequent transmission of information that occurs once they are made, are not the end of the communication event. On the other side of the bridge is the person for whom the message is intended—the recipient. In order for the communication to be completed, the recipient must also make a number of decisions:

1. *Do I want or need to obtain to this information?* The decision to listen to a message (or to ignore it) is often based on emotional considerations. A person who is stressed or distracted may simply tune out a communication, even one otherwise considered important, because of a need to limit the information overload being experienced. Alternatively, the person may perceive the information being transmitted as highly important and may drop everything in order to focus on the communication process—even when the person transmitting the information feels much less urgency about the need for communication.

2. *How do I feel about the information that has been transmitted?* The first decision represents the considerations around accepting information; this decision, which is similarly emotional in nature, is distinct from the first in that it focuses on *processing* the information that has been transmitted. A person can receive and comprehend information on an intellectual level, but may have trouble internalizing or coming to grips with the communiqué on an emotional level, particularly if the ramifications of what has been said create stress. A sudden loss, a frightening diagnosis or incident, and similar high-impact communications can cause the recipient to struggle with this particular decision.

3. *How do I feel about the person transmitting the information?* The previous two decisions are nearly always strongly affected by the recipient's feelings about the individual or source delivering the message. A trusted

or authoritative messenger will likely obtain more attention from the recipient regarding the message being communicated—although if there are too many positive feelings about the messenger, the recipient may focus on the messenger rather than the message! In contrast, an unknown or disliked messenger will receive less attention, or the message, once received, may be devalued—that is, regarded as unimportant or suspect.

As an educator, you must take conscious control of your own decision making on both sides of the communication bridge. When transmitting messages to clients, word choice, tone, body language, and emotional subtext must be carefully considered—preferably in advance—so that the intended message is transmitted clearly and unambiguously. When interviewing clients or obtaining feedback, examine your decision-making process so that the client's information can be received without impediment.

Create a relationship in which you establish with the client a belief that you are trustworthy, knowledgeable, and competent. Helping the client to feel positive about you is one factor. Another is the capacity to model the type of behavior you wish to obtain from the client: active, engaged listening and learning. See FIGURE 3-1.

Active Listening

Effective, active listening is one of the most difficult skills to learn because it requires the listener (the recipient of communication) to do more than simply hear the message being provided by the messenger (Aled, 2007; Camillo Sdo, Nóbrega Mdo, & Théo, 2010; Piotrowski, 2005). Friedman, Bowden, and Jones (2003) note that **active listening** requires the listener show empathy, focus on the other person's needs and desires, and avoid interrupting the sender's communication. This requires a conscious and continual effort to suppress the natural desire to pay attention to the client's own needs, desires, and wish to communicate. It also necessitates rapid processing of the information being provided by the person to whom the client is listening. In the context of a high-stakes conversation in which two people are not in agreement about a matter of great emotional importance to one or both (what Patterson, Grenny, McMillan, and Switzler [2002] call a crucial conversation), the emotional considerations of obtaining the other person's agreement contradict the desire to listen—unless the listener deliberately sets aside the emotional response he or she feels and focuses on obtaining the information being provided by the other participant. Similarly, in a casual conversation where the matter under discussion is not important to one or both, the listener's attention may be prone to wander, and information is likely to be missed as a result.

An active listener is one who exhibits engagement through expression, tone, and body language, responding to the messages sent by the communicating

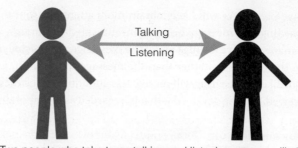

Two people who take turns talking and listening are more likely to have effective communication about a topic.

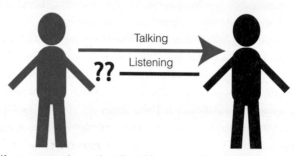

If one person is continually talking, it is difficult to obtain cues that show the other person is listening. Over time, the "listener" may start tuning out much of what the "talker" is saying.

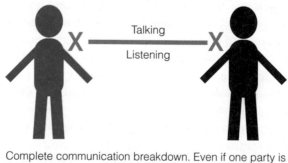

Complete communication breakdown. Even if one party is talking, the other is not listening. Or, neither party is talking. In either case, there is no communication occurring.

FIGURE 3-1   Communication is a two-way street

party in an appropriate fashion (feedback) that expresses an understanding and validation of the message (Friedman et al., 2003). Appropriate feedback acknowledges the content of the communication, whether spoken, unspoken, or both, and validation demonstrates that the content has been internalized and understood.

For example, imagine that you are helping a grieving client describe a recently deceased parent. You are leaning forward, looking directly at the client and saying, in a soft voice with a sympathetic tone, "I can see that talking about your late father makes you a feel sad." By doing these things, you have shown both that you heard what was said (feedback) and understood it (validation). In contrast, imagine that you say the exact same sentence in a dry, unemotional voice while sitting with your body turned away from the client, and your eyes looking at a computer screen instead of the client's face.

Although the same verbal response is offered, the message sent is very different. The feedback shows that you heard the message, but your body language does not validate the client's message. Your lack of engagement is obvious, and the client may respond accordingly by refusing to listen to you.

While simply modeling active listening for a client is a good way to establish positive feelings in the client (most people enjoy having a listener's full, unimpeded attention), it is also a good way to assess whether the client needs instruction in how to engage in similar behavior. A client who is not a skilled listener or who is stressed, fatigued, in pain, etc., may display inattentiveness, may not comprehend instructions or information being offered, or may speak continually without allowing you to respond. If your ultimate goal is to engage in health promotion activities with this client, then you must first take steps to ensure that the client is capable of receiving the instruction being offered.

Empathy can help make the client more receptive to your communication. **Empathy** means you communicate back to clients the feeling and meaning they express to you. There are five levels of communication.

Level 1: You do not focus on the client's communication and overlook expressed surface feelings.

Level 2: Your communication of client feelings is not congruent with what the client expresses.

Level 3: You paraphrase what the client said, but the meaning you provide is of a superficial nature.

Level 4: You believe you understand what the client is driving at and you add significantly to the client's expressions of feeling.

Level 5: You not only add significantly to the client's feeling expressions at more than one deeper level, you know you understand what the client is experiencing.

Example:

Client: "I don't like what the doctor told me."

Level 1 response: "Time for your walk now."

Level 2 response: "You'll learn to like what he says."

Level 3 response: "You don't like what the doctor told you?"

Level 4 response: "I see your face tensing up about what the doctor told you."

Level 5 response: "It's really upsetting when you hear something that isn't helpful to you."

Guidelines for communicating effectively with clients include:

1. Maintain eye contact and focus on what clients are saying and how they are saying it.
2. Mirror the degree of formality and word choice clients use.
3. Identify client feeling tone and use similar words when discussing a situation with clients.
4. Avoid simply sitting passively and listening. Actively and frequently respond to client communications.
5. Communicate client nonverbal expressions back to them.
6. Trust your feelings and be genuine in your communications.
7. Ask for specific details and instances, e.g., "Give me an example of what you mean," and "Tell me what you heard and saw so I can understand."
8. Only disclose personal information when it could benefit the client, e.g., how you felt when you experienced a situation similar to the one a client describes.
9. Point out what you observe about client behavior and how it is affecting your ability to be helpful to them: "When you don't answer or turn your back to me, it's difficult to understand you and how I could help."
10. State discrepancies in client verbal and nonverbal behavior, e.g., "You told me you're upset, but you're smiling."
11. State what clients are struggling to express, e.g., "I hear your anger about your situation and I'm going to help you with that."
12. Always communicate with respect; point out that clients know what is needed and by speaking with confidence about how you can teach clients to choose appropriate change goals and take action to accomplish them.
13. Explain what you can and cannot help with, e.g., "I can help you choose goals and learn ways to reach them, but I can't decide for you."
14. Encourage clients to problem solve by helping them specify reasonable goals, how they will know when they've met their goals, and when they plan to implement action toward their goals.
15. Teach clients to brainstorm by making comments such as, "Here's a piece of paper and a pen. Write down all the possible ways you could meet your goal."
16. Show clients how to evaluate alternate ways to meet their goals, e.g., "These are good ideas, but are there other ways you could meet your goal?"
17. Help clients to takes small steps to their goal, e.g., "It can be overwhelming to think about changing. Let's talk about how to break your goal into small steps that will be less stressful for you."

HEALTH PROMOTION CHALLENGE

Use the following statement by a community member to provide level 1, 2, 3, 4, and 5 empathic responses:

Client: "The school nurse is trying to force my daughter to have a whooping cough vaccination, even though the vaccine works no better than a placebo and even though my son died after receiving the vaccination. (Rage in her eyes). Is that fair? (Paces up and down the room). They might not let my daughter in school without the vaccination, but I'm not putting her in that position . . . not after my son (bangs her fist on the table). Do you believe it? These are people who are supposed to be concerned with health, and they're trying to force me to do something that killed my son!"

ACTIVE LISTENING TRAINING EXERCISE

A simple exercise to train yourself in active listening is to sit down with another student and practice giving information and then ask the other student to repeat what was heard before responding to it. Each of you must wait for confirmation before continuing. The benefit of this strategy is that it allows the originator of the message to correct misunderstandings, and it also slows the pace of communication down so that information is relayed in smaller, more readily processed packets. It also allows you time to consider the tone, body language, and expression used in communication. Practice active listening with at least two classmates and discuss your results with each other.

Personality Traits and Communication

No two people learn or communicate in the same ways. Learning and communication styles develop in an individual as a complicated interaction between personality traits (which themselves are determined by complex genetic, sociocultural, and environmental factors), life experience, and family and social environments. Modeling and teaching active listening can be a critical factor in helping clients change their communication style or pattern. Three other factors that are important to an individual's or family's communication style are the level of differentiation, the presence of (and respect for) clear boundaries, and assertiveness.

Levels of Differentiation

In the 1970s, psychiatrist Murray Bowen developed the concept of **differentiation** to define a person's ability to separate emotional stimuli from rational thought processes and actions (Bowen, 1972, p. 19). Bowen also used the term to explain the extent to which people intellectually distinguish themselves and their own needs from others in their emotional relationship system, e.g., a family (Miller & Winstead-Frey, 1982). The level of differentiation an individual displays reflects that person's capacity to identify and distinguish emotional input so that a response is undertaken, not in pure reaction to emotions, but with input from the rational, conscious mind as well.

The concept of differentiation draws on the fact that there are distinct emotional and intellectual systems in the brain. Each center responds virtually simultaneously to the same source of stimulus—a noise, a sensation, or a situation between people that links to a related experience, knowledge, or memory. For instance, if a person hears someone talking in a manner that reminds him of his father, he may think to himself, "Gosh, that guy sounds just like Dad." At the same time, he is undergoing physiological responses related to the experience of similarity between the speaker and his father, depending upon what emotions that experience triggers. If he has a difficult or distant relationship with his father, for instance, hearing someone who sounds like him may trigger a stress response—elevated heart rate, shallow breathing, sweatiness. If he has a close, loving relationship, he may have the opposite reaction—hearing a voice that reminds him of his father's may make him feel relaxed, happy, and confident. What matters is whether this person is able to act upon the intellectual recognition of the resemblance and comprehend that it is different from the emotional recognition of the resemblance—in other words, whether he is able to differentiate between the intellect and the emotions.

At a low level of differentiation, the intellectual center (which allows people to think about their lives and plan and control their behavior) is not well differentiated from the emotional center. People who are less well differentiated have a high level of fusion between their emotional and intellectual systems, which means that decisions and behavior are strongly influenced by emotional responses. Individuals with low differentiation are prone to acting impulsively, to reacting emotionally under stress, or to having difficulty foreseeing the consequences of their actions.

At a high level of differentiation, the intellectual center is well developed and screens stimuli from the emotional center. Individuals with high differentiation stay calm under high stress or in extremely emotional circumstances. This does not necessarily mean they are lacking in empathy or compassion, but simply that they are capable of discerning and separating an emotional response from an intellectual one. Let us suppose, for example, that the person in the previous example has a poor relationship with his father, who is over-bearing, hypercritical, and verbally abusive. He hears the voice and starts feeling nervous and stressed, but then says to himself, "Don't be silly. Dad is back home in Arizona. It's just someone who sounds like him." Because he is well differentiated, he is able to recognize and acknowledge his emotional response without letting it overwhelm him. If he were less well differentiated, he might become agitated or leave the room abruptly to escape the source of the emotional stimulus.

Although Bowen considered people to be on a continuum from low-level differentiation to high-level differentiation, it may be more useful to regard people as moving less well among various levels, depending on the amount of anxiety they are experiencing; in other words, an individual may function with a high level of differentiation under certain circumstances, but with a lower level of differentiation when under high stress or specific forms of stress. High levels of anxiety short-circuit the intellectual system and lead to overly emotional responses. Stress, fatigue, and burnout are associated with lower level of differentiation and may also be related to increased susceptibility to illness or infection (Callen, Mefford, Groër, & Thomas, 2010). Physiological correlates of high anxiety and lack of the relaxation response have been known for years. Some signs that are associated with low-level differentiation during stressful situations with clients include increased blood pressure, pulse, and respiration, and decreased ability to focus on the work at hand. Measures that enhance relaxation and decrease stress can enhance level of differentiation.

As a role model for health and wellness, learn to differentiate intellectual from emotional impulses, both in clients and in yourself, so that the guidance you offer is founded on knowledge rather than reaction. Use your understanding of the client's health and wellness value system and your own to develop a path that will be helpful to health promotion. On occasion, differences between you and the client in health-related ideas and goals may prove challenging and uncomfortable for you.

Support a high level of differentiation in yourself and the client by thinking through your responses and teaching clients to do the same. You will see this factor in action not only in clients, but also in colleagues, and even in yourself. For example, when experiencing anxiety, you or clients may over-react to a situation. When emotion and emotional systems take precedence over the intellect, self-talk similar to the following might occur: "Uh-oh, time to panic!" or "I can't handle this, I'd better get out of here" or "How dare she say that!" The task of the well-differentiated you is to recognize the emotional response for what it is, maintain a sense of groundedness as the situation unfolds, and avoid reacting to the client's emotions with an emotional response of your own.

Similarly, a well-differentiated you will be able to note your own emotional responses and take appropriate actions to prevent them from overcoming the intellectual response. For example, you can redirect emotional energies by breathing deeply before replying to a highly charged question, stepping out of a room for a time out to collect your thoughts, or even counting to 10 in your head.

Maintain awareness of your trigger points, those comments or situations that set off irrational reactions in you. This is a powerful method of preventing those buttons from being pushed. At a higher level of differentiation, the intellectual system screens noxious stimuli, and thoughts and perceptions may be more like the following: "Keep calm," "I can handle this," "What am I getting so excited about?" and "This isn't the end of the world; I can deal with this." It's helpful to think one or more of these comments to yourself even when you don't feel it because they can bring you out of an emotional state.

CASE STUDY Low versus High Levels of Differentiation

Jill is a new hire in the Portland City Hospital intensive care unit (ICU). Although this is her first staff position in an ICU, she trained for it in a teaching hospital that is renowned for its cutting-edge program that researches and develops new techniques. She was told when she was hired that her knowledge of the latest methods was something her supervisors wanted her to share with the hospital's veteran nurses.

Mary, an experienced staff nurse who has worked in this ICU for 15 years, was working with Mr. White, a man with pneumonia and Parkinson's disease, who was hospitalized on that unit. His family was visiting at the time, and his neurologist was also in attendance. Mr. White's muscles frequently became locked as an effect of his Parkinson's disease. Mary was performing a manipulation technique intended to help ease Mr. White's muscles so that he could change his position more easily, which would help his breathing. She used the technique she had been taught many years ago.

Upon entering the room where Mary was working, Jill saw that Mary was using a technique that she had been trained to avoid. Jill was taught that in the hands of an experienced person, the technique worked well, but if used incorrectly, it had the potential to injure a client. The alternate technique Jill had been taught was safer, but was sometimes less effective.

Because she was not experienced in its use, Jill could not assess whether Mary was using the technique correctly or not. How should Jill handle her concerns about Mary's technique?

A. Enter the room and say to Mary, "What are you doing? You're doing that wrong! Let me show you how to do it right."

(continues)

B. Leave the room quickly and go get a supervisor, telling her with great urgency that Mary's actions were endangering the client's welfare and requesting immediate intervention.

C. Enter the room and say to Mary, "May I watch? I wasn't trained to use that technique, so I'm interested to see what you're doing." Once she finished, Jill could plan to ask Mary to meet her for coffee so she could talk to Mary about the safety issues with her technique and offer to train her in a more updated method.

D. Enter the room, introduce herself, and simply observe what Mary does, taking unobtrusive notes. That way, Jill could document the client's well-being and intervene if Mary inadvertently injured him. Later, Jill could talk with a supervisor and describe her concerns—and suggest a training session between her and Mary to discuss the two different techniques.

Which of these responses reflect a low level of differentiation?
Which response is most professionally appropriate?

Analysis

Response A reflects a very low level of differentiation. It is a knee-jerk emotional response that demonstrates lack of forethought, lack of respect, lack of collegiality, and lack of consideration. Simply blurting out "You're doing it wrong!" to a senior colleague is not only unprofessional, but it is rude—and it creates a hostile environment in the client's sick room, in the presence of a physician responsible for the client's well-being. By responding in this manner, Jill may adversely affect:

- the client, who may be startled and disquieted by having his treatment interrupted so abruptly
- the family, who will likely be concerned at being told their relative is being mishandled
- the physician, who may have any of a number of negative responses depending on his relationship with Mary and his understanding of the technique she uses
- Mary, her coworker, whom Jill would have just criticized—perhaps unjustly—in front of both a client and a professional colleague

If Jill later must work with either this client and his family or either of these colleagues to engage clients in health promotion activities, her poorly differentiated response would probably affect their trust in her capabilities, and thus reduce her effectiveness.

Response B is not much better. While it may not have an impact on the client, his family, or his physician, Jill is suggesting to their mutual supervisor that Mary is doing harm to a client—which is founded on Jill's *emotional* response to seeing Mary's technique, not her reasoned response. Her accusation

(continues)

very likely is not true. The fact that Mary's technique is not *as safe* as the technique Jill knows does not mean it is *unsafe*, particularly when used by an experienced practitioner, which Mary is. Jill's reaction has created a problem where most likely none existed, and her response may cause workplace conflict between Jill and Mary or between Jill and her supervisor. Again, this will affect her colleagues' trust in Jill's capabilities during future collaborations.

Both response C and response D show high differentiation. Jill has concerns, but she does not react emotionally or with panic about the technique she sees Mary using. In both cases, Jill understands that she needs to trust in her colleague's experience and maintain her professionalism in the presence of the client, family, and physician. She thinks ahead to how she can address the situation in a way that will maintain collegiality and respect.

Of the two, however, response D is more professionally appropriate. Because client safety is the focus of Jill's concern, it is necessary that she formally present her issue and solution to the supervisor so that it can be resolved officially, not off the record, as Jill's solution in response C would do. By taking notes, Jill documents not only the situation, but also the technique she is observing—which may be useful down the line should Jill need to assess another practitioner's use of this unfamiliar technique in the future. Training between Jill and Mary may be mutually instructive, teaching Jill something she needs to know as well as bringing Mary's practice into line with current thinking.

HEALTH PROMOTION CHALLENGE

Evaluate your level of differentiation and set a goal for raising your level. Decide on a date for implementing your goal that's reasonable for you.

Boundaries

Boundaries are invisible crossing points where the self of one individual encounters that of another. In the physical sense, this is also sometimes referred to as "personal space," but boundaries are most commonly envisioned in non-physical terms; that is, they are felt as an emotional response to a perceived intrusion on the client's turf or a reduction of the client's personal dignity. Boundaries are often distinguished by the level of trust entailed in crossing them; that is, the rigidity or permeability of a boundary depends on the nature of the relationship between those individuals. The closer the relationship, the more permeable the boundary tends to be. But boundaries can change in response to changes in relationship dynamics.

An example would be a situation in which someone confides embarrassing information to a trusted friend, who then reveals that information to someone else. By disclosing the confidence, the friend crossed the boundary of trust and friendship implicit in the act of confiding. Upon learning of the indiscretion, the first individual is likely to experience emotions of hurt, anger, embarrassment, and loss of trust in the friend. As a result of the indiscretion and the subsequent emotions, a formerly fluid boundary between this individual and the friend will likely become more rigid. A boundary based on a level of trust that has been breached is often extremely difficult to restore to prior levels.

Boundaries are also instrumental in determining appropriate behaviors between two individuals based on the roles these people play in relation to one another. For example, actions that may be appropriate between two people in a parent–child or a spousal relationship (tight hugging or cuddling, for example) are not considered appropriate between strangers or casual acquaintances.

A well-differentiated person has a strong sense of self, and recognizes consciously as well as unconsciously where the outer limits of his or her tolerance lie. A poorly differentiated person lacks this delineation of boundaries, and may often be lacking awareness of others' boundaries (as well as his or her own). The fusion trait described earlier as characteristic of people with low differentiation can be alternately described as poor awareness of boundaries.

In a nurse–client relationship, it is important that you are aware of boundaries and able to identify potential boundary conflicts. Failure to do so can disrupt your role as teacher and motivator, and in extreme cases can prove emotionally or even physically harmful to you, the client, or both. You will see personal sides of clients, but it is important to maintain professional boundaries and not reveal too much information about yourself (Helming & Jackson, 2009). Keep your focus on the client's needs and desires, not your own.

Assertiveness

A third important element of effective communication is assertiveness. **Assertiveness** is the ability to clearly and willingly express thoughts, feelings, or desires in a respectful and cordial manner. It means being able to define and stand up for reasonable rights while respecting others' rights, setting goals for wellness, acting on these goals by following through consistently, and taking responsibility for the consequences of actions. Assertive behavior, by definition, requires a high level of differentiation and solid self.

Assertiveness is a useful communication skill for several reasons. Assertive individuals can

- Keep interactions focused and goal oriented
- Let both parties in a conversation know where they stand and free up energy to deal with the situation as it really is, instead of wasting energy trying to decipher what the other person really means
- Role model and encourage similarly assertive behavior in others with whom they are communicating.

Do not confuse assertiveness with aggressiveness. Being assertive requires taking a risk by clearly stating what is expected from others and what they can expect from the nurse. *I* messages are used, e.g., "I would like to . . . " or "I suggest we settle it by . . . " or "I feel angry when I'm called lazy." In contrast, **aggressiveness** has an element of control or manipulation. *You* messages, such as "Why didn't you . . . ?" or "You should have . . . " or "I think you are crazy" prevail when aggressiveness occurs. An aggressive interaction is one in which one party seeks to exert power or control over another; aggression has no place in health promotion, where the goal is to motivate and educate individuals to work toward their own health improvement.

☐ What Prevents Individuals from Being Assertive?

Clients and nurses alike often fear being assertive because they fear not being liked, being rejected, being retaliated against, and so forth. It is important to be aware of which of these fears (or others) may be preventing assertiveness and take action to dispel them. The same fears seem to operate regardless of gender. Women may be most fearful of rejection and tend to bend over backwards to please, but men also feel pressure to be strong and never show their feelings. Both of these reactions can be traced back to early family experiences in which girls are raised to be nice, not fight, not show anger, and (often) are judged on how they look or socialize, not on their competence in the task. As a result, many girls grow up to be women who underestimate their achievements, attribute their success to luck, and doubt their ability even when they are highly competent. Men assume they are competent and readily set out to prove it (Rivers, Barnett, & Baruch, 1979).

Early school experiences also influence the assertiveness of male and female nurses. Dweck (1975) found that teachers expect boys to be rowdy and inattentive about schoolwork, but girls are expected to be well-behaved, dutiful, and exerting their best effort. When boys fail, they are told to try harder (a motivation problem), but girls are just told they have done something incorrectly (which may be interpreted as a lack of ability).

Assertiveness appears to be situational. Some women feel more comfortable being assertive at work, while some men feel more comfortable being assertive at home. Perhaps one of the few generalizations that can be made is that everyone has some assertiveness issue to deal with; no one is totally unassertive nor totally assertive. Assertiveness is a continuum.

CASE STUDY   Assertiveness with Peers

Bob Smith was working to obtain his BSN. When assertiveness was discussed in a seminar, he shared the following comment: "Why is it that everyone expects you to be strong and handle every situation?" As the discussion group helped Bob explore the issue further, it became clear that Bob's female nursing peers gave him verbal and nonverbal messages to be strong and not show any uncertainty he felt about dealing with some nursing situations. It was suggested that Bob set up a time to talk with his female counterparts about how he felt and to share how difficult it was to always be the one who was expected to be strong and competent. The next week in class, Bob shared how he had met with his female peers and seemed surprised that they were surprised about how he felt. They decided to ask each time a stressful situation occurred how each one felt about taking responsibility in that situation. Bob reported feeling greatly relieved that "Things are now out in the open."

HEALTH PROMOTION CHALLENGE

Interview a nurse or nursing student of the opposite gender and find out which areas of assertiveness are a problem for him or her. Find a way to work together to help each other improve assertiveness skills.

☐ Assertiveness and Stress

Development of assertiveness is also useful as a stress reduction measure. Individuals who are unable to express their thoughts and feelings directly or who feel unappreciated or exploited often report having psychosomatic complaints such as headaches or stomach problems. Assertive individuals often report increased feelings of self-confidence, reduced anxiety, decreased bodily complaints, and improved communication and response from others. There are a number of strategies to use to become more assertive, which we will describe later in the chapter, but one key to reduce anxiety and fear about being assertive is to regularly practice relaxation exercises.

RELAXATION EXERCISES

Progressive Relaxation: This exercise is especially for clients who are not tuned into tension in their bodies.

1. Lie down in a comfortable spot or sit in a comfortable chair.
2. Close your eyes. Follow steps 3–10, tensing for 5–7 seconds and relaxing for 20–30 seconds. Allow yourself to deeply experience bodily changes.
3. Tense all the muscles of your hands, forearms, and upper arms.
4. Let all the tension out of the muscles of your hands, forearms, and upper arms.
5. Tense all the muscles of your head, face, throat, and shoulders, including the forehead, cheeks, nose, eyes, jaw, lips, tongue, and neck.
6. Release all the tension in your head, face, throat, and shoulders.
7. Tense all the muscles in your chest, stomach, and lower back.
8. Release all the tension in your chest, stomach, and lower back.
9. Tense all the muscles in your thighs, buttocks, calves, and feet.
10. Release all the tension in your thighs, buttocks, calves, and feet.

Taking a Trip in Your Mind's Eye: Especially useful for clients who use imagery or can picture items easily.

1. Find a comfortable, quiet spot and assume a relaxed position.
2. Close your eyes.
3. Let your breathing begin to move lower in your body, moving toward your abdominal area. Each time you exhale, move your breathing lower in your body toward your abdominal area.
4. Take yourself on a trip in your mind's eye to a place that is comfortable and relaxing, somewhere you have been or somewhere you would like to be. See all the sights associated with your quiet, relaxing place. Hear all the sounds, smell all the wonderful smells, taste any tastes associated with your quiet, relaxing place. Fully experience all the sensations associated with your peaceful, relaxing place.
5. Totally immerse yourself in your quiet, relaxing place until you are ready to return, then gradually return from your trip, keeping the relaxation and calmnness with you for as long as you wish. Then, gradually open your eyes, feeling refreshed and ready to resume your day.

Assertiveness requires teaching the client to present himself or herself in a confident, self-assured manner. When body musculature is tense and constricted, a self-confident presentation is difficult. A relaxed body increases the probability that others will be approached in a direct, open manner.

Communication Barriers

Even when two persons have direct interactions, there may be a number of potential stumbling blocks. Health promotion is, at heart, about teaching, training, and supporting—all of which require the communication of key health promotion messages from the nurse to the client(s). If communication is ineffective, the messages are not transmitted or are transmitted incorrectly—and the health promotion effort likely will fail. In this section, we will talk about how to identify problem areas in communication, and what to do about them.

Dysfunctional Communication

Functional communication occurs when individuals or groups are able to discuss matters of concern in a respectful, mutually supportive manner. Each party takes turns expressing a position, each party listens to the other party's points, and they negotiate a position that both can find satisfactory because both parties care about reaching a compromise and working through differences. Emotionally mature, well-differentiated people may not always communicate in a functional manner, but most of the time, they do. Unfortunately, many people do not learn how to communicate this way, and resort to a variety of dysfunctional tactics (see BOX 3-1).

Box 3-1   Dysfunctional Communication

In messenger dysfunction, the messenger:
- Makes assumptions
- Has an unclear expression of feelings or wishes
- Uses bait-and-switch (starts with one message when a second message is what is on his or her mind)
- Offers judgmental responses
- Cannot define his or her own needs
- Presents incongruent messages (i.e., body language does not match verbal statements)

In recipient dysfunction, the recipient:
- Does not listen
- Disqualifies the message ("Yes, but …")
- Responds with insults or defensiveness
- Refuses to explore message or cuts off communication
- Refuses to validate message
- Brings up unrelated or tangential issues

Source: Friedman, M. M., Bowden, V. R. & Jones, E. G. (2003). *Family Nursing: Research, Theory, and Practice* (5th ed.), Upper Saddle River, NJ: Prentice Hall.

❑ Listening Blocks

Make sure you're not engaging in any listening blocks such as:

- Comparing yourself to clients rather than listening to them.
- Trying to figure out what clients really mean rather than listening to what they say and observing what they do.
- Rehearsing your answer to the client rather than listening to what is said.
- Filtering out anything a client says or does that makes you feel uncomfortable.
- Judging what clients say or do rather than trying to understand and be helpful.
- Fantasizing instead of listening to clients.
- Focusing on your own feelings rather on the client's.
- Advising the client about what to do.
- Arguing with the client.
- Trying to be right rather than helpful.
- Joking or changing the subject rather
- than listening and observing clients.
- Agreeing with what clients say so they'll think your nice or pleasant.

The key to reducing the impact of such blocks is to train yourself to recognize they are occurring in you or the other person. To a certain extent, noting such tactics in another communicant helps resolve the issue by continually bringing the subject back to the matter under discussion. If use of these tactics appears to be habitual in a client (or in yourself), the pattern can be decreased or eliminated by increasing differentiation. Centering (see *Centering* later in this chapter) can also be helpful (McKay, Davis, & Fanning, 1983, pp. 1, 6–9).

❑ Avoidance and Aggression

Avoidance in the context of communication means taking steps to prevent a message from being delivered, either by impeding the messenger from transmitting it, or more commonly, simply refusing to receive it. **Aggression** in communication can mean two things: (1) communicating in a manner that directs overt hostility, anger, or other negative feelings toward other parties, or (2) communicating in a manner intended to promote similar feelings in other parties. In the context of health care, both of these methods are usually undertaken as a way of diverting attention from a topic the avoidant/aggressive party does not wish to discuss. **Passive aggression** means expressing hostility or anger through passivity or silence—such as sullenly refusing to acknowledge a speaker or failing to do something that has been agreed upon as a way of annoying others.

In healthcare settings, avoidance and aggression are often seen in tandem and are particularly common in family settings. An avoidance/aggression

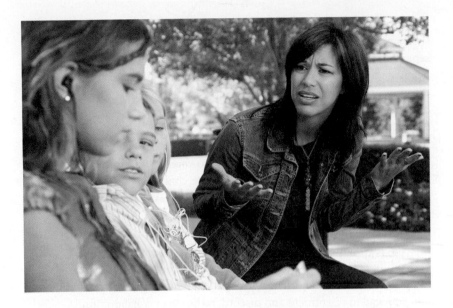

pattern may play out as follows: One family member may avoid a confrontation or wellness issue, which leads to buildup of resentment in other family members; this eventually fuels a blowup or angry outburst. Without intervention to break entrenched communication habits, family members may have feelings of guilt and recrimination that allow the avoidant person to return to their original pattern of avoidance, starting the cycle all over again.

Avoidant and aggressive behaviors are an outgrowth of an agenda that fundamentally seeks to establish power and control over a situation. Avoidance is a control behavior based in denial, e.g., *If I don't address this situation, I can make it not exist.* Aggression is a more direct expression of a desire for control; e.g., *Matters are not to my satisfaction, and I am going to make others uncomfortable in an effort to get my way.* Neither form of control seeking is healthy or helpful in a healthcare context, because they divert energy from the health issue for which an intervention takes place. You can reestablish a focus on the problem by simply acknowledging the underlying concern: "I know this is new territory for you, and it might be frightening. But let's agree to take it slow, and that you'll tell me when you are concerned or uncomfortable, and we'll get through it without any conflicts. OK?"

☐ Distinguishing Assertive from Aggressive Messages

As discussed earlier, assertive messages start from the *I* position. You assert your stance as coming from your solid self, staking a territory in the conversation where you ask (not demand) your counterpart to meet you. "This is where I am. Please come join me," is the tenor of an assertive interaction. Of course, if the counterpart in this interaction is also engaged in assertive behavior, he or she may simply respond with a similar proposition, staking a different position separate from yours. At this point, being well-differentiated people, you can negotiate to find common ground—a place in the middle that the two of you can agree upon. Or, if agreement is not an essential outcome, you can agree to disagree! As long as this is done in a respectful manner, the outcome is usually satisfactory for both parties.

Sometimes *you*-aggressive messages masquerade as assertive ones, e.g., "I think you're wrong!" or "I feel you ought to change" or "I want you to do as I say." In these messages, the speaker tries to control the listener by judging behavior or attempting to force change or action; these messages are aggressive and avoid the responsibility each person has for his or her behavior. Some *we* messages can also be assertive, especially if they imply collaboration, such as "We can meet and work this out."

Undifferentiated messages, such as, "Let's take our bath now," are not asser-tive or collaborative. They infantilize or patronize the object of the communica-tion and lead to resentment and discord, rather than collaboration.

You-blaming messages are apt to put others on the defensive; for this reason alone they ought to be avoided. In addition, they absolve the speaker of his or her responsibility in the issue at hand. Examples of this type of aggressive state-ment are: "Why didn't you take care of that?" "Why can't you do it right?" "I think this is your fault," and "Why are you going around upsetting everyone?" Some assertive messages do use the word *you*, but there is neither blame nor coercion attached to assertive *you* messages (e.g., "Would you like to tell me your point of view?" or "I want to thank you" or "I thought I heard you say . . .").

Recognize that while the point of your engagement in a conversation is to transfer your idea or thought to the other person, the other person in the conversation is simultaneously trying to accomplish the exact same goal. Com-munication is not one way—it must go in *two* directions in order to be effective. That means both parties must listen as well as talk. And listening is something that a surprising number of people do not know how to do. *I*-position state-ments in a conversation should also be interspersed with noncoercive, assertive *you* messages that show the other person that you are willing to listen—which is also conducive to helping this other person to relax and start listening to your message (Patterson et al., 2002).

❑ Triangulation

Triangulation is a situation in which two people who are involved in a rela-tionship of emotional significance experience anxiety or stress building up between them, and to alleviate this stress, one or both of the individuals calls upon another person, issue, or object to intervene or disrupt the conflict and thereby decrease discomfort (Bowen, 1972). Note that the creation of triangles does not mean the source of stress is resolved, only that stress is disrupted for the immediate term; unresolved tensions do not generally go away following these disruptions, but may actually increase over time. Triangulation is therefore most often a way of deferring conflict, rather than solving it.

CASE STUDY   Triangulation among a Husband, Wife, and Physician

Daniel is a 65-year-old man with multiple chronic ailments. He suffers from epilepsy, congestive heart failure, and late-stage Parkinson's disease. He is hospitalized with pneumonia, which requires intensive care. Daniel has a written do-not-resuscitate (DNR) order and has given his wife Annette a medical power of attorney to make decisions for him, both of which are noted in his file. Annette has explained to Daniel's own physician and to the nurses on the ward that Daniel does not like to make waves about his treatment, but that he has told her that he wants no heroic measures to be undertaken to keep him alive.

Overnight, after Annette has returned home, Daniel's blood oxygen levels start to deteriorate. The attending physician, who is reviewing Daniel's case for the first time, feels that Daniel should be intubated right away. In the doctor's opinion, intubation does not fall into the category of heroic measures. He speaks to Daniel, who is alert and awake at the time, and tells him what he wishes to do, and asks if intubation is acceptable to him. Daniel's response is, "You need to speak to my wife." When pressed to give a decision himself, he becomes agitated and refuses to communicate directly with the physician, who must then call Annette to come in to the hospital. After conferring privately with her husband, Annette steps out of the room and speaks with the physician in the hallway, explaining to him that Daniel is against the idea of being intubated, but feels unable to say so to the doctor. She then sits with the doctor and draws up a list of procedures that Daniel has told her are not acceptable to him.

Often, an individual brought in as arbiter between the two parties who are experiencing stress or tension in their relationship places his or her own interpretations or values on the message, which further muddies the intended communication from the first person to the second. This is the principal reason why avoiding triangles is important. Mixed messages often create misunderstandings and emotional disruptions that are not helpful in promoting health.

Triangles occur in all families as well as in other social and work situations in which there is high anxiety or stress. In a healthcare setting, we often see triangles in the context of the physician–client relationship. For example, a client may be anxious about getting answers from his physician, and may pull you into a triangle by asking or manipulating you to talk to the doctor on the client's behalf. Variants on this triangle are a nurse who questions her ability and triangles in the physician, or a physician who questions his ability to talk with the client about the client's impending death or other highly charged issues and triangles in the nurse to do his talking for him. Or, an adult child with an ailing parent forms triangles with the parent and caregivers, whether these are home health aides, nursing home staff, or a primary care physician. The parent may not want to complain about issues or discomfort to the caregivers, and instead raises these issues to the son or daughter, who then brings them up to the caregivers.

If triangulation (or attempts at creating triangles) happens in the setting of health promotion, it should be regarded as an opportunity to help the client increase differentiation and promote more direct, better differentiated interaction between stressed individuals—often spouses or parents/children. When you act as a mediator between two individuals who are both present, the conversation need not turn into a triangle. By being a facilitator of healthy, straightforward interactions, you can help increase differentiation in clients, and possibly in yourself.

ASK YOURSELF   `www`

Suppose a client is not convinced losing weight will help him with his back problems, his hip problems, his lung congestion, and his blood pressure. What would you tell him? What written information might you provide?

☐ Cultural Differences

Cultural differences in communication styles exist, and can become a barrier to communication if your expectations of how a conversation should be conducted conflict with the client's norms (Cuellar, Brennan, Vito, & de Leon Saintz, 2008). A variety of cross-cultural studies indicate that communication styles and mannerisms deemed appropriate in conversation vary widely. In an ideal world, people from all cultural backgrounds would have access to nurses who share their worldview, language, and cultural context, but this rarely occurs, particularly in a society as diverse as that of the United States. Various studies have shown that cultural disparities can lead to disparities in health care (Misra-Hebert & Isaacson, 2012). The remedy for this issue is for nurses (and other practitioners) to develop greater **cultural competence**—that is, skills in identifying cultural differences between themselves and their clients, and maintaining an attitude of flexibility when dealing with a situation in which the client's norms differ from their own.

Techniques for Enhancing Communication Skills

Techniques for Enhancing Assertiveness

Nurses may encounter clients who are not aware of how they come across to others. There are a number of strategies that can be used to provide feedback about presentation of self. **Mirror practice** gives feedback about facial expression, posture, and whether words fit with gestures and body position. It can also be helpful in rehearsing assertive statements prior to trying them with the real-life person. This kind of rehearsal can build confidence so that assertiveness in the real-life situation is more likely.

Audio, digital, and videotape recorders also provide excellent practice in assertion. All provide clues about whether there are sufficient pauses, whether tone of voice is assertive, whether statements are made too quickly, if words are said with sufficient firmness and authority, and whether the issue is stated clearly and adhered to. Tape and digital recorders are also useful for recording (and providing instant replay about) one's ability to limit interruptions, express feelings appropriately, take a stand on an issue, disagree, admit a mistake, reward or thank another person, give positive criticism, say no, express distress about the way a relationship is moving, and ask for collaboration.

Some statements to record and evaluate for effectiveness are:

- I cannot talk to you now. I'll talk to you at two o'clock.
- I feel really angry about this!
- I have made up my mind on this.
- I see your point, but I disagree.
- I did make an error.
- Let's sit down and work this out together.
- No, I will not reconsider this; this item is not negotiable.
- I'm upset about our relationship and I'd like to talk with you about it.
- I appreciate your help.
- We agreed your report would be on my desk yesterday. What happened?

Another use of recorders is to keep relaxing or rewarding messages that can be played back at a later time. Some rewarding messages to consider recording for yourself or clients are:

- You are working toward wellness in a useful, helpful way. Congratulations on your effort.
- Keep up the good work.
- Congratulations on not smoking. Give yourself a hug or find someone to hug. Be proud of yourself. Allow yourself to feel good about your accomplishment.
- Congratulations on meeting your fitness goal. Treat yourself to a reward and be sure to allow yourself to feel good about your accomplishment!

Videotape feedback adds the extra information of

1. Eye contact
2. Body posture and positioning
3. Gestures
4. Facial expressions
5. Verbal responses that are too quick or hesitant

6. Conciseness of statements
7. Confidence of presentation

Probably the best use of videotape is to enable role-playing or review of situations, whether past or upcoming. Scripts can be written for two people and then recorded and evaluated according to each of the information components. TABLE 3-1 provides a completed guide for assessing an assertive presentation of self that has been videotaped.

HEALTH PROMOTION CHALLENGE

Use Table 3-1 to evaluate your assertiveness skills.

Table 3-1 Evidence-Based Health Promotion: Assertiveness Assessments

Nonverbal Presentation of Self	Examples/Comments
Frequent and direct eye contact	"I kept looking at the ceiling when talking."
Speaking loudly enough and firmly enough	"I crossed my arms and looked angry when talking about being pleased."
Open, direct body communication	
Gestures match words said	

Verbal Presentation of Self	
Remain on the point of discussion without changing topics	"I let her lead me away from my goal and we started talking about her sore leg instead of my raise."
Use *I* messages, e.g., "I can't help you now," "I feel angry when . . .," "I'd like to talk with you about . . .," "I don't like to be shouted at . . .," "I realize you're concerned, but please don't make decisions for me," "I did make a mistake," "Thank you," "I'd like to do a joint evaluation with you," or "I think we can work this out."	"I used the following blaming messages: I think you should give me a raise. I feel you overlooked me."
Refrain from using *You*-blaming messages; e.g., "You didn't . . .," "You should have . . .," "It's your fault that . . .," "You aren't doing that right."	

Goal(s) for a Role Play

1. Maintain eye contact.
2. Uncross my arms.
3. Tell my partner I feel angry instead of giving an inconsistent message.
4. Get feedback from partner.

In the role-playing approach, one person tells the other about an upcoming or past situation. It is best to choose two-person situations, avoiding those with a long history of emotional overlay; strive for choices that are likely to end in a successful role-play, not in frustration because deep-seated issues are involved. For example, in an exercise that takes place between Angela and Chris, where Angela is seeking Chris's help in learning how to deal with aggressive clients or colleagues:

1. Angela gives Chris a description of what is to be said, which role each of them will take, how Chris should act to approximate the real-life situation, and how the interchange will end and begin. (A 3–5-minute script is suggested.)

2. Chris should be told that making it easy for Angela is not helpful. Being as aggressive or avoidant as a real-life person might be provides much better practice and will better prepare Angela for actual encounters.

3. Some directions that might be given are: "Be sure to try to make me feel guilty about saying no" or "Every time I try to stick to the issue, you change the subject" or "Use a really angry tone of voice, but tell me that you're not angry."

4. The goal of the role-playing exercise is to help Angela learn how to maintain emotional distance (differentiation) while sticking to her guns (assertiveness); if she loses her cool or becomes flustered, the two should take a break, discuss why Angela lost composure, and replay the exercise.

All of the procedures discussed are also appropriate when assisting clients to be more assertive and may prove invaluable if your initial interactions with the client show that lack of assertiveness is impeding effective communication.

Value Clarification

Value clarification can assist you and clients to develop larger portions of solid self and thus become more differentiated and open to health promotion actions. The process of value clarification is founded in effective communication, but that communication is not always between you and the client—it can also be between the client and him or herself. The steps of value clarification and their attendant processes are as follows (Kirschenbaum, 1976; Kirschenbaum & Simon, 1974; Raths, Harmin, & Simon, 1966):

Prizing

1. Prizing and cherishing. At this step in the process, nurses set priorities, become aware of what they are for or against, begin to trust their inner experiences and feelings, and examine why they feel as they do.

2. Clearly communicating the client's own values and actively listening to others' expressions of values.

Choosing

1. Choosing freely by examining values others have imposed on them.
2. Choosing thoughtfully between alternatives by examining the process by which they choose, and considering the possible consequences of each choice.

Acting

1. Trying out the value choice includes developing a plan of action and trying it out; contracts to act may be drawn up between the nurse and self or others.
2. Evaluating what happened when action was taken and making plans to reinforce actions that support their values.

CASE STUDY   Assisting a Client to Clarify His Values

Theresa, a community health nurse, was working with Mr. Thomas, who was recovering from a heart attack. Mr. Thomas was overweight and showing signs of prediabetes. Although Theresa's first impulse was to tell him to lose weight, she restrained herself and decided to try value clarification instead. One of their conversations follows:

Theresa:	What kinds of things about yourself concern you the most?
Mr. Thomas:	I'm afraid I'll have another heart attack.
Theresa:	Anything else?
Mr. Thomas:	My wife's nagging; she's always trying to get me to stay on a diet, but at the same time, she bakes cakes and pies.
Theresa:	Maybe the three of us can discuss this. [Theresa goes out to the waiting room and requests that Mrs. Thomas join the conversation.]
Theresa:	Your husband was just telling me about your concerns about his staying on a diet.
Wife:	The doctor told him to lose weight, and I try, but he's always sneaking goodies.
Theresa:	Are you interested in losing weight, Mr. Thomas?
Mr. Thomas:	Well, if it would make my wife happy … [poor differentiation]
Theresa:	I'm wondering what would make *you* happy.
Mr. Thomas:	Not having a heart attack again.
Theresa:	What do you know about preventing a heart attack?
Mr. Thomas:	The doctor says losing weight, exercising regularly, and eating more vegetables will help, but it seems like a lot to me.
Theresa:	What if you could choose one of those to begin with; which would it be?
Mr. Thomas:	Exercising. I've always been active in construction and baseball until this heart attack laid me low.
Theresa:	Suppose we find an exercise plan for you and your wife agrees to exercise with you? How does that sound?
Mr. Thomas:	Sounds good to me, but can you get her to stop nagging me?

(continues)

Theresa:	I can teach you both how to support each other without nagging. We can start by using assertiveness skills such as *I* messages and other communication skills that have been found useful by some of my other clients. How does the plan sound to you, Mrs. Thomas?
Mrs. Thomas:	OK, I guess.

Analysis

The conversation between Theresa and Mr. Thomas begins with the client's expressed desire to avoid another heart attack. By following up this expression with an open-ended invitation to the client to express other concerns on his mind, Theresa encourages Mr. Thomas to address other factors that may impede his success in this goal. While Mr. Thomas takes this as an opportunity to triangulate (blaming his wife for the lack of success in his dieting), it is evident that the mixed message of her nagging to stick to his diet coupled with baking sweets presents a real issue of concern to him. The nurse's act of bringing the wife into the room after the husband attempts to blame her for his inability to lose weight creates a barrier to triangulation by reintroducing direct communication between stressed parties. The triangulation does not stop completely—Mrs. Thomas's first act is to accuse her husband of sneaking goodies, deflecting blame from her own behavior—but Theresa's next response is effective in defusing the poor communication between the couple. Instead of getting involved in a wrangle over whether the wife is to blame for baking or the husband is to blame for eating what she bakes, she asks Mr. Thomas to express his wants—inviting him, in other words, to establish his *I* position. Initially, he does not take this opportunity, instead deferring to his wife, but Theresa redirects the question to once again obtain an *I* position from him. This time, he states his wants clearly. From here, Theresa now has the opportunity to give Mr. Thomas options on how to reach his stated goal. She offers Mr. Thomas a selection of choices regarding activities that can help him lose weight, and gives him control over which choice is most meaningful to him. When he picks exercise, she suggests an exercise program that involves his wife.

Bringing his wife into the selected program should provide Mr. Thomas with greater support in his weight loss efforts—support that his repeated comment about her nagging indicates he needs. The wife's limited, nonassertive verbal response may be a cue to lack of investment on her part. The husband has earlier complained that the wife sabotages his efforts at maintaining a healthy diet by baking cookies and pies, which the wife, in her turn, has accused him of sneaking. The disparity in their descriptions is significant and may point to a larger issue between them that has not been addressed—and that may be a continued obstacle to Mr. Thomas's success in losing weight.

If you were working with this couple, it would be important to note this and work to promote greater investment on the part of Mrs. Thomas. For example, asking Mrs. Thomas to agree to stop baking might not be realistic if baking is a hobby she enjoys. Asking her to bake less often, or to give her baked goods to friends, food pantries, or bake sales might be a way to negotiate a compromise—one which both Mr. and Mrs. Thomas can accept. Such a negotiation can reduce the sneaking of food and, in the long term, help support Mr. Thomas's efforts at weight loss. Discussion continues as the nurse proceeds through rest of the value clarification processes and makes plans with the couple to try out new behaviors and evaluate them.

HEALTH PROMOTION CHALLENGE

Read the case study that follows, choose a health promotion issue of importance to you, and follow the value clarification steps with at least one other student helping you through the process.

CASE STUDY

All students in a seminar were asked to write about an assertiveness issue that they wanted to work on and bring their papers to class (choosing freely). The instructor helped each student discuss when he or she might want or not want to be assertive in their situation (prizing and cherishing; examining alternatives and consequences of action). Students selected another student to pair up with to practice role playing the assertiveness situation. Some students decided to contract with one another to try out the situation in real life and to receive positive reinforcement from one another for doing so (trying out; contracting; reinforcing change). All students were encouraged to try their new assertive behaviors out in real life situations and to report back to the class by evaluating their performance (evaluating).

Techniques for Raising Self-Awareness

If you assess a client as lacking adequate differentiation or assertiveness, it is worthwhile to consider options for improving these qualities. A number of techniques have been developed to support an individual's abilities in this regard.

☐ Centering

Centering refers to finding within oneself an inner reference of stability, a sense of self-relatedness that can be thought of as a place of inner being, a place of quietude within oneself where one can feel truly integrated, unified, and focused (Krieger, 1979).

Centering is a powerful, easily achieved skill (see BOX 3-2) for enhancing differentiation of self and thereby freeing individuals from becoming too emotionally entangled in life issues—what might be regarded as living in the problem rather than living in the solution. Centering is a practice that can benefit the nurse just as much as the client; when nurses are not centered, they are apt to feel fatigued, stressed, depressed, or angry when working with a client who lacks the ability to differentiate. Centering allows the nurse to be separate from, yet open to input from clients—which enhances effective communication.

Learning to reach one's center takes little time once the idea is mastered, but it can have an important impact on practice. Nurses have reported to the author the following ways of using centering:

- "I take a moment, go to the rest room, and get centered between clients."
- "I center myself as I'm walking down the hall on the way to my next client."
- "I center myself when I'm with the client; I ask the client to center herself or himself, and we do it together. I find we both have a lot more energy to concentrate on the tasks ahead when we do."

Box 3-2   Centering

Centering can be achieved while standing or sitting, but beginning efforts produce the best results in a sitting position.

1. Sit in a comfortable chair with feet flat on the floor and hands resting quietly in your lap; close your eyes.
2. Check out your body for tension spots and relax these areas as you exhale.
3. Inhale easily, filling your body with relaxation.
4. Exhale, moving your breathing to your center, about the level of your navel.
5. Continue breathing in this manner until you feel calm, integrated, unified, and focused.
6. (Optional) Picture the body surrounded by a protective shield that allows positive energy in, but keeps negative energy out. The shield may be conceived as a color, light source, or in a spiritual sense.

As the third example shows, it can be effective to teach clients to use centering. For example, clients may find it helpful to use prior to any anxiety-provoking situation in the hospital, at home, in social situations, or at work. The steps in centering remain the same. Directions given for the nurse can be copied or adapted for use with clients.

Affirmations

Affirmations are a self-care strategy that can reduce anxiety and stress and lead to calm, productive behavior. An **affirmation** is a positive thought you consciously choose to immerse yourself in. Examples include: "I refuse to let this bother me," "I can stay calm and focused," "I can handle this," "I'm handling this now," and "I'm taking deep breaths and getting calmer every second." For nurses engaged in health promotion, affirmations can be used both to strengthen the nurse's practice or as a means of reinforcing behaviors in the client.

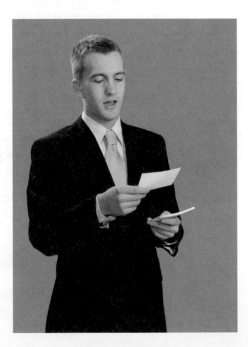

Write or say the affirmation at least 20 times a day to counter the effects of negative thoughts and provide a sense of empowerment. Jot affirmations down on 3 × 5 cards and carry them in a pocket, post on the refrigerator or bathroom mirror, or set them on the car seat to read at stoplights.

Refuting Irrational Ideas

We all talk to ourselves in our thoughts and sometimes in words. This is called **Self-talk**. When our thoughts and words are positive and realistic they can be helpful, but when they are negative and irrational, they can create unneeded stress.

- Statements that "awfulize" an experience, e.g., thinking silence is a negative criticism or that a momentary pain is a sign of cancer or a heart condition.
- The belief that inactivity and endless leisure can lead to happiness.
- The idea that it is easier to avoid difficulties and responsibilities rather than face them.
- The thought that misery is due to external events that trigger emotion.
- The belief that it is possible to be perfect at all times.
- The idea that it is horrible when things are not the way they should be.
- The belief that people can't live without love and approval from others.
- The thought that we have no control over what we feel or experience.
- The idea that new situations must lead to anxiety and fear.
- The belief that good relationships mean constant giving and sacrifice.
- The thought that people are fragile and cannot accept the truth.
- The idea that worth is dependent on producing and achieving things.
- The belief anger is bad.
- The thought that rejection and abandonment will result unless we always try to please others.
- The idea that there is one perfect relationship and one perfect love.
- The belief that going after what is wanted or needed is a bad thing.

Goodman (1974) added to Ellis and Harper's guidelines for changing irrational thoughts into more rational ones. When **refuting irrational ideas**, keep the following points in mind:

1. One person cannot argue; it takes at least two.
2. Everyone makes mistakes.
3. To believe things aren't as they are is magical thinking.
4. Thoughts come first, then feelings; it is our interpretation of what happens, not the events themselves, that leads to emotions.
5. We can never know that real cause of many problems, so it's best to focus on the here-and-now.

TABLE 3-2 provides an example of the use of Ellis and Harper's format for refuting irrational ideas.

HEALTH PROMOTION CHALLENGE

Use Table 3-2 as a model to refute one of your irrational ideas.

Table 3-2 Evidence-Based Health Promotion: Refuting Irrational Ideas

Steps Actions/Thoughts/Feelings

1. *Activating event:* My family complains about me.

2. *Rational ideas:* I know they're under a lot of stress now, so I should give them some slack.

3. *Irrational ideas:* I can't stand hearing them whisper and point at me. I'm out of control and I may scream at them or punch them.

4. *Main feelings:* Rage, anger, falling apart.

5. *Refuting the irrational idea(s):* Refuting the irrational idea(s): I may feel horrible, but I'm not falling apart. I can handle it and stay calm without overreacting.

6. *The worst thing that could happen:* The worst thing that could happen is I could scream and shout at them, but so what? I'm only human.

7. *Good things that could occur as a result of this incident:* I'll learn how to handle myself in an upsetting situation without overreacting; even if I do overreact, I'll see that my family can handle that because I don't do it that often.

8. *Alternate thoughts:* Maybe they're whispering about something or somebody other than me. I don't need to take everything so personally. Even if they are talking about me, I'm okay with it. I can handle being talked about and whispered about. I'm strong.

9. *Alternate emotions:* Just by writing all this down helps me feel more in control of myself. I can't control anyone else's feelings, but I can learn to control mine.

Assertive Strategies for Dealing with Criticism

Criticism is a fact of life in any profession. Constructive criticism can lead to improvement; feedback from others can help you learn not to repeat the error. For nurses, the goal is to extract the growth-promoting aspects of criticisms from others and use them to grow. To do this, the nurse must dispel irrational beliefs that criticism means failure or wrongness. Sometimes criticism is accurate, but not constructive; other times, criticism is unjustified. However, to determine what beneficial features are present in a critique, the nurse must be willing to face the criticism and assess its validity from an intellectual (well-differentiated) position, rather than responding emotionally.

Three strategies for assertively responding to criticism are acknowledging, clouding, and probing (McKay, Davis, & Fanning, 1983).

☐ Acknowledging

Whenever criticism is received, an assertive response includes **acknowledging** the critic's comment. Some examples are: "You're right, I am half an hour late for work," "You're right, I did misspell a lot of words," and "Yes, I am late in handing in this report."

Excuses and apologies are not part of an assertive response. Consider them automatic leftovers from childhood when excuses and apologies were demanded; parents and teachers expected an explanation and so one was offered—whether real or made up. As adults, individuals have the right to choose whether to give an explanation or not. Often, it is not advantageous to give an explanation because it provides further ammunition for the other person and does not present a picture of competence. Consider the two situations below; the first presents the individual as blame fixing, childlike, and incompetent. The second presents the individual as assertive and adult.

Situation 1: Nonacknowledging

Supervisor: You're late again! How long do you think I'm going to tolerate this?

Employee: Oh, I'm so sorry, the car broke down again and my husband wouldn't give me a lift.

Supervisor: You've always got an excuse, but this time I'm not buying it. I'm writing you up and docking you for 15 minutes.

Situation 2: Acknowledging

Supervisor: You're late again! How long do you think I'm going to tolerate this?

Employee: You're right, I am 15 minutes late.

Supervisor: I'm docking you for the 15 minutes.

The major difference between the two situations is that the nurse gives an excuse in the first instance and does not acknowledge error; in the second instance, the nurse acknowledges error and does not give an excuse. The supervisor lacks the impetus to make an accusatory statement and can simply state the consequence to be handed down—which limits the personalization and attacking nature of the response that is present in the first version.

☐ Clouding

Clouding is an assertiveness technique to use when receiving criticism of a manipulative nature (Eshelman, McKay, & Fanning, 2008). To use this technique, clients must listen carefully to determine which part of the criticism they agree with in part or in principle, but not to agree to change.

Situation 1: Agreeing in Part

Supervisor: You always have an excuse for not working overtime. What's the matter with you anyway?

Supervisee: Yes, I do have many reasons for not working overtime, but you know how it is when you have small kids at home.

Supervisor: You don't seem to care for your job at all.

Supervisee: I can see where you might conclude that, but it's not how I feel.

The initial critique offered by the supervisor is valid (even if rudely made); the supervisee does not work overtime much. However, the supervisee has valid reasons for refusing overtime; in agreeing, the supervisee has the opportunity to deflect the criticism by pointing out, gently, what the supervisor has overlooked—the fact that she/he has young children to care for. The second criticism, however, is unfair; working overtime (or not) has no relationship to the supervisee's commitment to the job. By suggesting that the supervisor's assessment may *seem* valid, but does not reflect the supervisee's *actual* level of commitment (I position), the supervisee again partly agrees and deflects the critique. Stating the *I* position here is key because the supervisor cannot contradict it; "This is how I feel" is a statement that only the person making it can assess for validity.

Situation 2: Agreeing in Probability

Supervisor: You know, this workstation is a disaster. You can't possibly work in such a mess. Why aren't you keeping it more organized?

Employee: Actually, my shift just started, but you may be right that the station needs to be organized better.

The supervisor's criticism is misplaced and rudely stated. The base concern, however, is valid—a poorly organized workstation is a hindrance to effective workplace functioning. Rather than entering into an argument over whether she should accept the blame for the problem, agreeing in probability with the (valid) underlying suggestion and letting the accusatory tone pass is the employee's best option; it is unlikely that the supervisor will pursue the point once it has been (apparently) accepted.

Situation 3: Agreeing in Principle

Faculty member: If you don't study more than you do, you're going to fail.

Student: You're right. If I don't study, I will fail.

The critique of the student's study habits might be valid, or it might not be; the faculty member is assuming that the student does not study enough, which may not actually be the case. The stated principle, however, is accurate: A student who does not study will likely fail. That is something the student can agree with without accepting the (probably false) premise that he/she is not studying enough. Agreeing deflects further criticism.

☐ Probing

Criticism is often used by others to avoid important feelings or wishes. Assertive **probing** assists in determining whether criticism is constructive or manipulative and clarifies unclear comments.

- The first step in assertive probing is to listen carefully and isolate the part of the criticism that seems most bothersome to the critic.
- The next step is to ask the critic, "What is it that bothers you about . . . ?"

Situation 1: Assertive Probing

Supervisor: You're not doing a very good job here. Your work is not up to par.

Employee: What is it about my work that bothers you?

Supervisor: Well, everyone else is working overtime, but you waltz out of here two out of three nights right at quitting time.

Employee: Why is it a problem that I leave on time when other people work overtime?

Supervisor: I don't like working overtime either, but the work has to be done. It's not right that you just work by the clock.

Employee: What is it that bothers you when I work by the clock?

Supervisor: When you leave, someone else has to finish your work. I want you to make sure your work is completed before you leave.

Employee: I see. Thanks for explaining the situation to me.

In this scenario, the problem as originally stated is not the actual problem at all. By continuing to question the supervisor for specifics, eventually the employee arrives at the *real* issue, stated in a way that he or she can accept, rather than an attack.

Additional Assertive Strategies

☐ Broken Record

This approach is useful when others do not seem to hear or accept what is being said, or when an explanation would provide the other person with an opportunity to continue a pointless discussion. It is especially useful for saying no to others' unreasonable requests.

The process for using broken record includes the following steps:

1. Clarify exactly what the limits of what will be done are.
2. Formulate a short, specific statement about what is wanted; avoid giving excuses or explanations because they give the other person ammunition to undermine the original statement.

3. Use consistent body language that supports the statement, including maintaining eye contact, standing or sitting erect, and keeping hands and arms quietly at the side of the body.

4. Calmly and firmly repeat the chosen statement as many times as necessary until the other person realizes there is no negotiation possible. The first few times a statement is made, the other person may given an excuse or attempt to derive a different answer.

5. (Optional) Briefly acknowledge the other's ideas, feelings, or wishes before returning to the broken record statement, e.g., "I hear you saying you're upset, but I don't want to work any more overtime."

Situation 1: Broken Record

Nurse 1: I just got an opportunity to fly to Aspen to ski. Won't you help me out and switch vacation schedules with me?

Nurse 2: How great for you. No, I don't want to switch schedules.

Nurse 1: You mean you're not going to help me? What kind of a friend are you?

Nurse 2: I understand that you're disappointed, but I don't want to switch schedules.

Nurse 1: But I have to go to Aspen, and you're the only one who can help me.

Nurse 2: No, I don't want to switch schedules.

Nurse 1: Boy, you're really hard hearted. What happened to you? You used to be so nice, now suddenly, you're Wanda the Witch.

Nurse 2: I appreciate your difficulty, but I don't want to switch schedules. That's not going to change.

☐ Content-to-Process Shift

When the focus or point of the conversation drifts away from the original topic, the content-to-process shift can be used to shift from the subject being discussed (the content) to what is occurring between the two speakers (the process), e.g., "We're off the point now, let's get back to what we agreed to discuss."

Content-to-process shift can involve self-disclosure of current thoughts or feelings, e.g., "I'm feeling uncomfortable discussing this now, and I notice we're both tense." This approach is especially useful when voices are raised and anger is present: "We seem to be getting into a battle about this." The trick is to comment neutrally about what is observed so the other person does not experience the comment as an attack.

☐ Momentary Delay

There is a compelling aspect to many social situations. There is often the implied command from another person that a question must be answered right away. Rather than being swayed by the emotion of the moment, take a deep breath and a momentary (or longer) delay. This procedure allows for further understanding and analysis of the pros and cons of each available response.

Situation 1: Momentary Delay

Supervisor: I'd like you to read the riot act to the aides; they aren't doing their work. You have to do something right now!

Nurse: [Takes a deep breath.] I'll need more information before I can act.

Situation 2: Momentary Delay

Supervisee: I think I deserve a break. I've been working nonstop for 7 hours, and if I wait any longer it will be time to go home!

Supervisor: You may be right, but I need to check the floor to make sure we won't be short-handed. Can you hang on for just a few more minutes?

☐ Time Out

When the conversation reaches an impasse, but the discussion is an important one, the conversation can be delayed to a later time; time out is only assertive if a specific time in the near future is set to continue the discussion.

Situation 1: Time Out

Teenager: I think you're blaming me unfairly.

Parent: We've been talking about this quite a while now, and I don't think we're getting anywhere. Let's sleep on it and I'll see you at 9:00 a.m. tomorrow to talk then.

☐ Joining and Circling the Attacker

The joining and circling the attacker approach is derived from the martial art of aikido, in which the attacked person accepts the attack and turns with it, letting the attacker pass in the direction he or she has chosen. According to Dobson and Miller (1994):

> One of the best ways to survive . . . is to . . . flow with them. Harmonize . . . Be the water, not the rock. The water has direction and flexibility. Eon by eon the rock is worn down, until halfway through eternity it has become a pebble. If the rock would turn with the force of the water, still retaining its place in the stream bed, the rock would lose nothing; the water would continue past. (p. 87)

As in the martial art, there is a pause the attacker takes just before a change in direction. That brief moment is when the attacker loses balance; it is at that precise moment that the defender takes charge and helps the attacker to a new, firmer, less aggressive balance. Most attackers are spoiling for a fight. They are overextended, and they need the victim to fight back and preserve their tenuous balance. So if you yell at a yeller, that helps him stay upright. With joining and circling, focus of energy is, instead, on the resolution of conflict, and problem solving, and the restoration of harmony. In each attacking or conflict situation, there are six alternative ways to respond:

1. Do nothing
2. Use diversion, deflection, or humor
3. Join with the attackers
4. Withdraw
5. Parley
6. Fight back

Do Nothing This is an appropriate response when time is needed, when more information is needed to find out what is behind the attack, when the attacked person does not want to dignify the attack by reacting (it is not necessary to answer charges unless the nurse chooses to do so), or when the attack makes no sense. Doing nothing must be a conscious choice, not a response to fear, in order to be an assertive response.

Use Diversion, Deflection, or Humor An appropriate response is to deflect or redirect an attack. "Most attacks . . . come at you along a fairly straight line. By employing . . . surprise, you can break that line and cause the attack to misfire." Changing the subject ("I see you're wearing a new suit.") or giving absurd explanations can be used to create a diversion or deflection.

Situation 1: Using Deflection/Humor
Supervisor: You forgot to get that report in!
Nurse: You're right. I'm sorry I didn't follow through on our agreement.
Supervisor: That's no excuse! What were you thinking?
Nurse: I was planning my zombie attack preparedness strategies.
Supervisor: Um. What?
Nurse: I found it on the CDC's website. No, seriously. They have a page on zombie preparedness.[1]

Join with the Attackers Agree with the attacker's right to feel as he or she does. (This is aikido, confluence, flowing with being the water, not the rock.)

Situation 1: Joining the Attacker
Supervisor: What have you done? You're the—worst nurse I've ever seen!

---

[1] The CDC's zombie preparedness page is at http://www.cdc.gov/phpr/zombies.htm

Nurse: I don't blame you.

Supervisor: What do you mean, I don't blame you?

Nurse: It's not up to me to blame anybody for feeling the way they do. You're not happy, and I can't quibble with that.

Supervisor: [Puzzled] But you think your work is up to par?

Nurse: It can't be if you're not happy with it. My job is to work with you.

Supervisor: [Confused] I don't understand.

Nurse: If you don't think I should be fired outright, let's see if we can't work together on this thing and make it mutually acceptable. What are some of your complaints?

The nurse's use of surprise combined with joining the attack led to the supervisor losing his balance. The nurse has joined the supervisor and is helping him; the nurse does not take the attack personally, but objectifies the conflict. This leads to confusion. The nurse then takes the lead in identifying and resolving the problem in her relationship with the supervisor. Note that the supervisor must have a genuine issue with her work that is simply not well expressed; by taking this tack, the nurse provides an opportunity for better communication, both now and in the future.

Withdraw Withdrawal is an appropriate choice when all else fails and an escape route is open or when the time and place for discussion is wrong. To use withdrawal well, it must be completed clearly and with a single intention. Being unclear about the right to leave the scene can result in confusion. It is important to withdraw with certainty, knowing that it is each person's right to stay out of destructive involvements. Appropriate techniques for withdrawal include statements such as, "I can see we're not going to reach agreement on this, so we'll have to agree to disagree, as I have somewhere else I need to be right now," or "Unfortunately, there isn't time for us to hash this out, so I'm going to have to leave on that note."

Parley Parley is most effective when involved in a no-win situation in which the other person has defined the encounter as a contest. In this case, the nurse or client can remain centered and turn the conflict around, offering a reasonable way out for both parties. Some parleying comments are:

- "Shall we see if we can work out a compromise?"
- "Let's see if we can't iron out the problem."
- "Maybe we can figure out a way to solve both our problems by working together."

Fight Back Fighting back is the response of choice when there is no other option. It is a question of life or death, or it is a question of serious priority. Fighting back could include expressing anger directly or standing up to an insult.

Situation 1: Fighting Back

   Surgeon: [He has just cornered the nurse in front of several other surgeons and physicians.] Listen, kid, my time is too valuable to spend chasing all over the place to find that room you assigned me to just because you're so inefficient you can't get the simplest things through your pinhead! And another thing, where is that new scalpel I ordered?

   Nurse: Excuse me, I am not willing to be blamed for someone else's room assignment and I don't order scalpels. Now, we can argue, or we can try to solve the problem together.

   Surgeon: I don't have to take this from you! I can have you fired!

   Nurse: This is not productive. If you want to solve the problem, why don't you work on figuring out the room assignment and I'll find out about the scalpel. [She exits.]

This response focuses the surgeon on the problem and its solution, yet allows the nurse to stand up for her rights, which she has already decided are a high priority for her with this surgeon who has just attempted to humiliate her in public. The nurse might lose her job (an unlikely but possible resolution), but she has already decided she has no intention of continuing to work under these conditions. Most likely the job will not be lost, and conditions could improve as the surgeon realizes he cannot bully the nurse.

When the decision to stand up for the client's rights has been made, it is important to make several assessments prior to acting, including:

1. Does this person have something to lose by being aggressive? (If the answer is yes, the person may choose to reconsider this response and choose another, since the other person may be irrational in the interchange.)

2. What is the minimum amount of energy needed in this situation to make the point? (Use the minimum energy needed to restore harmony.)

3. What is the best time and place for the confrontation?

4. What is the best way to stop an attacker's advance?

5. What is the best way to focus the conflict on the problem and not on generalities or personalities?

6. What does the respondent want his or her face to say and how can he or she ensure it says that?

7. What does the respondent want his or her body to say and how can he or she ensure it says that?

8. What spatial relationship to the other person is most likely to end in harmony?

□ Multiple Attack

An attack from several other people feels intimidating. Examining the geometry of forces, it can be seen that due to the nature of the force exerted by the attackers, they require one another's presence in order to continue the attack. Their forces create a balance due to focusing energy directly on the attackee. If the attackee keeps an attacker positioned between her or him and the rest of the attackers, the larger group will be unable to focus their attention on the victim, and the multiple attack will be defused. The nurse may still have to deal with the attacker nearest to the nurse's position, but handling one attacker is better than attempting to deal effectively with two or more.

Situation 1: Multiple Attack Sandra is a staff nurse who believes in wellness and health promotion. She tries to collaborate with her clients and help them to take responsibility for decisions about what happens to them. As a result, she spends more time talking with her clients than some of the other nurses. Her supervisor has noted her wasting time talking with clients a number of times and several physicians have demonstrated impatience waiting for her to make rounds or assist them.

Sandra is in a bind. She believes in what she is doing but knows she is being evaluated negatively. She knows this cannot go on indefinitely, so she moves in on a straight line to bring the attacks into direct confrontation. She calls a meeting of physicians and her supervisor to discuss the kinds of nursing plans she has implemented. Sandra centers herself, which helps her to remember the group is not there to get her. They are anxious about their work and worried about time pressures and being evaluated positively by their supervisors.

Ms. Bart, the nursing supervisor, is the most outspoken and demands that Sandra spend less time talking with clients and more time assisting physicians and completing her paperwork. Sandra pays attention to her breathing and keeps centered so she doesn't scream out, "Look here, I went to nursing school to learn these special skills I have, and I know that's the best way to practice nursing!" Sandra realizes that Ms. Bart, in the best tradition of attackers, has attacked with such force that she has almost lost her balance. Sandra decides to slide around Ms. Bart toward the other attackers. She asks for comments from the physicians, thanks them for their concern about clients, and asks if all the physicians agree with Ms. Bart about her spending less time providing care for their clients. The physicians disagree with one another and raise unrelated questions. Sandra refrains from becoming defensive and continues to go back to Ms. Bart's demands, keeping her between herself and the physicians. Sandra eventually offers to speak at the next grand rounds, sharing with the physicians her nursing interventions and outcomes for various clients they label as difficult.

Situation 2: Multiple Attack Sue Anderson, RN, is working with a client, Emily Weiss, who is constantly complaining that her teenage kids seem to be down on her lately. They argue about performing household tasks and complain about her cooking and nagging. As a result, Emily feels cut off and resentful. Sue suggests a family meeting to bring the attacks into direct confrontation. Emily resists at first, until Sue does some role-playing with her to help her decide exactly what she wants to say to her family.

Emily practices centering herself prior to the family meeting and resists becoming defensive when the complaints start. Emily pays attention to her breathing, thanks them for being so candid, slides around the children's attacks, and keeps her husband between herself and the kids. Emily offers to stop nagging them in exchange for their agreeing to each cook one meal a week. The next week she reports to Sue that things are better around the house.

RESEARCH BOX 3-1 examines the relationship between assertiveness and aikido.

RESEARCH BOX 3-1   Aikido Principles and Assertiveness Training

» BACKGROUND: Self-defense classes aim to prevent violence against women by strengthening women's capacity to defend themselves; however, little research has examined the effects of self-defense training on women's attempts to fight back during actual attacks. This study investigated the relationship of self-defense or assertiveness training and women's physical and psychological responses to subsequent rape attacks.

» SAMPLE (N = 1,623).

» METHODS: Multivariate analyses.

» RESULTS: Victims with preassault training were more likely to say that their resistance stopped the offender or made him less aggressive than victims without training. Women with training before their assaults were angrier and less scared during the incident than women without training, consistent with the teachings of self-defense training. Preassault training participants rated their degree of nonconsent or resistance as lower than did nonparticipants, perhaps because they held themselves to a higher standard.

Source: Brecklin, L.R., & Ullman, S. E. (2005). Self-Defense or Assertiveness Training and Women's Responses to Sexual Attacks. *Journal of Interpersonal Violence, 20*(6), 738–762.

HEALTH PROMOTION CHALLENGE

Using Research Box 3-1, come up with at least three ways to use the findings and promote health of the nurse and/or client.

☐ Hidden Agendas

Hidden agendas are unstated issues that are played out through interaction with others. Hidden agendas are excellent defensive maneuvers for low self-esteem. They protect against rejection by creating the desired impression at the expense of intimacy and authenticity. Nurses and clients use them to put up a smoke screen of carefully selected stories and calculated remarks. Clues that hidden agendas are operating include making the same point again and again while trying to prove something. The problem with hidden agendas is that they are obstacles to authentic, positive relationships. Therefore, it is important to assess the tendency for operating from a hidden agenda and take steps to devise self-instructions to counteract the pretense.

Eschelman, Davis, and Fanning (2008) list eight major hidden agendas:

1. *I Am Good.* Many of the statements from a person using this agenda demonstrate how caring and sensitive the person is; a fine character is created, but not an authentic self. No one is entrusted with the parts of the self that are less than wonderful. People who always present themselves as good, honest, loyal, generous, successful, powerful, strong, wealthy, self-sacrificing, etc., tend to bore other people, and an intimate relationship becomes difficult.

2. *I Am Good (But You Are Not).* In this agenda, the person attempts to raise his or her self-esteem by showing how stupid, incompetent, selfish, unreasonable, lazy, frightened, or insensitive others are. One nurse often complained, "Do you think I can ever get anyone around here to help me? I'm the only one doing the work!" This hidden agenda gives a temporary boost to self-esteem, but others feel threatened and put down and defensive maneuvers on their part soon follow.

3. *You Are Good (But I Am Not).* People who constantly flatter others have this agenda. More complex forms involve worship of smart, beautiful, or strong people. This agenda can also be used to ward off anger, rejection, and high expectations; who expects much of someone who is incompetent and self-berating?

4. *I am Helpless, I Suffer.* This agenda portrays the person as a victim who has suffered misfortune, injustice, and abuse. The implied message is that the person is helpless and not responsible for what happens. Variations include presenting a problem and then proving nothing will help resolve it, and sharing horror stories with another to form a bond of sympathy.

5. *I am Blameless.* This is the agenda of people who have innumerable excuses for their failures. The basic position is: "I didn't do it." (Variations include, "The doctor did it . . .," "The client did it . . .," "The family interferes . . .," and "My boss is the problem . . .") There is a basic

inability to accept responsibility for any actions that do not lead to success—although generally these people are happy to accept credit for success, whether it's due or not.

6. *I Am Fragile.* The basic stance is, "Don't hurt me; I can't take it." The person tells or shows others he needs protection from the truth. ("I don't want to talk about it; it upsets me," "You're giving me another of my headaches," and "This reminds me of my parents fighting; let's not get into it" are typical comments from this stance.) On most hospital units, there is one person who does not do his or her work but is not confronted by others because "She's fragile and couldn't take it."

7. *I Am Tough.* A variation is the super nurse whose communication is often a harried listing of things done or to do; the underlying message is "I work harder, longer, and faster than anyone." The purpose of the agenda is to ward off hurt and protect a fragile self-esteem.

8. *I Know It All.* This is the agenda of the perpetual instructor, constantly moralizing as a protection from reencountering early experiences of shame of being inadequate and ill-informed.

Eschelman, McKay, and Fanning (2008) suggest using self-instructions for overcoming hidden agendas. The statements can be said as mantras over and over again and can be taped to a bathroom mirror, the inside of a briefcase, or carried on 3 × 5 cards.

☐ Affirmations for Overcoming Hidden Agendas

"I'm a mixture of strengths and weaknesses; I can learn to be balanced."

"I don't have to put you down to make me feel good; I can feel good on my own."

"I can get attention for my strengths without making excuses."

"I experience joy as well as pain; I can allow myself to experience both."

"I'm responsible for what happens to me."

"I can learn to deal with upset."

"I can be safe without being tough."

"I can learn a lot from others if I listen, watch, and ask questions."

RESEARCH BOX 3-2 examines the identification of hidden agendas.

HEALTH PROMOTION CHALLENGE

Using the information in Research Box 3-2, identify at least three ways to use the findings to promote health.

RESEARCH BOX 3-2   Dealing with Hidden Agendas

» BACKGROUND: Most gynecologists lack the unique skills required for communication with female adolescent clients and with their parents. Years of clinical experience are required to develop communication skills that would facilitate the confidence of the young client during the first visit. Simulation-based medical education at the Israel Center for Medical Simulation (MSR) has become a powerful force in quality-care training for healthcare providers using empirical educational modalities, enabling controlled proactive experiential exposure to both regular and complex scenarios. Among the various MSR programs for various medical sectors, training programs have been developed to improve the skills of physicians, including primary care physicians and school doctors, in communicating with adolescents. This paper describes the first reported simulated client-based MSR training program for gynecologists in communication with adolescents who present with common complaints encountered in gynecology clinics.

» SAMPLE: Twenty gynecologists participated.

» METHODS: The researchers used eight individual simulated scenarios and conducted them at simulated physicians' offices which were equipped with audiovisual recording cameras and one-way mirrors for observation. Three physicians experienced in debriefing and in facilitating group discussions led the debriefing sessions, using the video recording of the simulated scenario following the simulation exercises. These discussions focused on communication techniques when facing adolescent clients with or without their parents, hidden agendas disclosed by using systematic physical and psychosocial reviews, the emotional load often associated with clinical problems, and the nonjudgmental and supportive approach to adolescent clients.

» FINDINGS: The clear recommendation that emerged from the high satisfaction of the program participants was to expand simulated client-based programs for gynecologists and to include it as an integrated part of the training curriculum in pediatric and adolescent gynecology.

Source: Beyth, Y., Hardoff, D., Rom, E., & Ziv, A. (2009). A simulated patient-based program for training gynecologists in communication with adolescent girls presenting with gynecological problems. *Journal of Pediatric and Adolescent Gynecology, 22*(2), 79–84.

Facilitating Movement Toward Health and Wellness

When you've established a high level of differentiation and professionalism, you will be able to use these attributes to create a method for facilitating clients' wellness without adversely impacting your own. This is an important consideration because being an effective role model is a key factor in teaching and motivating. A sure way to fail is to ask a client to do something that you yourself would find unpalatable or impossible; on the other hand, if you can show the client evidence that a strategy has been successful for you in the past (whether in your own health promotion or in other clients' efforts), it encourages trust and effort.

A highly differentiated nurse with solid self can support consistent client involvement in the assessment, implementation, and evaluation of client goals and can teach clients to perceive life experiences as manageable and meaningful by increasing self-responsibility and commitment to action. Facilitating client assertive and creative behavior and assisting clients to differentiate themselves from you and significant others will promote behaviors that support health. Likewise, facilitating clients' social supports and evaluating the effect of change toward health and wellness, as well as resistance to and readiness for change, can aid in developing effective strategies. Use of contracting, self-assessments, belief scales, imagery, structured relaxation, affirmations, and other health promotion procedures can reinforce goals and strategies for the client.

Evaluating the Effect of the Proposed Change

Movement toward health and wellness requires change. One reason people resist change is because new habits or ways of thinking are unfamiliar. If movement toward wellness is viewed as a threat to current status, existing ways of life, job or money, familiar habits, or autonomy or free will, resistance to change can be expected. When facilitating movement toward health and wellness, ask the following questions:

- What other factors will be affected as a result of changing?
- What forces are operating to inhibit change at this time?
- What information or experiences are needed to change?
- What new procedures or experiences will need to be developed as a result of the change?
- Who is likely to suffer from the change?
- How will power, influence, custom, or lifestyle be affected by the change?
- How aware is the client of the need for change or of its purpose?
- Is the client sufficiently involved in planning for the change?
- What past experiences between the nurse and the client might be influencing resistance to change now?
- How open has the client been to the introduction of change in the past?

A factor to assess when examining client responsibility is the level of dissatisfaction with current lifestyle and the readiness for change. Clients who may be most ready to change include:

- A client who is constantly slightly depressed and lacking in energy and who has tried all medical treatments may be dissatisfied enough to be ready to try jogging or another form of exercise as a treatment.

- Another client who has tried all the fad diets available in an effort to lose weight may be ready to try a long-term weight management program if it seems enticing and if support is provided.
- A client who is in chronic pain that is not touched by strong medication may be willing to learn self-hypnosis or other noninvasive pain control measures.

Clients are most open to taking responsibility for health and wellness during childhood, when values may still be forming, and again between ages 35 and 45, when people enter the midlife crisis and begin to see they are alone, mortal, and are searching for internal, not institutional, validation. This and other times of crisis may provoke a move toward self-fulfillment and openness to change.

Decreasing Resistance to Change

Once sources of resistance to change have been identified, steps can be taken to reduce it. If anxiety or threats are the source of resistance to change, teach clients to practice centering.

Resistance to change will be decreased if rewards for changing are given and problem solving is used. The first step in learning more effective behavior is to identify the behavior to be changed. Behavior is an action, not a feeling, attitude, or mood. Behaviors must be pinpointed and expressed in such a way that they can be counted. TABLE 3-3 shows examples of behaviors that can and cannot be counted.

Once the behavior is expressed in countable terms, baseline data can be gathered. These data consist of information gathered prior to treatment. The

Table 3-3 Examples of Behaviors That Can and Cannot Be Counted

Countable Behaviors	Noncountable Behaviors (General Behaviors or Internal States)
Jogging	Being neat
Brushing and flossing teeth	Being organized
Drinking fluids	Being motivated
Losing weight	Being depressed
Gaining weight	Being angry
Smoking a cigarette	Being guilty
Practicing relaxation exercises	Improving communication
Attending yoga class	Grieving
Eating complex carbohydrates	Being noncompliant

pinpointed behavior is counted or measured to see how often it occurs now. These data can be charted and hung in the client's home or elsewhere, and they can be recorded on the treatment chart, in the client's journal, or wherever agreed upon. Data from this before or baseline phase can be used later to check progress toward the goal. Behavior can be counted by

- Frequency
- Rate over time
- How long the behavior continues

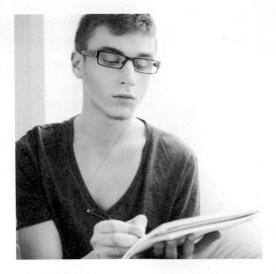

The method used to count depends on the behavior. For example, the frequency method might be best for participating in relaxation exercises, the rate over time to measure weight gain or loss, and the duration method to measure jogging. A notebook, graph, chart, or journal can be used to gather baseline data.

Using Rewards to Increase Desired Behavior

The next step in increasing desirable behavior is to find out what is rewarding and depriving to the particular client. TABLE 3-4 shows reinforcers for a student who was chronically late to class. Clients, too, can be asked to make such a list. There are some nearly universal rewards, such as attention, smiles, praise, candy, or other sweets. If the client is unable to state a reward, a universal reward can be used or the chart can be read to find hints. Of course, giving sweets to someone with diabetes or who wants to lose weight would be self-defeating; if a reward is something that will worsen, not improve, health, then it should not be used. A reward also cannot be used if control cannot be established over when the reinforcement is dispensed. For example, if a family lets a child watch TV whether or not the child participates in family meetings, watching TV cannot be used as a reward for the child's participation in family meetings. If the client is hospitalized, more rewards can be controlled. If the client is at home, fewer rewards are under nursing control. It is wise to enlist the aid of families, other personnel, and whoever it is who dispenses rewards; the best way to do this is to reward them for helping by giving them attention, not scolding them when they do not comply, and by using whatever other things seem to be rewarding to them.

When operating from a health promotion/wellness framework, keep in mind that self-modification or client choice in applying behavior modification principles and voluntary changes in selected aspects of behavior is the focus, not changing the behavior of others through the manipulation of rewards and punishments (Pender, Murdaugh, & Parsons, 2010).

Table 3-4 Reinforcers for One Student

Positive, Rewarding Reinforcers	Negative, Depriving Reinforcers
Eating ice cream	Watching cartoons
Seeing a movie	Working overtime
Sleeping late on weekends	Being told I'm late
Talking with other nurses	Doing dishes
Going dancing	Doing reports
Reading mysteries	Eating cottage cheese

❑ When to Reward Desired Behavior

To increase the occurrence of a goal-directed behavior, the reward must immediately follow movement toward that behavior. Giving praise 2 days after a client walked around the block is less likely to increase walking behavior than praising right after the walk.

In some cases it may be unrealistic or impossible to provide the reinforcement immediately following the occurrence of the goal-directed behavior. In that case, a written contract, wall chart, token system, or some other method can be used to indicate a reward is due. For example, a wall chart could be used to show participation in planned exercise. A mark could be used to indicate 30 minutes of TV time or crossword puzzle work that could be collected that evening or on the weekend for each time 30 minutes of exercise is accomplished. Or, clients can be given tokens to indicate completion of a behavior; a specified number of tokens can be used to purchase a reward.

Using Shaping Techniques

Some desired behaviors may occur at random or very rarely. In such cases, **shaping techniques** to reinforce approximations to the target behavior can be used. For example, telling the client the exact words to say and then praising the behavior, or asking the client to avoid smiling when talking are ways of shaping behavior. When shaping client behavior, nurses act as sculptors, helping clients to approximate the behavior that will be successful for them.

HEALTH PROMOTION CHALLENGE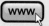

Read the case study that follows and decide what else the nurse could have done to promote health.

CASE STUDY Helping a Client
Start an Exercise Program

Mr. Sconce had just been discharged from the hospital and had been advised
to begin an exercise program by his physician. The client revealed his anxiety
about beginning such a program to the nurse, Ms. Joshua. The nurse began by
listing the steps in an exercise program (learn how to take pulse, learn warm-up
and cool down exercises, choose a suitable type of exercise, set up rewards and a
way to chart movement toward exercise goal).

Next, the nurse demonstrated the steps, ignoring any statements of
fear of failure and praising any positive attempts. (The use of the negative
reinforcement of not commenting verbally or nonverbally on fears will
extinguish that behavior in time, if used consistently.)

Ms. Joshua asked Mr. Sconce to copy what she did, and praised him for
each step successfully completed. Ms. Joshua also enlisted Mrs. Sconce in the
effort and both client and spouse soon were actively engaged in a walking
program together. Ms. Joshua taught the Sconces how to make a contract with
one another for changing behavior. FIGURE 3-2 shows the contract the Sconces
used.

Use Goal-Setting and Self-Contracting to Promote Health

Whether working with clients, peers/family members, or self-contracts to
achieve wellness goals, the **contracting** process remains the same.

☐ Mutual Exploration of Goals

Questions to ask include:

- Is this goal realistic for me now?
- Why is this goal being chosen now?
- Has this goal been chosen before and what were the results, things
  learned, barriers encountered? Does this goal have a high personal pri-
  ority or was it chosen to please others?
- How appropriate is this goal now?
- How specifically written is the goal?
- Has only one goal been chosen?

☐ Identification of Actions Needed to Accomplish the Goal

What countable behaviors are involved in meeting the goal? (The more clearly
and specifically actions are stated, the easier it is to evaluate progress toward
the goal.)

❏ Establishment of Reward(s) for Movement toward Goal

What is reinforcing and realistic as a reward?

❏ Division of Responsibilities

What responsibilities are involved? Who is responsible for which ones? What specific assistance will the facilitator give the other person; e.g., encouragement, phone calls, assertive asking about how the wellness goal is going, weekly meetings to discuss the goal?

❏ Time Limit

What mutually agreed upon time limit is set to accomplish the goal and/or evaluate movement toward the goal?

❏ Evaluation of Movement Toward Goal

How will movement toward the goal be evaluated? By whom? When? What consequences will accrue as a result? What additional assistance does the goal writer need from the facilitator in order to move toward goal attainment? What barriers are interfering with movement toward the goal and how can they be surmounted?

❏ Modification, Renegotiation, or Termination of the Contract

If a goal is met, a new one is reset. If a goal proves inappropriate, a new goal is found.

FIGURE 3-2 provides one client's contract.

Facilitators for wellness goals can be nurses, but they can also be peers, family members, other health professionals, or anyone who agrees to learn and follow the procedure for contracting. Self-contracting can also be used, but research and empirical knowledge have shown that people with low self-esteem or little perceived control over what happens to them may not take responsibility for carrying through on a contract (Pender, 1982, p. 190).

Using Self-Assessments to Promote Wellness

A wellness/health promotion framework implies that the responsibility for the client's body/mind/spirit resides with the client, unless there is a life-threatening situation in which the client cannot decide. It also implies that a health or wellness goal chosen by the client may not have high priority for the nurse. For example, an obese client may have set a high priority on stress manage-

A Behavioral Contract for Mr. Adolph and Mrs. Edith Sconce

Wellness goal: To walk briskly for 30 minutes every day.

I, Adolph Sconce, promise to walk briskly with Edith Sconce 30 minutes every day for a period of 2 weeks, whereupon my wife, Edith, and I will treat ourselves to a movie. I understand that if I do not fulfill this contract, the designated reward (movie) will be withheld.

Signed:

(Client)

(Facilitator)

(Nurse)

(Date)

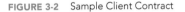

FIGURE 3-2   Sample Client Contract

ment, while the nurse thinks weight loss should be the first priority. A wellness framework assumes the client sets the goal, not the nurse.

Stepping out of the caretaking role may be difficult. However, consider the following. If the client takes self-responsibility for body/mind/spirit in one small issue, the process has been learned and it can be transferred to other issues, including those of high priority for the nurse. Also, if the nurse is able to demonstrate how success in attaining (life) goals can be accomplished, trust can be established and the client is more apt to agree to pursue a wellness goal of agreed-upon high priority. In some settings, such as the ICU, clients may not have a great deal of energy to invest in setting and striving toward wellness goals. It may not always be clear how health and wellness can be encouraged but even in these situations, clients can make decisions about when to have their bed, bath, what kind of juice to drink, and other simple choices.

A beginning step is to adapt nursing histories to fit a health promotion/wellness framework. Some questions that could be asked of clients on admission are:

1. What are the symptoms you are most concerned about?
2. What feelings and emotions are you concerned about?
3. What are the goals you would like to begin moving toward?
4. What are your strong points and special abilities?
5. What kind of help do you want from me?

6. What do you think is wrong with you?
7. Why do you think you are having this problem now in your life?
8. What does this disease (symptom, worry, etc.) mean in your life?
9. What would you have to give up or take on to get rid of this problem (disease, symptom, worry, etc.)?

The Health and Wellness Belief Scale

Another measure nurses can use to facilitate health and wellness includes assisting clients to examine their health and wellness beliefs. FIGURE 3-3 shows a health and wellness belief scale.

		Agree
These questions can be used to find out how different people feel about health and wellness. Each item consists of a pair of statements, A and B. Select the statement for each pair which you most strongly agree with or think is true, not the one you think you should choose. There are no right or wrong answers; this scale is a measure of what you believe. For some items, you may find you believe both statements or neither one. In such cases, be sure to select the one you most strongly believe by checking one "agree" for each number. Try not to be influenced by your previous choice.		
1.	A. I carry the key to my own health and well-being in the way I choose to live.	⊙
	B. Health and illness are both luck and beyond my control.	
2.	A. Being healthy and well is a lifelong effort.	⊙
	B. If I wait, medical science will develop cures for all illnesses.	
3.	A. It matters little whether my healthcare practitioner pursues health and wellness as long as he or she looks after mine.	
	B. I think it's important to steer clear of healthcare practitioners who are not pursuing their own health and wellness by not smoking, by keeping their weight down, etc.	⊙
4.	A. No matter how hard I try, I think I'll probably still get ill (or won't be able to quit smoking or lose weight), so I might as well do what I want to do.	
	B. I have faith in my ability to increase my health and wellness.	⊙
5.	A. I think that if I'm going to be ill, I'm going to be ill.	
	B. Trusting to fate about my health and wellness doesn't work. I find I have to take a definite course of action.	⊙
6.	A. Staying healthy and well is a matter of hard work, and luck has little or nothing to do with it.	⊙
	B. Staying well is a matter of being born under the right condition and being in the right place at the right time.	
7.	A. Environmental factors have little effect on whether I get ill or not.	
	B. Heredity is important, but I can take steps to counter it.	⊙

FIGURE 3-3   Health and Wellness Belief Scale
© Carolyn Chambers Clark, 2010.

8.	A. I can influence governmental decisions about health and wellness.	○
	B. Politicians, business people, and scientific experts make the decisions about my health and wellness.	___
9.	A. When I devise a health or wellness plan, I am pretty certain I can make it work.	○
	B. I don't make long-term plans for health or wellness because I don't think they work.	___
10.	A. Sometimes I don't think I can control my state of health.	___
	B. It is hard for me to believe that my state of health is always due to luck or chance.	○
11.	A. I might as well decide my wellness goals by flipping a coin.	___
	B. Getting what I want in terms of health and wellness has little or nothing to do with luck.	○
12.	A. With enough effort I think I can decrease the antihealth and antiwellness parts of my environment.	○
	B. I think it's difficult and perhaps impossible to decrease the antihealth and antiwellness factors in my environment.	___
13.	A. A good health insurance plan ought to include incentives for staying healthy and well.	___
	B. A good health insurance plan should be inexpensive, covering catastrophes like chronic illnesses and heart attacks.	○
14.	A. It doesn't really matter what I eat since health and wellness is unrelated to food.	___
	B. I should choose what I eat carefully, because it contributes to my health and wellness.	○
15.	A. I should work at being physically and mentally fit because both contribute to my wellness and health.	○
	B. It doesn't matter whether I'm fit or not because health and wellness are due to luck and my doctor's prescription.	___
16.	A. Stress is due to factors beyond my control.	___
	B. I can learn to reduce my stress level and thereby be healthier.	○
17.	A. If I heal when I'm hurt or ill, it's because something outside me helped me to heal, like an antiseptic or medicine.	___
	B. I can learn to use my own healing potential and thereby enhance my health and wellness.	○
18.	A. I think it's important to stand up for my rights when I feel others are trampling on them.	○
	B. It doesn't pay to stand up to others since they don't listen anyway.	___
19.	A. I think it's important to question healthcare practitioners, lawyers, and anyone from whom I purchase a service because I share the responsibility for what happens to me.	○
	B. I assume doctors, lawyers, nurses, and other authorities know what I need better than I do.	○
20.	A. Meeting new friends is a matter of luck and being in the right place at the right time.	___
	B. Meeting new friends is up to me to go places, introduce myself, and suggest we spend time together.	○
21.	A. Pain is something that has to be endured, and it will pass.	___
	B. When I am in pain, I can take action to reduce my pain.	○

FIGURE 3-3 (Continued)

The scale was modeled after Rotter's original work (1966) on internal locus of control or the degree to which people believe they have control over what happens to them. The purpose of the belief scale is to measure client responsibility for health and wellness, by measuring degree of internality. Those who score 21 are at a high point of internality.

Beliefs about health and wellness can influence the degree to which people take responsibility for their wellness. Numerous studies support the idea that people with strong beliefs about their ability to control destiny are more likely to be alert to information in the environment, place greater value on skills or achievement rewards, be more concerned about this ability (especially if the ability is lacking), and be resistive to subtle attempts to influence them. Rotter referred to these two basic stances as internal and external orientation. RESEARCH BOX 3-3 examines the use of locus of control with clients diagnosed with cancer.

RESEARCH BOX 3-3   Locus of Control and Well-Being in Older People Diagnosed with Cancer

» PURPOSE: To identify differences and similarities in health locus of control (HLC) and well-being between internalistic clients, recently diagnosed cancer clients, and healthy control subjects.

» SAMPLE: 110 clients with internal diseases, 196 cancer clients, and 80 healthy control subjects aged 60+ years

» METHODS: HLC was assessed with the Multidimensional Health Locus of Control Scales (MHLC), and well-being was assessed with the Positive and Negative Affect Schedule.

» FINDINGS: Clients with internal diseases scored highest on internal HLC. Scores on social externalism and fatalism MHCL subscales of internalistic clients were similar to those of cancer clients. Both client samples reported reduced positive affect. Higher levels of education, more social support, higher self-esteem, internal HLC, and daily functioning predicted positive affect in the total sample. In addition, an interaction effect of internal locus of control and daily functioning was found in cancer clients. There were no group-specific predictors of positive affect. Results suggest that high internal HLC is associated with positive affect in each of the three samples. However, an internal HLC only contributes to positive affect in cancer clients when they are in sufficient physical condition to exert control over their health.

Source: Knappe, S., & Pinquart, M. (2009). Tracing criteria of successful aging? Health locus of control and well-being in older patients with internal diseases. *Psychology, Health and Medicine, 14*(2), 201–212.

To request a copy of the entire study, contact Dr. Knappe at knappe@psychologie.tu-dresden.de

HEALTH PROMOTION CHALLENGE

Read the information in Research Box 3-3. What strategies would you take to promote health with this population?

People who are internally oriented are more likely to take responsibility for wellness; others are apt to let a healthcare practitioner or fate determine level of wellness. Most people fall along a range from externality (0: take little responsibility for their own wellness) to internality (21: take a great deal of responsibility for their own wellness).

Gender may be a factor in locus of control. In one study, males and normal-weight students showed higher affective motivation and overall intrinsic motivation compared to females and overweight students (Furia, Lee, Strother, & Huang, 2009). In another study that focused on healthy participants, overweight was associated with increased harm avoidance and decreased self-directedness in women but not in men (Suzuki et al., 2009). Some evidence suggests that acceptance is a promising approach for reducing body dissatisfaction in females, who are characteristically more dissatisfied with their bodies and may revert to over- or undereating as a result.

In a series of interviews, nine mothers related their beliefs and ideas about strategies utilized to maintain a perceived sense of wellness. The mothers used three main strategies: (1) obtaining help, (2) having a plan, and (3) taking time out. Discovery of a successful strategy led to a mother feeling greater confidence in the efficacy of her selected method, calmer, and in greater control.

Once the client completes the belief scale, a discussion about what the answers mean to the client's health and wellness can ensue. Writing down what is peripherally known can often clarify thoughts and feelings and can be the basis for change. When responses are discussed in a group, lively debates and (sometimes) changes in beliefs can occur.

Promoting Health in Multicultural Populations

When promoting health in multicultural populations, it is essential to understand traditional health beliefs, practices, and folk healers used by various population groups. To promote health across cultures, a nurse must attempt to enter the client's world to understand pertinent beliefs, values, attitudes, and feelings. The attitudinal aspects of transcultural nursing are the most difficult to learn because students must overcome their own ethnocentric tendencies and stereotypical beliefs (Andrews & Boyle, 2007).

TABLE 3-5 contains some of the explanatory models for health and illness in various cultural communities.

Table 3-5 Traditional Models of Health and Illness

Cultural Group	Beliefs
Brazilians	Illness may be attributed to divine intervention, fate, changes in temperature, food ingestion, activity, or strong emotions (Hilfinger Messias, 1996).
Guatemalans, Salvadorans, Nicaraguans	Illness may be the result of an imbalance among the individual, the environment, and outside forces, including the evil eye, ghosts, a witch's curse, and other similar agents, that may affect health and illness.
Cubans	The germ theory is accepted, but stress, extreme nervousness, evil spells, and voodoo-type magic may also explain illness (Boyle, 1996).
Mexican Americans	Ill health is an imbalance between the individual and the environment; emotional, social, physical, and spiritual factors can account for sickness (De Paula, Lagana, & Gonzalez-Ramirez, 1996).
Puerto Ricans	Illness may be attributed to heredity, lack of personal attention to health, punishment from God for a sin, or evil or negative environmental forces (Juarbe, 1996).
African Americans	Illness may be natural (caused by stress; drinking or eating too much; fighting with friends or neighbors; impurities in air, food, or water; cold air or winds; or punishment from God), or unnatural (caused by evil influences induced by witchcraft that require a voodoo practitioner) (Spector, 1991).
Asian Americans	The forces of yin and yang, and the five elements (wood, fire, earth, metal, water) are employed. Yin conditions include cancer, pregnancy, and postpartum care and are treated with yang foods such as chicken, beef, eggs, and spicy foods. Yang conditions include infections, hypertension, and venereal diseases and are treated with pork, fish, fresh fruits, and vegetables. Acupuncture, acupressure, meditation, acumassage, moxibustion, cupping, coining, herbology, shamanistic rituals, and Western medicine may be used. Mild illnesses may be attributed to organic causes, while more serious diseases are believed to be caused by supernatural forces including spirit attacks, soul loss, and other metaphysical manifestations that can only be treated by a shaman who uses rituals such as tying strings around the wrist to symbolically keep protective spirits within the body (Chan, 1992).
Native Americans	All things are connected (Joe & Malach, 1992). Health is closely linked to spirituality. The focus is on lifestyle and behavior. American Indians and Alaska Natives may see no conflict in using both Western medicine and traditional medicine practices (Lyon, 1996).
Pacific Islanders	Illness is related to the breaking of rules for how one is to live and is related to both the spiritual and physical worlds.

HEALTH PROMOTION CHALLENGE

Choose one culture that is dissimilar from yours. Devise a plan for learning more about how to understand beliefs, discover what is wrong, why it happened, and what should be done to promote health based on a client from that culture.

Taking Action on Political and Health Promotion Policy Issues

National and local political and policy issues affect the practice of nursing. They provide the larger picture for practice focused on health promotion. Avoid assuming that because healthcare reform has passed that all problems with health will be solved. The list of health promotion issues that follows will still require input and action from you:

1. Hypertension, overweight/obesity, and diabetes are on the upswing in children. What health promotion actions need to be taken to reduce these increases (World Health Organization, 2010)?

2. Fewer than half of all Americans exercise regularly (Kruger & Kohl, 2007). What health promotion actions need to be taken to increase this number?

3. The United States is one of two countries in the world that allows drug advertising on TV. What health promotion actions need to be taken to disallow these ads?

4. Firearms injuries remain a leading cause of death in the United States, particularly among youth (Branas, Richmond, Culhane, Ten Have, & Wiebe, 2009). What health promotion actions need to be taken to reduce this cause of death?

5. *Healthy People 2020* posted a list of objectives for promoting health in America. These objectives still require input from citizens, including nursing students, and assistance in implementation.

HEALTH PROMOTION CHALLENGE

Choose one of the Healthy People objectives (or find one of your own). Devise an action plan, take action, and report your findings to at least three other nursing students.

☐ Facilitating Health Promotion via the Internet

Many clients now use the Internet to obtain information about their condition and medications and to obtain support. Is the Web now positioned to replace health professionals or provide important information for them? To help decide, read RESEARCH BOX 3-4.

RESEARCH BOX 3-4   Is the Internet Replacing Health Professionals?

» BACKGROUND: People with mental disorders often report unmet medicines information needs and may search for information on medicines from sources including the Internet, telephone services, books, and other written materials.

» OBJECTIVE: This study aimed to identify and describe the sources of medicines information used by people with and without mental disorders.

» METHODS: A cross-sectional postal survey was mailed to a nationally representative sample (n = 5,000) of Finns aged 15–64 years in spring 2005. Completed responses were received from 3,287 people (response rate 66%), of whom 2,348 reported using one or more sources of medicines information during the past 12 months. Of those who reported one or more sources of medicines information, 10% (n = 228) reported being diagnosed with or treated for a mental disorder. The main outcome measures were the sources of medicines information used by people who did and did not report being diagnosed with or treated for a mental disorder.

» RESULTS: Among respondents with and without a mental disorder, physicians (83% vs. 59%), pharmacists (56% vs. 49%) and client information leaflets (53% vs. 43%) were the most common sources of medicine information. After adjusting for age, gender, level of education, working status, and number of chronic diseases, respondents with mental disorders were more likely to use client information leaflets (OR 1.47, 95% CI 1.06–1.98) and the Internet (OR 1.64, 95% CI 1.02–2.64) as sources of medicines information than respondents without mental disorders.

» CONCLUSIONS: The results indicate that physicians and pharmacists are the most common sources of medicines information among people both with and without mental disorders. However, client information leaflets and the Internet were more commonly used by people with mental disorders. There may be an opportunity for clinicians to better exploit these sources of medicines information when developing medicines information services for people with mental disorders.

Source: Pohjanoksa-Mäntylä, M., Bell J., Helakorpi, S., Närhi, U., Pelkonen, A., & Airaksinen, M. S. (2010, March 12). Is the Internet replacing health professionals? A population survey on sources of medicines information among people with mental disorders. *Social Psychiatry and Psychiatric Epidemiology, 46*(5), 373–379.

To request a copy of the full study, e-mail: Division of Social Pharmacy, Faculty of Pharmacy, University of Helsinki, Helsinki, Finland, marika.pohjanoksa@helsinki.fi.

HEALTH PROMOTION CHALLENGE

After reading Research Box 3-4, devise a health promotion tip to provide to clients.

The Web provides an inexpensive, relatively easy, and accessible format for health promotion. For information on the use of the Internet to reduce stress, read RESEARCH BOX 3-5 concerning a website stress reduction program.

RESEARCH BOX 3-5   Workplace Use of Website Stress Program

» BACKGROUND: In web-based health promotion programs, large variations in participant engagement are common. The aim was to investigate determinants of high use of a worksite self-help web-based program for stress management.

» METHODS: Two versions of the program were offered to randomly selected departments in IT and media companies. A static version of the program including a health screening tool, diary, and information about stress was offered to the control group. Additional materials, i.e., interactive, cognitive-based and classical stress management exercises, and a chat room, were offered to the intervention group. Baseline data regarding participants' demographics, health (self-ratings and biological measures), lifestyle, work-related factors, and group membership were analyzed to study determinants of employees' participation in the program during a period of 12 months. Multiple logistic regression analysis was used.

» FINDINGS: Intervention group membership, being a woman, having at most a secondary education, regular physical exercise habits, and having positive expectations of the program were significant predictors of high use. The findings demonstrate that the interactivity of a web-based program is an important factor for determining participation in a web-based worksite stress management program.

Source: Hasson, H., Brown, C. & Hasson, D. (2010). Factors associated with high use of a workplace web-based stress management program in a randomized controlled intervention study. *Health Education Research.* http://her.oxfordjournals.org/cgi/content/abstract/cyq005

HEALTH PROMOTION CHALLENGE

Use the information in Research Box 3-5 to identify important elements in a website health promotion program.

Summary

Effective communication is a necessity in health promotion. Active listening can enhance client learning and success in the client's health promotion goals; it includes thinking of the client's needs and avoiding disruption of the client's flow of communication and using an interested tone of voice and a positive body language. Empathy is the communication of at least as much feeling and meaning as the client communication. High differentiation implies the ability to respond to clients without reacting impulsively or irrationally, but by remaining calm under high stress. To be helpful to clients, it is important to maintain clear and rational boundaries. Assertiveness is the ability to clearly and willingly express thoughts, feelings, or desires in a respectful and cordial manner. Communication barriers include dysfunctional communication and listening blocks. Triangulation is a two-person situation in which one or both individuals calls upon a third person, issue, or object to intervene or disrupt the conflict as a way to decrease discomfort. Clarifying values is a process that can help clients move toward higher levels of health. Centering is a way to find the client's inner reference of stability. Affirmations are a self-care strategy that can reduce stress and lead to calm, productive behavior. Refuting irrational ideas is a method of helping clients to take responsibility for their behavior. Hidden agendas are obstacles to authentic, positive relationships. Evaluating and decreasing resistance to change are two ways to implement change. Shaping techniques are ways to reinforce approximations to a health promotion goal. Contracting is a method to help clients reach their health promotion goals.

REVIEW QUESTIONS

1. A person with a high level of differentiation is most likely to:
   a. Act impulsively
   b. Stay calm under high stress
   c. Have a high capacity for aggressiveness
   d. Engage in self-talk

2. Using *I* messages is a form of:
   a. Assertiveness
   b. Aggressiveness
   c. Self-talk
   d. Dysfunctional communication

3. Calling on a third person to disrupt a conflict between two parties is known as
   a. Affirmation
   b. Setting boundaries
   c. Centering
   d. Triangulation

4. Finding an inner reference of stability within oneself is known as
   a. Balancing
   b. Centering
   c. Yoga
   d. Goal setting

5. Which of the following is an affirmation?
   a. I can do this.
   b. I will stay calm.
   c. I will not let this bother me.
   d. Both a and b.
   e. All of the above.

6. Which of the following is not a strategy for assertively responding to criticism?
   a. Acknowledging
   b. Apologizing
   c. Clouding
   d. Probing

7. What is the purpose of the belief scale?
   a. To measure client responsibility for health and wellness
   b. To refute irrational ideas
   c. To decrease resistance to change
   d. To use rewards to increase desired behavior

EXERCISES

www.

1. Use FIGURE 3-4 Health Wellness Self-Assessment, and Figure 3-3, the Health Wellness Belief Scale, and see where you stand. Choose at least one health wellness goal to pursue for the next 6 months. Share your findings with at least three students and ask for feedback and support in achieving your goal. Find another student who agrees to work as your health/wellness buddy to provide support for you and vice versa.

2. Evaluate your level of differentiation and devise a plan to become more differentiated. Share your plan with at least one other student and ask for feedback and support.

3. Evaluate your level of assertiveness. Develop a program to help yourself become more assertive. Share your plan with at least one other student and work together to help support each other in becoming more assertive. Keep a diary of your progress and reevaluate your assertiveness skills each month. If needed, add more assertiveness approaches to enhance your assertive behavior.

Directions: Read the statements for each dimension of wellness; circle the number which most appropriately resembles the importance of each statement to you and your well-being and current interest in changing your lifestyle:				
1. I am already doing this. (Congratulate yourself!)				
2. This is very important to me and I want to change this behavior now.				
3. This is important to me, but I'm not ready to change my behavior right now.				
4. This is not important in my life right now.				
Nutritional Wellness				
I maximize local fresh fruits and uncooked vegetables in my eating plan.	1	2	3	4
I minimize the use of candy, sweets, sugar, and simple carbohydrates.	1	2	3	4
I eat whole foods rather than processed ones.	1	2	3	4
I avoid foods that have color, artificial flavor, or preservatives added.	1	2	3	4
I avoid coffee, tea, cola drinks, or other substances that are high in caffeine or other stimulants.	1	2	3	4
I eat high-fiber foods daily.	1	2	3	4
I have a good appetite, but I eat sensible amounts of food.	1	2	3	4
I avoid crash diets.	1	2	3	4
I eat only when I am hungry and relaxed.	1	2	3	4
I drink sufficient water so my urine is light yellow.	1	2	3	4

FIGURE 3-4   Health and Wellness Promotion Self-Assessment
© Carolyn Chambers Clark, 2010.

I avoid foods high in saturated fat, such as beef, pork, lamb, soft cheeses, gravies, bakery items, fried foods, etc.	1	2	3	4
I use a reverse osmosis water filtration system or drink distilled water to ensure safe drinking water.	1	2	3	4

Fitness and Wellness

I weigh within 10% of my desired weight.	1	2	3	4
I walk, jog, or exercise for more than 20 minutes at least 3 x/week.	1	2	3	4
I seem to digest my food well (no gas, bloating, etc.).	1	2	3	4
I do flexibility or stretching exercises daily and always prior to and following vigorous exercise.	1	2	3	4
I am satisfied with my sexual activities.	1	2	3	4
When I am ill, I'm resilient and recover easily.	1	2	3	4
When I look at myself nude, I feel good about what I see.	1	2	3	4
I use imagery to picture myself well and healthy every day.	1	2	3	4
I use affirmations and other self-healing measures when ill, injured, or to enhance my fitness.	1	2	3	4
I avoid smoking and smoke-filled places.	1	2	3	4

Stress and Wellness

I sleep well.	1	2	3	4
I have a peaceful expectation about my death.	1	2	3	4
I live relatively free from disabling stress or painful, repetitive thoughts.	1	2	3	4
I laugh at myself occasionally, and I have a good sense of humor.	1	2	3	4
I use constructive ways of releasing my frustration and anger.	1	2	3	4
I feel good about myself and my accomplishments.	1	2	3	4
I assert myself to get what I need instead of feeling resentful toward others for taking advantage of or intimidating me.	1	2	3	4
I can relax my body and mind at will.	1	2	3	4
I feel accepting and calm about people or things I have lost through separation.	1	2	3	4
I get and give sufficient touch (hugs, etc.) daily.	1	2	3	4

FIGURE 3-4   (Continued)

Wellness Relationships and Belief				
I have at least one other person with whom I can discuss my innermost thoughts and feelings.	1	2	3	4
I keep myself open to new experiences.	1	2	3	4
I listen to others' words and the feelings behind the words.	1	2	3	4
What I believe, feel, and do are consistent.	1	2	3	4
I allow others to be themselves and to take responsibility for their thoughts, actions, and feelings.	1	2	3	4
I allow myself to be me.	1	2	3	4
I live with a sense of purpose.	1	2	3	4
Wellness and the Environment				
I have designed a wellness support network of friends, family, and peers.	1	2	3	4
I have designed my personal living, playing, and working environments to suit me.	1	2	3	4
I work in a place that provides adequate personal space, comfort, safety, direct sunlight, fresh air; limited air, water, or material pollutants; or I use nutritional, exercise, or stress reduction measures to minimize negative effects.	1	2	3	4
I avoid cosmetics and hair dyes that contain harmful chemicals.	1	2	3	4
I avoid pesticides and the use of harmful household chemicals.	1	2	3	4
I avoid X-rays unless serious disease or injury is at stake, and I have dental X-rays for diagnostic purposes only every 3 to 5 years.	1	2	3	4
I wear protective clothing when exposed to the sun for more than 15 minutes (light-skinned) or 45 minutes (dark-skinned)	1	2	3	4
I use the Earth's resources wisely.	1	2	3	4
Commitment to Wellness and Health				
I examine my values and actions to see that I am moving toward health and wellness.	1	2	3	4
I take responsibility for my thoughts, feelings, and actions.	1	2	3	4
I keep informed on the latest health/wellness knowledge rather than relying on experts to decide what is best for me.	1	2	3	4
I wear seat belts when driving and insist that others who ride with me also do.	1	2	3	4
I ask pertinent questions and seek second opinions whenever someone advises me.	1	2	3	4
I know which chronic illnesses are prominent in my family and take steps to avoid incurring these illnesses.	1	2	3	4
I work toward achieving a balance in all wellness and health promotion efforts.	1	2	3	4

FIGURE 3-4   (Continued)

REFERENCES

Aled, J. (2007). Putting practice into teaching: An exploratory study of nursing undergraduates' interpersonal skills and the effects of using empirical data as a teaching and learning resource. *Journal of Clinical Nursing 16*(12), 2297–2307.

Andrews, M. M., & Boyle, J. S. (2007). *Transcultural Concepts in Nursing Care*. Philadelphia, PA: Wolters Kluwer/Lippincott Williams & Wilkins.

Bowen, M. (1972). *Toward the differentiation of self in one's family of origin*. Garden City Park, NY: Avery Publishing Group, Inc.

Branas, C. C., Richmond, T. S., Culhane, D. P., Ten Have, T. R., & Wiebe, D. J. (2009). Investigating the link between gun possession and gun assault. *American Journal of Public Health, 99*(11), 2034–2040.

Callen, B. L., Mefford L., Groër M., & Thomas S. P. (2010, October 29). Relationships among stress, infectious illness, and religiousness/spirituality in community-dwelling older adults. *Research in Gerontological Nursing*, pp. 1–12.

Camillo Sde, O., Nóbrega Mdo, P., & Théo, N. C. (2010). Nursing undergraduate students' view on listening to patients during care delivery. [Article in Portuguese.] *Revista da Escola de Enfermagem da U S P, 44*(1), 99–106.

Carkhuff, R. (1969). *Helping & human relations. Vol. I & II*. New York, NY: Holt, Rinehart and Winston, Inc.

Cuellar, N. G., Brennan, A. M., Vito, K., & de Leon Siantz, M. L. (2008). Cultural competence in the undergraduate nursing curriculum. *Journal of Professional Nursing, 24*(3), 143–149.

Dobson, T., & Miller, V. (1994). *Aikido in everyday life: Giving in to get your way*. New York, NY: North Atlantic Books.

Dweck, C. S. (1975). The role of expectations and attributions in the alleviation of learned helplessness. *Journal of Personality and Social Psychology, 31*, 674–685.

Ellis, A., & Harper, R. A. (1961). *A guide to rational living*. Upper Saddle River, NJ: Prentice Hall.

Eshelman, E., McKay, M., & Fanning, P. (2008). *The relaxation and stress reduction workbook*. Oakland, CA: New Harbinger.

Friedman, M. M., Bowden, V. R., & Jones, E. G. (2003). *Family nursing: Research, theory, and practice* (5th ed.). Upper Saddle River, NJ: Prentice Hall.

Furia, A. C., Lee, R. E., Strother, M. L., & Huang, T. T. (2009). College students' motivation to achieve and maintain a healthy weight. *American Journal of Health Behavior, 33*(3), 256–263.

Goodman, D. (1974). *Emotional well-being through rational behavior training*. Springfield, IL: Charles C. Thomas.

Helming, M. B., & Jackson, C. (2009). Relationships. In B. M. Dossey & L. Keegan (Eds.), *Holistic nursing: A handbook for practice* (5th ed., pp. 367–391). Sudbury, MA: Jones and Bartlett.

Kirschenbaum, H. (1976). Clarifying values clarification: some theoretical issues and a review of research. *Group and Organization Studies, 1*(1), 99–115.

Kirschenbaum, H., & Simon, S. (1974). Values and the future movement in education. In A. Toffler, (Ed.), *Learning for tomorrow: The role of the future in education* (pp. 257–271). New York, NY: Vintage Books.

Krieger, D. (1979). *The therapeutic touch*. Englewood Cliffs, NJ: Prentice-Hall.

Kruger, J., & Kohl, H. W. R. (2007). Prevalence of regular physical activity among adults—United States, 2001 and 2005. *Morbidity and Mortality Weekly Report, 56*(46), 1209–1212.

McKay, M., Davis, M., & Fanning, P. (1983). *Messages, the communication book.* Oakland, CA: New Harbinger.

Miller, S. R., & Winstead-Frey, P. (1982). *Family systems theory in nursing practice.* Reston, VA: Reston Publishing Co.

Misra-Hebert, A. D., & Isaacson, J. H. (2012). Overcoming health care disparities via better cross-cultural communication and health literacy. *Cleveland Clinical Journal of Medicine, 79*(2), 127–133.

Patterson, K., Grenny, J., McMillan, R., & Switzler, A. (2002). *Crucial conversations: Tools for talking when the stakes are high.* New York, NY: McGraw-Hill.

Pender, N. (1982). *Health promotion in nursing practice.* Norwalk, CT: Appleton-Century-Crofts.

Pender, N., Murdaugh, C. L., & Parsons, M. A. (2010). *Health promotion in nursing practice.* Upper Saddle River, NJ: Prentice-Hall.

Piotrowski, M. B. (2005, January/February). Are you listening? Tips on improving your communication skills. *Biomedical Instrumentation & Technology*, pp. 1–2.

Raths, L., Harmin, M., & Simon, S. B. (1966). *Values and teaching* (pp. 63–65). Columbus, OH: Charles E. Merrill Books.

Rivers, C., Barnett, R. C., & Baruch, G. K. (1979). *Beyond sugar and spice: How women grow, learn, and thrive.* New York, NY: Putnam.

Rotter, J. (1966). Generalized expectations for internal vs. external control of reinforcement. *Psychological Monographs, 80*(1), 1–28.

Suzuki, A., Kamata, M., Matsumoto, Y., Shibuya, N., & Otani, K. (2009). Increased body mass index associated with increased harm avoidance and decreased self-directedness in Japanese women. *Journal of Nervous and Mental Disease, 197*(3), 199–201.

World Health Organization. (WHO). (2010). Childhood overweight and obesity. Retrieved from http://www.who.int/dietphysicalactivity/childhood/en/

INTERNET RESOURCES

For a full suite of assignments and learning activities, use the access code located in the front of your book to visit this exclusive website: **http://go.jblearning.com/healthpromotion**. If you do not have an access code, you can obtain one at the site.

PART 2

Health Promotion In Action

LEARNING OBJECTIVES

Upon completing this chapter, you will be able to:

1. Describe key aspects that define good physical health.

2. Discuss methods of removing or working with obstacles to client engagement.

3. Analyze different strategies for identifying and promoting health goals in an individual client.

4. Discuss six key questions to answer to help a client create a health promotion plan.

5. Identify factors that limit client ability to maintain health.

6. Analyze principal areas of concern stated in the Healthy People 2020 initiative.

KEY TERMS

Adaptability

Goals

Health disparities

Interventions

Motivational interviewing

Objectives

Physical health

Physiologic healing

Priorities

CHAPTER 4

Promoting Physical Health

- Introduction
- Physical Health and Well-Being In Individuals
- Topic Areas
- Summary

http://go.jblearning.com/healthpromotion

For a full suite of assignments and learning activities, use the access code located in the front of your book to visit the exclusive website: http://go.jblearning.com/healthpromotion If you do not have an access code, you can obtain one at the site.

Introduction

In a previous chapter, we defined *health* and *health promotion*, discussed some theories that explain how individuals learn new habits or behaviors, and talked about your role in guiding people to learn new health-related attitudes or habits. This section seeks to put into practice what was discussed in prior chapters. We will talk about the real-world situations in which you, as nurse, can facilitate health in clients.

Because health manifests itself across physical, mental/emotional, and familial/community dimensions, we need to address each dimension These are artificial distinctions, but for our purposes we will discuss them as if they occur independently—beginning with **physical health** in individuals, and continuing on to mental and family health. Keep in mind that these are factors that affect one another, so in the practice setting, try to assess all three factors at once.

Physical Health and Well-Being In Individuals

What constitutes a physically healthy person? There are a great many potential answers to that question, but certain aspects may be readily agreed upon. A physically healthy person is one who:

- Maintains bodily tissues, organs, and systems in a well-functioning state at both the cellular and macro level (that is, has no significant, long-term impairments to pulmonary function, nutrient absorption, endocrine/metabolic function, cardiovascular function, etc.)
- Eats, digests, and eliminates without impairment
- Is able to obtain sufficient oxygen, nutrients, fluids, and sleep to satisfy daily and long-term requirements without difficulty
- Has developmentally appropriate neurological function and transitions through developmental stages normally
- In general, experiences no significant pain or weakness upon moving muscles or limbs in a manner consistent with average activity levels, and heals quickly and thoroughly from occasional injuries or minor physical ailments
- Has the immunological responses necessary to meet the challenges posed by infectious agents, toxins, injuries, and other bodily harm that all individuals encounter during their lives
- Is capable of normal reproductive and sexual activity consistent with developmental stage and/or age

- Obtains and processes sensory input without significant impairment
- Has the ability to heal from or adapt to significant physical or psychological injuries

At minimum an individual needs to have a majority of these factors in place to be considered physically healthy. Individuals with some impairment (e.g., a person who is deaf or who has a food allergy) can still enjoy good overall physical health. **Adaptability**, or the ability to compensate for a loss of function in one area, can offset factors that might otherwise suggest or lead to poor health.

No one goes through life without obtaining wounds of some kind, whether physical or emotional. The ability to heal from these wounds—or to adapt physically and emotionally in the event that healing is not possible—is a key factor in maintaining health.

A prime example is found in the story of Aron Ralston, a hiker whose arm was trapped by a fallen boulder. Ralston was obliged to amputate his own arm in order to survive. Despite the loss of his arm—an injury from which he cannot fully heal—Ralston is today a physically healthy individual. He has obtained a prosthetic arm that partly restores some of his physical capacity, and having adapted to the loss of one arm to the greatest extent possible, continues to live his life in the manner he prefers without it (Ralston, 2010).

The other health problems that developed during his crisis—dehydration, blood loss, nutritional deficits—are all fully healed, and his body functions normally. His lost limb notwithstanding, an argument can be made that Ralston satisfies all categories listed previously—even the first one, because the sacrifice of his trapped arm was necessary to preserve the function of all remaining bodily tissues.

The effort needed to restore function after an injury is what we commonly refer to as **physiologic healing**. Maintaining a capacity for physiologic healing is one important aspect of physical health, but it is not the sole factor. A client whose physiologic healing mechanisms function appropriately can still suffer tremendous (physical) ill health if social, psychological, and even spiritual facets of existence are disturbed.

The Nurse's Role in Health Promotion: Working with Individual Clients

Many clients are not looking to necessarily obtain *good* physical health, but instead are seeking *better* physical health. Either of these **goals** is legitimate. Your job is to help clients reach the level of health they want to achieve.

Without their active participation, your efforts will only succeed in frustrating clients. Work with clients to assess their current general state of health and to identify the obstacles to health improvement. Find places where clients can make changes to improve health, and help them learn how to make those changes.

HEALTH PROMOTION CHALLENGE

Use the questions in the Motivational Interviewing section later in this chapter for ideas on how to motivate clients to change.

It is in this last arena that the variety of health-related theories and models can be put to practical use in developing a health promotion plan or program by addressing each of these key questions:

1. What are the key health issues?
2. What knowledge or understanding is needed to improve health status?
3. What is the client's capacity to learn or accept new ideas, habits, or methods ?
4. How motivated is the client to make changes for health promotion, and if motivation is absent or low, how can it be increased?
5. What forms of family and social support are available to the client to aid in health promotion activities?
6. What are the client's health goals?

Learning the answers to these questions requires you interview the client. But of all the questions on the list, the last question is by far the most crucial in working with an individual client. Client ideas about and goals for changing may differ radically from factors you consider important. For example, a person who is overweight and a smoker may regard losing weight as the more important issue to be addressed, and, based on this priority, may even refuse to consider smoking cessation options on the grounds that quitting smoking will cause further weight gain. The client's goal will always trump yours because the client is the person who must put the plan into action. Your challenge is to not only help address the weight problem, but also to help the client see that smoking cessation is equally important, if not more important, but only when the client is ready to discuss it.

Be open minded and nonjudgmental in guiding the client, and above all, use honest motivational tactics—manipulation, pressuring, and being dismissive of a client's decisions about her or his health goals will likely prove counterproductive.

Identifying Obstacles to Health Promotion

The primary obstacles to health promotion include:

- Lack of information, incorrect information, or lack of concern regarding the health condition being addressed
- Fear, anger, or other strong emotions about the diagnosis (includes having experienced or believing stigmas and stereotypes about the disease or condition)

- Physical inability to make necessary changes
- Psychological or cultural barriers to making necessary changes
- Low or absent motivation to make needed changes
- Low or absent familial/social support for making needed changes; may also include lack of personal control over health circumstances
- Reluctance to engage with the nurse in developing and implementing a health promotion plan

Motivational Interviewing

Motivational interviewing (see FIGURE 4-1) is a way of joining with clients to see their world, their fears, their accomplishments. It is a way to work with

Motivational interviewing includes:

1. *Empathy.* Talking about the world as the client sees it. "So, you're looking for a way to lose weight first. Let's talk about that because it's something I can help you with."

2. *Collaboration, not confrontation or forcing.* "Let's see how we can work together on your goal of losing weight."

3. *Drawing out the client to speak about goals, skills, and dreams.* Some questions to ask:

   - What will losing weight do for you and your lifestyle?

   - Let's talk about how you think losing weight will be helpful.

   - How have you tried to lose weight, and what experiences have you had?

   - Tell me some more about what you learned from your dieting experiences.

   - When you picture losing weight, what do you picture yourself doing?

4. *Encouraging autonomy.* "There is no single right way to lose weight, and I'm going to help you develop a menu of options for you to try."

This format can be used to help clients with any health promotion goal. Just change the words *losing weight* to *stop smoking, stop drinking,* or whatever the client's goal is. Work on one goal at a time. After the client has achieved success in one goal, you can move on to the client's next goal, but not until the client signals readiness.

A free and much more detailed article about motivation interviewing is available at http://www.stephenrollnick.com/index.php/all-commentary/69-motivational-interviewing-article-published-in-the-british-medical-journal

FIGURE 4-1 Motivational Interviewing to Help Clients Change

clients that was developed by Miller and Rollnick (2002) and Rollnick, Miller, & Butler (2008). At first, you focus on building a rapport with clients so trust can evolve. To do that, you have to be willing to listen to their thoughts and feelings and to acknowledge and encourage even the slightest movement toward health.

Everyone is resistant to change because it brings with it the unknown. By offering yourself as a person who can accompany clients on their journey and not force them to do something they're afraid of, resistance to change will decrease.

HEALTH PROMOTION CHALLENGE   [www]

Read Dr. Rollnick's article at the website mentioned in Figure 4-1 and role play a health promotion problem with another student who takes the role of nurse. Once you've worked through it as client, switch and take the role of nurse for another health promotion problem. Write up your findings and share them with your class.

☐ Lack of Information

A variety of factors affecting physical health may be present, but the client may be unaware of them or lack understanding of their importance. Careful questioning of the client about pain, eating habits, sleeping habits, toilet habits, and other key physical indicators may help uncover the client's **priorities** for health. Use some of the motivational interviewing questions in Figure 4-1.

Some clients simply need guidance in assessing their health concerns and developing goals. Others may simply know too little about the health circumstances in which they find themselves to consider them worthy of attention. For example, a young woman diagnosed with HPV may not understand that it represents increased risk of cervical cancer. Here, your role is as much an educator as health promoter, yet you must avoid putting value judgments on the information that gets passed along. If a nurse starts lecturing about promiscuity, chances are good the information will be ignored; if, on the other hand, the nurse couches her advice in terms of long-term prevention, it may be better received.

Make an effort to be aware of your biases when passing on information to others. Engebretson and Headley (2009) noted that "recognition of personal cultural attitudes requires conscious effort; most people are unaware of their cultural beliefs because their beliefs are so integrated into their perception of the world" (p. 575).

Ask your best friend to tell you about your biases and be open to what you hear. Avoid stereotyping based on ethnicity, age, gender, or religion. Clients recognize and resent the implications of stereotypes—and such negative evaluations by the client will spell the end of any success in your health promotion efforts.

☐ Emotions, Judgments, and Stigma

Be cognizant of value judgments the client may put on the information being offered, particularly when it comes to diseases or conditions that are subject to stereotypes or social stigma. For example, despite many public health campaigns seeking to educate the public about HIV and AIDS, there is still considerable stigma and misinformation associated with the virus (Bunn, Solomon, Miller, & Forehand, 2007), both in rural communities where prevalence of the disease is relatively low (Groft, Robinson, & Vollman, 2007; Zukoski, Thorburn, & Stroud, 2011) and in urban areas where one might expect better dissemination of facts among a more deeply affected populace (Aggleton, Yankah, & Crewe, 2011; Gonzalez, Miller, Solomon, Bunn, & Cassidy, 2009; Saleh, Operario, Smith, Arnold, & Kegeles, 2011). The popular misperceptions that characterized the discovery of the virus in the 1980s are still expressed in certain sectors of society—that HIV/AIDS is a disease of gay men, drug users, and sexually promiscuous or deviant individuals; as well as the extreme views that HIV represents a punishment or judgment upon particular subgroups in society (Muturi & An, 2010). A new set of myths and misperceptions have developed, including the idea that confining the client to sexual partners of a race different than the client's own will help to avoid HIV infection (Millett et al., 2011). Barriers to undertaking HIV prevention and/or seeking care for HIV infection may vary depending on demographic factors (James et al., 2011; Moore, 2011). Clients receiving retroviral treatments may also experience physical changes that affect their view of their own bodies, which can further inhibit their motivation and attitudes regarding compliance with treatment protocols (Cabrero, Griffa, & Burgos, HIV Body Physical Changes Study Group, 2010).

HIV and AIDS do not, of course, target people based on sexual orientation, race, ethnicity, economic status, religion, age, or even moral character. Clients need to be aware of such truths to take the stigma—particularly that which is self-inflicted—out of their path to wellness (Sengupta, Banks, Jonas, Miles, & Smith, 2011). It is not uncommon for individuals with HIV to believe, or to have been told, that they caused their condition by virtue of risky behaviors or the choice of sexual partners or orientation. At the same time they receive and often believe messages laying the blame for their illness squarely on their own shoulders. They may be unable to locate accurate, judgment-free, practical information that they can use to help them maximize health. A client who feels defensive, victimized, guilty, angry, or frustrated is a client who may have difficulty hearing your recommendations, or indeed learning any means of coping with the ramifications of the disease. Using motivational interviewing techniques, especially building rapport, may be helpful in these situations.

☐ Physical Incapacity to Engage in Health Promotion Activities

It is not unusual that the very health problem for which a client wants a solution represents an obstacle to finding that solution. This is particularly true in relation to mobility issues. A client who has had a stroke and wants to relearn how to walk and write is hampered in doing so by the damage to the brain that reduced these skills. You will be challenged to identify methods and resources for this client that have a realistic chance of being successful. Try to ensure that the client's goals are reasonable—although it is worth keeping in mind that motivated people have managed to accomplish astonishing, "impossible" recoveries with the right support. Again, refer to motivational learning resources for assistance with this issue.

☐ Psychological or Cultural Barriers to Undertaking Health-Promoting Actions

Client sociocultural and educational background and opinions about health can lead to resistance to taking steps that might otherwise promote health. An example would be a male client with back pain who hesitates to take up yoga because he believes it is not manly, despite being advised that yoga works well for relieving back pain, or a client who expresses an unwillingness to take recommended medication because of a preference for complementary therapies.

In either case, you have the option of either working to overcome the barrier or helping the client find more satisfactory alternatives. The male client who hesitates to try yoga might be more inclined to agree to a t'ai chi (martial arts) class or a Pilates class, or he may agree to try yoga if provided with a class taught by a male instructor that has other male students.

☐ Low or Absent Motivation to Make Needed Changes

Bear in mind that motivation toward health is something not all clients have. Lack of motivation may be grounded in many things—poor self-esteem; a fatalistic outlook; denial that the health issue exists; the presence of other, seemingly higher priorities than health; or a thousand other possibilities. Your task is to make use of the concepts and models discussed in the earlier chapters to identify ways to increase motivation. Motivational interviewing is nearly always the best place to start.

☐ Low or Absent Familial or Social Support for Health Promotion Activities

It is very uncommon that a client lives and works in isolation from others; most people have some sort of social network and/or family members that they rely on. There are, of course, exceptions: A single adult who has just moved to a new city to take a job, an older adult who lives alone and has no family or friends nearby, and a young teenage runaway are examples of people who may lack these sorts of connections and support, or who may have only tenuous, unreliable community or family bonds.

Even where such bonds exist, though, the presence of family and friends in a client's life does not mean those people will be supportive and encouraging of health-related changes the client is trying to make. A man whose friends are his drinking buddies may get highly negative responses if he decides he wants to quit drinking, for instance. Some individuals may also lack personal control over their access to activities that will help with health circumstances they wish to change. For example, a wheelchair-bound person wishing to participate in physical therapy intended to help him strengthen and rehabilitate his injured legs or back may have difficulty finding transportation if his family members are not willing to drive. It is not unusual that family members simply lack interest in providing encouragement to a concern that is not a priority to them, even it if is a priority to the client. In such cases, you may be called upon to assist the client in finding alternate support for the client's health goal—whether it be locating support groups or sources of transportation, or simply helping the client to identify all the alternative sources of encouragement.

☐ Reluctance to Engage with the Nurse in Developing and Implementing a Health Promotion Plan

A client may be unwilling to work with you or may even be downright hostile. There can be a variety of reasons for this, including suspicion that you are a representative of someone else's agenda (e.g., "I'm here because my wife insisted, not because I think you can help."), a desire to maintain control (e.g., "I'm going to do this my way."), and a belief that you have nothing to offer the client (e.g., "There's nothing you can tell me I don't already know, so this is really a waste of my time.").

Maintaining a professional demeanor and attempting to engage with the client to determine, at the very least, whether the client's resistance can be decreased or diminished is your goal. The best way to accomplish it is to communicate the message that you are there to support the client, rather than to oppose, direct, or enforce behavior. Establishing the client's self-efficacy and ownership of the process is crucial. Some useful responses might be: "Well, this is between me and you, not me and your wife. I'm here to help *you*; what do *you* want to accomplish?" or "That's fine, but can we talk about what it is you want to achieve, just so I know? It may be that I can give you some ideas about how to get there faster," or "I love having a well-informed client. But I'm a terrific organizer, so maybe we can put your time to good use by working together to develop a plan. Who knows? Maybe I can use your insights to help someone else."

For more useful ways around client resistance, refer to the section on Motivational Interviewing in this chapter.

Working with the Client: Respecting the Client's Assessments

Even when the client is not reluctant, make an effort to engage the client. It is all too easy to decide that you know what will be best for the client and present your decisions as the plan—only to find that the client is hesitant about participating. Asking, "What are your [the client's] key health issues?" requires you to take both an objective and subjective response simultaneously, because this question encompasses aspects of client beliefs and priorities.

Here is an example: Suppose you are working with a client who has been diagnosed with prediabetes, psoriasis, and atherosclerosis—all serious issues that affect quality of life and longevity. This client is aware of all of these diagnoses, but she may tell you that the most serious problem, in her view, is her poor sleep. She describes frequent waking, inability to get back to sleep on many occasions, tossing and turning for hours—she is exhausted, and she wants to do something about this problem more than any other. She believes that dealing with her frequent bouts of insomnia must come first because, she tells you, she is just too tired all the time to exercise, to shop for healthy foods, or to do any of the other things she has been told will help her fend off diabetes and heart disease. To the untrained eye, this seems bizarre; insomnia may be unpleasant, but is it life threatening?

In fact, the client may be correct about prioritizing her sleep issues above the other three. Not only is she accurate in her assessment that poor sleep acts as an inhibitor of the mental and emotional processes she needs to follow through on a plan of action; lack of good sleep can increase insulin resistance and promote susceptibility to diabetes (Darukhanavala et al., 2011). Factors that interrupt sleep—including obstructive sleep apnea—occur relatively more often in individuals with psoriasis (Gowda, Goldblum, McCall, & Feldman, 2010). Sleep apnea has been linked with systemic inflammation, which can promote all of the conditions for which the client is at risk: diabetes, autoimmune diseases such as psoriasis, and cardiovascular diseases (Ryan, Taylor, & McNicholas, 2009).

On paper, the disease processes might seem more important, but the client's self-identified issue is key. Referring her to a sleep study or teaching her relaxation procedures with an eye toward solving her insomnia will not, of course, be the cure-all for every issue facing her, but doing so *is* an important facet of the overall health-promotion plan. Acting on the client's principal health consideration enhances trust, making it more likely she will continue to invest in the process as you seek to address her other health issues. Helping the client recover good quality of life by addressing the sleep issue sets the stage for subsequent efforts to address, for example, dietary changes necessary to support improvements in diabetes and cardiovascular risk.

Evidence-Based Recommendations

When developing a plan for a client or community, base your teaching strategies on research evidence about what works best for a given condition. An easy place to start is at www.pubmed.gov, which gives up-to-date research results. Just type in one or two terms—for example, *nutrition cancer*, or *exercise heart*—in the top Search box, and many studies will be listed. It's not necessary to type in conjunctions or prepositions such as *and* or *for* or to type *treatment*, which may result in fewer studies listed.

HEALTH PROMOTION CHALLENGE

Choose nutrition, cancer or exercise for one condition and see how many research studies you can find to help develop evidence-based recommendations for a client with that health issue.

Topic Areas

Although it is beyond the scope of this chapter to address health promotion procedures for specific physiologic conditions, there are particular areas of health that are of higher concern that we can discuss in general terms. These areas, identified as part of the *Healthy People 2020* initiative, have been noted as affecting large numbers of individuals in the United States. They are likely to be issues of concern in clients that you see in practice. Remember that different populations have differing priorities. Topic areas are listed in alphabetical order, recognizing that you may need to prioritize these topics depending on the communities you serve.

The topic areas are:
- Access to health services
- Adolescent health
- Arthritis, osteoporosis, and chronic back conditions
- Blood disorders and blood safety

- Cancer
- Chronic kidney disease
- Diabetes
- Disability and secondary conditions
- Early and middle childhood
- Environmental health
- Family planning
- Food safety
- Genomics
- Hearing and communication disorders
- Heart disease and stroke
- HIV
- Immunization and infectious diseases
- Injury and violence prevention
- Maternal and infant health
- Mental health disorders (physical impacts)
- Nutrition and weight status
- Older adults
- Oral health
- Physical activity and fitness
- Sexually transmitted diseases
- Substance abuse
- Tobacco use
- Vision

Topic Area: Access to Health Services

A key obstacle to health promotion is the lack of access to one or more of the following: health insurance, a usual primary care provider, and coverage for clinical preventive services (Kottke & Isham, 2010). Each or all of these factors contributes to an individual experiencing difficulty in, or delaying, obtaining necessary medical care, dental care, or prescription medicines. Each or all of them is also frequently (though not always) related to a combination of cost and local availability; many people may have hospitals, private practices, and teaching hospitals nearby but are unable to afford care from these providers, while some people who can afford the cost of health care still cannot get it because they are located far from areas that offer the specific care they need (for example, oncology or gastroenterology specialists). Access to evidence-based clinical preventive services and primary care providers is already limited in many nonurban communities, but a number of medical organizations have warned that a more widespread shortage of primary care providers is looming (Bodenheimer, 2006; American College of Physicians, 2006).

A client's ability to obtain services needed to assist with health promotion activities is a factor that needs your attention. Lack of physical activity and fitness programs, nutrition guidance for weight issues, substance abuse programs, and community-based educational programs can affect health and health promotion efforts. Familiarity with the range of services available at the local, state, and national level is crucial if you hope to direct clients to resources that will assist them in obtaining needed services.

Clients who wish to start health promotion programs can do so without a building or community program. You can be instrumental in helping clients in these cases by using the information in this book to help them develop their own health promotion program.

The issue of access can affect acute care. For example, if an individual's hospital emergency department visit wait exceeds the recommended time frame, that can negatively affect the outcome of the acute health concern (Ackroyd-Stolarz, Guernsey, Mackinnon, & Kovacs, 2011; Bernstein et al., 2009; Guttman, Schull, Vermeulen, & Stukel, 2011). Working with an individual who has frequent episodes of acute health issues (for example, repeated acute episodes of obstructed breathing, as in asthma or COPD), but who lacks ready access to an uncrowded emergency facility in an acute health event, can be challenging. You can help the client to either find alternative services, recognize the onset of acute symptoms earlier, or, ideally, take actions that will prevent acute events and thereby limit the need for the acute-care services that are in short supply.

In the case of the asthma example, this may involve helping clients to determine the triggers for acute episodes and learn how to limit exposure to such triggers. Alternately, teaching clients to be aware of the initial signals of a crisis could be a key factor in helping them avoid the need to access critical care services.

Topic Area: Adolescent Health

It is not surprising that several of the Healthy People 2020 **objectives** for adolescents focus on adolescent sexuality. Two specific goals are to increase the percentage of adolescents who have been tested for HIV and increase the percentage of middle and high schools that prohibit harassment based on a student's sexual orientation or gender identity. Teen pregnancy and STD transmission continue to be of great concern, with the United States having the highest rates of teen pregnancy and STD infections among developed nations. The physical health of adolescents focuses on sexuality because the prospect for poor health is far greater in those individuals who are prone to engage in risky behaviors. Your work to educate teens and reduce their likelihood of taking sexual risks can greatly impact their physical health.

But as large as sexual issues loom in adolescents, they are not the sole cause of poor physical health in teens. Nutrition—or the lack of it—is a major health issue, particularly among teen girls, who may skip meals or eat poorly in order to address perceived or real considerations of excess weight, or as a product of self-esteem or emotional issues. A tendency to skip breakfast is particularly correlated with the development of weight-related health issues (Deshmukh-Taskar et al., 2010).

It is no accident that the Healthy People 2020 objectives include expanding access of teens to school breakfast programs. Similarly, screen time (the amount of time teens spend watching television, using a computer, or using a video-game machine) has a direct impact on physical welfare. Teens who have a lot of screen time per day show a tendency to develop poor exercise habits and significant metabolic effects in insulin regulation, particularly among adolescent boys (Foltz et al., 2011; Hardy, Denney-Wilson, Thrift, Okely, & Baur, 2010). Providing teens with extracurricular activities that draw them away from computers and videos, promoting good nutrition plus regular exercise, and making connections between teens and a parent or other positive adult caregiver are central points to promoting adolescent health (Patrick et al., 2004).

Topic Area: Arthritis, Osteoporosis, and Chronic Back Conditions

Painful joints, backaches, and brittle bones are often viewed as inevitable hallmarks of aging. These misconceptions offer tremendous opportunity for health promotion. The following areas are prime targets for health promotion efforts:

- reducing the mean level of joint pain among adults with doctor-diagnosed arthritis;
- reducing the percentage of adults with arthritis who have difficulty in performing two or more personal care activities, thereby preserving independence;
- reducing the percentage of adults with osteoporosis (thus lowering the risk of debilitating hip fractures); and,
- reducing activity limitation due to chronic back conditions.

Key factors in addressing these conditions include (1) exercise and physical therapies that improve joint flexibility and strengthen bones (Chyu et al., 2011; Selfe & Innes 2009; Sinaki et al., 2010), (2) assessment and improvement of weight and nutrient status (Christensen et al., 2011; Garriguet, 2011; Riecke et al., 2010), and (3) reduction of inflammation, either in the joint or systemwide (Rai & Sandell, 2011).

Topic Area: Blood Disorders and Blood Safety

Because blood disorders and blood safety is a new topic area to the Healthy People initiative, so are most of the objectives. The Universal Data Collection

Project from the Centers for Disease Control and Prevention [CDC] and the Registry and Surveillance in Hemoglobinopathies within the National Institutes of Health and the CDC offer primary sources of data. One goal in this area is increasing the percentage of persons who donate blood. Research into factors that work both for and against blood donation—including the level of self-efficacy experienced by donors (Veldhuizen, Ferguson, de Kort, Donders, & Atsma, 2011) and anxiety related to the paraphernalia and context of donation (Clowes & Masser, 2011)—may prove helpful in addressing the behavioral factors that tip an individual's decision against donating.

Similarly, advances in screening donated blood for infectious diseases such as HIV, HCV, and other blood-borne diseases continue, with West Nile virus and others under investigation (Dodd, 2009; Goodnough, 2011). You may encounter concerns about blood safety in clients who require transfusions or who are scheduled for surgery, so keeping in touch with safety advances (as well as encouraging practices such as familial donation or autologous blood-banking prior to surgery) can help reassure clients. Other goals include:

- decreasing hospitalizations for sickle cell disease among children aged 9 years,
- the increased use of penicillin with sickle cell disease from 4 months to 5 years of age,
- reducing the incidence of venous thromboembolism, and
- increasing the rate of accurate diagnosis of such diseases as inherited bleeding disorders and von Willebrand's disease.

Multiple other objectives cover developmental milestones of those with hemoglobinopathies.

Topic Area: Cancer

Many of the objectives from the topic area of cancer focus on the continued reduction of site-specific cancer death rates, but include counseling about cancer prevention through mammograms, Pap tests, programs to educate about the risks associated with sunburn and sun exposure, and increased screening rates for colorectal, cervical, and breast cancers.

Prevention activities represent a key opportunity for health promotion. Assessing risk factors and educating clients about how to reduce risk may form the basis of many of your health promotion actions. Likewise, activities undertaken to address cancer survivors' quality of life, including decreasing the risk of recurrence of invasive colorectal, uterine, cervical, and late-stage breast cancers, offer many opportunities for health promotion. Providing information about the importance of exercise, nutrition, sunlight (or another source of vitamin D), and stress reduction can also provide health promotion and disease prevention motivation for clients (Anzuini, Battistella, & Izzotti, 2011; Erinosho, Moser, Oh, Neberling & Yaroch, 2012; Krishnan, Trump, Johnson & Feldman, 2012; Tsai et al., 2012).

ASK YOURSELF   www.

Suppose you have decided to become active in your community in the area of toxic environmental waste and its effect on health. How would you approach the topic and the institutions in your area? What role would you be interested in playing in this field?

Topic Area: Chronic Kidney Disease

Healthy People 2020 goals for chronic kidney disease include:
- reducing the rate of new cases of end-stage renal disease,
- reducing deaths in persons with end-stage renal disease,
- increasing the percentage of chronic kidney disease clients who receive care from a nephrologist at least 12 months before the start of renal treatment,
- increasing the percentage of dialysis clients < 70 years of age who are on a waiting list and/or who receive a donor kidney transplant within 1 year of being diagnosed with end-stage renal disease,
- ensuring that all clients on dialysis receive a transplant within 3 years of registration on a waiting list,
- decreasing kidney failure due to diabetes;
- increasing medical screening of persons with diabetes and chronic kidney disease;
- improving cardiovascular care in persons with chronic kidney disease; and,
- decreasing the percentage of the U.S. population with chronic kidney disease.

Kidney disease can stem from a number of issues, but its correlation to cardiovascular disease is clear, even in the absence of diabetes, with which kidney disorders are commonly associated (Ito, 2011). Vascular complications in turn have a significant impact on the microscopic blood vessels of the kidneys, setting up a vicious downward spiral where the cardiovascular disease reinforces kidney dysfunction and vice versa. Working to support good cardiovascular health in persons with kidney disease, whether diabetes related or not, is an essential aspect of health promotion.

Topic Area: Diabetes

Diabetes is a surprisingly complex topic area. On the one hand, diagnoses of all forms of diabetes are on the rise, with a variety of contributing factors involved in the increase—above and beyond the poor diet and sedentary lifestyle so commonly, and often inaccurately, cited in popular media as the principal culprits. Increased awareness of the risk factors and symptoms of diabetes has increased the rate of diabetes diagnoses and promoted early detection of this silent killer, helping to reduce the rate of diabetic complications such as lower extremity amputations.

Many people (and even some healthcare providers) do not grasp the nature of diabetes as a multifaceted disease in which genetic risk factors, unavoidable exposures, and modifiable lifestyle factors all contribute (Fradin & Bougnères, 2011; Morgan, 2011; Qi, Cornelis, Zhang, van Dam & Hu, 2009). This lack of knowledge can lead to considerable misinformation and even stigma in relation to a diabetes diagnosis.

Stigma related to obesity and weight bias also contribute. A common popular perception is that obese individuals who develop diabetes deserve their disease because of a perceived lack of self-control regarding food (Spero, 2006). Even more problematic, the client sometimes confronts weight bias—an attitude of condescension or disrespect for those who are overweight—in healthcare providers from whom the client is seeking care (Teixeira & Budd, 2010). The experience of stigma related to diabetes, obesity, or overweight often causes clients to avoid healthcare services, which can be detrimental to the effort to teach diabetic or prediabetic clients about diet, exercise, insulin regulation (through medications and/or injected insulin regimens), and glycemic control (Earnshaw & Quinn, 2011; Mold & Forbes, 2011).

These issues relate to a key aspect of diabetes management that differs from many disease interventions: Diabetes is explicitly a self-managed disease, yet learning to manage diabetes requires regular interaction with healthcare professionals. Because blood glucose levels must be monitored daily, with measurements taken every few hours (particularly in pediatric type 1 diabetes clients), it is not possible for a physician or nurse to be the primary caregiver. The client (or parents, in the case of children) must assume responsibility for the task of monitoring blood glucose and taking action to address high or low blood glucose values. Establishing a comfort level with self-managing the disease is a key factor in success—defined as maintaining normal overall glucose levels and limiting risk of long-term complications. At the same time, close contact with diabetes clinicians can assist the client in identifying and incorporating methods to reduce long-term blood glucose and HbA_{1c} values. Identifying other needs through the use of specific client-centered tools can enhance the success of an intervention.

Diabetic clients have a variety of barriers to maintaining good glycemic control that can be addressed through training, specific **interventions** (e.g., use of medications to improve insulin sensitivity or devices to monitor blood glucose levels), and screening exams. Education about how to reduce risk of long-term complications should focus on using complications as motivating factors promoting good glycemic control, instead of focusing on complications as something the client should expect to happen.

Topic Area: Disability and Secondary Conditions

Disability and secondary conditions cover a broad range of health issues. Most of the objectives in the *Healthy People 2020* document relate to mental health and access issues. For example, one objective is decreasing the percentage of children and adolescents with disabilities who are reported to be sad, unhappy, or depressed. A related objective is increasing emotional support and eliminating disparities, including decreasing environmental barriers, among people with disabilities and the wider community. A key aspect of this, in which health promotion activities can focus, is increasing the percentage of adults with disabilities who participate in social, recreational, community, and civic activities to the degree that they wish, as well as decreasing the number of those with disabilities in congregate care facilities (with 16 beds or more).

Topic Area: Early and Middle Childhood

The early and middle childhood topic area is new to the Healthy People initiative, and thus so are the objectives—five in all. They include decreasing the percentage of children who have poor quality of sleep, increasing the percentage of schools that require health education, increasing early intervention services in children up to age 2, and increasing the percentage of parents who use positive parenting and communicate this with their child's healthcare provider.

Topic Area: Environmental Health

Environmental health has moved to the forefront in recent years as the impact of pollutants and other environmental factors on human health has attracted greater interest from scientists and activists. Contamination of water and air in the home, workplace, school, and healthcare settings are all matters that affect an individual's physical health and well-being, sometimes in small ways (e.g., mild allergy symptoms related to an airborne contaminant such as dust) and sometimes in significant, even debilitating ways (e.g., carbon monoxide poisoning from a poorly maintained heating system). Exposure to excessive heat, cold, and damp conditions (which foster growth of molds and fungi that can trigger allergies) represents another form of environmental hazard that may affect clients with health issues, particularly those who lack sufficient income to install heating/air conditioning systems or dehumidifiers. Toxic chemicals, radiation, and other environmental exposures that cause injury or illness are less widespread, but still common problems.

☐ Water

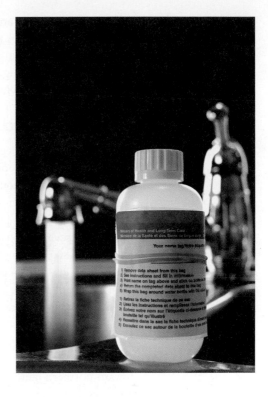

Aging urban infrastructure and high use of agricultural pesticides are two culprits in concerns about safe drinking water and sanitation (Ritter et al., 2002), and objectives in the report include reducing waterborne disease outbreaks, pesticide exposures, and the number of housing units with moderate or severe physical problems. For individuals with health issues, especially those who live in older housing or older neighborhoods (that is, units constructed prior to the 1970s, when lead pipes were phased out of use), one facet of health promotion may be assessing the quality of tap water and drinking water to avoid heavy metal exposures or other contaminants. Concerns about chemicals leaching from plastics, especially estrogenic compounds such as bisphenol A and phthalates, among many others (Wagner & Oehlmann, 2011), are not to be disregarded, particularly in female clients who are at risk from estrogen-receptor positive breast and ovarian cancers. Women should avoid drinking from plastic water bottles labelled #1 or #7 (Gurd, 2007). Clients may need information about how to purify drinking water using filters or reverse osmosis systems, how to distill water, how to test for common well-water or water-system contaminants, and how to address contaminants if found.

☐ Air

Air pollution has long represented a significant source of physical harm for Americans and is particularly relevant in relation to asthma and COPD; reducing the number of days the air quality index exceeds 100 and lowering overall toxic emissions into the air remain key goals in promoting general public health. On an individual level, exposure to airborne contaminants can range from household and occupational incidences of potentially lethal carbon monoxide poisoning (Graber, Macdonald, Kass, Smith, & Anderson, 2007) to industrial and transportation-related air pollution in urban centers, which has been linked to a variety of diseases ranging from asthma and COPD to cancer (Laumbach & Kipen, 2012; Wei, Davis, & Bina, 2011). Mitigating these health effects is an important and increasingly common challenge to health promotion efforts. Medication is one obvious method, but strategies to help avoid exposures can be helpful as well; for instance, recommending a HEPA-filtered air purifier and teaching a client how to check local ozone levels and pollen counts can reduce the effects of allergic asthma.

❏ Heat and Cold

National Weather Service statistics from the past decade indicate that on average, every year, 162 people die of heat-related complications—a number that does not take into account the many thousands of people who suffer such complications but do not die. The variability in heat-related deaths is quite significant, however; in particularly hot years, spikes of anywhere from several hundred to several thousand have been reported, including an extreme incidence of 14,800 deaths reported in France in the 2003 heat wave (Dhainaut, Claessens, Ginsburg, & Riou, 2004). Older adults and the very young are at greatest risk of adverse health conditions related to heat, particularly if they live in low economic circumstances and/or have preexisting health conditions.

Cold-related deaths outstrip this number by a considerable margin; the average annual number of deaths due to cold weather in the United States is estimated at 14,380, although incidence of cold-related fatalities is skewed toward northern latitudes (Deschenes & Moretti, 2007). Again, older adults and very young individuals living in impoverished conditions are at higher risk. At especially high risk are individuals with preexisting conditions and homeless persons.

Education on how to best cope with extreme temperatures is a principal focus of health promotion activities for at-risk individuals. Examples of simple but effective strategies include teaching clients how to choose more appropriate clothing for the extreme weather and helping the clients find financial aid resources to obtain heating fuel in winter, or offering guidance about maintaining adequate hydration and providing access to cooling stations during summer heat emergencies.

❏ Damp Conditions and Fungal Contaminants

Buildings located in damp areas (e.g., near a wetland or low-lying area) or that are subject to wet conditions (e.g., high annual rainfall) may be prone to high interior humidity, which can promote the growth of molds, mildews, and fungal species. Many of these release toxins that cause allergic or immune responses in the buildings' inhabitants. Scientists studying sick building syndrome (SBS) have identified a variety of potential sources of the illness, including molds that produce mycotoxins, although the association between particular molds and symptoms of SBS is still unclear.

In clients who suffer from allergy symptoms related to fungal contamination of their home or work place, health promotion involves both treating the allergic response in the client *and* reducing the source of the problem by means of a variety of mold-remediation measures (Sauni et al., 2011).

Topic Area: Family Planning

Family planning encompasses the prevention of pregnancy in those who do not want children and supporting women who become pregnant (whether by choice or inadvertently). In both instances, aiding women in obtaining reproductive health services is a crucial factor, as well as providing pregnant women with supportive care so that they deliver a healthy baby and are well prepared to care for their infant (or, alternatively, have access to adoption agencies should they wish to give up an unwanted child).

Unintended pregnancies, particularly in people who do not want or are not emotionally/financially ready for children, are a complex and often emotionally difficult issue. Increasing a client's knowledge of and access to contraception (both standard and emergency methods) can be one important facet of health promotion activities in this area. Options for contraception, e.g. condoms, spermicides, intrauterine devices (IUDs), and hormone-based birth control pills, should be discussed with clients so that the client has a good knowledge of the pros and cons of each method. Where contraception is not acceptable to the client for religious or cultural reasons, educating both partners on identifying the woman's ovulatory cycle (in order to avoid sexual activity during the days on which her fertility is at its maximum) can be an appropriate alternative. Clients should be warned that natural contraception is not as effective as barrier methods or hormonal contraceptive pills.

Family planning services may include obtaining access to abortion, which (it should go without saying) is controversial and a difficult subject for both clients and nurses alike. It is a topic with which many people are uncomfortable, even those who do not have strong opinions on the subject. Abortions are sometimes medically necessary in women who have health issues that make supporting a pregnancy through two or even one trimester dangerous, and they are also frequently recommended for women whose fetuses are diagnosed with several specific defects that are incompatible with life or that have a high likelihood of death within days of birth (e.g., anencephaly) (Cook, Erdman, Hevia, & Dickens, 2008).

Medically necessary abortions are likely to be extremely traumatic for women whose pregnancy was planned, but even women pregnant unintentionally may have strong reactions to learning that an abortion is recommended. Depending on the state, abortions that are not medically necessary (elective abortions) may be subject to certain legal restrictions, such as waiting periods of 1 to several days, denial of coverage for abortion for women on Medicaid, or requirements that parents be notified when the woman seeking the abortion is a minor (the age of majority can be defined differently in different states).

When working with a client who is seeking or considering an abortion, a nonjudgmental attitude and conscious effort to help the client reach her own decision are crucial. The client needs to reach a place of peace with her choice no matter what she decides, as she is the person who is most intimately connected (physically and emotionally) to the outcome of the decision. The physiologic sequelae of abortion should be explained to her as straightforwardly as possible.

Whether she decides to abort or retain a pregnancy, the client will need supportive services, whether they be postprocedure counseling (both mental health counseling and counseling about prevention of future pregnancy/safe sex may be required) or perinatal, obstetrical, and postpartum support if she decides otherwise. Postpartum support includes access to adoption agencies if the client chooses not to raise her infant. A woman who decides to continue the pregnancy and raise her infant may also need the services of a lactation consultant and parenting training, if she is a first-time mother.

Topic Area: Food Safety

Two key objectives pertaining to food safety in the Healthy People 2020 initiative are (1) to reduce severe allergic reactions to food among adults with a food allergy diagnosis and (2) to improve employee food preparation practices that directly relate to food-borne illnesses in retail food establishments.

☐ Food Allergies

Allergic responses to food occur on a spectrum ranging from mild (e.g., symptoms of stomach upset, diarrhea, urticaria (hives), or sinusitis) to life-threatening (anaphylaxis). Common sources of allergic responses include wheat (gluten), dairy, egg, peanut/tree nut, soy, fish, or shellfish, but allergies to a wide range of other foods have been documented (Waserman & Watson, 2011). Identifying and mitigating (avoiding) foods that cause allergic responses, plus educating clients about how to identify and address symptoms of an allergic episode in case of accidental exposure, are important points in health promotion activities for food allergies.

☐ Food-Borne Illnesses

Goals related to reducing food-borne infections focus on key pathogens transmitted through food (*Campylobacter* species, Shiga toxin-producing *Escherichia coli*, *Listeria* monocyte genes, and *Salmonella* species). A related factor focuses attention on preventing an increase in percentage of *Salmonella* and *Campylobacter jejuni* isolates resulting from humans' resistance to antimicrobial drugs (quinolones, third-generation cephalosporin, gentamicin, ampicillin, and erythromycin). With regard to working with individuals, the key to health promotion in this area relies on education, specifically teaching clients to follow key food safety practices (called clean, separate, cook, and chill processes).

Clients need to be aware of the nature of contamination in specific food groups (beef, dairy, fruits/nuts, leafy vegetables, and poultry) so that they understand how to decrease exposures to contaminated meat, poultry, and vegetables.

Topic Area: Genomics

Genomics is discipline that is expanding rapidly. While genetic counseling for certain disease states has been available for some time (e.g., Huntington's disease, BRCA-related breast and ovarian cancers), testing for other conditions is new. The Healthy People 2020 initiative includes two new objectives based on testing advances. The first new objective is to increase the percentage of persons with newly diagnosed colorectal cancer who receive genetic testing to identify Lynch syndrome (or familial colorectal cancer syndromes). The second is to increase the percentage of women with a family history of breast/ovarian cancer who receive genetic counseling. In both instances, the goal is to encourage genetic testing to assess risk factors and identify ways to mitigate risk.

HOT TOPICS

Here are some topics to explore:
- Healthcare-associated infections
- Social support and health
- Quality of life and well-being
- Genomics
- Global health
- Health disparities
- Adult immunization
- MRSA
- School-sponsored physical activity
- Autism spectrum disorder
- Work-related stress
- Theory of planned behavior

With many clients, suggestion of genetic testing based on familial risk factors can be stressful. Some clients will state emphatically that they do not want to know their risk of developing a disease that is common in their family. Others may pursue testing eagerly, but express concerns about whether there will be financial ramifications (e.g., loss of insurance coverage) related to positive test results. The benefits and costs for genetic testing (including emotional costs) should be weighed carefully with each client.

Topic Area: Hearing and Other Sensory or Communication Disorders (Ear, Nose, Throat, Vision, Speech, and Language)

A wide variety of hearing and other sensory or communication disorders were included in the Healthy People 2020 recommendations, including:

- Decrease otitis media in children
- Decrease adult hearing loss
- Increase hearing screening and use of assistive devices, cochlear implants, and hearing protection
- Increase the percentage of newborns who are screened for hearing loss by no later than age 1 month, have audiologic evaluation by age 3 months, and are enrolled in appropriate intervention services by age 6 months
- Address problems of tinnitus, dizziness/balance problems, and potential adverse outcomes
- Address smell and taste disorders
- Address communication/speech problems and language delays

Health promotion in these areas centers around obtaining testing and medical care to identify the cause of a hearing, speech, or other disorder and determining appropriate therapies with the specialist and the client. Linking clients to rehabilitation services, device suppliers, supplemental insurance, etc., are additional aspects of health promotion for many of these conditions.

Topic Area: Heart Disease and Stroke

Hypertension, coronary heart disease, and stroke are three major killers of Americans. Happily, they are three conditions that respond well to behavioral changes, and the opportunities for health promotion activities in these areas are boundless. Important aspects of health promotion for individuals include:

- Increasing knowledge of the risk factors related to hypertension and heart disease, including smoking, family history, cholesterol levels, exercise levels, overweight/obesity, high stress levels, and diabetes/prediabetes. Raising awareness of early warning signs and symptoms of stroke and heart attack and educating those at risk on what to do in the event of the onset of symptoms are also important points.

- Increasing adherence to medical and lifestyle approaches for reducing hypertension, high low-density lipoprotein levels, and recurrence rates in survivors of heart disease and stroke
- Supporting changes to diet and lifestyle to improve quality of life and reduce risk

RESEARCH BOX 4-1: A Review of: Fruit/Vegetable Intake and Physical Activity among Adults with High Cholesterol

» PURPOSE: The Division for Heart Disease and Stroke Prevention, National Center for Chronic Disease Prevention and Health Promotion, Centers for Disease Control and Prevention, Atlanta, Georgia, undertook a study to determine whether hypercholesterolemic adults followed healthy eating habits and appropriate physical activity.

» METHODS: The researchers used the 2007 Behavioral Risk Factor Surveillance System and measured ≥ 5 servings of fruits and vegetables/day and Healthy People 2010 recommended physical activity.

» RESULTS: Of 363,667 adults ≥ 18 years, 37.3% had hypercholesterolemia. The percentages of healthy eating and physical activity were lower among those with hypercholesterolemia than among those without (23.8% versus 27.9% for healthy eating [P < 0.001], 43.1% versus 51.7% for physical activity [P < 0.001]).

» CONCLUSION: Hypercholesterolemic adults are less likely to practice healthy eating and to engage in physical activity than are those without hypercholesterolemia.

Source: Fang, J., Keenan, N. L., & Dai, S. (2011). Fruit/vegetable intake and physical activity among adults with high cholesterol. *American Journal of Health Behavior, 35*(6), 689–698.

HEALTH PROMOTION CHALLENGE

How could you use the findings of the hypercholesterolemia study to promote health in your work?

Topic Area: HIV

Individual health promotion related to HIV/AIDS focuses on two factors: reduction of risky behaviors (e.g., intravenous drug use, failure to use condoms during sexual activity) for those who are at risk for infection, and provision of medical treatment and emotional support to individuals diagnosed with the virus. The nature of such interventions may differ when addressing individuals from specific ethnic, racial, demographic, or religious groups, based on social and cultural perceptions about the disease. HIV is a highly charged topic for some individuals and (as discussed earlier) is often subject to significant stigma. The presence of substance abuse issues frequently complicates therapeutic efforts, even when intravenous drug use is not involved.

Identifying those at risk requires the nurse to look beyond popular myths and misconceptions. At minimum, assume that all sexually active persons who have had more than one partner (or whose partner has had prior partners) have some level of risk, irrespective of whether the client is heterosexual, homosexual, or bisexual. How high that risk might be depends on a variety of factors, including the number of partners and frequency with which partners change; the level of education about, and willingness to use, safe sex practices; and the use of illicit drugs, particularly intravenous drugs.

Health promotion activities for clients diagnosed with HIV center around supportive care for medical and emotional needs. Compliance with antiretroviral therapies and establishment of a support network for the client are two key goals in health promotion. Clients should also be encouraged to consider developing healthy eating, exercising, stress-reduction, and sleeping habits and learn methods of avoiding exposure to infectious agents that might exceed the capabilities of a compromised immune system.

Topic Area: Immunization and Infectious Diseases

The infectious disease topic area includes a number of different objectives. Some of these relate to the reduction of specific infectious agents, many of which have experienced a recent increase due to the development of resistance to antibiotics in certain strains (e.g., MRSA, tuberculosis, influenza viruses). Of particular concern are diseases for which vaccines exist, but which are increasing in incidence due to public refusal to vaccinate resulting from concerns, valid or otherwise, about vaccine safety and effectiveness (such as measles and whooping cough). Educating clients about excessive antibiotic use and increasing vaccination are activities that you may undertake, particularly with clients who have young children. You can also assist clients to assess risk factors for infection and help them to undertake basic measures to prevent disease transmission by improving hygiene (e.g., hand washing, maintaining clean surfaces in kitchens and bathrooms, and regularly cleaning light switches and doorknobs to reduce the prevalence of infectious microbes).

Topic Area: Injury and Violence Prevention

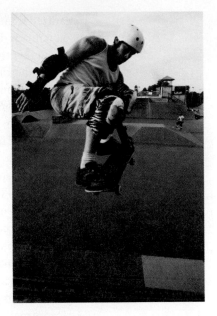

Injury encompasses a wide range of areas. Included in the Healthy People 2020 objectives were such diverse goals as:

- A decrease in homicides and firearm-related deaths/injuries
- Review of children's deaths (those 17 and under) by a child fatality review team
- A decrease in pedestrian deaths/injuries
- An increase in safety belt use and vehicle restraint systems for small children
- An increase in the use of helmets and other safety equipment on recreational vehicles, including motorcycles, bicycles, and ATVs, as well as in sports such as skiing, snowboarding, and equestrian activities, with a related goal of decreasing incidence of traumatic brain injuries and/spinal cord morbidity and mortality
- Decreases in general sport and recreational injuries
- A decrease in residential fire deaths
- A decrease in poisoning and unintentional injury, suffocation deaths, nonfatal child maltreatment, and violence among intimate partners

While these objectives encompass a wide range of circumstances, the common thread among many of them is awareness. Prevention of most of these injuries hinge on individual awareness of risk and knowledge of risk mitigation strategies, including safety equipment, appropriate licensing and training, and precautionary habits to avoid risky circumstances. With respect to the majority of these goals, you can discuss the client's risk for such injuries as seems appropriate, and offer appropriate educational materials to assist with increasing risk mitigation knowledge. This can include training in firearm safety, conflict resolution strategies, anger management, and the use of devices and equipment that prevent injury.

Topic Area: Maternal, Infant, and Child Health

One area of health that the United States as a whole manages poorly is infant mortality. The most recently updated CIA Online Factbook page (n.d.) on infant mortality places the United States 175th of 222 on the list of countries organized from highest to lowest rate of infant mortality, with an average rate of 6.06 infant deaths per 1,000 live births (estimated) for 2011. (Reverse the order so that the best rate is on top, and the United States ranks 47th.) This rate puts the United States well behind the level of other developed nations, which have considerably lower rates of infant deaths, and behind even much less wealthy countries like Cuba (4.9/1,000) and Greece (5.0/1,000). Maternal death rates per 100,000 live births are no better; the United States ranks 39th, equal with the former Yugoslavian province of Macedonia, with 17 deaths per 100,000 births (Hogan et al., 2010). Wide race-based disparities in access to care, lower maternal education levels, and presence of comorbidities such as HIV infection have been cited as factors that exacerbate infant and maternal mortality. A Congressional Budget Office assessment of the problem in 1992 pinpointed access to prenatal care, complications of low birth weight, and improved access to health care (particularly for minority women and younger, rural, and economically disadvantaged women) as key factors in reducing the rate of maternal and infant deaths. All of these factors are still in place; indeed, the disparity in care between white women and minority women, particularly African American women, has grown in the interim.

CULTURAL RESEARCH STUDY

A review of: Health Characteristics of American Indian or Alaska Native Adult Population: United States, 2004–2008

BACKGROUND: The ability to measure the success of Healthy People 2020 objectives requires baseline information to measure from. The following article provides such a baseline and is also relevant in its reporting of **health disparities** that exist for minority groups.

METHOD: This was a study comparing health status indicators, health behaviors, health care utilization, health conditions, immunizations, and HIV testing status for American Indian or Alaskan Native (AIAN) adults. The group was compared to white, black, Asian, and Hispanic adults. Data came from the 2004–2008 National Health Interview Surveys conducted by the CDC.

FINDINGS: The non-Hispanic AIAN community was found to have higher rates of risky health behaviors, poorer health status and conditions, and lower utilization of health services.

Source: Barnes, P. M., Adams, P. F., & Powell-Griner, E. (2010). Health characteristics of American Indian or Alaska Native adult population: United States, 2004–2008. *National Health Status Report, 9*(20), 1–22.

Pregnancy outcomes are greatly improved when women have early, consistent access to prenatal care (including prepregnancy healthcare that helps women achieve a more optimal health state before attempting to become pregnant). Health promotion opportunities in this area are abundant, but particular activities need to be tailored to demographic factors and risk factors affecting the client.

Also included are objectives to increase:

- the percentage of healthy, full-term infants who sleep on their backs;
- abstinence from alcohol, cigarettes, and illicit drugs in pregnant women;
- mothers who breastfeed; and
- access to a medical home and comprehensive coordinated systems for children with special needs.
- Reducing maternal illness and complications due to pregnancy, reducing the incidence of cesarean births among low-risk women, and addressing risk factors for preterm births are also important goals.

In terms of child health, many objectives focus on providing screening services and care for infants and young children in relation to conditions such as Down syndrome, sickle-cell disease, autism spectrum disorders, and other conditions that benefit from intensive early intervention.

Topic Area: Mental Health and Mental Disorders

The connections between physical health and mental health deserve mention in the context of physical health promotion. A client who suffers from untreated or poorly managed mental health issues, whether relatively mild ones such as seasonal affective disorder or severe functional illnesses such as schizophrenia, has a preexisting barrier to engaging in health promotion efforts aimed at physical health. This is especially true if the mental health condition is exacerbated by substance abuse, a not-uncommon circumstance. Working with a client to promote physical health is generally unsuccessful if existing mental health issues are not addressed either simultaneously with, or in advance of, physical health issues. The interrelationship between mental and physical health is such that serious emotional or mental health issues may manifest themselves in physical illness, so addressing the mental health problem helps resolve the physical illness. Certain health promotion activities focused on physical wellness can help reduce the severity of some mental health concerns; for example, encouraging a client who suffers from depression to participate in a mindful exercise program on a regular basis can improve both physical and mental health and wellness (Gill, Womack, & Safranek, 2010).

Topic Area: Nutrition and Weight Status

Nutrition and weight are significant factors affecting physical health and wellness for a large proportion of the American population. Goals of the Healthy People 2020 initiative include the following:

- Increase the percentage of adults who are at a healthy weight and reduce the percentage of adults who are obese (CDC statistics on 4/20/12 place this percentage at about 33.9% of the adult population)
- Reduce the percentage of children and adolescents who are overweight or obese
- Reduce iron deficiency among young children, females of childbearing age, and pregnant females
- Reduce the consumption of saturated fat and sodium in the population aged 2 years and older
- Increase the variety and contribution of fruits, vegetables, and whole grains to the diets of the population aged 2 years and older
- Increase the contribution of fruits to the diets of the population aged 2 years and older, the variety and contribution of vegetables to the diets of the population aged 2 years and older, the contribution of whole grains to the diets of the population aged 2 years and older
- Increase the consumption of calcium in the population aged 2 years and older
- Increase the percentage of work sites that offer nutrition or weight management classes or counseling
- Eliminate very low food security among children in U.S. households

☐ Overweight and Obesity

Most people are by now aware that being overweight is an important risk factor for many diseases. While that concern may be among those driving a client's wish for weight loss, psychological and self-image factors may be as or more important than health as motivational factors for weight loss. Clients may have already attempted to lose weight using popular diet and/or exercise programs; in many cases, such clients either found that they could not adhere to the program they selected, that the program did not cause the expected weight loss, or that although they achieved success, they regained the weight shortly after completing the program. Such prior experiences tend to leave clients feeling frustrated, anxious, and lacking in self-efficacy.

Weight loss is not a one-size-fits-all prospect. No single mode of eating or exercising will work for all individuals (Dale et al., 2009). The standard of taking in fewer calories than you expend that most people use as the basis of weight loss efforts is unhelpful for those with long-term, entrenched weight problems. These include clients whose excess weight is a metabolic issue, or even a genetic one (Farooqi, 2011; Grimm, & Steinle, 2010; Kim, 2008; Lev–Ran, 2001; Walsh, 2010) rather than an imbalance between calorie input/utilization.

Some caloric restriction plans cause rapid weight loss initially, but trigger the body's starvation responses (e.g., slowdown of metabolic processes to conserve energy in the face of a perceived food stress) so that weight loss slows over time. When these dieters become frustrated and resume normal eating habits, they experience a rapid regain of weight as a consequence—even if still exercising regularly. Some research also suggests that it matters just as much where the calories come from (e.g., protein, fats, carbohydrate, etc.) as the total calorie count (Manninen, 2004).

The popular belief that weight gain and weight loss relate solely to energy exchange (where food = energy in and exercise = energy out) is a gross oversimplification of how the body's energetic system works. Poor sleep, stress, and genetic and metabolic factors all may promote weight gain or impair the efficacy of weight loss efforts (Foster et al., 2005; Spiegel, Tasali, Leproult, & Van Cauter, 2009). Nutritional deficits can also adversely affect metabolism (Chacko et al., 2011; Parra, Palou, & Serra, 2010; Shahar et al., 2010).

Even the concept of exercising for weight loss is oversimplified. Different types of exercise have different effects on metabolism. While most exercise programs focus on cardiovascular exercise to promote increased metabolic rate/caloric output, strength training to build muscle mass is also important, but often overlooked (Churilla, Magyari, Ford, Fitzhugh, & Johnson, 2011). The plateau that many people reach in using exercise for weight loss is well documented and results from a number of factors, but principally from using only aerobic exercise and not muscle-building methods. The body also adapts to consistent levels of exertion, so that if a client is doing the same type of exercise at the same rate all the time, metabolic processes become more efficient and use less energy (Fahey, 1998; Peterson, Pistilli, Haff, Hoffman, & Gordon, 2011). Interval training and alternating exercise methods—mixing it up by walking one day, doing weight training the next, and attending a yoga class the third day—can limit this adaptation. When a plateau is reached, continued weight loss requires continued progression to more intense/more frequent exercise levels.

A factor in success that weight-loss programs such as Jenny Craig and Weight Watchers have put to good use is social support. Clients who have a personal trainer, weight-loss buddy, or a group of peers supporting their efforts do better than people attempting to lose weight on their own. One study found that over a 2-year period, an inexpensive program providing nurse support was as effective as a more resource-intensive program for weight maintenance despite using diets of different macronutrient composition (Dale et al., 2009).

When working with clients to develop a weight-loss plan intended to provide safe, lasting weight loss, use motivation interviewing techniques with the client regarding all of the following factors:

1. The amounts and types of foods that are eaten over a 2-week period
2. Exercise habits and daily energy outputs

3. Family history of obesity/overweight or other weight-related conditions
4. Amount and distribution of body fat
5. Sleep and snack patterns
6. Current stress factors
7. Metabolic dysfunctions (e.g., hypothyroidism or insulin resistance) that may contribute to weight gain and impede weight loss
8. Other health issues (e.g., alcohol use, mental health issues) that may impede weight loss efforts
9. Amount of social support available for a weight-loss program

The information gained from the interview can be used in conjunction with the client to formulate a plan of dietary, exercise, and behavioral changes that can alter a multitude of factors affecting weight loss. Keep in mind that developing such a program may mean educating the client about the errors in some of his or her assumptions about weight. Aside from the very common mistake of believing that calorie counting is all that matters, clients may have unrealistic ideas about how much weight they can lose and how fast they can lose it; many may not appreciate the safety issues with too-rapid weight loss. Also, implementing a comprehensive plan all at once may be overwhelming for clients; instead, ask the client to set a reasonable timeline for achievement of specific goals.

For example, a client who needs to start exercising and change to a low-carb diet may be more successful if a goal is set that allows commitment to a half hour of exercise 3 days a week, with a deadline of 4 to 6 weeks to establish

RESEARCH BOX 4-2   Successful Weight Loss Maintenance

A study conducted at the Nutritional Epidemiology Program, National Institute of Health and Nutrition in Tokyo, Japan, examined behavioral factors related to successful weight maintenance.

Participants were 90 middle-aged participants who attended a weight loss program and were followed for 1 year.

» FINDINGS: Compared to unsuccessful weight maintainers (USWM), successful weight maintainers (SWM) showed a greater improvement in their regularity of eating, walked more, and felt less stress regarding their increased physical activity than the USWM. During the follow-up period, significantly more SWM participants had self-efficacy (for measuring weight, practicing dietary objectives, and assessing the practice and keeping records), actually kept records, and measured weight more than the USWM participants. In contrast, more USWM participants felt stress about measuring weight.

» CONCLUSIONS: The researchers concluded that an increased amount of physical activity, having a higher self-efficacy, and consistently keeping records of the client's activities, as well as regularly weighing themselves, may be important for successful weight maintenance.

Source: Nakade, M., Aiba, N., Morita, A., Miyachi, M., Sasaki, S., Watanabe, S. (2012). What behaviors are important for successful weight maintenance? *Journal of Obesity*. 2012:202037. doi: 10.1155/2012/202037

this exercise regimen as a regular pattern. Once the client has succeeded in reaching that commitment, a new goal—adding two or three more half-hour sessions a week within 4 weeks' time—is added. Upon reaching that goal, a dietary goal—perhaps eliminating white sugar and flour from the client's diet to help reduce carb intake—might be added, with another 4-week deadline for completing that change. Success in reaching a goal means formulating a more advanced goal. This allows the client to make changes gradually, yet also offers the client the reward of feeling success upon completion of each goal.

Suggest the client work with a significant other to provide support for a weight loss plan and identify alternative activities to eating and snacking. See FIGURE 4-2.

Food Composition and Nutrient Content Many of the goals in the *Healthy People 2020* document relate to uneven distribution of nutrition. Hunger and malnutrition are much more common in the United States than many realize; at the same time, there are some people who have plenty to eat, but are still lacking in the base nutrients needed for good health simply because they do not get a varied diet. The USDA food pyramid has been altered frequently

---

Share these activities with clients who hope to lose weight.

- Examine each food before eating it and ask, "Am I hungry now or am I tired, angry, lonely, or stressed?"
- Keep track of activities, exercise, and food intake in a daily diary.
- Review the diary with the nurse.
- Identify situations that promote eating and find alternative activities.
- Work with a significant other or a buddy who provides support for weight loss.
- Set rewards for changing eating behaviors, such as money, praise, prizes, a weekend trip, or whatever is rewarding to the client.
- Use imagery to picture the client as slim and happy.
- Role play with the nurse or buddy how to handle pressure to eat.
- Learn relaxation techniques or purchase a relaxation CD and use diversionary tactics, such as drinking a glass or two of water, taking a walk, or deep breathing, when eating urges occur.
- Don't eat while watching TV or doing some other activity; when eating, concentrate on the taste, the sensations of eating, and food smells.
- Cut way back on appetite stimulants such as coffee, spices, chocolate, sugar, sodas, and salt.

FIGURE 4-2   Activities That Can Help in Losing Weight

in recent years to reflect this, and was finally exchanged for a food plate in an attempt to give greater guidance to consumers and to offer advice about nutrition that is more tailored to particular demographic groups (Harmon, 2011; Haven, Burns, Herring, & Britten, 2006; Shelnutt, Bobroff, & Diehl, 2009).

Ensuring that clients have access to and an understanding of good basic nutrition is a foundation of health promotion efforts. A client with a poor diet, whether a result of not having access to enough food or having a diet composed of nonnutritious food or a limited variety of foods, is a client who either already lacks good health or who is on the road to poor health.

Clients may not recognize that food quality (fresh versus prepared) matters, and many may not know how to read labels and assess ingredient content (e.g., sodium, sugars, or additives), so basic training in identifying better options may be required to help teach clients what to buy. Clients who cannot cook or prepare food should be encouraged to learn so that they do not rely exclusively on prepared frozen, dried, or packaged foods, which sometimes have lower nutrient content and higher calories (even when the labeling suggests otherwise) (Urban et al., 2010).

Providing supplemental nutrition via vitamin and mineral supplements may be a short-term option to boost nutrient status in clients with clear-cut deficiencies (which should be identified by testing rather than assumed). For long-term wellness, changing dietary habits, educating clients on what constitutes a healthy diet, and improving client access to healthy foods are better routes to nutrient sufficiency.

Bear in mind that women may need to take calcium/magnesium supplements as they age, especially after menopause, when it is difficult to get the recommended 1,200–1,500 mg/day via food alone:

> After menopause, a woman's calcium needs go up to maintain bone health. Women 51 and older should get 1,200 milligrams (mg) of calcium each day. Vitamin D also is important to bone health. Women 51 to 70 should get 600 international units (IU) of vitamin D each day. Women ages 71 and older need 800 IU of vitamin D each day. (U.S. Department of Health and Human Services [DHHS], 2010)

Topic Area: Older Adults

There are a number of health challenges and life issues unique to older adults. Many of these are physical aspects associated with aging: declines in nutrition status (particularly protein intake) and muscle strength; bone loss and related fracture risk (osteoporosis); mobility issues; vision, hearing, and other sensory impairments; sleep disturbances; and neurological deterioration. Often, where such issues affect an older adult, there are social and mental health issues that exacerbate the condition, so that what would otherwise be a nuisance becomes a serious health problem. For example, many older adults experience an unmet need for caregiver support services, particularly older adults with disabilities. Ironically, improvements in medical management of chronic illness that have resulted in a greater longevity have also created a critical shortage of facilities and support systems to assist older adults with one or more chronic health conditions. Unpaid caregivers, usually family members, sometimes subject elder relatives to maltreatment and neglect. The lack of assistance may cause an individual who would otherwise be reasonably independent and functional to experience worsening health, greater morbidity, and earlier death. Health promotion for older adult clients (and their caregivers) therefore hinges on identifying needs for assistance and support intended to help the older adult maintain independent functioning to the greatest extent possible.

Eating is often an issue with older adults when they have difficulty chewing or food doesn't taste the same any more. Certain medicines can make food tasteless. Encourage clients to ask their physician or nurse practitioner to prescribe a medicine that does not interfere with taste. Suggest clients use lemon juice and spices such as oregano, thyme, rosemary, turmeric (also called curcumin), and garlic to spice up their meals. Each of these also has healing qualities; for example, curcumin is known to inhibit cancer cells (Sundram, Chauhan, Ebeling, & Jaggi, 2012; Lee, Li, Tsao, Fong, & Tang, 2012).

HEALTH PROMOTION CHALLENGE

Go to www.pubmed.gov and look up studies that provide evidence that oregano, thyme, rosemary, cinnamon, clove, and garlic have healing qualities. Share your information with at least one classmate and trade references.

FIGURE 4-3 provides some tips to give older clients that may help them eat more nutritious food. Consider making a copy and providing it to older clients.

Topic Area: Oral Health

For many individuals, oral health is simply about having clean teeth, a bright smile, and avoiding bad breath. However, maintaining good oral health is an important factor in supporting overall health. Studies show that poor oral health, particularly loss of teeth, is a predictor of cardiovascular and respiratory disease mortality (Aida et al., 2011; Belstrøm, Damgaard, Nielsen, & Holmstrup, 2011; Holmlund, Holm, & Lind, 2010).

Chronic periodontal disease also correlates to Alzheimer's disease, possibly as a result of systemic inflammation (Watts, Crimmins, & Gatz, 2008). Individuals who get regular dental checkups are also more likely to have oral and pharyngeal cancer detected at the earliest stage.

- Eat many different colors and types of vegetables and fruits.

- Make sure at least half of your grains are whole grains.

- Eat only small amounts of solid fats, oils, and foods high in sugars. Limit saturated fat (found mostly in foods that come from animals) or *trans* fats (found in foods like some margarines, shortening, cookies, and crackers).

- Every day, eat the following foods and amounts:

  Fruits—1.5 to 2.5 cups
  What is the same as a half cup of cut-up fruit? One medium whole fruit or a quarter cup of dried fruit.

  Vegetables—2 to 3.5 cups
  What is the same as a cup of cut-up vegetables? Two cups of uncooked leafy vegetables.

  Grains—5–10 ounces
  What is the same as an ounce of grains? One roll; a small muffin; a slice of bread; 1 cup of flaked, ready-to-eat cereal; or a half cup of cooked rice, pasta, or cereal.

  Meat/beans—5–7 ounces
  What is the same as an ounce of meat, fish, or poultry? One egg, a quarter cup of cooked beans or tofu, a half ounce of nuts or seeds, or 1 tablespoon of peanut butter.

  Milk—3 cups of fat-free or low-fat milk
  What is the same as 1 cup of milk? One cup of yogurt or 1.5 to 2 ounces of cheese. One cup of cottage cheese is the same as a half cup of milk.

- Drink enough liquids so your urine is pale yellow, not dark yellow.

- It is better to get fiber from food than dietary supplements. Start adding more fiber slowly. That will help avoid unwanted gas. Here are some tips for adding fiber: Eat cooked dry beans, peas, and lentils often. Leave skins on your fruit and vegetables if possible. Choose whole fruit over fruit juice. Eat whole-grain breads and cereals. Drink plenty of liquids to help fiber move through your intestines.

- *Here's a tip:* Stay away from empty calories. These are foods and drinks with a lot of calories but not many nutrients—for example, chips, cookies, sodas, and alcohol.

FIGURE 4-3   Eating Tips for Older Adults
Source: http://www.nia.nih.gov/health/publication/healthy-eating-after-50

In addition to health issues related to teeth and gums, structural issues with the oral/craniofacial area can have a significant adverse impact on health. These include respiratory problems related to jaw malformation, micrognathia, temporomandibular joint (TMJ) dysfunction, and soft-tissue structural defects such as cleft lip or palate, many of which require surgical intervention or, in the case of TMJ, the use of dental appliances to relieve symptoms.

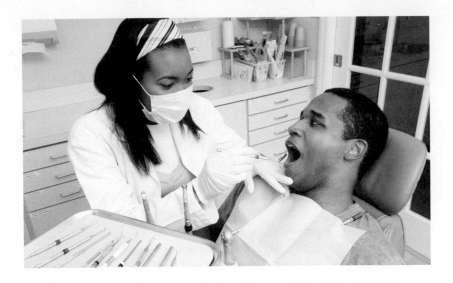

Objectives in the *Healthy People 2020* document pertaining to oral health are:

- Reduce the percentage of children and adolescents who have dental caries in their primary or permanent teeth, as well as the percentage of children, adolescents, and adults with untreated dental decay and periodontitis
- Increase the percentage of adults who have never had a permanent tooth extracted due to caries or disease
- Increase the percentage of children who have received dental sealants on their molar teeth
- Increase the percentage of long-term care residents who use the oral healthcare system each year
- Increase the number of school-based health centers with an oral health component
- Increase the number of local health departments and federally qualified health centers that have an oral health component
- Increase the percentage of referral of children with cleft lips and palates to craniofacial teams

Topic Area: Physical Activity and Fitness

Exercise was discussed at length in the section on weight loss, but fitness is about more than just weight maintenance. It relates to cardiovascular and pulmonary health, muscle strength, flexibility and joint function, and even neurologic function. Mental health benefits of physical activity are well documented. In sum, promoting fitness activities to individual clients generally will help with nearly every health concern; however, some clients will need their exercise programs tailored to suit physical limitations.

In the physical activity and fitness area, the objectives in *Healthy People 2020* include the following:

- Increasing the number of the nation's public and private schools that require daily physical education for all students, the percentage of adolescents who participate in daily school physical education, and the percentage of adolescents who spend at least 50% of school physical education class time being active
- Increasing the number of public and private schools that provide access to physical activity spaces and facilities for all persons outside of normal school hours
- Reducing the number of adults who engage in no leisure-time physical activity
- Increasing the percentage of adults and adolescents who meet current guidelines for aerobic physical activity and for muscle strength training
- Increasing the percentage of children and adolescents who meet guidelines for television viewing and computer use
- Increasing the percentage of employed adults who have access to and participate in employer-based exercise facilities
- Increasing the number of trips made by walking and bicycling
- Increasing the percentage of physician office visits for chronic health diseases or conditions that include counseling or education related to exercise

Use FIGURE 4-4 to help clients increase their strength through exercise. Even small changes in muscle strength can make a real difference in getting up from a chair, climbing stairs, carrying groceries, opening jars, and playing with children. Lower-body strength exercises will improve balance.

- Use a 1-pound can of food or a 1-pound weight the first week, then gradually add more weight. Starting out with weights that are too heavy can cause injuries.

- It should feel somewhere between hard and very hard for you to lift or push the weight. It shouldn't feel very, very hard. If you can't lift or push a weight 8 times in a row, it's too heavy for you. Reduce the amount of weight.

- Take 3 seconds to lift or push a weight into place, hold the position for 1 second, and take another 3 seconds to return to your starting position. Don't let the weight drop; returning it slowly is very important.

- Try to do each exercise 10 to 15 repetitions. Think of this as a goal. If you can't do that many at first, do as many as you can. You may be able to build up to this goal over time.

FIGURE 4-4   Exercise Ideas to Enhance Strength

Source: http://www.nia.nih.gov/health/publication/exercise-physical-activity-your-everyday-guide-national-institute-aging/sample

- Want to be able to lift your carry-on bag into the overhead bin of the airplane or get in and out of the car more easily? Keep doing those strength exercises, and you'll get there.

Safety

- Talk with your doctor or nurse practitioner if you are unsure about doing a particular exercise. For example, if you've had hip or back surgery, talk about which exercises might be best for you.
- Don't hold your breath during strength exercises. Holding your breath while straining can cause changes in blood pressure. This is especially true for people with heart disease.
- Breathe regularly. Breathe in slowly through your nose and breathe out slowly through your mouth. If this is not comfortable or possible, breathe in and out through either your nose or mouth.
- Breathe out as you lift or push, and breathe in as you relax. For example, if you're doing leg lifts, breathe out as you lift your leg, and breathe in as you lower it. This may not feel natural at first, and you probably will have to think about it for a while as you do it.

Proper form and safety go hand in hand. For some exercises, you may want to start alternating arms and work your way up to using both arms at the same time. If it is difficult for you to hold hand weights, try using wrist weights.

- To prevent injury, don't jerk or thrust weights into position. Use smooth, steady movements.
- Avoid locking your arm and leg joints in a tightly straightened position. To straighten your knees, tighten your thigh muscles. This will lift your kneecaps and protect them.
- For many of the sample exercises in this guide, you will need to use a chair. Choose a sturdy chair that is stable enough to support your weight when seated or when holding on during the exercise.
- Muscle soreness lasting a few days and slight fatigue are normal after muscle-building exercises, at least at first. After doing these exercises for a few weeks, you will probably not be sore after your workout.

Progressing

Here's an example of how to progress gradually: Start out with a 1-pound weight that you can lift only 8 times. Keep using that weight until you become strong enough to lift it easily 10 to 15 times. When you can do 2 sets of 10 to 15 repetitions easily, add more weight so that, again, you can lift it only 8 times. Keep repeating until you reach your goal, and then maintain that level as long as you can.

FIGURE 4-4   (Continued)

- If you feel sick or have pain during or after exercise, you're doing too much.

- Exhaustion, sore joints, and painful muscle pulling mean you're overdoing it. None of the exercises should cause severe pain.

- Overexercising can cause injury, which may lead to quitting altogether. A steady rate of progress is the best approach.

Working with Weights

You don't have to go out and buy weights for strength exercises. Find something you can hold on to easily. For example, you can make your own weights from the following unbreakable household items:

- Fill a plastic milk jug with sand or water and tape the opening securely closed.

- Fill a sock with dried beans, and tie up the open end.

- Use common grocery items, such as bags of rice, vegetable or soup cans, or bottled water.

Hand grip

This simple exercise should help if you have trouble picking things up or holding on to them. It also will help you open things like that pickle jar more easily. You can even do this exercise while reading or watching TV.

1. Hold a tennis ball or other small rubber or foam ball in one hand.

2. Slowly squeeze the ball as hard as you can and hold it for 3–5 seconds.

3. Relax the squeeze slowly.

4. Repeat 10–15 times.

5. Repeat 10–15 times with other hand.

6. Repeat 10–15 times more with each hand.

Wrist curl

This exercise will strengthen your wrists. It also will help ensure good form and prevent injury when you do upper body strength exercises.

1. Rest your forearm on the arm of a sturdy chair with your hand over the edge.

2. Hold a weight with palm facing upward.

3. Slowly bend your wrist up and down.

4. Repeat 10–15 times.

5. Repeat with other hand 10–15 times.

6. Repeat 10–15 more times with each hand.

FIGURE 4-4   (Continued)

Overhead arm raise

This exercise will strengthen your shoulders and arms. It should make swimming and other activities such as lifting and carrying grandchildren easier.

1. You can do this exercise while standing or sitting in a sturdy, armless chair.
2. Keep your feet flat on the floor, shoulder-width apart.
3. Hold weights at your sides at shoulder height with palms facing forward. Breathe in slowly.
4. Slowly breathe out as you raise both arms up over your head keeping your elbows slightly bent.
5. Hold the position for 1 second.
6. Breathe in as you slowly lower your arms.
7. Repeat 10–15 times.
8. Rest; then repeat 10–15 more times.
9. As you progress, use a heavier weight and alternate arms until you can lift the weight comfortably with both arms.

Front arm raise

This exercise for your shoulders can help you put things up on a shelf or take them down more easily.

1. Stand with your feet shoulder-width apart.
2. Hold weights straight down at your sides, with palms facing backward.
3. Keeping your arms straight, breathe out as you raise both arms in front of you to shoulder height.
4. Hold the position for 1 second.
5. Breathe in as you slowly lower your arms.
6. Repeat 10–15 times.
7. Rest; then repeat 10–15 more times.

As you progress, use a heavier weight and alternate arms until you can lift the weight comfortably with both arms.

Side arm raise

This exercise will strengthen your shoulders and make lifting groceries easier.

1. You can do this exercise while standing or sitting in a sturdy, armless chair.
2. Keep your feet flat on the floor, shoulder-width apart.
3. Hold hand weights straight down at your sides with palms facing inward. Breathe in slowly.

FIGURE 4-4   (Continued)

4. Slowly breathe out as you raise both arms to the side, shoulder height.

5. Hold the position for 1 second.

6. Breathe in as you slowly lower your arms.

7. Repeat 10–15 times.

8. Rest; then repeat 10–15 more times.

As you progress, use a heavier weight and alternate arms until you can lift the weight comfortably with both arms.

Arm curl

After a few weeks of doing this exercise for your upper arm muscles, lifting that gallon of milk will be much easier.

1. Stand with your feet shoulder-width apart.

2. Hold the weights straight down at your sides, palms facing forward. Breathe in slowly.

3. Breathe out as you slowly bend your elbows and lift weights toward your chest. Keep your elbows at your sides.

4. Hold the position for 1 second.

5. Breathe in as you slowly lower your arms.

6. Repeat 10–15 times.

7. Rest; then repeat 10–15 more times.

As you progress, use a heavier weight and alternate arms until you can lift the weight comfortably with both arms.

Wall push-up

These push-ups will strengthen your arms, shoulders, and chest. Try this exercise during a TV commercial break.

1. Face a wall, standing a little farther than arm's length away, feet shoulder-width apart.

2. Lean your body forward and put your palms flat against the wall at shoulder height and shoulder-width apart.

3. Slowly breathe in as you bend your elbows and lower your upper body toward the wall in a slow, controlled motion. Keep your feet flat on the floor.

4. Hold the position for 1 second.

5. Breathe out and slowly push yourself back until your arms are straight.

6. Repeat 10–15 times.

7. Rest; then repeat 10–15 more times.

FIGURE 4-4   (Continued)

Elbow extension

This exercise will strengthen your upper arms. If your shoulders aren't flexible enough to do this exercise, try the chair dip.

1. You can do this exercise while standing or sitting in a sturdy, armless chair.

2. Keep your feet flat on the floor, shoulder-width apart.

3. Hold a weight in one hand with palm facing inward. Raise that arm toward the ceiling.

4. Support this arm below your elbow with your other hand. Breathe in slowly.

5. Slowly bend your raised arm at the elbow and bring the weight toward your shoulder.

6. Hold position for 1 second.

7. Breathe out and slowly straighten your arm over your head. Be careful not to lock your elbow.

8. Repeat 10–15 times.

9. Repeat 10–15 times with the other arm.

10. Repeat 10–15 more times with each arm.

If it's difficult for you to hold hand weights, try using wrist weights.

Chair dip

This pushing motion will strengthen your arm muscles even if you are not able to lift yourself up off the chair.

1. Sit in a sturdy chair with armrests with your feet flat on the floor, shoulder-width apart.

2. Lean slightly forward; keep your back and shoulders straight.

3. Grasp the arms of the chair with your hands next to you. Breathe in slowly.

4. Breathe out and use your arms to push your body slowly off the chair.

5. Hold the position for 1 second.

6. Breathe in as you slowly lower yourself back down.

7. Repeat 10–15 times.

8. Rest; then repeat 10–15 more times.

Back leg raise

This exercise strengthens your buttocks and lower back.

1. Stand behind a sturdy chair, holding on for balance. Breathe in slowly.

2. Breathe out and slowly lift one leg straight back without bending your knee or pointing your toes. Try not to lean forward. The leg you are standing on should be slightly bent.

3. Hold the position for 1 second.

4. Breathe in as you slowly lower your leg.

FIGURE 4-4   (Continued)

5. Repeat 10–15 times.

6. Repeat 10–15 times with the other leg.

7. Repeat 10–15 more times with each leg.

As you progress, you may want to add ankle weights.

Side leg raise

This exercise strengthens hips, thighs, and buttocks.

1. Stand behind a sturdy chair with your feet slightly apart, holding on for balance. Breathe in slowly.

2. Breathe out and slowly lift one leg out to the side. Keep your back straight and your toes facing forward. The leg you are standing on should be slightly bent.

3. Hold the position for 1 second.

4. Breathe in as you slowly lower your leg.

5. Repeat 10–15 times.

6. Repeat 10–15 times with the other leg.

7. Repeat 10–15 more times with each leg.

As you progress, you may want to add ankle weights.

Knee curl

Walking and climbing stairs are easier when you do both the knee curl and leg straightening exercises.

1. Stand behind a sturdy chair, holding on for balance. Lift one leg straight back without bending your knee or pointing your toes. Breathe in slowly.

2. Breathe out as you slowly bring your heel up toward your buttocks as far as possible. Bend only from your knee, and keep your hips still. The leg you are standing on should be slightly bent.

3. Hold the position for 1 second.

4. Breathe in as you slowly lower your foot to the floor.

5. Repeat 10–15 times.

6. Repeat 10–15 times with the other leg.

7. Repeat 10–15 more times with each leg.

As you progress, you may want to add ankle weights.

Leg straightening

This exercise strengthens your thighs and may reduce symptoms of arthritis of the knee.

1. Sit in a sturdy chair with your back supported by the chair. Only the balls of your feet and your toes should rest on the floor. Put a rolled bath towel at the edge of the chair under thighs for support. Breathe in slowly.

FIGURE 4-4   (Continued)

2. Breathe out and slowly extend one leg in front of you as straight as possible, but don't lock your knee.

3. Flex your foot to point your toes toward the ceiling. Hold the position for 1 second.

4. Breathe in as you slowly lower leg back down.

5. Repeat 10–15 times.

6. Repeat 10–15 times with the other leg.

7. Repeat 10–15 more times with each leg.

As you progress, you may want to add ankle weights.

Chair stand

This exercise, which strengthens your abdomen and thighs, will make it easier to get in and out of the car. If you have knee or back problems, talk with your doctor before trying this exercise.

1. Sit toward the front of a sturdy, armless chair with your knees bent and your feet flat on the floor, shoulder-width apart.

2. Lean back with your hands crossed over your chest. Keep your back and shoulders straight throughout the exercise. Breathe in slowly.

3. Breathe out and bring your upper body forward until sitting upright.

4. Extend your arms so they are parallel to the floor and slowly stand up.

5. Breathe in as you slowly sit down.

6. Repeat 10–15 times.

7. Rest; then repeat 10–15 more times.

People with back problems should start the exercise from the sitting upright position.

Toe stand

This exercise will help make walking easier by strengthening your calves and ankles, and as you progress, the exercise will help your balance.

1. Stand behind a sturdy chair, feet shoulder-width apart, holding on for balance. Breathe in slowly.

2. Breathe out and slowly stand on your tiptoes, as high as possible.

3. Hold the position for 1 second.

4. Breathe in as you slowly lower your heels to the floor.

5. Repeat 10–15 times.

6. Rest; then repeat 10–15 more times.

As you progress, try doing the exercise standing on one leg at a time for a total of 10–15 times on each leg.

FIGURE 4-4   (Continued)

Topic Area: Sexually Transmitted Diseases

The earlier discussion of HIV/AIDS touched upon a number of issues relevant here. Promotion of safe sex tactics and education of clients about the prevalence of STDs are key points to risk reduction. Many STDs will be unfamiliar to clients at risk for them, including pelvic inflammatory disease and congenital syphilis. Reduction of *Chlamydia*, gonorrhea, syphilis, genital herpes, and human papillomavirus infection are specific goals of the Healthy People 2020 initiative.

Topic Area: Substance Abuse

Substance abuse is a large and complex topic. Use of alcohol and illicit drugs and misuse of legally or illegally obtained prescription medications are all encompassed in this category. Individuals may have an addiction problem, or they may use drugs recreationally without awareness of the health impacts. Adolescent drug use may impair brain development (Winters, 2008). Health can be directly affected by conditions brought on by substance abuse, including liver damage, overdose, neurologic damage related to drug–drug and drug–alcohol interactions, withdrawal symptoms, and drug-related deaths. Indirect health effects include risks associated with driving while intoxicated (or riding with an intoxicated driver); transmission of HIV, hepatitis C virus, and other infectious diseases by intravenous drug users who share needles; vulnerability to violence while obtaining or using drugs; and heightened risk of sexual assault for intoxicated individuals. Drug or alcohol use may also significantly affect a client's ability to make changes or engage in health promotion activities related to other health issues. Addressing addiction problems is one key factor in helping the client move to greater health and wellness.

The objectives of Healthy People 2020 pertaining to substance abuse include:

- Increasing the number of those who need alcohol/drug treatment who actually receive treatment
- Increasing the number of those who are referred for follow-up care for alcohol problems, drug problems after diagnosis, or treatment for one of these conditions in a hospital emergency department
- Decreasing the number of adults who drank excessively in the previous 30 days
- Reducing nonmedical use of prescription drugs
- Reducing the rate of impaired driving

Topic Area: Tobacco Use

Tobacco use (cigarettes, cigars, and chewing and pipe tobacco) has become widely known as a major risk factor for a wide range of health concerns, most particularly lung and oral cancers. Nevertheless, it continues to be widespread despite high-profile antismoking campaigns. Familial and peer behaviors tend to be strong influencing factors in an individual's decision to take up smoking, whether the addictive nature of tobacco (and the related health concerns) are known or not (Giovino, Henningfield, Tomar, Escobedo, & Slade, 1995; Kennedy, Tucker, Pollard, Go, & Green, 2011). Some of the same factors that motivate people to start can also motivate them to quit tobacco use, particularly when coupled with concern for health and sociocultural factors favoring nonsmoking (Bowen & Kurz, 2011).

Smoking cessation is difficult. Particularly in women, concerns about weight gain, nicotine cravings, irritability, insomnia, anxiety, and depression are frequently expressed or used as a rationale for not quitting (Allen, Allen, & Pomerleau, 2009; Perkins 2001; Perkins, Levine, Marcus, & Shiffman, 1997). Smokers who have attempted to quit and failed previously may be discouraged by past failure and reluctant to try again, not realizing that a majority of those who quit successfully usually must fail at least once, if not multiple times, before succeeding (American Lung Association, 2009). Using motivational interviewing (discussed earlier in this chapter) may be helpful, and FIGURE 4-5 provides some tips for helping clients quit smoking.

1.	Keep a notebook of current and past successes. Use the list as a reminder of your ability to succeed in new ventures.
2.	Identify a personal reason for quitting, not something the client should do because it's bad for him or her.
3.	Make a list of things that are personally pleasurable. Choose one as a reward (instead of a cigarette) when you are feeling uncomfortable or bored.
4.	Make a list of reasons you began smoking and compare that with a list of current reasons for smoking.
5.	Write down all the missed opportunities that you regret; choose one that is reachable and take action on it.
6.	Keep a log of each cigarette lit, including purpose (to get up, get to work, to relax, to appear calm, to celebrate, to quell hunger, after sex, after eating, etc.), focus on smoking the cigarette and the sensations that occur during and after smoking.
7.	Write a list of stress enhancers. Learn structure relaxation and stress reduction approaches or buy a stress reduction tape and listen to it at least twice a day (when you get up and when you go to bed) to deal with each stressor.

FIGURE 4-5 Quitting Smoking   *(continues)*
© Carolyn Chambers Clark, 2012.

8.	When using cigarettes as an energizer, substitute six small high-protein meals, sufficient sleep, a glass of milk, a piece of fresh fruit, fruit or vegetable juice, exercise, or movement, or dance or listen to a relaxation CD.
9.	End all meals with foods not associated with smoking; e.g., a glass of milk or half a grapefruit rather than a cup of coffee or a drink.
10.	Switch to noncaffeinated coffee or a cereal beverage by mixing caffeinated coffee with either one and then gradually over a week or two, adding more decaffeinated beverage.
11.	Eat a couple of sunflower seeds or chew licorice instead of having a cigarette.
12.	Eat more foods that leave the body alkaline and reduce the urge to smoke, such as vegetables, seeds, and fruits.
13.	Use affirmations, such as "I no longer smoke," "I can quit," "It's getting easier and easier to quit smoking," or "It's getting easier and easier to think about quitting smoking."
14.	Use deep breathing (from the abdomen) when the urge for a cigarette occurs.
15.	Work with a peer who can be called for positive feedback when the urge for a cigarette occurs. Ask that person to say the affirmations in No. 13 to you over and over until you believe them.
16.	Stay away from friends who smoke and from places where people smoke.
17.	Buy different brands of cigarettes and avoid smoking two packs of the same brand in a row.
18.	Buy cigarettes only by the pack, not by the carton.
19.	Smoke with the opposite hand from the one you usually use.
20.	Brush your teeth right after eating.
21.	Put your cigarettes in unfamiliar places.
22.	Every time you reach for a cigarette, ask, "Do I really want this cigarette?" "Do I really need a cigarette?" "What can I do instead of smoking this cigarette?"
23.	Develop and practice responses to peer pressure to smoke, including comments such as, "Come on, one won't hurt," "Smoking makes you independent, like an adult," "Here, have one," "Are you a sissy?"
24.	Take an assertiveness course online or at a community center to develop the skill of saying, "No!"
25.	Tell six people, "I quit smoking, and it was easy."

FIGURE 4-5   (Continued)

26.	Ask friends and coworkers not to leave cigarettes around or offer them to you.
27.	When the urge to smoke occurs, picture the word *STOP* in big red letters.
28.	Ask for a hug instead of having a cigarette.
29.	Choose a moment to quit smoking when peak mental or physical performance is not expected.
30.	Write and sign a contract with a trusted person so continuing to smoke will prove embarrassing or will result in great loss.
31.	Read articles and books by people who have successfully quit smoking or helped others to do so.
32.	To prevent weight gain, switch to low-fat foods, and eat fresh fruit or a handful of raw nuts or a tablespoon of peanut butter for snacks.
33.	When feeling depressed, talk with people who have successfully quit smoking and ask for information about why they are glad they quit.
34.	Chew gum or suck on xylitol-sweetened mints to quell the urge to smoke.
35.	Go to the morgue and look at someone who died from lung cancer.
36.	Talk to someone in the hospital who has incurable lung cancer about the course of the disease; get to know what that individual is like as a person.

FIGURE 4-5   (Continued)

Topic Area: Vision

The final topic area is vision, with objectives in *Healthy People 2020* focusing on increasing the percentage of individuals who receive comprehensive vision screening, reducing blindness and visual impairment in children 17 and under, reducing occupational eye injuries by increasing the use of personal protective eyewear in recreational and home activities, and increasing vision rehabilitation. Other objectives seek reduction in uncorrected visual impairment due to refractive error and in visual impairment overall.

Many of these objectives are related to the need for regular eye care—something many people who do not require corrective lenses often do not get. While those who wear corrective contact lenses must get a vision exam in order to receive a prescription, individuals who choose glasses can go years without follow-up examinations, which can result in incorrect prescriptions if they continue to have eye changes but do not receive new lenses. But eye exams are not simply about making sure a nearsighted or farsighted person gets corrective lenses—they are also opportunities to detect conditions such as macular

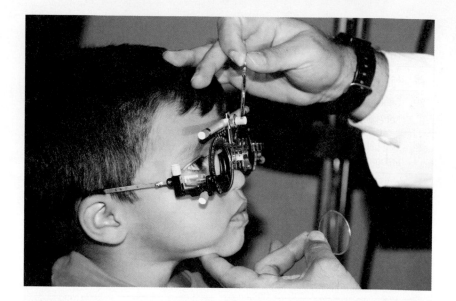

degeneration, glaucoma, cataracts, or retinopathies that offer an acute threat to vision. Individuals who do not receive regular care may be at risk of these disorders without realizing it. Educating and encouraging clients to visit an optometrist annually are primary factors in promotion of vision health.

Summary

Good physical health can be defined in accordance with the correct functioning of organs and tissues as well as the ability of individuals to support this functioning. When promoting physical health, promote client engagement in identifying and developing health goals and respect client input.

Key questions you should answer to help a client create a physical health plan are:

1. What are the client's key health issues?
2. What knowledge or understanding is needed to help improve client health?
3. What is the client's capacity to learn or accept new ideas, habits, or methods for self-management of health?
4. How motivated is the client to make changes for health promotion, and if motivation is absent or low, how can it be increased?
5. What forms of family and social support are available to the client to aid in health promotion activities?
6. What are the client's health goals?

Identify factors that limit an individual's ability to maintain health so that obstacles to health promotion planning can be addressed. Such obstacles include lack of information, incorrect information, or lack of concern regarding the health condition being addressed; strong emotions about the diagnosis; experiencing or believing stigmas and stereotypes about the disease; physical inability to make necessary changes; psychological or cultural barriers to making necessary changes; low or absent motivation to make needed changes; lack of familial/social support for making needed changes; and reluctance to engage in developing and implementing a health promotion plan. Use motivational interviewing to help clients succeed with their health goals.

The Healthy People 2020 initiative identifies a number of areas of concern for health promotion efforts, including:

- Access to health services
- Adolescent health
- Arthritis, osteoporosis, and chronic back conditions
- Blood disorders and blood safety
- Cancer
- Chronic kidney disease
- Diabetes
- Disability and secondary conditions
- Early and middle childhood
- Environmental health
- Family planning
- Food safety
- Genomics
- Hearing and communication disorders
- Heart disease and stroke
- HIV
- Immunization and infectious diseases
- Injury and violence prevention
- Maternal and infant health
- Mental health disorders (physical impacts)
- Nutrition and weight status
- Older adults
- Oral health
- Physical activity and fitness
- Sexually transmitted diseases
- Substance abuse
- Tobacco use
- Vision

REVIEW QUESTIONS

www

1. Health disparities are
   a. Adverse effects on groups of people who have significantly greater obstacles for health than the general population
   b. The results of specific activities or outcomes to be achieved over a stated period of time; they are specific, measurable, and realistic
   c. Campaigns and services that promote individual and community health

2. Objectives are
   a. Adverse effects on groups of people who have significantly greater obstacles for health than the general population
   b. The results of specific activities or outcomes to be achieved over a stated period of time; they are specific, measurable, and realistic
   c. Campaigns and services that promote individual and community health

3. Health is
   a. An approach that covers measures not only to prevent occurrence of disease, but also to arrest its progress
   b. A condition of well-being, free of disease or infirmity, and a basic human right
   c. Alternatives ranked according to feasibility, value, and/or importance

4. One of the new topic areas for Healthy People 2020 is
   a. HIV
   b. Family planning
   c. Genomics

5. All of the following are overarching goals of Healthy People 2020 except
   a. Attain high quality, longer lives free of preventable disease, disability, injury, and premature death
   b. Create social and physical environments that promote good health for all
   c. Achieve access to preventive services for all Americans

6. Concepts included in the Healthy People 2010 conceptual map include
   a. Biology
   b. Physical environment
   c. Policies and interventions
   d. All of the above

EXERCISES

1. Conduct a literature review on the relationship between social support and health. Summarize what you find in a brief paper.

2. Contact the health department in your county and the local hospital about the types and incidence of healthcare-related infections. Present this information to your class.

3. Visit your local blood bank and ask them about input into the *Healthy People 2020* document. Summarize the current issues of concern for blood banks.

4. Select a focus area of the *Healthy People 2020* document that you are especially interested in. Investigate the progress in refining of objectives which has occurred for this area.

REFERENCES

Ackroyd-Stolarz, S., Guernsey, J. R., Mackinnon, N. J., & Kovacs, G. (2011). The association between a prolonged stay in the emergency department and adverse events in older patients admitted to hospital: A retrospective cohort study. *British Medical Journal of Quality and Safety 20*, 564–569.

Aggleton, P., Yankah, E., & Crewe, M. (2011). Education and HIV/AIDS-30 years on. *AIDS Education and Prevention, 23*(6), 495–507.

Aida, J., Kondo, K., Yamamoto, T., Hirai, H., Nakade, M., Osaka, K., . . . Watt, R. (2011). Oral health and cancer, cardiovascular, and respiratory mortality of Japanese. *Journal of Dental Research, 90*(9), 1129–1135.

Allen, S. S., Allen, A. M., Pomerleau, C. S. (2009). Influence of phase-related variability in premenstrual symptomatology, mood, smoking withdrawal, and smoking behavior during ad libitum smoking, on smoking cessation outcome. *Addictive Behaviors, 34*(1), 107–711.

American College of Physicians. (2006). The impending collapse of primary care medicine and its implications for the state of the nation's health care. Retrieved from http://www .acponline.org/advocacy/events/state_of_healthcare/statehc06_1.pdf

American Lung Association. (2009, September 30). Most smokers make multiple quit attempts before they quit smoking for good. [Press release.] Retrieved from http:// www.lungusa.org/press-room/press-releases/lung-assn-launches-quitter-in-you.html

Anzuini, F., Battistella, A., & Izzotti, A. (2011). Physical activity and cancer prevention: A review of current evidence and biological mechanisms. *Preventive Medicine & Hygiene, 52*(4), 174–180.

Belstrøm, D., Damgaard, C., Nielsen, C. H., & Holmstrup, P. (2011). Does a causal relation between cardiovascular disease and periodontitis exist? *Microbes and Infection, 14*(5), 411–418.

Bernstein, S. L., Aronsky, D., Duseja, R., Epstein, S., Handel, D., Hwang U., . . . Asplin, B. R. (2009). The effect of emergency department crowding on clinically oriented outcomes. *Academic Emergency Medicine, 16*(1), 1–10.

Bodenheimer, T. (2006). Primary care—will it survive? *New England Journal of Medicine, 355,* 861–864.

Bowen, S., & Kurz, A. S. (2011). Smoking, nicotine dependence, and motives to quit in Asian American versus Caucasian college students. *Nicotine and Tobacco Research*, doi: 10.1093/ntr/ntr281

Bunn, J. Y., Solomon, S. E., Miller, C., & Forehand, R. (2007). Measurement of stigma in people with HIV: A reexamination of the HIV Stigma Scale. *AIDS Education and Prevention, 19*(3), 198–208.

Cabrero, E., Griffa, L., & Burgos, A., for the HIV Body Physical Changes Study Group. (2010). Prevalence and impact of body physical changes in HIV patients treated with highly active antiretroviral therapy: Results from a study on patient and physician perceptions. *AIDS Patient Care STDS, 24*(1), 5–13.

Chacko, S., Sul, J., Song, Y., Li, X., LeBlanc, J., You, Y., . . . Liu, S. (2011). Magnesium supplementation, metabolic and inflammatory markers, and global genomic and proteomic profiling: A randomized, double-blind, controlled, crossover trial in overweight individuals. *American Journal of Clinical Nutrition, 93*(2), 463–473. Abstract retrieved from http://www.ncbi.nlm.nih.gov/pubmed/21159786

Christensen, P., Bartels, E. M., Riecke, B. F., Bliddal, H., Leeds, A. R., Astrup A., . . . Christensen, R. (2011). Improved nutritional status and bone health after diet-induced weight loss in sedentary osteoarthritis patients: A prospective cohort study. *European Journal of Clinical Nutrition, 66*(4), 504–509.

Churilla, J. R., Magyari, P. M., Ford, E. S., Fitzhugh, E. C., & Johnson, T. M. (2011). Muscular strengthening activity patterns and metabolic health risk among U.S. adults. *Journal of Diabetes, 4*(1), 77–84.

Chyu, M. C., von Bergen, V., Brismée, J. M., Zhang, Y., Yeh, J. K., & Shen, C. L. (2011). Complementary and alternative exercises for management of osteoarthritis. *Arthritis.* 2011:364319.

Clowes, R., & Masser, B. M. (2011). Right here, right now: The impact of the blood donation context on anxiety, attitudes, subjective norms, self-efficacy, and intention to donate blood. *Transfusion.* Advance online publication. doi:10.1111/j.1537-2995.2011.03486.x

Congressional Budget Office, United States Congress. (1992). *Factors contributing to the infant mortality ranking of the United States.* Washington, DC: Author. Retrieved from http://www.cbo.gov/ftpdocs/62xx/doc6219/doc05b.pdf

Cook, R. J., Erdman, J. N., Hevia, M., & Dickens, B. M. (2008). Prenatal management of anencephaly. *International Journal Gynaecology and Obstetrics, 102*(3), 304–308.

Dale, K., McAuley, K. A., Taylor, R. W., Williams, S. M., Farmer, V. L., Hansen, P., . . . Mann, J. (2009). Determining optimal approaches for weight maintenance: A randomized controlled trial. *Canadian Medical Association Journal, 180*(10), E39–E46. Retrieved from http://www.cmaj.ca/cgi/content/full/180/10/E39

Darukhanavala, A., Booth, J. N., 3rd, Bromley, L., Whitmore, H., Imperial, J., & Penev, P. D. (2011). Changes in insulin secretion and action in adults with familial risk for type 2 diabetes who curtail their sleep. *Diabetes Care, 34*(10), 2259–2264.

Deschenes, O., & E. Moretti. (2007). Extreme weather events, mortality, and migration. NBER working paper No. w13227. Retrieved from http://www.econ.berkeley.edu/~moretti/weather_mortality

Deshmukh-Taskar, P. R., Nicklas, T. A., O'Neil, C. E., Keast, D. R., Radcliffe, J. D., & Cho, S. (2010). The relationship of breakfast skipping and type of breakfast consumption with nutrient intake and weight status in children and adolescents: The National Health and Nutrition Examination Survey 1999–2006. *Journal of the American Dietetic Association, 110*(6), 869–878.

Dhainaut, J.-F., Claessens, Y.-E., Ginsburg, C., & Riou, B. (2004). Unprecedented heat-related deaths during the 2003 heat wave in Paris: Consequences on emergency departments. *Critical Care, 8*(1), 1–2.

Dodd, R. (2009). Managing the microbiological safety of blood for transfusion: A US perspective. *Future Microbiology, 4*(7), 807–818.

Earnshaw, V. A., & Quinn, D. M. (2011). The impact of stigma in healthcare on people living with chronic illnesses. *Journal of Health Psychology, 17*(2), 157–168

Engebretson, J. C., & Headley, J. A. (2009). Cultural diversity and care. In B. M. Dossey & L. Keegan. (Eds.), *Holistic nursing: A handbook for practice* (pp. 573–597). Sudbury, MA: Jones and Bartlett.

Erinosho, T. O., Moser, R. P., Oh, A. Y., Nebeling, L. C., & Yaroch, A. L. (2012). Awareness of the Fruits and Veggies—More Matters campaign, knowledge of the fruit and vegetable recommendation, and fruit and vegetable intake of adults in the 2007 Food Attitudes and Behaviors (FAB) Survey. *Appetite.* Advance online publication.

Fahey, T. D. (1998). Adaptation to exercise: Progressive resistance exercise. In T. D. Fahey (Ed.), *Encyclopedia of sports medicine and science.* Retrieved from http://sportsci.org

Farooqi, I. S. (2011). Genetic, molecular and physiological insights into human obesity. *European Journal of Clinical Investigation, 41*(4), 451–455.

Foltz, J. L., Cook, S. R., Szilagyi, P. G., Auinger, P., Stewart, P. A., Bucher, S., & Baldwin, C. D. (2011). UA adolescent nutrition, exercise, and screen time baseline levels prior to national recommendations. *Clinical Pediatrics (Phila), 50*(5), 424–433.

Foster, G., Makris, A. P., & Bailer, B. A. (2005). Behavioral treatment of obesity. *American Journal of Clinical Nutrition, 82*(Suppl.), 230S–235S. Retrieved from http://www.ajcn .org/cgi/content/full/82/1/230S

Fradin, D., & Bougnères, P. (2011). T2DM: Why epigenetics? *Journal of Nutrition and Metabolism*, 2011:647514.

Garriguet, D. (2011). Bone health: Osteoporosis, calcium and vitamin D. *Health Reports, 22*(3), 7–14.

Gill, A., Womack, R., & Safranek, S. (2010). Clinical inquiries: Does exercise alleviate symptoms of depression? *Journal of Family Practice, 59*(9), 530–531.

Giovino, G. A., Henningfield, J. E., Tomar, S. L., Escobedo, L. G., & Slade, J. (1995). Epidemiology of tobacco use and dependence. *Epidemiologic Reviews, 17*(1), 48–65.

Gonzalez, A., Miller, C. T., Solomon, S. E., Bunn, J. Y., & Cassidy, D. G. (2009). Size matters: Community size, HIV stigma, & gender differences. *AIDS and Behavior, 13*(6), 1205–1212.

Goodnough, L. T. (2011). Operational, quality, and risk management in the transfusion service: Lessons learned. *Transfusion Medicine Reviews.* Advance online publication.

Gowda, S., Goldblum, O. M., McCall, W. V., & Feldman, S. R. (2010). Factors affecting sleep quality in patients with psoriasis. *Journal of the American Academy of Dermatology, 63*(1), 114–123.

Graber, J. M., Macdonald, S. C., Kass, D. E., Smith, A. E., & Anderson, H. A. (2007). Carbon monoxide: The case for environmental public health surveillance. *Public Health Reports, 122*(2), 138–144.

Grimm, E., & Steinle, N. (2010). Genetics of eating behavior: Established and emerging concepts. *Nutrition Reviews, 69*(1), 52–60. Retrieved from http://onlinelibrary.wiley .com/doi/10.1111/j.1753-4887.2010.00361.x/full

Groft, J. N., & Robinson Vollman, A. (2007). Seeking serenity: Living with HIV/AIDS in rural western Canada. *Rural Remote Health, 7*(2), 677.

Gurd, V. (2007). Which plastic bottles don't leach chemicals? Retrieved from http://trusted.md/blog/vreni_gurd/2007/03/29/plastic_water_bottles#axzz1wP0cckBp

Guttman, A., Schull, M. J., Vermeulen, M. J., & Stukel, T. A. (2011). Association between waiting times and short term mortality and hospital admission after departure from emergency department: Population based cohort study from Ontario, Canada. *British Medical Journal, 342*, d2983.

Hardy, L. L., Denney-Wilson, E., Thrift, A. P., Okely, A. D., & Baur, L. A. (2010). Screen time and metabolic risk factors among adolescents. *Archives of Pediatrics and Adolescent Medicine, 164*(7), 643–649.

Harmon, K. (2011, June 2). Pyramid versus plate: What should the USDA's food chart look like? *Scientific American*. Retrieved from http://www.scientificamerican.com/article.cfm?id=usda-food-plate

Haven, J., Burns, A., Herring, D., & Britten, P. (2006). MyPyramid.gov provides consumers with practical nutrition information at their fingertips. *Journal of Nutrition Education and Behavior, 38*(6 Suppl), S153–S154.

Hogan, M. C., Foreman, K. J., Naghavi, M., Ahn, S. Y., Wang, M., Makela, S. M., . . . Murray, C. J. (2010). Maternal mortality for 181 countries, 1980–2008: A systematic analysis of progress towards millennium development goal 5. *The Lancet, 375*, 1609–1623.

Holmlund, A., Holm, G., Lind, L. (2010). Number of teeth as a predictor of cardiovascular mortality in a cohort of 7,674 subjects followed for 12 years. *Journal of Periodontology, 81*(6), 870–876.

Ito, S. (2011). Cardiorenal connection in chronic kidney disease. *Clinical and Experimental Nephrology*. Advance online publication.

James, C. A., Hart, T. A., Roberts, K. E., Ghai, A., Petrovic, B., & Lima, M. D. (2011). Religion versus ethnicity as predictors of unprotected vaginal intercourse among young adults. *Sex Health, 8*(3), 363–371.

Kennedy, D. P., Tucker, J. S., Pollard, M. S., Go, M. H., & Green, H. D., Jr. (2011). Adolescent romantic relationships and change in smoking status. *Addictive Behaviors, 36*(4), 320–326.

Kim, B. (2008). Thyroid hormone as a determinant of energy expenditure and the basal metabolic rate. *Thyroid, 18*(2), 141–144. Abstract retrieved from http://www.ncbi.nlm.nih.gov/pubmed/18279014

Kottke, T. E., & Isham, G. J. (2010). Measuring health care access and quality to improve health in populations. *Preventing Chronic Disease, 7*(4), A73.

Krishnan, A. V., Trump, D. L., Johnson, C. S., & Feldman, D. (2012). The role of vitamin D in cancer prevention and treatment. *Rheumatic Disease Clinics of North America, 38*(1), 161–178.

Laumbach, R. J., & Kipen, H. M. (2012). Respiratory health effects of air pollution: Update on biomass smoke and traffic pollution. *Journal of Allergy and Clinical Immunology, 129*(1), 3–11.

Lee, H. P., Li, T. M., Tsao, J. Y., Fong, Y. C., & Tang, C. H. (2012). Curcumin induces cell apoptosis in human chondrosarcoma through extrinsic death receptor pathway. *International Immunopharmacology, 13*(2), 163–169.

Lev–Ran, A. (2001). Human obesity: An evolutionary approach to understanding our bulging waistline. *Diabetes Metabolism, 17*(5), 347–362. Abstract retrieved from http://onlinelibrary.wiley.com/doi/10.1002/dmrr.230/abstract

Manninen, A. (2004). Is a calorie really a calorie? Metabolic advantage of low-carbohydrate diets. *Journal of the International Society of Sports Nutrition, 1*(2), 21–26. Retrieved from http://www.pubmedcentral.nih.gov/articlerender.fcgi?artid=2129158#B9

Miller, W. R., & Rollnick, S. (2002). *Motivational interviewing: Preparing people for change (2nd ed.)*. New York, NY: Guilford Press.

Millett, G. A., Ding, H., Marks, G., Jeffries, W. L., 4th, Bingham, T., Lauby, J., . . . Stueve A. (2011). Mistaken assumptions and missed opportunities: Correlates of undiagnosed HIV infection among black and Latino men who have sex with men. *Journal of Acquired Immune Deficiency Syndromes, 58*(1), 64–71.

Mold, F., & Forbes, A. (2011). Patients' and professionals' experiences and perspectives of obesity in health-care settings: A synthesis of current research. *Health Expectations.* Advance online publication. doi:10.1111/j.1369-7625.2011.00699.x

Moore, R. D. (2011). Epidemiology of HIV infection in the United States: Implications for linkage to care. *Clinical Infectious Diseases, 52*(Suppl 2), S208–S213.

Morgan, A. R. (2011). Determining genetic risk factors for pediatric type 2 diabetes. *Current Diabetes Reports.* Advance online publication.

Muturi, N., & An, S. (2010). HIV/AIDS stigma and religiosity among African American women. *Journal of Health Communication, 15*(4), 388–401.

Parra, P., Palou, A., & Serra, F. (2010). Moderate doses of conjugated linoleic acid isomers mix contribute to lowering body fat content maintaining insulin sensitivity and a noninflammatory pattern in adipose tissue in mice. *Journal of Nutritional Biochemistry, 21*(2), 107–115. Abstract retrieved from http://www.ncbi.nlm.nih.gov/pubmed/19195867

Patrick, K., Norman, G. J., Calfas, K. J., Sallis, J. F., Zabinski, M. F., Rupp, J., & Cella, J. (2004). Diet, physical activity, and sedentary behaviors as risk factors for overweight in adolescence. *Archives of Pediatric and Adolescent Medicine, 158*(4), 385–390.

Perkins, K. A. (2001). Smoking cessation in women. Special considerations. *CNS Drugs, 15*(5), 391–411.

Perkins, K. A., Levine, M. D., Marcus, M. D., & Shiffman, S. (1997). Addressing women's concerns about weight gain due to smoking cessation. *Journal of Substance Abuse Treatment, 14*(2), 173–182.

Peterson, M. D., Pistilli, E., Haff, G. G., Hoffman, E. P., & Gordon, P. M. (2011). Progression of volume load and muscular adaptation during resistance exercise. *European Journal of Applied Physiology, 111*(6), 1063–1071.

Qi, L., Cornelis, M. C., Zhang, C., van Dam, R. M., & Hu, F. B. (2009). Genetic predisposition, Western dietary pattern, and the risk of type 2 diabetes in men. *American Journal of Clinical Nutrition, 89*(5), 1453–1458.

Rai, M. F., & Sandell, L. J. (2011). Inflammatory mediators: Tracing links between obesity and osteoarthritis. *Critical Reviews in Eukaryotic Gene Expression, 21*(2), 131–142.

Riecke, B. F, Christensen, R., Christensen, P., Leeds, A. R., Boesen, M., Lohmander, L. S., . . . Bliddal, H. (2010). Comparing two low-energy diets for the treatment of knee osteoarthritis symptoms in obese patients: A pragmatic randomized clinical trial. *Osteoarthritis Cartilage, 18*(6), 746–754.

Ritter, L., Solomon, K., Sibley, P., Hall, K., Keen, P., Mattu, G., & Linton, B. (2002). Sources, pathways, and relative risks of contaminants in surface water and groundwater: A perspective prepared for the Walkerton inquiry. *Journal of Toxicology and Environmental Health. Part A, 65*(1), 1–142.

Rollnick, S., Miller, W. R., & Butler, C. (2008). *Motivational interviewing in health care: Helping patients change behavior.* New York, NY: Guilford Press.

Ryan, S., Taylor, C. T., & McNicholas, W. T. (2009). Systemic inflammation: A key factor in the pathogenesis of cardiovascular complications in obstructive sleep apnoea syndrome? *Postgraduate Medical Journal, 85*(1010), 693–698.

Saleh, L. D., Operario, D., Smith, C. D., Arnold, E., & Kegeles, S. (2011). We're going to have to cut loose some of our personal beliefs: Barriers and opportunities in providing HIV prevention to African American men who have sex with men and women. *AIDS Education and Prevention, 23*(6), 521–532.

Sauni, R., Uitti, J., Jauhiainen, M., Kreiss, K., Sigsgaard, T., & Verbeek, J. H. (2011). Remediating buildings damaged by dampness and mould for preventing or reducing respiratory tract symptoms, infections and asthma. *Cochrane Database System of Reviews.* 9:CD007897.

Selfe, T. K., & Innes, K. E. (2009). Mind-body therapies and osteoarthritis of the knee. *Current Rheumatology Reviews, 5*(4), 204–211.

Sengupta, S., Banks, B., Jonas, D., Miles, M. S., & Smith, G. C. (2011). HIV interventions to reduce HIV/AIDS stigma: A systematic review. *AIDS and Behavior, 15*(6), 1075–1087.

Shahar, D. R., Schwarzfuchs, D., Fraser, D., Vardi, H., Thiery, J., Fiedler, G. M., . . . Shai, I., DIRECT Group. (2010). Dairy calcium intake, serum vitamin D, and successful weight loss. *American Journal of Clinical Nutrition, 92*(5), 1017–1022.

Shelnutt, K. P., Bobroff, L. B., & Diehl, D. C. (2009). MyPyramid for older adults. *Journal of Nutrition Education and Behavior, 41*(4), 300–302.

Sinaki, M., Pfeifer, M., Preisinger, E., Itoi, E., Rizzoli, R., Boonen, S., . . . Minne, H. W. (2010). The role of exercise in the treatment of osteoporosis. *Current Osteoporosis Reports, 8*(3), 138–144.

Spero, D. (2006). *Diabetes: Sugar-coated crisis.* Gabriola Island, BC, Canada: New Society Publishers.

Spiegel, K., Tasali, E., Leproult, R., & Van Cauter, E. (2009). Effects of poor and short sleep on glucose metabolism and obesity risk. *Nature Reviews. Endocrinology, 5*(5), 253–261. Retrieved from http://www.ncbi.nlm.nih.gov/pubmed/19444258

Sundram, V., Chauhan, S. C., Ebeling, M., & Jaggi, M. (2012). Curcumin attenuates ß-catenin signaling in prostate cancer cells through activation of protein kinase D1. *PLoS One, 7*(4),e35368.

Teixeira, M. E., & Budd, G. M. (2010). Obesity stigma: A newly recognized barrier to comprehensive and effective type 2 diabetes management. *Journal of the American Academy of Nurse Practitioners, 22*(10), 527–533.

Tsai, M. H., Hsu, J. F., Chou, W. J., Yang, C. P., Jaing, T. H., Hung, I. J., . . . Huang, Y. S. (2012). Psychosocial and emotional adjustment for children with pediatric cancer and their primary caregivers and the impact on their health-related quality of life during the first 6 months. *Quality of Life Research.* Advance online publication.

Urban, L., Dallal, G., Robinson, L., Ausman, L., Saltzman, E., & Roberts, S. (2010). The accuracy of stated energy contents of reduced-energy, commercially prepared foods. *Journal of the American Dietetic Association, 110*(1), 116. doi:10.1016/j.jada.2009.10.003

U.S. Central Intelligence Agency. (n.d.). Country comparisons: Infant mortality rate. In *The world factbook.* Retrieved from https://www.cia.gov/library/publications/the-world-factbook/rankorder/2091rank.html

U.S. Department of Health and Human Services. (2010). Do I need a special diet as I approach menopause? Retrieved from http://www.womenshealth.gov/publications/our-publications/fact-sheet/menopause-treatment.cfm

Veldhuizen, I., Ferguson, E., de Kort, W., Donders, R., & Atsma, F. (2011). Exploring the dynamics of the theory of planned behavior in the context of blood donation: Does donation experience make a difference? *Transfusion, 51*(11), 2425–2437.

Wagner, M., & Oehlmann, J. (2011). Endocrine disruptors in bottled mineral water: Estrogenic activity in the E-Screen. *Journal of Steroid Biochemistry and Molecular Biology, 127*(1–2), 128–135.

Walsh, E. (2010). Interleukin Genetics, Inc., and Stanford University report genetic test improves weight loss success. Retrieved from http://www.ilgenetics.com/content/news-events/newsDetail.jsp/q/news-id/213

Waserman, S., & Watson, W. (2011). Food allergy. *Allergy, Asthma, and Clinical Immunology, 7*(Suppl 1), S7.

Watts, A., Crimmins, E. M., & Gatz, M. (2008). Inflammation as a potential mediator for the association between periodontal disease and Alzheimer's disease. *Neuropsychiatric Disease and Treatment, 4*(5), 865–876.

Wei, Y., Davis, J., & Bina, W. F. (2011). Ambient air pollution is associated with the increased incidence of breast cancer in US. *International Journal of Environmental Health Research*, pp. 1–10.

Winters, K. C. (2008). Adolescent brain development and drug abuse: A special report commissioned by the Treatment Research Institute. Philadelphia, PA: TRI. Retrieved from http://www.tresearch.org/archives/2008Jan_TeenBrain.pdf

Zukoski, A. P, Thorburn, S., & Stroud, J. (2011). Seeking information about HIV/AIDS: A qualitative study of health literacy among people living with HIV/AIDS in a low prevalence context. *AIDS Care, 23*(11), 1505–1508.

INTERNET RESOURCES

For a full suite of assignments and learning activities, use the access code located in the front of your book to visit this exclusive website: **http://go.jblearning.com/healthpromotion**. If you do not have an access code, you can obtain one at the site.

www.

Upon completion of this chapter, you will be able to:

1. Define mental health.

2. Explain how mental and physical health interrelate.

3. Discuss the importance of evidence-based research in mental health promotion.

4. Describe four common threads found in approaches to mental health.

5. Compare variables that affect mental health.

6. List elements to be included in a mental health promotion assessment.

7. Develop nursing interventions to promote mental health.

Evidence-based research

Meditation

Mental health

Mental health promotion

Music therapy

Self-esteem

Socioecologic approach

CHAPTER 5

Mental Health Promotion

http://go.jblearning.com/healthpromotion

www.

For a full suite of assignments and learning activities, use the access code located in the front of your book to visit the exclusive website: http://go.jblearning.com/healthpromotion If you do not have an access code, you can obtain one at the site.

Introduction

The purpose of this chapter is to identify what mental health is and explore strategies for integrating mental health promotion concepts into your practice as a health promotion role model.

What Is Mental Health?

In an online Q&A, the World Health Organization (WHO) answered the question, *What is mental health?* as follows:

> Mental health is not just the absence of mental disorder. It is defined as a state of well-being in which every individual realizes his or her own potential, can cope with the normal stresses of life, can work productively and fruitfully, and is able to make a contribution to her or his community. (WHO, 2007, p. 1)

In an earlier publication (WHO, 2004, p. 1), spirituality and healthy public policy were mentioned as important variables in individual, family, and/or community mental health.

It also issued this statement: "Mental health promotion is meant to foster activities in the field of mental health, especially those affecting the harmony of human relations." In the same manuscript, WHO participants noted that mental health can be affected by non-health policies such as education, housing, and child care. They also stated that it is impossible to be mentally healthy without a climate of safety and basic civil, political, cultural, economic, and social rights.

These objectives and functions of World Health Organization are at the core of our commitment to mental health promotion.

HEALTH PROMOTION CHALLENGE

Choose either spirituality or healthy public policy and develop a program to enhance mental health. Base it on evidence you find at www.pubmed.gov as well as Googling for mental health programs that address your choice. Share your findings with at least two other students and request feedback. If possible, implement at least one portion of your program and write up your results.

Variations on this theme can be found in other definitions. For example, a definition published on the University of Leeds Ahead4health website is:

> 'Mental health' properly describes a sense of well-being: the capacity to live in a resourceful and fulfilling manner, having the resilience to deal with the challenges and obstacles which life presents. (University of Leeds, 2006, p. 1)

Based on these definitions, **mental health** is part of a client's health and well-being, and it can have an impact on or be affected by physical illnesses. It may be difficult to determine where the mental health aspect starts and the physical health aspect ends. There is good reason for this difficulty: Mental health encompasses not only the structure and proper physiologic functioning of the brain, but also the psychological factors that shape behavior.

What Variables Affect Mental Health?

Many variables affect mental health. One variable important in many mental health promotion efforts is assertiveness/advocacy. Clients who are involved in the decision process about their own health can reap benefits (Pickett et al., 2012) found that clients involved in a peer-led education program that empowered mental health consumers increased their assertive/advocacy skills.

Exercise is correlated with positive mental health. In one study, participants in a four-week exercise program reported a beneficial decrease in perceived stress (Stavrakakis, de Jonge, Ormel, & Oldehinkel, 2012).

In another study (Mason & Holt, 2012) that examined why physical exercise is so helpful to mental health, the researchers found a high degree of congruence in support of the themes of social interaction and social support; feeling safe; improved symptoms; a sense of meaning, purpose, and achievement; identity; and the role of the facilitating personnel. They concluded that exercise

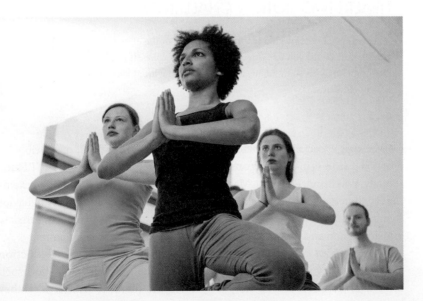

interventions deserve greater emphasis both theoretically and clinically, as many service users experience them as socially inclusive, non-stigmatising, and, above all, effective.

Yoga can also enhance mental health. Smith, Greer, Sheets, and Watson (2011) compared the physical and mental benefits of an exercise-based yoga practice to that of a more comprehensive yoga practice (one with an ethical/ spiritual component). They found that over time, participants in both the integrated and exercise yoga groups experienced decreased depression and stress, an increased sense of hopefulness, and increased flexibility compared to the control group. Only the integrated yoga group experienced decreased anxiety-related symptoms and decreased salivary cortisol (an indicant of reduced stress) from the beginning to the end of the study.

Exercise can even help individuals hospitalized in a forensic setting. In one study (Wynaden, Barr, Omari, & Fulton, 2012), a healthy lifestyle program, which included a formal exercise component, was introduced at the service. Participants reported that the program assisted them in managing their psychiatric symptoms, as well as improving their level of fitness, confidence, and self-esteem. In addition, all participants received education about the importance of regular exercise to their mental health and the role exercise plays in preventing chronic illness and obesity. While the benefits of exercise on mental health outcomes for people with depression and anxiety are well established, this research adds to the evidence that such programs provide similar benefits to individuals diagnosed with a psychotic illness who are hospitalized in an acute secure setting.

HEALTH PROMOTION CHALLENGE   ⭐   (www)

Based on what you learned from these studies of the effect of exercise on mental health, how could you use this information for yourself and with your clients?

Come up with some ideas, then share them with at least two classmates and ask for feedback.

Massage, especially combined with lavender aromatherapy, may help with emotional distress in clients in cancer/palliative care. According to the ToT Study (Serfaty, Wilkinson, Freeman, Mannix, & King, 2012), a controlled trial to examine the clinical effectiveness of aromatherapy massage versus cognitive behavior therapy, massage/aromatherapy produced significant results in reducing anxiety and depression and was as well-received as cognitive behavioral therapy.

One form of **meditation** called Mindfulness-Based Stress Reduction (MBSR) has a favorable influence both on biomarkers of stress regulation, such as cortisol secretion, and on sleep. MBSR teaches clients to witness what they are feeling or thinking, but not to immerse themselves in it. By stepping back from painful thoughts and feelings, relaxation and calm can reign and sleep can occur (Brand, Holsboer-Trachsler, Naranjo, & Schmidt, 2012)

Nutrition can affect mental health. Sugar can affect ability to think clearly and function. Ye, Gao, Scott, and Tucker (2011) investigated intake of added sugars. Intake of mainly fructose is associated with metabolic syndrome and type 2 diabetes. The objective of their analysis was to examine whether habitual intakes of total sugars, added sugars, sugar-sweetened beverages, or sweetened solid foods are associated with cognitive function. Greater intakes of total sugars, added sugars, and sugar-sweetened beverages were significantly associated with lower mental state score on the Mini-Mental State Examination (MMSE), indicating that sugar can affect mental health.

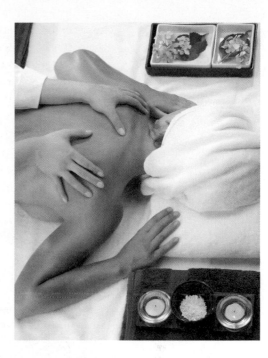

Hypovitaminosis D is associated with cognitive decline among older adults. The relationship between vitamin D intakes and cognitive decline is not well understood. A study conducted by Annweiler, Fantino, Schott, Krolak-Salmon, Allali, and Beauchet (2012) examined whether the dietary intake of vitamin D was an independent predictor of the onset of dementia within 7 years among women aged 75 years and older. They found that women with the lowest vitamin D dietary intakes were more likely to develop Alzheimer's Disease (AD). Women who ingested the highest level of vitamin D foods had a lower risk of AD.

An Australian study (Forsyth, Williams, & Deane, 2012) examined the nutrition status of primary care clients with depression and/or anxiety. The researchers found that although some participants were low in folate and calcium intake, only magnesium intakes were significantly associated with depression. The researchers concluded that nutrition recommendations for clients with depression and anxiety should be based on the Australian Guide to Healthy Eating, with particular attention to increasing intake of fruit, vegetables, and whole grains.

HEALTH PROMOTION CHALLENGE

Choose to either use the nutritional evidence presented here and plan a way to use it with clients or search www.pubmed.gov for more nutritional effects on mental health studies. Either way, share your findings with at least two other classmates and ask for feedback.

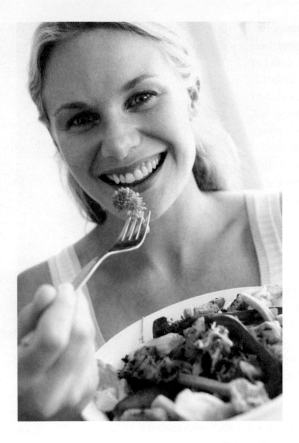

Another nutritional element important to mental health is the omega-3 family of fatty acids. Observational studies suggest an association between low concentrations of omega-3 family fatty acids (good sources include sardines, salmon, flax seeds, and walnuts) and greater risk for postpartum depression (PPD). The objective of a Brazilian study (da Rocha & Kac, 2012) was to investigate the effect of unbalanced dietary intake of omega-6/omega-3 (ratio >9:1) in the prevalence for postpartum depression. The results verified an association between omega-6/omega-3 ratio above 9:1, the levels recommended by the Institute of Medicine, and the prevalence of PPD. The results add to the evidence regarding the importance of omega-6 and omega-3 fatty acids in the regulation of mental health mechanisms.

Music therapy can improve the mental health of depressed clients. It may be effective because active music-making within a therapeutic frame offers clients the opportunity for new aesthetic, physical, and relational experiences (Maratos, Crawford, & Procter, 2011).

Reading a self-help manual can reduce psychological distress in people with depression. In one study, participants in psychological distress were assigned randomly to an intervention or control group. The intervention group participants were given a self-help manual in addition to standard care and treatment while the control group received standard care and treatment. Psychological distress was measured with the Kessler Psychological Distress Scale. The findings affirm the benefits of bibliotherapy or self-help therapy in book form in helping to reduce psychological distress in people with moderate depression. The approach is easy to use and can be incorporated as an adjunct to standard care and treatment. Bibliotherapy can be used by community mental health nurses and other clinicians to reduce psychological distress and self-control.

In a series of four experiments, Rounding, Lee, Jacobson, and Ji (2012) tested the idea that religion was a cultural adaptation necessary for promoting self-control, which in turn may be a psychological pillar of support for numerous psychological and behavioral actions. If this proposal is true, the researchers reasoned, then subtle reminders of religious concepts should result in higher levels of self-control. The researchers consistently found that when religious themes were made implicitly salient, people exercised greater self-control, which augmented their ability to make decisions in a number of behavioral domains. When self-control resources were minimized, making it difficult for people to exercise restraint on future unrelated self-control tasks, they found that by making implicit reminders of religious concepts, participants refueled their ability to exercise self-control.

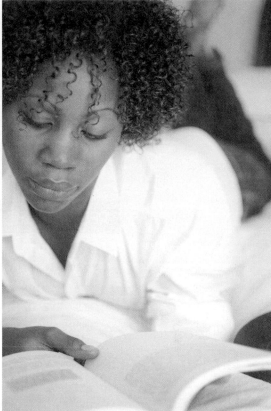

Self-efficacy is the belief you can achieve a task or goal. Individuals with high self-efficacy believe in themselves and their ability to function, a trait correlated with mental health. Bandura (1977), who originated the term, described four ways to improve self-efficacy:

1. Successful experiences
2. Observing other's successful experiences
3. Remembering positive encouragements from other people
4. Interpreting signs of distress, e.g., "butterflies in the stomach," as normal and unrelated to ability

A study in *Complementary Therapies in Clinical Practice,* by Dellmann and Lushington (2012), focused on how natural therapists enhance positive expectations in their clients by stressing their personal strengths and ability to achieve their goals (self-efficacy).

HEALTH PROMOTION CHALLENGE

How can you use Bandura's theory and Dellmann and Lushington's research to enhance self-efficacy in yourself and clients? Write down your ideas and then share them with at least two classmates. Ask for feedback.

Another important variable in mental health is **self-esteem**, "a positive or negative orientation toward oneself; an overall evaluation of one's worth or value. People are motivated to have high self-esteem and having it indicates positive self-regard, not egotism" (Rosenberg, n.d., p. 1). Clients with low self-esteem do not have the confidence to feel good about themselves and what they are doing.

Self-esteem is part of a broad-spectrum approach for mental health promotion. Self-evaluation is crucial to mental and social well-being because it influences aspirations, personal goals, and interaction with others. Self-esteem is a protective factor and can lead to better health and social behavior. Poor self-esteem is associated with depression, suicidal tendencies, eating disorders, anxiety, violence, and substance abuse (Mann, Hosman, Schaalma, & de Vries, 2004, p. 1). More recently, bullying has been found to correlate with low self-esteem.

RESEARCH BOX   SELF-ESTEEM AND BULLYING

» BACKGROUND: Bullying is an important and increasing problem for nurses. Recent research has suggested a possible association between bullying and low self-esteem.

» OBJECTIVE: To determine the prevalence of bullying at work in a sample of Spanish nurses, to examine the association between bullying and self-esteem, and to investigate factors that determine bullying at work.

» DESIGN: A descriptive survey study was used to answer the research question.

» PARTICIPANTS: The sample consisted of 538 nurses who met the inclusion criteria of having worked for a minimum of 1 year in adult or pediatric services in the public or private healthcare system of Principado de Asturias-Spain.

» METHODS: The Rosenberg Self-Esteem Scale (RSE) and the Negative Acts Questionnaire (NAQ) standardized for Spain were used to measure self-esteem and bullying behaviors.

» RESULTS: Nearly one in five nurses (17%) experienced subjective bullying, and 8% of these cases reported weekly or daily bullying. The negative acts reported most frequently in bullied and non-bullied nurses were work-related bullying behaviors, such as "Being given tasks with unreasonable or impossible targets or deadlines" (2.71, SD = 1.33). Bullied nurses reported significantly higher rates in all questions of the NAQ, and self-reported bullying was significantly related to low self-esteem ($\chi2 = 109$; $p<0.001$).

» CONCLUSION: Prevalence of self-reported bullying is high among Spanish nurses and is clearly associated with higher exposure to bullying behaviors at work and lower levels of self-esteem.

Source: Iglesias, M.E. & Vallejo, R. B. (2012, February 10). Prevalence of bullying at work and its association with self-esteem scores in as Spanish nurse sample. *Contemporary Nurse* [Epub ahead of print], http://www.ncbi.nlm.nih.gov/pubmed/22551268

HEALTH PROMOTION CHALLENGE

Answer the questions on the Rosenberg Self-Esteem Scale and see how you rate. Find it at http://www.bsos.umd.edu/socy/research/rosenberg.htm If your self-esteem is lower than you wish it to be, use some of the interventions discussed in this section to boost it.

Low self-esteem is a symptom of depression and may predict relapse, while high self-esteem seems to buffer against depression. Competitive Memory Training (COMET) has shown to be effective for the enhancement of self-esteem in several conditions. In a new study, COMET is also an effective intervention for clients with depression (Korrelboom, Maarsingh, & Huijbrechts, 2012).

Compared to the patients who received only therapy as usual, patients in the COMET plus therapy as usual condition showed significant improvement with large effect sizes on indices of self-esteem, depression, and depressive rumination and remained stable after 3 and 6 months on all outcome measures or improved even more.

COMET for low self-esteem seems to be an effective intervention for depression. One Hour Cards are an example of COMET. The goal is to commit to memory and recall as many separate packs (decks) of 52 playing cards as possible. Other tasks include committing to memory and recall as many fictional numerical historic/future dates as possible and link them to the right historic event and to commit to memory and recall as many names as possible and link them to the right face. For more information on COMET, go to http://www.worldmemorychampionships.com

Sleep is also important to mental or psychological health. Nurse researchers studied the effect of sleep on self-esteem, depression, and perceived obesity stress in overweight and obese children. They found that sleeping less than seven hours a night was particularly detrimental to the investigated psychological variables in overweight, but not obese children (Kim, Ham, Kim, & Park, 2011).

Supportive relationships can also affect mental health. Research conducted at the Seoul Women's College of Nursing (Yoon, Kim, & Kim, 2011) examined the effect of teaching interpersonal relationship skills to students and then measuring the program's effect on interpersonal relationships, self-esteem, and depression. Ninety-minute group sessions were held 10 times over a period of 10 weeks. The researchers found that compared to a control group, the interpersonal relationship program had a positive effect on improving interpersonal relationships and self-esteem, and decreasing depression in nursing students.

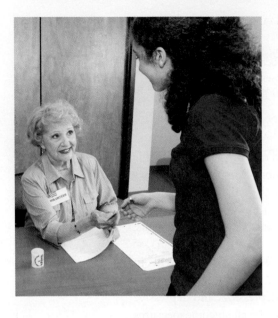

Volunteering is another activity that can improve mental health, especially in older women. By volunteering to help others, participants can raise their quality of life, enhance self-esteem by increasing a sense of contributing, and find social support (McDonnall, 2011; Parkinson, Warburton, Sibbritt, & Byles, 2010; Tang, Choi, & Morrow-Howell, 2010).

Writing that is positive and expressive can help clients deal with stressful events. Expressive writing—writing about traumatic, stressful, or emotional events—often leads to improvements in physical and psychological health in non-clinical and clinical populations. Studies have shown that positive writing may also be beneficial. Research has not yet investigated whether either expressive writing or positive writing offers benefits for people with mood disorders.

In one study (Baikie, Geerligs, & Wilhem, 2012), the expressive writing, positive writing, and time management control writing groups all reported significantly fewer mental and physical symptoms for at least 4 months post-writing. When expressive and positive writing groups were combined, the resulting "emotional writing group" showed significantly lower scores on the DASS stress subscale than the control writing group at all time-points.

HEALTH PROMOTION CHALLENGE

Choose either bibliotherapy or positive/expressive writing and plan a program for yourself or a client. Discuss your ideas with at least two other students and ask for feedback. If possible, implement your plan.

Mental Health Promotion Assessment

Nursing mental health promotion assessment is in its infancy stage. The DSM-IV provides psychiatric diagnoses based on opinion. Here we present a newly-developed mental health promotion assessment for nurses. As more evidence accumulates, new questions will be added.

Mental health promotion assessment in nursing includes many lifestyle questions and engages the client as collaborator. FIGURE 5-1 presents some questions that can help to evaluate the mental health of clients.

Below you will find a list of suggested questions to ask clients about their mental health. Revise the wording or add to them depending on your style of speaking and your experience.

1. What would you like to tell me about your mental and emotional health?
2. What are your strengths as a person?
3. What is your usual diet?
4. What are your sleep patterns?
5. How often do you listen to calming music or sing?
6. How often do you volunteer to help others?
7. What activities help you keep your mind active?
8. Everybody talks to themselves in their thoughts. What do you say in your head when you talk to yourself?
9. What do you do to cope when things get stressful?
10. How assertive are you? Are you an advocate for your own mental health?
11. Do you meditate?
12. Do you read?
13. Do you write in a journal or diary regularly?
14. What would you like to learn to do?
15. What kind of exercise do you do and how often?
16. What kinds of things do you usually think about or worry about?
17. What do you believe is your life purpose?
18. What do you think led up to your current state of mental and emotional health?
19. Who is the one person you can talk to about your feelings and feel understood?
20. How has this person helped or hindered you in getting mentally healthy?
21. What would be a sign to you that you are emotionally healthy?
22. What are your goals in relation to being mentally and emotionally healthy?
23. What goals do you have that you need help to achieve?
24. What do you need to learn to achieve your goals?
25. What can I do specifically to help you achieve your goals?
26. What story can you tell me about your life journey and struggle?
27. What kind of self-health approaches have/haven't worked for you?

(Ask about each of the activities below. Put a *yes* if it helped; *no* if didn't help. Use *NA* if not tried.)

___ acupressure	___ affirmations	___ aromatherapy	___ reading
___ energy therapy	___ guided imagery	___ hypnosis	___ puzzles
___ massage	___ prayer	___ relaxation therapy	___ yoga
___ touch therapies	___ reframing	___ exercise	___ tai chi
___ nutrition/supplements	___ music	___ writing	___ other: describe

FIGURE 5-1 Mental Health Assessment Questions

Mental Health Promotion

Mental health promotion is the same as health promotion itself in that it includes concepts of not only promotion, but also prevention. **Mental health promotion** should focus on the positive aspects of mental health and improving quality of life by building strengths and resources. In addition, prevention is key to reducing incidence and prevalence of a targeted illness, morbidity, and mortality.

Box 5-1	Common Misconceptions about Mental Illness

MYTH   "Young people and children don't suffer from mental health problems."

FACT   It is estimated that more than 6 million young people in America may suffer from a mental health disorder that severely disrupts their ability to function at home, in school, or in their community.

MYTH   "People who need psychiatric care should be locked away in institutions."

FACT   Today, most people can lead productive lives within their communities thanks to a variety of supports, programs, and/or medications.

MYTH   "A person who has had a mental illness can never be normal."

FACT   People with mental illnesses can recover and resume normal activities. For example, Mike Wallace of *60 Minutes*, who had clinical depression, received treatment and led an enriched and accomplished life.

MYTH   "Mentally ill persons are dangerous."

FACT   The vast majority of people with mental illnesses are not violent. In the cases when violence does occur, the incidence typically results from the same reasons as with the general public, such as feeling threatened or excessive use of alcohol and/or drugs.

MYTH   "People with mental illnesses can work low-level jobs but aren't suited for really important or responsible positions."

FACT   People with mental illnesses, like everyone else, have the potential to work at any level depending on their own abilities, experience, and motivation.

Source: © 2012 Mental Health America. http://www.nmha.org/go/action/stigma-watch

If client mental health affects the sense of well-being and quality of life, it can have two significant negative effects on efforts at promoting health. First, mental health issues can themselves be risk factors for physical health issues if they affect the individual's self-care ability. Second, mental health issues can obstruct efforts by the individual and by healthcare providers to take actions to promote or improve health.

An example would be a client with clinical depression who is unable to leave the house to obtain treatment due to their depression. If this person lives in a nice home, has a high income and a good education, eats well, and is generally physically fit and healthy, by some measures quality of life is high. In terms of health-related quality of life, this person experiences poor quality of life by any measure. Severe depression by itself is manifest by poor quality of life; lack of treatment and the inability to obtain treatment extend and increase this problem and may eventually impact physical health. If this individual's condition results in the loss of a good job and leads to inability to sustain financial and family well-being, then the impact spreads to other family members and to the community at large.

HEALTH PROMOTION CHALLENGE

What options can you come up with for homebound clients who require mental health care? Investigate online treatment, home visits, self-study books, and any other formats you can find by Googling *mental health treatment for homebound clients*. Share your findings with at least two other classmates and ask for feedback.

In reviewing any approach to mental health, common threads are evident. These include that the concepts (1) be positive and constantly changing, (2) be multidisciplinary, (3) build on the principles of health promotion, and (4) be rooted in the socioecologic approach.

A Socioecologic Approach to Mental Health Promotion

The **socioecologic approach** to mental health promotion evolves from the philosophy that change needs to start at the individual level, which causes a chain reaction in affecting the family, then the community, and ultimately the society. The approach recognizes that individuals do not exist in a vacuum. They influence, and are influenced by, the social groups with which they interact, whether that means family, friends, neighbors, coworkers, teachers, or the community at large. Programs for mental health promotion need to influence these environments in which the individual, family, group, or community functions. This can mean developing a plan not only to work with the individual in support of mental health, but also developing plans to create supportive environments in individual homes, or community settings of schools, workplaces, and health-care services.

Examples could include:

- a community-based program that assists developmentally disabled adults to obtain job training and placement
- a school program that teaches students self-esteem and stress reduction measures
- a work program that provides mental health promotion information and skill practice
- outreach programs for depressed adults or children
- outreach programs for clients suffering from posttraumatic stress disorder due to rape, school or work shootings, war, natural disasters, etc.
- a family-based plan developed to provide supportive care for a parent in the early stages of dementia, a pregnant or abused woman, or a client stopping smoking or taking drugs

HEALTH PROMOTION CHALLENGE   www

Choose one of the examples above and develop a mental health treatment plan. Use the Internet (www.pubmed.gov) to find examples of studies/programs as well as Google for ideas. Share your completed program with at least two other students and ask for feedback.

In all of these cases, interventions are targeted not only to the needs of the client, but also to alter the environment in which the client works and lives in order to accommodate mental health needs. Principles of mental health promotion build on empowerment philosophy by engaging the participants, building on their strengths, and enhancing their perspective of having control over their lives.

The Nurse's Role in Mental Health Promotion

There are two situations in which nurses work with individuals with mental illness. One occurs in a setting where an individual client is referred for health promotion activities and is not diagnosed with any form of mental issue, but displays characteristics of a mental health issue (as discussed in the section on identifying different forms of mental illness). Another is in the setting where the client has a formal diagnosis and is working with a nurse to address a diagnosed mental health concern. In the first case, the nurse may not have been specifically trained to work with patients with mental health issues; in the second, it is likely that the nurse has advanced mental health training.

Why do these distinctions matter? There are several reasons. First, if you work with a client and identify a mental health issue that is outside your scope of practice, there may be legal and ethical ramifications. A licensed practical nurse who is helping a client with reducing pain from rheumatoid arthritis, for instance, may not have the authority to intervene for that client should she suspect clinical depression. Also, it would be unethical and irresponsible to attempt to address an issue for which you have not been trained (Ballard, 2008).

Second, when a physically ill client presents signs of lack of mental health, it has implications for how the health promotion activity undertaken to address the physical problem can proceed. A person with untreated or overlooked mental health issues may not have the capacity to engage in health promotion activities until the mental health issue is dealt with. Likewise, health promotion activities may prove more successful following intervention for mental distress. That is why referral to appropriate mental health services is an important part of health promotion.

In mental health promotion, the relationship between the nurse and the client takes on an important therapeutic dimension—and it is important to get that relationship right as a result. Taylor (2008) explains that:

> [t]o be truly helpful to clients, you need to understand the difference between professional and social relationships. Social relationships are interactions in which the needs of both persons are of equal importance. In contrast, professional relationships are those in which the needs of the client are paramount. To engage in professional relationships with clients, nurses must have a highly developed degree of self-awareness. Self-awareness means that nurses know those areas in which they are emotionally vulnerable . . . Nurses need to be aware that boundaries are critical in maintaining a professional therapeutic relationship. At the beginning of the relationship, an agreement or contract between the nurse and client should be established. This is an excellent opportunity to establish the rules and behaviors or boundaries that are expected between the nurse and client, such as the time and frequency of meetings; reimbursement for services; contact with family members, significant others, and other therapists; and prohibition against socialization. (p. 18)

The orientation phase of a nurse–client relationship begins when you take steps to learn about the client's biosocial history (e.g., social, cultural, spiritual, family, developmental, and occupational history as well as medical, psychiatric, and substance abuse history), the history of the present illness or complaint, and current mental and physical state (Moran, 2008). Although all of these facts are important for your understanding of the client's situation, the key goal at this stage is to establish trust between you and the client. The best way to do this is to be consistent and professional, to be available when you say you will be available, and to focus on the client's needs. During this phase, and depending on the client, you may wish to ask some of the questions that appear in Figure 5-1 Mental Health Assessment Questions.

After trust is solidified, the relationship moves into a second phase, the working phase, in which the particulars of the client's circumstance are taken into account as you work to develop a strategy for helping the client. During this phase you can begin to work in collaboration with the client to plan interventions for the variables that appear in TABLE 5-1, Variables Affecting Mental Health.

The final phase, conclusion phase, occurs when the relationship comes to an end. The conclusion phase may happen either because you must refer the client on to services you cannot provide, or because the health promotion activities you and client have undertaken together have proven sufficiently successful that the client no longer needs your services.

Taylor (2008) notes that "[p]aradoxically, the more successful the relationship, the more emotionally painful is the termination" (p. 18). You and the client must let go of what is necessarily a high degree of intimacy and go your separate ways. Development of a personal relationship between a nurse and client after the working relationship is unethical, because it represents a changing of firmly established and healthy boundaries. At this stage, you know more about this client's personal experience than even close friends. Because you may be called upon to resume a professional interaction with the client in the future, you cannot risk developing a social interaction with the client, even after a successful intervention.

If you work with clients striving to become mentally healthy, you will be held accountable to various codes of ethics formulated by professional organizations and state licensing boards. It is your responsibility to know these codes and maintain close familiarity with their standards so your practice is in compliance with them.

Resources for Mental Health Promotion

TABLE 5-1, Variables Affecting Mental Health, is a good starting point for planned interventions. The Centers for Disease Control and Prevention (CDC) is in an excellent position to support the efforts of health agencies in promoting mental health (Safran, 2009). The efforts include collection of data through surveillance of mental illness, assessment of risk behaviors, and analysis of associated comorbidities of mental illness and chronic disease. The CDC also collaborates with the World Federation for Mental Health to address the stigma associated with the mental illness diagnosis, the primary barrier that prevents one from seeking effective treatment. This effort is evident through public

Table 5-1 Variables Affecting Mental Health

FINDINGS	VARIABLES
Assertiveness/ Advocacy	Pickett et al. (2012) found that using a peer-led educational group approach with mental health consumers increased their self-advocacy/assertiveness skills.
Exercise	Stavrakis et al. (2012) found that group exercise reduces perceived stress. Mason and Holt (2011) found that exercise improves social interaction and social support; increases feelings of safety; and provides a sense of meaning, purpose, and achievement. Smith et al. (2011) found that exercise decreases anxiety and stress when integrative yoga is used.
Massage	Serfaty et al. (2012) found that massage combined with lavender aromatherapy decreases anxiety and depression.
Meditation	Brand et al. (2012) found that meditation improves sleep and reduces stress.
Music	Maratos et al. (2011) found that music therapy can improve the mental health of depressed individuals.
Nutrition	Ye et al. (2011) found that the intake of sugars detrimentally affects mental functioning. Annweiler et al. (2012) found that eating foods high in vitamin D (especially cod, salmon, sardines, and shrimp) lowers the risk for Alzheimer's Disease. Forsyth et al. (2012) found that a low intake of magnesium from fruits, veggies, and grains is associated with depression. da Rocha and Kac (2012) found that a low intake of omega-3 fatty acids from food like (sardines, salmon, flax seeds, and walnuts) is associated with a greater risk for postpartum depression.
Reading	Songprakunp and McCann (2012) found that reading a self-help manual can reduce psychological distress in depressed clients.
Religion/Spirituality	Rounding et al. (2012) found that subtly reminding clients of religious concepts can increase self-control and the ability to make better decisions.
Self-efficacy	Bandura (1977) and Delmann and Lushington (2012) found that to enhance self-efficacy in clients, you should model success in reaching the client goal, stress client personal strengths, and use positive encouragement that the client can succeed.

(continues)

Table 5-1 *(Continued)*

FINDINGS	VARIABLES
Self-esteem	Menn et al. (2004) found that low self-esteem correlates with depression, suicidal tendencies, eating disorders, anxiety, violence, and substance abuse.
	Iglesias & Vallejo (2012) found that low self-esteem correlates with bullying.
	Korrelboom et al. (2012) found that competitive memory training can enhance self-esteem.
Sleep	Kim et al. (2011) found that sleeping less than 7 hours/night is correlated with obesity.
Supportive IPRs	Yoon et al. (2011) found that learning interpersonal relationship skills in a group had a positive effect on interpersonal relationships, self-esteem, and decreased depression.
Volunteering	Parkinson et al. (2010); McDonnall (2011) and Tang et al. (2010) found that volunteering to help others can reduce depression and increase social support and a sense of contribution.
Writing	Baikie et al. (2012) found that writing about trauma or difficult situations in an expressive, positive way can reduce stress.

© Carolyn Chambers Clark, 2012.

awareness campaigns and by supporting efforts of other agencies in consistent surveillance of mental illness as well as risk behaviors.

In 2002, the WHO published a document called *Prevention and Promotion in Mental Health*. The document was a result of the World Health Organization Meeting on Evidence for Prevention and Promotion in Mental Health: Conceptual and Measurement Issues, which was held in the WHO headquarters in Geneva, Switzerland, in 2001. It was attended by participants who were mental health experts from WHO regions. The role of WHO in the area of prevention and promotion in mental health includes the following:

1. To foster activities in the field of mental health, especially those affecting the harmony of human relations,

2. To promote maternal and child health and welfare and to foster the ability to live harmoniously in a changing total environment,

3. To study and report on, in cooperation with other specialized agencies where necessary, administrative and social techniques affecting public health and

medical care from preventive and curative points of view, including hospital services and social security. (WHO, 2002, p. 25)

The underlying theme of the conference was that "prevention and promotion in mental health are essential steps in reducing the increasing burden due to mental disorders" (WHO, 2002, p. 1). The document is key in mental health promotion in that it is based on the deliberations of the WHO meeting and additional sources, with special emphasis on evidence-based references. The beginning of the document outlines the rationale for the emphasis on mental health promotion,

The World Health Organization website contains excellent information about the organization's efforts to promote mental health in all countries. Go to http://www.who.int/topics/mental_health/en/ WHO initiatives are categorized according to regions, such as African Region or the Eastern Mediterranean Region; mental health resources/publications are available on the site, as well as statistical information.

The CDC provides information about mental health organizations by state plus links for governmental and nongovernmental resources. Go to http://www.cdc.gov/mentalhealth/resources.htm

HOT TOPICS

Here are some topics to explore:
- Autism
- Bibliotherapy
- Meditation
- Self-efficacy
- Self-esteem
- Nutrition and mental health

To these effects we would add:

1. Elevated instance of emotional/psychological suffering or physical dysfunction
2. Discrimination and stigma, including self-stigma (Sharac, McCrone, Clement, & Thornicroft, 2010)
3. Poor self-care, including failure to seek health care
4. Decreased quality of life

Mental health prevention strategies work best when implemented before the onset of the mental disorders. (WHO, 2002, p. 8). Mental health promotion is geared towards improving the coping skills of the individual and addressing underlying causes, not eliminating symptoms and deficits as in the medical model.

Teaching clients good nutritional habits and assertiveness skills, as well as the other activities in Table 5-1, can provide a start toward preventing mental disorders.

One of the most compelling aspects of *Prevention and Promotion in Mental Health* is the section covering the importance of **evidence-based research** in the area of mental health promotion. The premise is that "evidence not only provides validity for effectiveness of strategies, but also stimulates decisions and actions" (WHO, 2002, p. 12). The arguments in favor of evidence-based prevention and promotion in the field of mental health are also summarized. They include:

1. Growing awareness of the epidemiology of mental disorders and mental health-related problems and of their large financial and social burden on society has urged governments and nongovernment organizations to develop and implement effective preventive measures.

2. Societal pressure for increased accountability for spending public funds calls for both evidence of effectiveness and cost-effectiveness. This calls for information on what works best and under what conditions.

3. The pressure to shift governmental funds from health care or other budgets to prevention and promotion has evoked resistance. Skepticism about the possibilities of effective prevention in mental health, criticism of its weak scientific base, and the need to protect healthcare budgets have raised a call for proof that such interventions can be effective.

4. Growing numbers of preventive programs and strategies have urged policy makers, health managers, and program providers to select best practices, which requires objective standards for comparison. Given the existing diversity in efficacy and effectiveness of prevention programs, consumers have to be informed about the best available preventive services and be alerted as to possible negative side effects.

5. Evaluations of the outcomes of preventive interventions and mental health promotion are subject to a variety of possible biases, leading to incorrect conclusions. Solid evidence and standards for evidence are needed to prevent such incorrect conclusions. Available resources for preventive interventions being scarce, evidence of the program's outcomes will lead to more efficient use of resources.

6. Frequently, preventive and promotional interventions are addressed at large population groups using indirect intervention strategies and are aimed at assessing long-term outcomes. These features hinder their proper assessment; specific monitoring systems are needed to make the effects visible.

7. Mental health promotion, like other sectors of health promotion, requires intersectoral action; i.e., participation and investments by sectors outside mental health. Sustainable investments can only be expected when such partners can be confident that these will generate outcomes that are also relevant to their interests (e.g., social or economic benefits).

In addition, the WHO document emphasizes that before starting the process of designing promotion and preventive programs, a needs assessment should be initiated on the following issues:

1. Prevalence and incidence of mental disorders or mental ill health
2. Populations and individuals at risk
3. Health, social, and economic outcomes of problems or disorders
4. Community perceptions of risk and the need for preventive actions
5. Biologic, psychologic, and social risk and protective factors

6. Developmental trajectories of health and disease
7. Comorbidity and multiproblem trajectories

Strategies for Promoting Mental Health

Strategies for mental health promotion depend in large part on understanding the varying places where there are opportunities for intervention. A great many factors contribute to reduced mental health, ranging from learned behaviors, lack of exercise, low self-esteem, nutritional deficits (e.g., vitamin D or B-vitamin deficiency contributing to depression in older adults), poor interpersonal skills, or lack of knowledge about helpful self-care measures, to biochemical imbalances, toxic exposures, posttraumatic stress disturbances, poverty, and genetic and functional alterations to the brain.

Interventions can include a combination of lifestyle modifications (exercise, nutrition, and other approaches detailed in Table 5-1) and talk therapy for concerns like depression, anxiety, and anger issues; and nursing and/or occupational therapies and low-level psychological intervention needed for moderate functional issues like personality disorders, ADHD or OCD.

For many clients, mental health promotion may require input from the client's family. Activities may need to be planned not only with the client, but also with the client's family members, particularly in the case of an individual with a significant mental disability. Family dynamics that have developed to protect or control a family member identified as the problem may prove to be obstacles to the client's ability to self-promote mental wellness and independence.

Here's an example: Imagine a large family with eight children in which the youngest son, Jeff, is diagnosed with schizophrenia at the age of 12. When he takes his medication, Jeff's symptoms are usually well controlled, but like many adolescents, he resents being different and sometimes forgets or refuses to take his medications. He also complains the medicine makes him feel like he's in a mental straitjacket. Because both of his parents work, Jeff's three oldest siblings, who have graduated high school but live and work nearby, are sometimes called upon to intervene when his condition causes Jeff to have problems in school. As a result, Jeff's siblings have developed a pattern of protecting and watching over their baby brother. This pattern lasts well past adolescence and into adulthood, with Jeff's siblings providing their brother with transportation, housing, food, and clothing from the mistaken belief or their private agendas that the young man's diagnosis prevents him from taking on these tasks himself. If Jeff wants to obtain independence and manage his own mental health once he reaches maturity, the siblings may impede him from doing so, because of an entrenched dynamic that compels them to exercise control over his activities.

A nursing intervention for this client may require working not only with Jeff to help him develop better compliance with his treatment regimens and improve his life skills, but also with his family to develop healthier systems of interaction between Jeff and his oldest siblings. Be aware that a system, such as a family, struggles to maintain balance. When one individual changes behavior, the others will exert pressure to reverse the change, so build in special supports for Jeff's healthier behaviors.

Summary

Mental health encompasses complex biological, physiological, emotional, and psychosocial interactions. You can aid in mental illness prevention by helping people identify and monitor their own risk factors, assessing levels as well as their perception of stress with the effectiveness of their coping strategies, and to view the person in terms of their overall function and not just by their signs and symptoms.

Mental conditions contribute much to the worldwide disease burden; the World Health Organization estimated in 2001 that 450 million people suffered from mental disorders. According the U.S. Department of Health and Human Services, in 2000, costs related to mental illness were estimated at $150 billion annually.

In 2002, the World Health Organization published *Prevention and Promotion in Mental Health*. The roles of WHO in prevention and promotion in mental health include (1) fostering activities in the field of mental health, especially those affecting harmony in human relations; (2) promoting maternal and child health and welfare and fostering the ability to live harmoniously in a changing total environment; and (3) studying and reporting on in cooperation with other specialized agencies where necessary, administrative and social techniques affecting public health and medical care from preventive and curative points of view, including hospital services and social security. The negative effects of mental illness listed in *Prevention and Promotion in Mental Health* included extended treatment periods, absence due to sickness, unemployment, increased labor turnover, loss of productivity, disability that can last for years, emotional and socioeconomic toll on families, and an overall increase in costs.

Mental health promotion differs from general health promotion in that it is geared toward improving the coping skills of the individual instead of eliminating symptoms and deficits, as in the medical model. The WHO document also stresses the importance of evidence-based research in mental health promotion and the need for a thorough assessment prior to designing promotion and prevention programs.

Common threads found in approaches to mental health include concepts that (1) are positive and constantly changing, (2) are multidisciplinary, (3) build on the principles of health promotion, and (4) are rooted in the socio-ecologic model.

Variables affecting mental health that nurses can develop interventions for, based on evidence already, available include: assertiveness/advocacy, exercise, massage/aromatherpy, meditation, music, nutrition, reading, religion/spirituality, self-efficacy, self-esteem, sleep, supportive interpersonal relationships, volunteering, and writing.

REVIEW QUESTIONS

1. Mental illness costs the United States an estimated
   a. $150 million annually
   b. $150 billion annually
   c. $450 million annually
   d. $450 billion annually

2. Mental health promotion is geared toward:
   a. Primary prevention
   b. Secondary prevention
   c. Improving coping skills
   d. Tertiary prevention

3. Evidence-based practice:
   a. Relies on solid research studies that provide validity for effectiveness of strategies
   b. Builds on practice patterns handed down from older practitioners
   c. Does not require studies utilizing scientific methods.

4. Threads or concepts that are commonly found in approaches to mental health are all of the following except:
   a. Multidisciplinary
   b. Positive and constantly changing
   c. Static and unchanging

5. Negative effects of mental illness include all of the following except:
   a. Increased labor turnover
   b. Reduced cost of health care
   c. Extended treatment periods

6. Before starting the process of designing promotion and preventive programs:
   a. An assessment of needs should be initiated
   b. A search for funding sources should be undertaken
   c. An assessment of local professionals and their qualifications should take place

EXERCISES

1. Do some research on the Bright Futures national health promotion initiative. Summarize the various areas of focus in the program and gather detailed information about the Public Health Approach to Mental Health section.

2. Review the *Healthy People 2010* document portions related to mental health and then review the activities of the National Center for Mental Health Promotion and Youth Violence Prevention. In what ways does the work of this group support the goals of Healthy People?

3. Compile a literature search on an area of mental health promotion that interests you. Write up a brief summary of your findings.

REFERENCES

Annweiler, C., Fantino, B., Schott, A. M., Krolak-Salmon, P., Allali, G., & Beauchet, O. (2012). Vitamin D insufficiency and mild cognitive impairment: cross-sectional association. *European Journal of Neurology, 19*(7), p. 1023-1029.

Balkie, K. A., Geerligs, L., & Wilhelm, K. (2012). Expressive writing and positive writing for participants with mood disorders: an online randomized controlled trial. *Journal of Affective Disorders 136*(3), 310–319.

Ballard, K. A. (2008). Issues and trends in psychiatric-mental health nursing. In P. G. O'Brien, W. Z. Kennedy, & K. A. Ballard (Eds.), *Psychiatric mental health nursing: An introduction to theory and practice* (pp. 21–38). Sudbury, MA: Jones and Bartlett.

Bandura, A. (1977). Self-efficacy: Toward a unifying theory of behavioral change, *Psychological Review 84*(2), 191–215.

Brand, S., Holsboer-Trachsler, E., Naranjo, J.R., & Schmidt, S. (2012). Influence of mindfulness practice on cortisol and sleep in long-term and short-term meditators. *Neuropsychobiology, 65*(3), 109–118.

da Rocha, C. M. & Kac, G. (2012). High dietary ratio of omega-6 to omega-3 polyunsaturated acids during pregnancy and prevalence of post-partum depression. *Maternal and Child Nutrition 8*(1), 36–48.

Dellmann T., & Lushington, K. (2012). How Natural Therapists enhance positive expectations of patients. *Complementary Therapies in Clinical Practice, 18*(2), 99–105.

Demyttenaere, K., Bruffaerts, R., Posada-Villa, J., Gasquet, I., Kovess, V., Lepine, J. P., . . . Chatterji, S.; WHO World Mental Health Survey Consortium. (2004). Prevalence, severity, and unmet need for treatment of mental disorders in the World Health Organization World Mental Health Surveys. *JAMA, 291*(21), 2581–2590.

Forsyth, A. K., Williams, P. G., & Deane, F. P. (2012). Nutrition status of primary care patients with depression and anxiety. *Australian Journal of Primary Health, 18*(2), 172–176.

Hopkins, M. E., Caroline Davis F., Vantieghem, M. R., Whalen, P. J., & Bucci, D. J. (2012, April 30). Differential effects of acute and regular physical exercise on cognition and affect. *Neuroscience*. Retrieved from http://www.ncbi.nlm.nih.gov/pubmed/2255478

Iglesias, M. E., & Vallejo, R. B. (2012, February 10). Prevalence of bullying at work and its association with self-esteem scores in a Spanish nurse sample [Epub ahead of print]. *Contemporary Nurse*. Retrieved from http://www.ncbi.nlm.nih.gov/pubmed/22551268

Kim, H. S., Ham, O. K., Kim, J. W., & Park, J. Y. (2012, March 28). Association between sleep duration and psychological health in overweight and obese children in Korea. *Nursing and Health Science*. Retrieved from http://www.ncbi.nlm.nih.gov/pubmed/22462655

Korrelboom, K., Maarsingh, M., & Huijbrechts, I. (2012). Competitive memory training (comet) for treating low self-esteem in patients with depressive disorders: a randomized clinical trial. *Depression and Anxiety, 29*(2), 102–110.

Mann, M., Hosman, C. M. H., Schallma, H., & de Vries, N. K. (2004). Self-esteem in a broad-spectrum approach for mental health promotion. *Health Education Research, 19*(4), 357–372.

Maratos A., Crawford, M. J., & Procter, S. (2011). Music therapy for depression: It seems to work, but how? *British Journal of Psychiatry, 199*(2), 92–93.

Mason, O. J., & Holt, R. (2012, April 25). Mental health and physical activity interventions: A review of the qualitative literature. *Journal of Mental Health*. Retrieved from http://www.ncbi.nlm.nih.gov/pubmed/22533784

McDonnall, M.C. (2011). The effect of productive activities on depressive symptoms among older adults with dual sensory loss. *Research in Aging, 33*(3), 234–255.

Moran, C. C. (2008). The psychiatric nursing assessment. In P. G. O'Brien, W. Z. Kennedy, & K. A. Ballard (Eds.), *Psychiatric mental health nursing: An introduction to theory and practice* (pp. 39–64). Sudbury, MA: Jones and Bartlett.

National Institutes of Mental Health. (n.d.a). Post-traumatic stress disorder. U.S. Department Of Health and Human Services, National Institutes of Health Publication No. 08 6388. Retrieved from http://www. nimh. nih. gov/health/publications/post-traumatic-stress-disorder-ptsd/nimh_ptsd_booklet. pdf

National Institutes of Mental Health. (n.d.b). Statistics: Leading categories of diseases/disorders. Retrieved from http://mentalhealth. gov/statistics/2LEAD_CAT. shtml

National Institutes of Mental Health. (n.d.c). Statistics: Leading causes of death ages 18–65 in the U. S. Retrieved from http://mentalhealth. gov/statistics/3AGES1865. shtml

National Institutes of Mental Health. (n.d.d). Suicide in the U. S. Statistics and prevention. Retrieved from http://www.nimh.nih.gov/health/publications/suicide-in-the-us-statistics-and-prevention/index.shtml#factors

Parkinson, L., Warburton, J., Sibbritt, D., & Byles, J. (2010). Volunteering and older women: psychosocial and health predictors of participation. *Aging and Mental Health,14*(8), 917–927.

Perlick, D. A., Nelson, A. H., Mattias, K., Selzer J., Kalvin, C., Wilber, C. H., Huntington, B., . . . Corrigan, P. W. (2011). In our own voice-family companion: Reducing self-stigma of family members of persons with serious mental illness. *Psychiatric Services, 62*(12), 1456–1462.

Rosenberg, M. (n.d.) The Rosenberg Self-Esteem Scale. Retrieved from http://www.bsos .umd.edu/socy/research/rosenberg.htm

Rounding, K., Lee, A., Jacobson, J. A., & Ji, L. J. (2012, May 2). Religion replenishes self-control [Epub ahead of print]. *Psychology and Science*. Retrieved from http://www.ncbi. nlm.nih.gov/pubmed/22555969

Rüsch, N., Angermeyer, M. C., & Corrigan, P. W. (2005). Mental illness stigma: Concepts, consequences, and initiatives to reduce stigma. *European Psychiatry, 20*(8), 529–539.

Safran, M. (2009). Achieving recognition that mental health is part of the mission of the CDC. *Psychiatric Services, 60*(11), 1532–1534.

Serfaty, M., Wilkinson, S., Freeman, C., Mannix, K., & King, M. (2012). The ToT Study: Helping with Touch or Talk (ToT): a pilot randomised controlled trial to examine the clinical effectiveness of aromatherapy massage versus cognitive behaviour therapy for emotional distress in patients in cancer/palliative care. *Psychooncology 21*(5), 563–569.

Sharac, J., McCrone, P., Clement, S., & Thornicroft, G. (2010). The economic impact of mental health stigma and discrimination: A systematic review. *Epidemiologia e Psichiatria Sociale, 19*(3), 223–232.

Smith, J. A., Greer, T., Sheets, T., & Watson, S. (2011). Is there more to yoga than exercise? *Alternative Therapies in Health and Medicine, 17*(3), 22–29.

Songprakun, W., & McCann, T.V. (2012, March 1). Evaluation of a bibliotherapy manual for reducing psychological distress in people with depression: a randomized controlled trial [Epub ahead of print]. *Journal of Advanced Nursing.* Retrieved from http://www.ncbi.nlm.nih.gov/pubmed/22381065

Stavrakakis, N., de Jonge, P., Ormel, J., & Oldehinkel, A. J. (2011). Bidirectional prospective associations between physical activity and depressive symptoms. *The TRAILS Study. 50*(5), 503–508.

Tang, F., Choi, E., & Morrow-Howell, N. (2011). Organizational support and volunteering benefits for older adults. *Gerontologist, 50*(5), 603–612.

Taylor, C. M. (2008). Introduction to psychiatric-mental health nursing. In P. G. O'Brien, W. Z. Kennedy, & K. A. Ballard (Eds.), *Psychiatric mental health nursing: An introduction to theory and practice* (pp. 3–20). Sudbury, MA: Jones and Bartlett.

Toblin, R. L., Riviere, L. A., Thomas, J. L., Adler, A. B., Kok, B. C., & Hog, C. W. (201U.S. Department of Health and Human Services. (2000). *Healthy people 2010.* Washington, DC: Author.

University of Leeds/Ahead4health. (2006). *What is mental health?* Retrieved from http://www. leeds. ac. uk/ahead4health/mental_health. htm

U.S. Department of Health and Human Services. (2010). Healthy People 2020. *Mental Health and Mental Disorders.* Retrieved from http://aspe.hhs.gov/health/reports/physicalactivity/

World Health Organization [WHO]. (2001). *The world health report: Mental health; new understanding, new hope.* Geneva, Switzerland: Author.

World Health Organization [WHO]. (2002). *Prevention and promotion in mental health.* Geneva, Switzerland: WHO. Retrieved from http://www. who. int/mental_health/media/en/545. pdf

World Health Organization [WHO]. (2004). *Promoting mental health: Concepts, emerging evidence and practice.* Retrieved from http://www.who.int/mental_health/evidence/en/promoting_mhh.pdf

World Health Organization [WHO]. (2007). *What is mental health?* Retrieved from http://www. who. int/features/qa/62/en/index. html

Wynaden, D., Barr, L., Omari, O., & Fulton, A. (2012). Evaluation of service users' experiences of participating in an exercise programme at the Australian State Forensic Mental Health Services. *International Journal of Mental Health Nursing, 21*(3), 229–235.

Ye, X., Gao, X., Scott, T., & Tucker, K. L. (2011). Habitual sugar intake and cognitive function among middle-aged and older Puerto Ricans without diabetes. *British Journal of Nutrition, 106*(8), 1423–1432.

Yoon, H. S., Kim, G. H., & Kim, J. (2011). Effectiveness of an interpersonal relationship program on interpersonal relationships, self-esteem, and depression in nursing students. *Journal of the Korean Academy of Nursing 41*(6), 805–813.

INTERNET RESOURCES

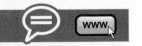

For a full suite of assignments and learning activities, use the access code located in the front of your book to visit this exclusive website: **http://go.jblearning .com/healthpromotion**. If you do not have an access code, you can obtain one at the site.

LEARNING OBJECTIVES

Upon completion of this chapter, the reader will be able to:

1. Describe at least five different definitions of family.

2. Critique at least three common assumptions about the family.

3. Assess two different family composition models.

4. List two assumptions of systems theory.

5. Determine three broad influences in Pender's family health promotion model.

6. Provide real-world examples of each of the elements in Pender's health promotion model.

7. Differentiate between each of five key components used in assessing family health promotion.

8. Analyze the traits that help define a healthy family.

9. Explain the difference between role strain and role stress.

10. Distinguish five informal family roles.

11. Differentiate between a genogram and an ecomap.

12. Assess the different components of the Calgary family intervention model.

13. Discuss some rules for conducting a family interview.

14. Describe three family interventions.

KEY TERMS

www

Blamer

Bystander

Caretaker

Coordinator

Dominator

Double bind

Ecomap

Emotional cut-off

Encourager

Family

Family composition

Family health promotion model

Family theory

Follower

Genogram

Harmonizer

Healthy family

Martyr

Opposer

Role ambiguity

Role conflict

Role incongruity

Role overload

Role strain

Role stress

Scapegoat

Systems theory

CHAPTER 6

Family Health Promotion

- Introduction
- What Is a Family?
- Systems Theory
- Putting It All Together: Health Promotion In Families
- Summary

http://go.jblearning.com/healthpromotion

For a full suite of assignments and learning activities, use the access code located in the front of your book to visit the exclusive website: http://go.jblearning.com/healthpromotion If you do not have an access code, you can obtain one at the site.

Introduction

Most individuals have family relationships, and whether they live with these family members or not, the relationships have an effect on health. Where individuals in a family live together (couples, parents and children, or even extended multigenerational families), each one interacts with and affects the other. Health behaviors are nearly universally taught and learned in family environments, making it even more of a priority for you to understand family systems and to promote health to families as well as individuals.

What Is a Family?

It may seem silly to ask such a question, because every one of us probably thinks we know the answer, but we all may have a different picture of what comprises **family**. In reality, family can mean different things to different people. Bomar (2004) compiled a list of various definitions of family, which included:

1. A fundamental social group in a society consisting of a man and woman and their offspring, a group of persons sharing a common ancestry, lineage, especially distinguished lineage, and all of the members of a household under one roof (American Heritage dictionary, college. 1982).

2. A group of two or more persons residing in the same household who are related by blood, marriage, or adoption (U.S. Census Bureau, 2002).

3. Two or more persons who are committed to each other and who share intimacy, resources, decisions, and values (Olson & DeFrain, 1994).

4. Two or more persons who are joined together by bonds or sharing and emotional closeness and who identify themselves as being part of the family (Friedman, Bowden, & Jones, 2003).

5. A group of individuals who are bound by emotional ties, a sense of belonging, and a passion for being involved in one another's lives (Wright, Watson, & Bell, 1996).

6. Two or more individuals who depend on one another for emotional, physical, and economical support (Hanson, 2001).

These definitions are diverse, but they have the common thread of involving two or more people. Beyond that, though, is a huge variety of options.

Political rhetoric during elections tends to focus on the idea of a typical nuclear family comprised of husband and wife with their 2.2 children. Reality shows that model to be anything but typical in the United States today—and it may have *never* been representative of families outside of the popular imagination. **Family composition** has changed over the last 50 years, and families themselves often change over time as older members die, new members are born, and marriages, divorces, and cohabitation occur.

CULTURAL RESEARCH STUDY

A review of: Structural and Cultural Factors in Successful Aging among Older Hispanics

This article focused on barriers to optimal aging for Hispanics, especially those of Mexican origin. This research had two major objectives: (1) to identify the cultural and structural factors that account for relatively favorable morbidity and mortality experiences among immigrants, and (2) account for high rates of chronic disease and disability in older Mexican-origin individuals.

The Mexican-origin population has a lower mortality rate than African Americans in the United States but higher morbidity due to chronic diseases. Though this population has nearly universal Medicare coverage, they are less likely than non-Hispanics to have private Medigap policies. Use of health care may be limited by language issues, as older Hispanics are less likely to be fluent in English. The history of exclusion and social marginality also place them in more vulnerable situations with economic issues and healthcare access, thus they may not receive chronic disease care.

Source: Angel, R. (2009). Structural and cultural factors in successful aging among older Hispanics. *Family and Community Health, 32*(1), S46–S57.

A variety of other factors has caused a change in family organization. These factors include changes in national demographics, such as an aging population that is now living longer and the infusion of immigrants, legal and otherwise, who bring with them their own notions about families. Recent decades have seen an evolution of cultural/religious beliefs in relation to marriage, childbearing, and same-sex relationships. Economic and financial variables have also affected the ability of individuals to live outside of a family-oriented household, where in years past such independence may have been taken for granted (e.g., seniors or recent college grads). Such factors, among others, have led individuals to redefine who is part of their family along unfamiliar and nontraditional lines in some cases. For example:

1. *Legally married without children*—Many couples are postponing having children until their careers have been established. Some may decide not to have any children.

2. *Cohabitating unmarried adults*—These adults could be in a romantic and/or sexual relationship and living together, or could be living together out of convenience and not personally involved, other than as friends. (We do not include roommates who live together strictly to limit financial burdens, but who otherwise have limited social interactions with one another, in this definition of *family*.)

3. *Single parent*—A single adult may be a parent through divorce, death of the co-parent, or adoption. The child may live with the single parent or

HOT TOPICS

Here are some topics to explore:
- Blended families
- Families with HIV/AIDS
- Grandparents raising grandchildren
- Gay and lesbian marriage
- Health promotion in families
- Family resiliency
- Genograms and ecomaps
- Family management style
- Childhood obesity
- Frail elders
- Social media and family nursing
- Families in other cultures

not. Single parents who live alone are considered a family with their live-away child if they actively participate in the child's life.

4. *Blended families*—A parent who has children forms a family with another adult, who may or may not also have children. The relationship of the child to the adult who is not the child's parent is that of stepchild to stepparent. If both adults have children, the children become stepsiblings. If the newly paired adults have a child together, the children are related as half-siblings. In some instances, children of adults who have gone through multiple relationships may have extensive and complex social and biological interrelationships with a variety of current (and former) stepparents, stepsiblings, and half-siblings.

5. *Extended families*—In addition to the nuclear family, aunts, uncles, grandparents, and cousins may reside in the household.

6. *Gay and lesbian couples*—A couple of the same sex are together, and in some states may be recognized as being married as well. Such families also include children who are either the biological offspring of one parent or adoptive children of both parents.

BOX 6-1 shows a very complicated hypothetical family. Bear in mind many blended families will not be this complex.

These are just a few examples; some of the families may be of multiple types, such as a gay couple living together with a child from a previous heterosexual relationship. Another example is a blended and extended family with stepchildren, children, and one of the adult's parents (a grandfather or grandmother) residing in the same home.

The preferred definition of family is however the family describes it.

RESEARCH BOX 6-1

Are you interested in international family health? Family Health International is an organization founded in 1971 whose aim is to bring lasting change to the world's most vulnerable people.

Visit its website http://www.fhi.org/en/index.htm

The World Health Organization has a family and community health department, which focuses on the health and development of individuals and families.

Visit its website at http://www.who.int/en

Box 6-1   Portrait of a Complex Blended Family

Eve married Dan at age 18 and had three children, two boys and a girl. The marriage broke up when Eve was 23 years old, and her children still very small. Raising her children took all of Eve's time, so she did not date for several years. However, Dan remarried a year after the divorce. Dan's new wife, Sarah, had a son from a prior relationship, and together Dan and Sarah had two children, both daughters.

About 4 years after her divorce, when she was 27 years old, Eve met Jim, a single man who had no children. She married him a year later upon finding herself pregnant. Eve and Jim had two children, a boy and a girl, in addition to raising Eve's children from her first marriage. But Eve was dissatisfied in the marriage, and when her youngest child was 2 years old, she left Jim for another man, Charles. Eve's three school-age children from her first marriage left with her, but the two children she had with Jim continued to live with their father. Eve married Charles when she was 32 years old, became pregnant almost immediately, and had three 3 children, two girls and a boy, with Charles in the subsequent 8 years. Jim, in the meantime, met another woman five years after his marriage with Eve ended. His new wife, Beth, had no children; together, Jim and Beth raised Jim's two children from his marriage with Eve, and had two more, both boys.

In this complex blended family, there are past or current relationships between 6 adults and 13 children, but Eve's relationships are at the core of the family milieu.

Eve's current family relationships include her husband, Charles, and eight biological children, while Charles's family consists of his wife, Eve, three biological children, and five stepchildren.

Eve's first husband, Dan, has a wife, a stepson, and five stepchildren.

Eve's second husband, Jim, has a wife and four biological children, while Jim's wife, Beth, has two stepchildren and two biological children.

Each of Eve's children has differing numbers of siblings, both step- and biological. For example, her daughter from her marriage with Dan has five brothers (two full-siblings, two half-brothers, and one step-brother) and five half-sisters (all half-siblings) while Eve's daughter from her marriage with Jim has six brothers (one full-sibling, five half-sisters. Depending on whether relations between Eve and her ex-husbands are cordial, these children may all know one another and consider one another to be family regardless of blood relationship, or they may have limited contact or no interactions at all. There are significant age differences between half-siblings as well. The oldest of Eve's children could plausibly be an independent adult when Eve's youngest child was born.

It is not unusual in such scenarios for different generations to become intertwined in terms of age groupings. For instance, if Eve's oldest daughter follows her mother's example and has children at a young age, Eve's eldest grandchild could be fairly close in age to Eve's youngest child.

How Families Affect Health

Family members affect one another's health in many ways. One obvious way is biological. Families transmit illness from one member to another, whether in terms of infections (colds, flu, or athlete's foot) or in terms of genetics. The transmission of diseases with a genetic component can involve either passing on a predisposition for health issues that have known or unknown environmental mediating factors (obesity, dementia, and arthritis are some examples) or can be a distinct genetic flaw that results in an extremely high likelihood of disease (e.g., cystic fibrosis, hemophilia, or BRCA1 breast cancer) regardless of other inputs. Yet another way families influence one another is emotional. Families develop specific ways of defining health and work to keep their definitions in place. Family members consciously or unconsciously agree to take on specific roles, some of which may be dysfunctional and unhealthy.

Families affect members' health in other ways, too, and these effects strongly influence health promotion activities among family members. Bomar (1996) generated a list of key points for family health promotion, reviewing published articles (Anderson, 2000; Young & Hayes, 2002):

1. Individuals are unique, and so families are as well.
2. Many variables affect decisions made by the family about health, including orientation to life and biological, social, economic, cultural, psychological, and spiritual variables.
3. Family decisions are made independently of the healthcare professional.
4. Transformation of family health is best achieved when the family has the power as the primary decision maker.
5. Family health is dynamic, multidimensional, and always in flux.
6. Families will engage in health behaviors by what they have determined to be the highest priority to their careers and social lives.
7. Family health is systematic and process based.
8. Family health is not just the health of each individual family member.
9. All families have the ability to transform their quality of life and thus family health.

Health promotion activities may best be undertaken in the family setting for three reasons. First, obtaining investment in the process from a family group may be an important factor in promoting the health of a particular family member with health issues (e.g., a child with a disability or an adult who needs to make a major behavioral or lifestyle change, such as quitting smoking or altering dietary habits). Second, interdependencies in the family may be overriding factors supporting (or blocking) health promotion actions on the part of one or more members. Third, when you, as nurse, visit a family on its turf, you avoid trampling on their power and may be more likely to engage them in needed change processes.

Marilyn Ford-Gilboe, RN, PhD, of the University of Western Ontario, describes family health promotion as:

> a process undertaken by the family to sustain or enhance the emotional, social, and physical well-being of the family group and its members. This orientation focuses on the strength and potential for growth within families and recognizes the ways in which social and political realities may restrict choices for healthy living. We are concerned with better understanding how families and their members work together to realize their full potential for health and development. With this basis, effective strategies can be identified to assist families in developing behaviours and beliefs necessary for healthy living. (Ford-Gilboe, 2000, p. 1)

To work effectively with a family, you must understand family dynamics This is best done in the context of systems theory.

Systems Theory

The most influential theory for understanding how families work is **systems theory**. The theory originally was described by von Bertalanffy (1950), and was derived from systems theories originally developed for the sciences of physics and biology (Hanson & Kaakinen, 2001). The assumptions of systems theories include:

1. A system is composed of a set of elements that interact with one another.
2. Each system is a unique entity from the environment.
3. An open system exchanges matter and energy with the environment, while a closed system does not and causes isolation from the environment.
4. Systems depend on both positive and negative feedback to maintain homeostasis.

A family system grows out of the interactions of its members. As described by Friedman, Bowden, and Jones (2003), a family system:

> is a unique, small group of closely interrelated and interdependent individuals who are organized into a single unit in order to attain family functions or goals. . . . [The] family cannot be considered as merely the sum of its parts. The family viewed as a whole . . . is something more than parent(s) plus child(ren).

Look upon a family as an organic entity with specific qualities, which operate above and beyond the actions and behaviors of individual members. As with individuals, a family's well-being depends on its ability to meet basic needs of the individual members as well as the needs of the family unit as a whole, adapt to changing circumstances, cope with stresses and loss, and process information from both internal and external sources.

Family systems theory was extrapolated from systems theory and has its own assumptions, including:

1. Family systems are greater than and different from the sum of the whole.
2. Family systems are seen as a whole, where individuals are parts of the system and are interdependent and interactive.
3. Boundaries between individuals may be evident and can be described as open, closed, or random, but no family is ever completely closed or completely open.
4. There may be hierarchies evident as well as subsystem dyads (two-person alliances), for example mother–son, father–daughter, etc.
5. The family is in a constant state of change in response to stress from the external environment.
6. When one member of the family is affected by change, the family as a whole is also affected.
7. Every family system has characteristics designed to aid in stability, which may be adaptive or maladaptive.
8. The patterns of family interaction are circular, indicating interventions need to be directed to the cycle, not just to a cross-sectional event.
9. Family members send each other non-explicit messages to control or induce guilt in each other. The victim of **double bind** receives contradictory injunctions or emotional messages on different levels of communication (for example, love is expressed by words, and hate or detachment by nonverbal behavior; or a child is encouraged to speak freely, but criticized or silenced whenever he or she actually does (Bateson & Jackson, 1964).

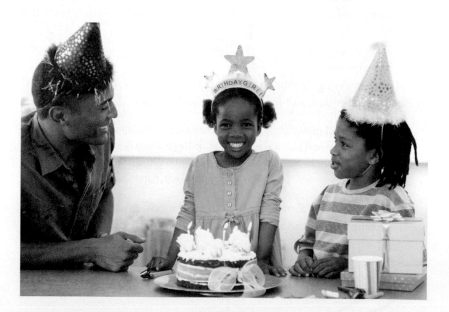

10. Triangles occur due to stress or anxiety when two people (often the parents) "triangle in" a third. This contributes significantly to the development of clinical problems. Two parents intensely focusing on what is wrong with a child can trigger serious rebellion in the child.

11. Family members with a poorly differentiated "self" depend so heavily on the acceptance and approval of others that either they quickly adjust what they think, say, and do to please others or they dogmatically proclaim what others should be like and pressure them to conform. (Bowen, 1966; 1971.)

ASK YOURSELF   `WWW.`

Suppose you are working with a family in which two of four children have childhood obesity. The parents and children are all being interviewed and assessed. What might your assessment and intervention plan consist of?

Key Components for Assessing Families

Key components for assessing family health promotion include family interaction, supportiveness, resilience, and nurturance; spirituality, rituals, celebrations, and routines; physical activity, recreation, and play; stress control and management; and the family's level of concern/responsibility for the health behaviors of its members, including nutrition, sleep patterns, sexuality, and living environment (Bomar & Baker-Word, 2001; Denham, 2003; Pender, Murdaugh, & Parsons, 2010)

All the concepts described in previous chapters involving health and health promotion for the individual can be applied to the family as well, including health and wellness, level of prevention, and theoretical frameworks.

Pender developed a **family health promotion model** (Pender et al., 2010). The model is portrayed in FIGURE 6-1, and represents the complex factors involved in family health behaviors.

In this model, Pender hypothesizes that there are three broad influences in the family's behavioral outcome of health-promoting behaviors. The influences include general influences, health-related influences, and behavior-specific influences.

◻ General Influences

General influences have three divisions, including family system patterns, demographic characteristics, and biologic characteristics. Each one of these directly influences health-promoting behaviors and health-related influences. The model

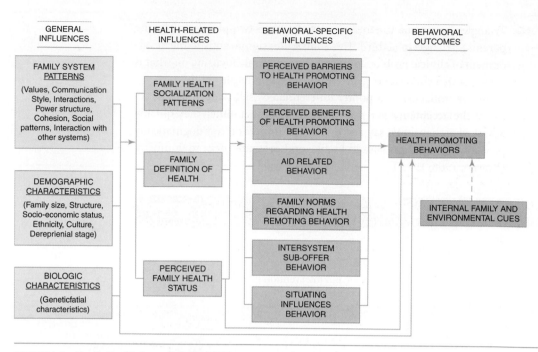

FIGURE 6-1   Family Health Promotion Model.

Source: Pender, Nola J.; Murdaugh, Carolyn L.; Parsons, Mary Ann, *Health Promotion in Nursing Practice, 6th Edition,* © 2011. Printed and Electronically reproduced by permission of Pearson Education, Inc., Upper Saddle River, New Jersey.

lists the patterns and characteristics under each heading. Family system patterns include values, communication style, interactions, power structure, cohesion, socialization patterns, and interaction with other systems. Demographic characteristics include family size, structure, socioeconomic status, ethnicity, culture, and development state. Finally, biologic characteristics include genetic factors and characteristics of biological relationships between individuals, e.g., sexual interaction between partners or parent–child emotional bonding.

☐ Health-Related Influences

Health-related influences include family health socialization patterns, family definition of health, and perceived family health status. These also directly affect health-promoting behaviors and behavioral-specific influences.

☐ Behavioral-Specific Influences

Behavioral-specific influences include perceived barriers to health-promoting behavior, perceived benefits of health-promoting behavior, prior related behavior, family norms regarding health-promoting behavior, intersystem support for behavior, and situational influences on behavior. These also directly impact health-promoting behaviors. Internal family and environmental cues may or may not have an influence on health-promoting behavior.

When working with a family, promote effective communication between you and the family as well as among family members. This can be particularly challenging if family dynamics are unhealthy (e.g., if individuals in the family treat other individuals disrespectfully or abusively), as we will discuss later in this chapter.

Traits of a Healthy Family

Health promotion for the family starts by understanding what exactly a **healthy family** is. According to DeFrain (1994), three categories define family health: unity, flexibility, and communication.

☐ Unity

Unity is evidenced by the level of interpersonal commitment and time spent together. In a healthy family, commitment is generated when a family member develops a sense of trust in other family members, teaches or learns respect for others, exhibits a sense of shared responsibility, and shares simple and quality time with other individuals in the family. Time spent together among family members enables them to share family rituals and traditions, enjoy each other's company, and share leisure time.

☐ Flexibility

Flexibility reflects a number of characteristics exhibited by and supported by family members. The first characteristic is the ability to deal with stress. Dealing well with stress is characterized by adaptability—the ability to see crises as a challenge and opportunity, show openness to change, seek help with problems, and grow together in crisis. Teamwork in solving problems and the ability to assume or relinquish leadership roles is an important component of family flexibility.

☐ Communication

In a healthy family, members speak and listen respectfully to each other and make an effort to understand the messages others are sending. When individuals communicate in this way, they are able to compromise and disagree without blaming or accusing one another. They are also able to share feelings and engage in family conversation on a broad range of issues. Disagreements are handled through negotiation rather than fighting, and disputes or arguments focus on the subject at hand rather than bringing in outside factors.

Family Roles

When working toward family health promotion, it is important to understand concepts of family roles. Family roles are established patterns of behavior of family members (Wright & Leahey, 2000). Roles are learned behaviors, not instinctive or automatic ones. Each member of the family usually does not just have one role, but multiple roles. Individuals may have different expectations for how this role should be played based on what they learned in their family of origin combined with what they learn from other family members. The expectations and understanding of each person's family role, if not clearly defined and agreed to by all parties, can be a source of conflict.

For example, consider a couple who have just had their first child. The father comes from a large family where everyone in the household looked after the children. Mother is the younger of two children born in a wealthy household where her mother worked and had live-in nannies undertake childcare tasks. Both parents may conceptualize childcare as a job done by more than one person, but they may identify their own position in regard to the role of caregiver differently.

The mother's family of origin experiences may leave her with limited ability to identify herself in the role of caregiver, while the father's may give him an expectation that both he and his spouse will take turns and be equally involved. If both parents are able to express their expectations about caregiving before the child's birth, or if the father is perceptive about his wife's childcare role models in her family of origin, the couple may be able to either reach a compromise position on caregiving roles, or one of the two could also adopt the other's model, with alterations to suit their circumstances. If such compromises are not reached, it is likely that the two views regarding roles will reach a point of conflict fairly quickly, given the stresses associated with child rearing.

If, for example, the mother in this couple accepts that she is responsible for handling some of the child care duties but finds herself unable to soothe her teething infant when it is her turn to take care of the child, she may feel **role strain**—the difficulty felt in fulfilling role obligations (Goode, 1960, p. 483).

Role strain contrasts with **role stress**, which is caused by difficulties outside of the individual or by the environment. An example could be that the parents agree upon their respective roles regarding childrearing, but a demanding job or a health crisis prevents one or the other from fulfilling that role.

Role stress may be the outcome of the following problems:

1. **Role ambiguity**—A vague and insufficiently defined role causing the individual to have disharmony or insecurity around performance of the role (e.g., "Am I doing this right? I don't really know how to manage my family's budget.")

2. **Role conflict**—Inconsistent expectations in the role set, usually caused by incompatible interaction by two or more roles, yielding unmet demands (e.g., "I can cook dinner for us, or I can pick the kids up at daycare. You can't expect me to do both at the same time.")

3. **Role incongruity**—Similar to role conflict with incompatibility, but it is evident between the role and the person who holds it. ("Look, I'm not comfortable advocating with the hospice staff—I'm just not able to look after Mom by myself. I need some help here.")

4. **Role overload**—Inability to meet the role obligations or failing to meet them in a specified period of time (e.g., "I know Jimmy has baseball practice, but Dad is in the hospital and I was supposed to get that project finished this evening—I'm a terrible mother!").

Roles can be informal or formal. Formal roles are dictated and defined by societal norms (e.g., mother, husband, boss, coworker, etc.), while informal roles are specific behaviors evident in certain settings. It is important to recognize that the same individual may take on different roles under different circumstances.

Informal roles are important in that the healthcare professional needs to direct interventions to that characteristic. Informal roles include:

1. **Harmonizer**—Tries to keep peace within the family by acting as mediator
2. **Opposer**—Is negative to family ideas and suggestions
3. **Martyr**—Sacrifices everything for the sake of the family
4. **Blamer**—Dictator who knows it all, thus is always finding fault
5. **Follower**—Passively accepts family decisions made by other family members
6. **Bystander**—Stands along the sideline with little involvement in family activities (even those in which he/she is actively involved in deciding to undertake)
7. **Coordinator**—Planner and organizer of family activities
8. **Scapegoat**—The one who is blamed for problems
9. **Encourager**—Motivates others by making them feel important
10. **Caretaker**—One who is called on the most for help and assistance; may also be called the nurturer
11. **Dominator**—Manipulates the family to be the primary authoritarian

These informal roles need not be dysfunctional all the time, but it is clear from the descriptions that there is an element of dysfunction inherent in some of them. The roles of blamer, scapegoat, martyr, and dominator are dysfunctional by nature. A family member who consistently takes the role of fault finder or authoritarian, for example, is by definition disrespectful of other members' needs for support, encouragement, self-efficacy, and affection.

Suppose you are involved in the care of a family in which a 5-year-old has been hospitalized due to burns suffered during a small family fire. The 5-year-old had 10% second-degree burns on his leg and lower back and his condition is stable. The family consists of a father, mother, and a brother and sister, ages 10 and 15, respectively. The fire was started by the 10-year-old boy who was playing with matches, while the 15-year-old daughter was babysitting. The family is quite disruptive in the visitor's lounge.

The father is insisting that the incident was the fault of the daughter, who should have been paying attention to both children. The mother seems to concur with this assessment, though it seems in part to be an appeasement to her husband. No one seems to be focusing on the 10-year-old who was actually responsible.

The unit social worker spends some time with the family and hears the mother and father blame the daughter for most of the problems that occur with the younger siblings. The father is the most vehement and insists that his opinions are usually correct. The daughter does not defend herself and seems accepting of her parents' pronouncements. From the brief encounter with this family, the social worker formed the following opinions about informal roles in this family.

The father was
a.   The coordinator
b.   The blamer
c.   The opposer

The mother was
a.   The harmonizer
b.   The follower
c.   The martyr

The daughter was
a.   The dominator
b.   The scapegoat
c.   The caretaker

The daughter could also be the caretaker. As more information about the family dynamics and situation emerges, it becomes apparent that both parents work long hours, leaving the 15-year-old in charge. Her silence in the midst of accusations may also suggest she believes herself to be the martyr. It is important to keep in mind how complex the family unit may be and that roles can be in continual flux.

A scapegoat family member who is continually taking the blame for problems is, in essence, offering an opportunity for other family members to avoid taking responsibility for their own actions. The martyr role is unhealthy for the individual as well as the family; a martyr does not get any needs met other than an unhealthy one—the need to feel superior to other family members. The common martyr's complaint, "I do *everything* for you, and you do *nothing* for me," is a martyr's way of saying "I'm a better person than you are."

Even healthier roles, such as encourager and coordinator, can be engaged in unhealthy ways if the person who steps into the role uses it to manipulate,

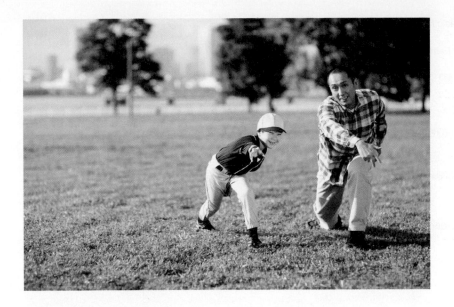

hide, or otherwise change the family dynamic in a way that is not beneficial to the family as a whole. An encourager who motivates family members to take actions that are not wise or that will not benefit their well-being may be placing personal goals ahead of what is best for the family. An example might be a parent who obsessively encourages the family's children to take up activities, such as theater or competitive sports, because the parent wants the children to make up for goals the parent never accomplished.

Identifying such roles (and which individuals in the family take them on) is an important step in promoting family health. Train family members to recognize when they are undertaking roles that are unhealthy, or when they are using particular roles in an unhealthy way.

HEALTH PROMOTION CHALLENGE

Identify your role in your family. Is it a role you like taking? If not, decide on a way to resist taking that role in the future. Get feedback on your plan from a trusted friend.

Genograms and Ecomaps

A **genogram** (FIGURE 6-2) is a visual representation of family structure, with symbolic representations of the family composition, health history, and

Symbol to describe basic family membership and structure

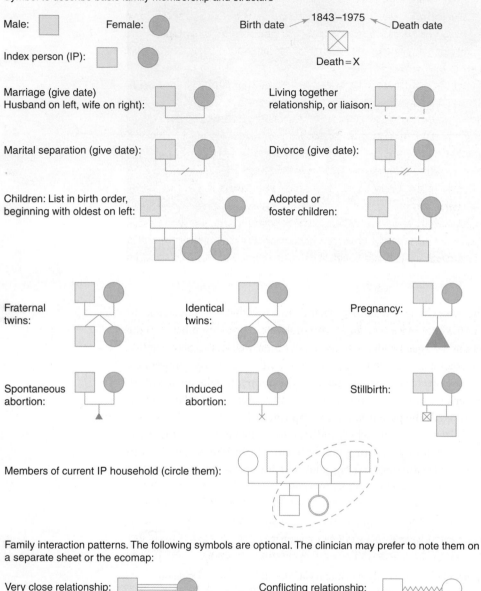

Members of current IP household (circle them):

Family interaction patterns. The following symbols are optional. The clinician may prefer to note them on a separate sheet or the ecomap:

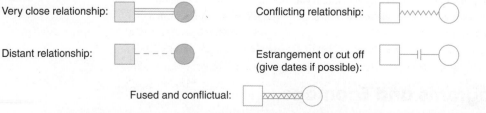

FIGURE 6-2   Standard Symbols for Genogram

Source: McGoldrick, M., Gerson, R., & Shellenberg, S. (1999). *Genograms: Assessment and intervention* (2nd ed.). New York, NY: WW Norton.

relationships with other members (McGoldrick, Gerson, & Shellenberg, 1999). There are many formats that are used to construct a genogram, but the most common ones are represented in family health promotion nursing literature (Hanson, 2001; Murray, Zenter, Brockhaus, Brockhaus, & Sullivan, 2001; Roth, 1996; Wright & Leahey, 2000).

Many times the genogram is constructed during the initial meeting. Take a large drawing pad with you and as you talk with a family, add in the relationships between family members, starting with mother and father at the top and then their offspring below that. The genogram process serves as an icebreaker between you and the family and also can help you gather important information about what grandfather died of and what chronic illnesses grandmother or the other family members have. The source of information is the family, so the process engages family members in discussion. The usual format constructs the relationships for three generations. Symbols are made for males and females, with lines depicting certain types of relationships between the individuals. An X is used to symbolize death. See Figure 6-2 for how to construct a genogram.

RESEARCH BOX 6-2

Interested in knowing more about genograms? Here is a website full of information and diagrams to show you how they work: http://www.genopro. com/genogram

Another type of drawing that is useful in family health promotion is the **ecomap** (FIGURE 6-3). This type of map is useful in providing a visual overview of how the family interacts with different systems in the environment, such as work, church, school, social networks, and community. In the center is the family that comprises the household, and around them are outer circles that consist of the systems in the environment, specifically ones that are significant.

Lines are drawn to connect the family to the different circles to denote the strength of connectedness. A straight line represents a strong relationship. More than one type of straight line may be drawn; for example a heavy, bold, straight line signifies a very strong connectivity. Broken lines, on the other hand, signify weak connections. Arrows represent the energy flow of family and the systems.

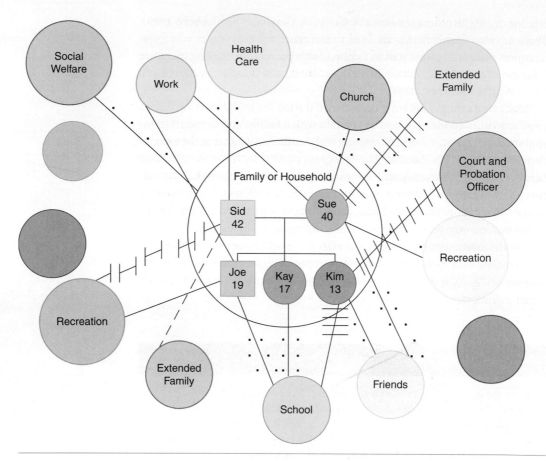

FIGURE 6-3 Sample Ecomap

Source: Reprinted with permission from the National Resource Center for Family Centered Practices, The University of Iowa School of Social Work, Iowa City.

Putting It All Together: Health Promotion In Families

The preceding information on how to understand a family system—dynamics, roles, and healthy versus unhealthy behaviors—offers a foundation for working with a family, but the practical application of this information is another matter. To address a problem in a family system, you must examine all areas of function and identify problems in each or all of them. Nursing diagnoses can be made in accordance with one or several diagnostic systems—the NANDA classification system and the Omaha system are two key diagnostic tools.

Having diagnosed issues in the family's function, you then identify interventions that might help the family function better. For example, the Calgary family intervention model identifies three domains of family functioning: the cognitive domain (e.g., ideas, opinions, information, education), the affective domain (emotional responses and coping) and the behavioral domain (habits, activities, rituals, etc.).

Addressing cognitive issues may require you to act as an educator, teaching family members about the illness or condition that affects one (or more) members. Addressing affective problems may require a different form of education—instruction on developing attitude changes and developing better differentiated emotional responses. Both cognitive and affective interventions are usually necessary to create behavioral changes that promote health in the family and its individual members.

For example, suppose you are asked to work with a family composed of two parents and five children ranging in age from 6 to 19. The youngest child, a 6-year-old girl, has been diagnosed with severe allergic asthma. The child's symptoms are so severe that exposure to any of several environmental triggers—cat dander, grass pollen, and cigarette smoke—is likely to require use of a rescue inhaler. On three occasions in recent weeks, exposures have resulted in an emergency department visit, which is why the family has been referred for a nursing intervention.

The parents have already taken several steps toward reducing their daughter's exposures by giving away the family cat, purchasing an air purifier for the daughter's bedroom, and undertaking smoking cessation programs. The father has been smoke-free now for several months, but the mother has been less successful, although she takes pains to smoke outdoors, away from where her daughter might be exposed.

More disconcerting is the fact that the oldest son still smokes and has explicitly refused to quit, saying he does not understand why such a huge fuss is being made just because his sister needs an inhaler. According to the parents, his sister's most recent emergency department visit occurred because the oldest son had been smoking in his bedroom against his parents' wishes. His refusal has sparked conflict in the family between him and his father, with the mother attempting to mediate between them.

The two middle children, a boy, age 15, and a girl, age 10, have expressed resentment for having to give up their cat. The 10-year-old girl has taken to picking on her little sister as a result, and recently her school has called the parents to say she has engaged in bullying of another student. The 15-year-old boy has become more protective of his youngest sister, making sure that her air purifier is always turned on at night and using his computer to check pollen levels each morning. He frequently intervenes on her behalf when the older girl picks on her.

In the initial interview, it becomes apparent that only the parents and the 15-year-old comprehend the fact that the little girl's bad cough is a serious, potentially life-threatening condition. The youngest child herself is shy and withdrawn, saying little when her siblings are present. In a separate interview with only the child and her parents, the little girl tells the nurse that she misses the cat, too, and does not understand why her sister is so mad at her for the cat's departure. The parents react differently to this statement: The father tells the child that her sister is just being bratty and assures her that she will get over it, while the mother quickly tells the little girl that the cat's departure is not her fault. Neither parent directly addresses the emotional content of the child's statement. The nurse notes that the mother's response has an underlying note of anxiety, while the father's seems irritable.

HEALTH PROMOTION CHALLENGE   (www.)

Draw a genogram for this family, using the information you learned from visiting the genogram website mentioned above. Pretend you are talking with the family and drawing the genogram. What would you do if the youngest daughter says, "What are you doing? Can I draw on it?"

In this hypothetical case, there is more than one problem facing this family's health. The family shows several of the factors that Wright and Leahey (2000) identify as indications for intervention: (1) a family member has presented with an illness that is having a detrimental effect on other family members; (2) family members are contributing to the symptoms or problems of the individual; (3) children/adolescents in the family have developed emotional and behavioral problems in the context of their sibling's illness (Friedman et al., 2003). Using the NANDA diagnostic classification, a number of potential diagnoses are evident (see TABLE 6-1). On the other hand, the family displays certain strengths; for example, the parents display a unity of purpose in their immediate and direct response to their child's diagnosis. Both parents have taken immediate steps to protect their child's health—the fact that the mother is less successful than the father at quitting smoking in no way detracts from the fact that she is nonetheless undertaking major behavioral changes on her daughter's behalf. Family support systems and problem-solving skills are evident in the willingness of both parents and one sibling to focus on protecting the youngest child's health and well-being, but they need to be expanded to encompass the oldest son and middle daughter, who are clearly having difficulty engaging with the family's goal of promoting the youngest member's health.

Table 6-1 2012–2014 NANDA-Approved Nursing Diagnoses Applicable to the Example

- Attachment, parent/infant/child, risk for impaired
- Caregiver role strain
- Caregiver role strain, risk for
- Communication: impaired, verbal
- Communication, readiness for enhanced
- Coping, defensive
- Coping: family, compromised
- Coping: family, disabled
- Coping, ineffective
- Decisional conflict
- Decision making, readiness for enhanced
- Denial, ineffective
- Family processes, readiness for enhanced
- Health behavior, risk-prone
- Health-seeking behaviors (specify)
- Knowledge, deficient (specify)
- Knowledge (specify), readiness for enhanced
- Parenting, readiness for enhanced
- Role performance, ineffective
- Self-care, readiness for enhanced
- Self-esteem, situational low
- Self-esteem, risk for situational low
- Stress, overload
- Therapeutic regimen management: family, ineffective
- Therapeutic regimen management, readiness for enhanced

Source: NANDA International Nursing Diagnoses: Definitions and Classification 2012–2014, © 2011 Wiley-Blackwell.

In summary, the little girl's asthma is the acute crisis that has brought them to the intervention, but it is not the only problem, nor is it necessarily the most difficult problem to address. Health promotion for a family cannot simply focus on the little girl's asthma. Because the interactions with family members and the functioning of the family as a whole may prove a critical factor in the individual's health, it is important to focus on helping the family to create a well-functioning unit that will support everyone's health. This means simultaneously addressing individual health promotion needs as well as family unit dysfunctions. In this case, you face several challenges in promoting this family's health:

1. Bringing all family members to the same level of understanding of the nature and severity of the health problem faced by its youngest member, including the importance of helping her to avoid allergic triggers such as smoke (cognitive domain)
2. Assisting the children through their emotional responses (resentment, anger, and sadness) stemming from the changes this health crisis has initiated in the family's daily life and interactions (affective domain)
3. Assisting the parents to learn more effective ways of communicating with their children (behavioral domain) and acknowledging both the children's and their own emotions regarding the health crisis (affective domain)
4. Developing a strategy to promote behavioral changes in individuals (e.g., the oldest brother's smoking and the older sister's aggressive acting out).
5. Developing a strategy for the family unit as a whole (e.g., increased family cohesion and better crisis management), and to reduce the youngest child's exposures to asthma triggers and ensure that she does not take on an unhealthy role in the family system, such as the scapegoat role (behavioral domain)

An intervention for a family dealing with a health crisis in one member may require a variety of approaches, depending on the functionality of the family. In this instance, the family is moderately dysfunctional. Although the parents and one child are acting in support of he sick family member, two of the siblings are at odds with the family's goals, in part because the nature of the problem and the goals and tasks related to solving it have not been clearly explained.

Educating the family, particularly the parents, in effective communication techniques may prove helpful. Individual counseling for more troubled members (the older girl and oldest son) may be helpful in addressing their affective and cognitive disturbances in relationship to their sister's health problem. Family counseling would likely also be useful, so that healthier interpersonal relationships among and between family members can be established. Goal-setting exercises and having the family group develop their own contract for lifestyle modification are possible techniques for promoting greater family health in all domains.

HEALTH PROMOTION CHALLENGE

Write a script for a session with this family. Role play it with a couple of other students. Get their feedback on your performance and the process everyone observed.

Some ideas to keep in mind:

Make sure to introduce yourself to each family member and make a connection with each one.

Pay attention to process (what is happening in the interview) more than the words said; observe the reactions of everyone to whoever is speaking;

To identify the family spokesperson, ask, "Can anyone tell me what the main problem in this family is?"

If there is a child problem, the adults are usually in disagreement about how to deal with the child.

Make sure to get everyone's viewpoint of the problem; begin to notice slight disagreements in the way family members see the problem; when parents begin to talk about the identified patient, notice how much the child is an issue between them and think about ways to help them resolve that issue.

Be neutral; don't take sides; point out positives and strengths of each family member.

When anxious, avoid turning to the identified patient (the one everyone says has the problem); instead, talk to the parents or the one least involved in the problem.

Ultimately, everyone should talk to everyone else. If some members are silent or don't speak to certain family members, ask them, "Could you help your parents with this? Talk to them."

Look for alliances and sub-groups as the family members speak.

When there is a problem child, one adult in the family has violated a generational boundary by becoming over-involved and overly concerned with a child. If mother is overly involved, ask Dad to talk to his child about the problem. If Mom says Dad never helps with the children, ask Dad to help the "problem child" draw a picture.

Give a task to the family at the end of the interview, but keep it simple, e.g., Talk to one family member this week you usually don't talk to and ask them what they like to do to feel good.

If parents have emotionally cut themselves off from their parents (**emotional cut-off**), ask them to visit their parents and ask them to talk about their kin and family history.

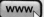
Summary

The definition of family has evolved since the early 1980s. In 1982, the family was defined as a social group consisting of a man and woman and their offspring, all living under the same roof. By 2003, Friedman et al. defined the family as two or more persons joined together by bonds or sharing and emotional closeness who identify themselves as being part of the family. The common thread for all the definitions was the presence of two or more individuals. Ten assumptions about families include the following: (1) families are unique; (2) family decisions are affected by a variety of factors; (3) family decisions are made independent of the healthcare professional; (4) health changes occur when the family has the power as the primary decision maker; (5) family health is dynamic, multidimensional, and always in flux; (6) engaging in health behaviors is guided by the highest priority to career and social lives; (7) family health is systematic and process based; (8) family health is not just the health of each individual family member; (9) families have the ability to transform their quality of life and family health; and (10) the role of the nurse is active listening and working as an advocate for informed decision making.

Family composition has changed over the last 50 years. Examples seen currently include legally married without children, cohabitating unmarried adults, single parents, blended families, extended families, and gay and lesbian couples.

The most influential theory about family is the systems theory, originally described by von Bertalanffy in 1950. The assumptions of system theory include the following: a system is composed of a set of elements that interact with one another; each system is a unique entity from the environment; an open system exchanges matter and energy with the environment, and a closed system causes isolation from the environment; and systems depend on both positive and negative feedback to maintain homeostasis. **Family theory** was extrapolated from systems theory and has its own assumptions. Family theory views the family within the larger community and subsystems and is holistic.

Pender's family health promotion model developed from her original health promotion model. In the model there are three broad influences in the family's behavioral outcome of health-promoting behaviors. These are general, health related, and behavioral specific. General includes family system patterns, demographic characteristics, and biological characteristics. Health-related influences include family health socialization patterns, family definition of health, and perceived family health status. Behavioral-specific influences include perceived barriers to health-promoting behavior, perceived benefits of health-promoting behavior, prior related behavior, family norms regarding health-promoting behavior, intersystem support for behavior, and situational influences on behavior. Pender has developed a format for assessment of family health promotion.

Identified necessary key components to include when assessing family health promotion include nutrition; family interaction and nurturance; spirituality; sleep patterns; sexuality; environment; family physical activity, recreation, and play; stress control and management; health responsibility; family resilience and resources; family support; and family rituals, celebrations, and routines. A variety of tools have been developed by those in the sociology, psychology, and nursing fields to evaluate the dimensions of family health promotion.

Three categories of traits exist in a healthy family. These are unity, flexibility, and communication. Family roles are established patterns of behavior of family members and are learned behaviors. Usually family members have multiple roles. Role strain is the difficulty in fulfilling role obligations. Role stress is caused by difficulties outside the individual or the environment and may be caused by role ambiguity, role conflict, role incongruity, and role overload. Some informal family roles are the following: harmonizer, opposer, martyr, blamer, follower, bystander, coordinator, scapegoat, encourager, caretaker, and dominator.

A genogram is a process for constructing a visual representation of family structure, with symbolic representations of the family composition, health history, and relationship with other members. An ecomap is a drawing used in family health promotion that provides a visual overview of how the family interacts with different systems in the environment, such as work, church, school, social networks, and community.

Health promotion in families requires diagnosing problems in the family system and identifying the domains in which health promotion activities can take place. The NANDA classification system and the Omaha system are two diagnostic systems commonly used for identifying individual and family health problems. Nursing interventions that follow the Calgary family intervention model identify issues in three domains of family function: cognitive, affective, and behavioral.

Important family problems include triangling, emotional cut-off, and lack of self-differentiation.

REVIEW QUESTIONS

1. All of the following are assumptions about the family except:
   a. Families are unique
   b. Family health is dynamic
   c. Family decisions depend on the healthcare professional

2. The following are family composition models except:
   a. Single parent
   b. Single adult
   c. Blended family

3. A system:
   a. Does not depend on feedback to maintain homeostasis
   b. Is composed of a set of elements that interact with one another
   c. Is part of its environment

4. Contained within the broad influence category of health-related, within Pender's family health promotion model, is:
   a. Family definition of health
   b. Biological characteristics
   c. Prior related behavior

5. Contained within the broad influence category of general, within Pender's family health promotion model, is:
   a. Family definition of health
   b. Biological characteristics
   c. Prior related behavior

6. Key components to include when assessing family health promotion include all of the following except:
   a. Sleep patterns
   b. Family resilience
   c. Ancestry

7. Role strain is:
   a. Caused by difficulties outside the individual or environment
   b. The informal family role of one who stands along the sideline without involvement
   c. Difficulty in fulfilling role obligations

8. The encourager is the informal family role in which:
   a. One motivates others by making them feel important
   b. One is a dictator who knows it all, thus finding fault
   c. One tries to keep peace within the family by acting as mediator

9. The harmonizer is the informal family role in which:
   a. One motivates others by making them feel important
   b. One is a dictator who knows it all, thus finding fault
   c. One tries to keep peace within the family by acting as mediator

10. An ecomap is:
   a. A visual overview of how the family interacts with different systems in the environment, such as work, church, school, etc.
   b. A visual representation of family structure
   c. A tool developed by Nola Pender

EXERCISES

`www`

1. Research the concept of resilience. Find instruments that have been developed to study resilience. Find studies in which families have been evaluated for resilience and summarize your findings.

2. Choose an area of family health that you are especially interested in. Find literature about this subject and create a subject bibliography. Keep this list and consider using it for a future project/paper.

3. Practice with genograms by constructing one about your family. Interview some of your family members to assist in accuracy.

4. Select an ethnic group that lives in your community. Read about the typical family structure/health patterns for this group.

REFERENCES

American Heritage dictionary, college. (1982). Boston, MA: Houghton Mifflin.

Anderson, K. (2000). The family health system approach to family systems nursing. *Journal of Family Nursing, 6*, 103–119.

Bateson, G. & Jackson, D. (1964). Some varieties of pathogenic organization. *Research Publications—Association for Research in Nervous and Mental Disease, 42*, 270–290.

Bomar, P. (1996). *Nurses and family health promotion* (2nd ed.). Philadelphia, PA: FA Davis.

Bomar, P. (2004). *Promoting health in families: Applying family research and theory to nursing practice.* Philadelphia, PA: Saunders.

Bomar, P., & Baker-Word, P. (2001). Family health promotion. In S. Hanson (Ed.), *Family health care nursing: Theory, practice and research* (2nd ed., pp. 197–219). Philadelphia, PA: FA Davis.

Bowen, M. (1966). The use of family theory in clinical practice. *Comprehensive Psychiatry, 7*(5), 345–374.

Bowen, M. (1971). Toward the differentiation of self in one's own family. In J. Framo (Ed.) *Family interaction* (pp. 111–173). New York, NY: Springer.

Curran, D. (1983). *Stress and the healthy family.* Minneapolis, MN: Winston Press.

Denham, S. (2003). *Family health: A framework for nursing.* Philadelphia, PA: FA Davis.

Ford-Gilboe, M. (2000). *Family health promotion research program.* Retrieved from http:// publish. uwo. ca/~mfordg/family.html

Friedemann, M. (1991). An instrument to evaluate effectiveness in family functioning. *Western Journal of Nursing Research, 13*, 220–241.

Friedemann, M. (1995). *The framework of systemic organization: A conceptual approach to families and nursing.* Thousand Oaks, CA: Sage.

Friedman, M. M., Bowden, V. R., & Jones, E. G. (2003). *Family nursing: Research, theory, and practice* (5th ed.). Upper Saddle River, NJ: Prentice Hall.

Goode, D. (1960). A theory of role strain. *American Sociological Review, 25*, 483–496.

Hanson, S. (2001). *Family health care nursing: Theory, practice, and research* (2nd ed.). Philadelphia, PA: FA Davis.

Hanson, S., & Mischke, K. (1996). Family health assessment and intervention. In P. Bomar (Ed.), *Nurses and family health promotion* (2nd ed., pp. 165–202). Philadelphia, PA: Saunders.

Hanson, S., & Kaakinen, J. (2001). Theoretical foundations for family nursing. In S. Hanson (Ed.), *Family health care nursing: Theory, practice and research* (2nd ed., pp. 36–59). Philadelphia, PA: FA Davis.

McCubbin, M., & McCubbin, H. I. (1987). Families coping with illness: The resiliency model of family stress, adjustment and adaptation. In H. McCubbin & A. Thompson (Eds.), *Family assessment inventories for research and practice* (2nd ed., pp. 3–232). Madison: University of Wisconsin Press.

McGoldrick, M., Gerson, R., & Shellenberg, S. (1999). *Genograms: Assessment and intervention* (2nd ed.). New York, NY: WW Norton.

Murray, R., Zenter, J., Brockhaus, J., Brockhaus, R., & Sullivan, E. (2001). The Family: Basic Unit for the Developing Person. In R. Murray & J. Zenter (Eds.), *Health promotion strategies through the life span* (7th ed., pp. 157–212). Upper Saddle River, NJ: Prentice-Hall.

Olson, D., & DeFrain, J. (1994). *Marriage and the family.* Mountain View, CA: Mayfield Publishing.

Olson, D. H., Porter, J., & Lavee, Y. (1985). *Family adaptability and cohesion evaluation scales* (3rd ed.). St. Paul: University of Minnesota.

Pender, N., Murdaugh, C., & Parsons, M. (2010). *Health promotion in nursing practice* (6th ed.). Upper Saddle River, NJ: Prentice-Hall.

Pless, I. B., & Satterwhite, B. (1973). A measure of family functioning and its application. *Social Science & Medicine, 7*(8), 613–621.

Roth, P. (1996). Family social support. In P. J. Bomar (Ed.), *Nurses and family health promotion: Concepts, assessment, and intervention* (2nd ed., pp. 107–138). Philadelphia, PA: WB Saunders.

Smilkstein, G. (1978). The family APGAR: A proposal for family function test and its use by physicians. *Journal of Family Practice, 6*(6), 1231–1239.

U. S. Census Bureau. (2002). *Current population survey CPS*. Retrieved from http://www. census. gov/population/www/cps/cpsdef. html

Von Bertalanffy, L. (1950). The theory of open systems in physics and biology. *Science, 111*, 23–29.

Wright, L., & Leahey, M. (2000). *Nurses and families: A guide to family assessment and intervention* (3rd ed.). Philadelphia, PA: FA Davis.

Wright, L., Watson, W., & Bell, J. (1996). *Beliefs: The heart of healing in families and illness.* New York, NY: Basic Books.

Young, L., & Hayes, V. (2002). *Transforming health promotion practice*. Philadelphia, PA: FA Davis.

INTERNET RESOURCES

For a full suite of assignments and learning activities, use the access code located in the front of your book to visit this exclusive website: **http://go.jblearning.com/healthpromotion**. If you do not have an access code, you can obtain one at the site.

Upon completion of this chapter, you will be able to:

1. Define health policy.

2. Analyze the factors affecting how healthcare policy is created.

3. Differentiate the different levels of healthcare policy—local, state, federal, and global.

4. Examine the role you can play in formulating and implementing health promotion policy.

5. Identify key advances in legislative healthcare policy, including the Patient Protection and Affordable Care Act of 2010.

6. Identify the roles of federal agencies that have jurisdiction over health promotion policy implementation.

7. Analyze the evolution of the *Healthy People* documents and developmental process.

8. Take action on one health promotion policy issue.

Genetic Information Nondiscrimination Act (GINA)

Genome

Health policy

Medicare Act

Nursing Workforce Development programs

Patient Protection and Affordable Care Act

Social Security Act Amendments

CHAPTER 7

Health Policy and Health Promotion

http://go.jblearning.com/healthpromotion

For a full suite of assignments and learning activities, use the access code located in the front of your book to visit the exclusive website: http://go.jblearning.com/healthpromotion If you do not have an access code, you can obtain one at the site.

Introduction

Everything you will do as a nurse is affected by government health policy. The main focal points of healthcare reform in the 21st century are health promotion and illness prevention. These policies form the basis of many health promotion programs.

Policies and laws regarding nurse practice standards constrain your interactions with clients. An understanding of healthcare policy—the factors that influence it, how policy affects practice, and how you can (and should) work to influence policy decisions—is vital to health promotion.

This chapter provides a brief overview of some of the significant health policies related to health promotion to help you understand the concepts involved in health policy creation and implementation. It also highlights the areas where you can work to help shape policies at the community, state, and national levels by serving as a political activist, developing policies for best practice in health promotion for individuals, families, and communities.

What Is Health Policy?

Health policy is defined by the World Health Organization (WHO) as follows:

> Health policy refers to decisions, plans, and actions that are undertaken to achieve specific health care goals within a society. An explicit health policy can achieve several things: it defines a vision for the future which in turn helps to establish targets and points of reference for the short and medium term. It outlines priorities and the expected roles of different groups; and it builds consensus and informs people. (WHO, 2012, p. 1)

For the purpose of this book, the best definition of *health policy* is this: decisions made by government bodies that are intended to support or improve the health of citizens. Health policy focuses on issues that affect individual health, for example by funding efforts to support individuals' health promotion activities. Examples are policies that support programs intended to help individuals lose weight, quit smoking, obtain prenatal care, or obtain clean drinking water and clean air.

Health policy also focuses on public health, which is an expression of the overall health status of the general population, including specific health issues experienced by the general population or by subgroups within the general population. Two examples of public health policies you can participate in with clients are: (1) Smoking cessation, and (2) Women, Infant, & Children (WIC) nutrition programs aimed at ensuring low-income mothers with young children have adequate food for their families.

Global health policy is policy undertaken by multiple nations (by means of agencies such as the World Health Organization or various United Nations programs such as UNICEF or UNAIDS) that seeks to affect the overall incidence of particular widespread health concerns over time. An example of a global health policy initiative would be reduce the infant and maternal death rate in countries with high death rates for women and young children.

Global health policy can include issues important in the United States. For example, babies in the United States have a higher risk of dying during their first month of life than do babies born in 40 other countries, according to a World Health Organization (2011) report. Some of the countries that outrank the United States in terms of newborn death risk are South Korea, Cuba, Malaysia, Lithuania, Poland and Israel, according to the study. "We know that solutions as simple as keeping newborns warm, clean and hold them close while properly breast-feeding them can keep them alive," said study researcher Joy Lawn of the Save the Children Foundation, which worked with the WHO on the report. "It isn't that you have to build invasive care units to halve your neonatal mortality."

Also important is ensuring that all pregnant clients receive preterm attention and counseling (Trippel, 2011).

HEALTH PROMOTION CHALLENGE ⭐ (www.)

What can you do to help lower the infant death rate in this country? Consider a letter to the editor of your local paper, Tweeting about this shocking statistic, placing information on your Facebook page, offering a class for pregnant women about the importance of breastfeeding while holding them close and keeping their infants warm and clean, or using some other way to institute change. Find out how many pregnant women in your community are not receiving preterm care and take action. Share your ideas and findings with your classmates.

Although the concept of global public health has changed over the past half century, the current goal as expressed by the World Health Organization is to promote health among all individuals such that each person reaches full health potential (Irvine, Elliott, Wallace, & Crombie, 2006). Reaching such goals requires addressing individual health challenges such as obesity, smoking, and alcohol and substance dependency. It also requires policies that tackle the economic, social, and environmental determinants of health, such as inequalities in health access, poverty, and exposure to industrial pollution.

How Are Health Policies Created?

Health policies generally develop out of combined efforts by individuals, organizations, and interest groups. For example, *Wilk v. American Medical Association*, 895 F.2d 352 (7th Cir. 1990), was a federal antitrust suit brought against the American Medical Association (AMA) and 10 co-defendants by chiropractor Chester A. Wilk, DC, and four co-plaintiffs. It resulted in a ruling against the AMA and third party payments for chiropractors.

These individuals and organizations advise legislators or international bodies on what actions to take to improve public health. The advice may be based on a variety of data, including:

- New scientific information regarding causes of health problems
- Sociological studies about demographic and cultural aspects of health
- An individual's personal experience with health care (e.g., an individual writing to a congressional representative to express an opinion in support of insurance reform based on a personal experience with coverage denials)

Input from a range of areas (see FIGURE 7-1) is gathered during the policy's formulation phase, where policy makers identify the problem they are trying to solve, review data on what causes the problem, and develop a range of

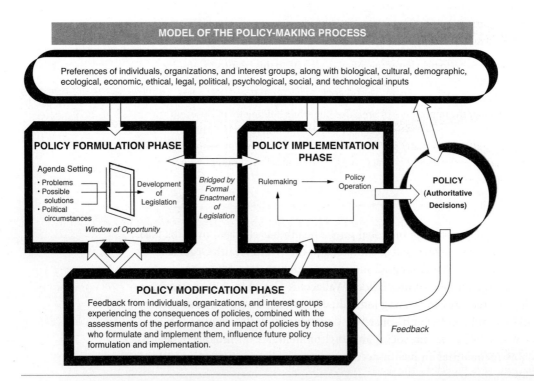

FIGURE 7-1 Model of the policy-making process.
Source: Reprinted with permission from Beaufort B. Longest, Jr., PhD

potential solutions to the problem. The focus of this chapter will be on national and local policies.

The creation of legislation intended to address a problem requires a great deal of debate and discussion. Priorities, costs versus benefits, and means of implementing changes are argued and weighed (usually in committees or sub-committees that focus on the topic at hand). Legislation developed in this process must then be made available for public comment and review—and it is nearly always scrutinized carefully by interest group lobbyists (insurance, healthcare professionals, unions, pharmaceutical companies, and so forth). Comments and objections are taken into account by the authors of the legislation, and the policy—if passed and funded—is either vetoed or signed by the president or governor. If signed, the law or policy is then implemented by government agencies (federal or state departments of health and human services), which must communicate to healthcare providers what their new responsibilities or limitations are under the law.

In an ideal world, policy would be developed based on evidence about the factors and conditions that affect both the causes and the solutions of health problems. In the real world, political and economic considerations often sway the process away from evidence-based research. The agendas of particular interest groups may bias the direction of either identifying the source of a problem or identifying potential solutions. You work daily with the people affected by policy changes, and are ideally situated to help legislators learn about the latest research, the real needs of clients, and the practical applications of data in supporting and promoting public health.

POLICY COLLISION: Federal And State Laws Leave Diabetic Children Vulnerable

Policies at the state and federal level do not always intersect well. A case in California illustrates the problem dramatically.

Students with medical disabilities are covered under three federal laws: Americans with Disabilities Act, the Rehabilitation Act of 1973, and the Individuals with Disabilities Education Act. This body of laws contains language that requires that public schools accommodate the students' medical needs or risk losing federal funding. Among the conditions covered by these laws is type 1 diabetes, a chronic autoimmune disease in which the insulin-producing cells of the pancreas are attacked and killed by the immune system. There is no cure for type 1 diabetes; a person with this disease can only manage it by injecting insulin with a syringe or via an insulin pump. For children with this disease, adult supervision is a must, because calculating insulin doses, delivering an injection or insulin pump bolus, and monitoring blood glucose are tasks that may be too complex for children under the age of 13. Federal law provides for parents and school officials to create a 504 plan (named for Section 504 of the Rehabilitation Act of 1973, which explicitly mandates accommodation of disabled students) that identifies responsible individuals at the school and describes what steps are to be taken to support the child's medical well-being while in school.

(continues)

In many school districts, the task of overseeing the child's diabetes care falls to a school nurse. Where nurses are not available, most states allow for another designated individual, such as a teacher or classroom assistant, to receive training on how to manage a child's blood sugar throughout the school day. In California, however, certain medical activities, including administration of injected medications, such as insulin, must be performed by a licensed medical practitioner or a nurse, according to a state law called the California Nursing Practices Act. The conflict between California law and federal law came about when budget cuts in the state made it impossible for every school to have a nurse on staff. Children who attended schools that lacked a school nurse could not get the diabetes care that federal law mandated. The seriousness of the problem was illustrated by an incident in which a 5-year-old girl on an insulin pump had a severe episode of hypoglycemia on a day when no nurse was present at the school. Because there was no one else on staff who could manage her diabetes, the girl's mother was called. The mother arrived at the school to find her daughter, semiconscious, out in the playground, where she had been sent by a teacher to await her mother's arrival despite the fact that it was a hot day. The teacher had been unaware that hypoglycemia could be exacerbated by heat exposure. The parents subsequently removed their child from the school system and home schooled her out of concern for her safety.

When this incident occurred in 2005, approximately 1 in 400 California public school students had type 1 diabetes, but the ratio of nurses to students was 1 nurse for every 2,777 students. Because diabetic students were not getting their medical needs met, a class action civil rights lawsuit was filed against California's superintendent of schools, the Department of Education, and the state's board of education. The goal of the lawsuit was to force the school system to live up to the provisions of the federal laws. The defendants in the case—California's public school system—eventually settled with the plaintiffs by issuing a rule that allowed individuals other than a registered nurse to administer diabetes care.

In response to this rule, the American Nurses Association filed a countersuit in 2008, arguing that this rule violated California law. Its point was that under California's own statutes defining who could and could not administer insulin, the only legal solution to the civil rights suit was to hire more nurses, so that each school had a nurse available to supervise care for children with diabetes—a path the state was financially unable to take because of severe budget shortfalls. The nurses' countersuit was upheld by California's Superior Court, and in 2010, the appeals court confirmed the original judgment. The decision was stayed pending appeal to California's Supreme Court, and as of 2012, was awaiting review.

Sources and Suggested Reading

Supreme Court of California. *ANA v. O'Connell*, Amicus Curie Brief (full description of legal background and findings of the case). Retrieved from http://www.justice.gov/crt/about/app/briefs/anavoconnell.pdf

Disability Rights Education & Defense Fund. 2012. "Diabetes Care in California Public Schools" (time line of lawsuit progress). Retrieved from http://www.dredf.org/diabetes/

Lopez, S. 2008. "Kids Pay Price in Medical Turf War." *Los Angeles Times*, November 23. Retrieved from http://articles.latimes.com/2008/nov/23/local/me-lopez23

Discussion

1. What are the benefits and risks of California's policy that requires trained nurses to provide certain kinds of medical care?

2. Given budget realities, what policy changes might the school system and the American Nursing Association suggest to reach a compromise that will support the health of children with diabetes?

3. If you were a nurse in California, what position would you take and why?

For example, suppose lobbyists from the dairy industry present scientific studies of calcium intake in relation to osteoporosis prevention. The lobbyists' goal is to convince a legislator that the solution to the problem of osteoporosis is to advocate for greater calcium intake among senior citizens. The data presented seems convincing, so the legislator promotes a policy to support programs that offer senior citizens discounts or rebates for buying milk. Unless someone points out to the legislator that exercise (Gómez-Cabello, Ara, González-Agüero, Casajús, &Vicente-Rodríguez, 2012), healthy meals (Yamaguchi, 2012), and other factors are equally important in osteoporosis prevention, this policy—which may have little or no effect on osteoporosis incidence—may be implemented. Implementation means that tax dollars and other resources will be used to support it. In the interest of efficient use of limited resources, it is important that policies have a sound underpinning of data and evidence supporting the actions called for by the legislation.

The most important factor in health policy creation is decision making, because goals, priorities, and methods for implementing policies all reflect the decisions of the person or people who create the policy. Different people will have different ideas about what is important, and they may also have conscious or unconscious biases for or against particular types of health promotion activities. When policies are created by small groups of people (e.g., a committee, town or city council, or a state legislature) to set goals and priorities around health, those policies not only affect the people who create them, but they affect the larger society as well. If the policy makers do not represent diverse perspectives, significant sectors of society may be left out of the decision-making process.

For example, suppose a majority of the people elected to a community or state legislature have religious or ideological beliefs that frown upon sex and childbearing outside of marriage. Such individuals often work against healthcare policies that promote family planning services for unmarried women and girls. They do so because they believe that offering such services would promote immoral behavior, which they feel causes harm to society in general. In a democracy, these individuals have the right, or even the duty, to promote policies that they believe will benefit society, so their actions are proper. If others who believe differently do not also run for election or otherwise contribute to the health policy decision-making process, the agenda and priorities of the first group determines the community or state policies around family planning. If the general population of the community is largely in agreement with this perspective, the policy may be acceptable for the community as a whole. Not everyone may agree, and the community may find that the policy creates unintended outcomes, such as a rise in teen pregnancy.

Ideally, enough individuals with differing opinions would be involved to develop a compromise policy that gives everyone some of the things they want. For example, the policy may promote availability of some services, such as pregnancy prevention education or birth control for women over 18, but not others, such as abortion services or birth control for minors without parental consent. Decision making does not always work this way in practice, which is why different states, and even different communities within the same state, have widely varying health policies in place.

How Are Health Policies Implemented?

Once a legislative body decides to enact a health policy into law, the executive branch of government puts the law into action. In the federal government, the executive branch is represented by the president and the various agencies that report to the executive, such as the Food and Drug Administration (FDA), the National Institutes of Health (NIH), the Centers for Disease Control and Prevention (CDC), and so forth.

At the state level, the executive consists of the state governor and agencies such as the department of human services, department of public health, state CDC branches, and so on. Different states organize their agencies differently; in some states, there may be a separate agency for public health and mental health, whereas in others, both may be under the supervision of the same agency.

HEALTH PROMOTION CHALLENGE   www

Choose one of the following topics (check with your classmates and make sure you are choosing different topics or pair up with another student to develop your project). If you still run out of topics, develop your own based on a search for health promotion issues.

- What policies should nursing organizations be pursuing to enhance the health of nurses?
- What additional protections are needed to ensure we all have safe drinking water?
- What additional protections are needed to ensure we all have clean air to breathe?
- Should corporations be allowed to place untested genetically-engineered components in food without listing them in the ingredients?
- Should there be better policies to protect women and men from being sexually and physically abused?
- Should there be stricter laws to punish people who abuse women and children?
- Should adults who want to have children have to pass a test to prove they know how to be parents?
- Should drug advertisements be allowed on television?
- Should people be allowed to have assault weapons and handguns in their homes?
- Should poverty exist in the United States?
- Should we have a choice whether we eat genetically-engineered foods or not?
- Should farmers be forced to only use pesticides developed by large corporations?
- Should new drugs have a longer testing period and be tested by someone other than the drug companies before they are deemed acceptable by the FDA?
- Should oil companies be allowed to sully our oceans?

- Should tropical rain forests that protect us against climate changes and outbreaks of tropical diseases (e.g., Ebola and Lassa Fever) and that provide renewable resources and protection for surrounding crops be allowed to be destroyed?
- Should the United Nations global warming framework be tightened so our species will survive?
- Should a global movement toward renewable energy sources be increased and an end put to the use of fossil fuels, especially oil that dirties the environment, makes breathing more difficult, and can kill important sources of nutrients, i.e., fish?
- Should parents be held partially responsible when their children take guns from the house and go to school and kill people?
- Should genetically-engineered corn be banned by the United States, as it has in Poland, now that there is evidence the corn kills honey bees that most of our crops depend on for pollinization?
- Should everyone be forced to buy into the President's new health insurance program or be fined?

Do a survey of at least 20 other nursing students and find out what they think. At the very least, get a yes, no, I don't know, or need more information. Make sure you are well-versed in the debate by Googling your topic online before you start your survey. When you have your findings, share them with your classmates. If possible go online to share them at http://ushealthpolicygateway.wordpress.com/ or a relevant blog.

Massachusetts, for example, has three agencies directly involved in health policy: the Division of Health Care Finance and Policy, the Department of Public Health, and the Executive Office of Health and Human Services. Colorado, on the other hand, has only one: the Department of Public Health and Environment. At the local level, communities may have city or town health services that implement health policies, or policies may be implemented directly by ordinances (for example, a city ordinance outlawing the use of pesticides within 50 feet of a school playground). These agencies are directed with setting rules and working with local communities, hospitals, healthcare providers, and insurers to implement and comply with new laws and policies.

Health promotion policies may be enacted to improve access to a desired health promotion activity or tool. Construction of walking or bicycle paths is one way that communities or states promote exercise for the general populace, for instance.

State or federal mandates for insurance reimbursement are often used to promote healthcare activities that lawmakers wish to see increased in the general populace for reasons that may have nothing to do with health promotion. Besides increased health risks, there are other drawbacks to states forcing insurers to support specific actions. First, some insurers may decide that the cost of providing the service outweighs the financial benefit obtained by serving consumers in that state; as such, insurers may stop doing business as a result of the mandate, and may change the conditions associated with reimbursement to put more costs on the shoulders of consumers. Second, the mandate to support the activity may not change even when new science shows that the activity is unnecessary or potentially harmful. For example, lawmakers established mandatory reimbursement for annual mammograms among women over 40 years old (Fenton, Foote, Green, & Baldwin, 2010). However, studies showed that an annual mammogram is of no benefit, and may cause additional cancers in, the majority of women whose actual risk for breast cancer is relatively low (Mandelblatt et al., 2009; Nelson et al., 2009; Stefanek, Gritz, & Vernon, 2010). Even the National Cancer Institute (2010) cautions against the dangers of mammograms including overdiagnosis, overtreatment, and radiation exposure.

Your Role in Health Policy Decisions

You can be politically active in policy making. Mason, Leavett, and Chafee (2007) described four spheres of political influence where you may contribute: (1) the workplace, (2) government, (3) professional organizations, and (4) the community. FIGURE 7-2 shows how these spheres are interrelated and interdependent.

☐ The Workplace

Workplace policies where you practice, for example in the home care or the acute care setting, are generally found in a policy and procedure book. Ideally, these would be located at a central place that can be easily accessed in any

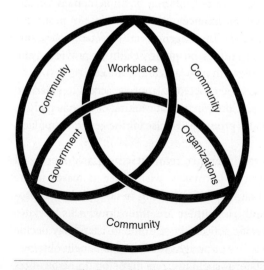

FIGURE 7-2   The Four Spheres of Political Influence in Which Nurses Can Effect Change

Source: Mason, D., Leavitt, J., and Chafee, M. 2007. *Policy and Politics in Nursing and Health Care* (5th ed.). St. Louis, MO: Saunders.

nursing practice setting, but it does not always happen that way. Other policies govern the workplace, including occupational and health standards for the use of needles, disposal of biohazard waste, and the use of gowns and masks when preparing to care for a patient who has a communicable disease. These are examples of policies that affect primary prevention for you, and in some cases, the client. Such policies may come from government mandates placed on healthcare facilities, or they may be best practices established by nursing or medical professional organizations.

You can affect workplace policies by checking www.pubmed.gov for recent studies and working with supervisors and staff in the workplace to generate procedures that support best practices. When the workplace is not supportive of nurses' policy recommendations or improvement suggestions, you can vote with your feet by leaving jobs at such facilities after making sure that human resources officers know the reason behind leaving the job.

HEALTH PROMOTION CHALLENGE

Read the workplace policies at your clinical sites. Do they support nurses? Talk with your clinical group and instructor about what could be done to enhance health policy so nurses are better protected.

☐ Government

You can influence policies at federal, state, and local levels by advocating for policy change to legislators and community leaders at each level. As healthcare providers working directly to promote health in individuals, you are in a front-line position to observe and identify concerns that might be addressed by policy changes. Your clinical expertise and experience offer a certain amount of authority when discussing health policy matters with government leaders about laws relating to health promotion. Examples of health promotion policy that you could influence include laws prohibiting the sale of tobacco products or alcohol to persons under the legal age, policies that identify students contemplating suicide and/or homicide, and policies supporting sex education in the schools.

You may be the distributor of services mandated by health promotion legislation, and the government indirectly influences the organization of your practice. It is up to you to keep apprised of (and stay involved in) government policy-making activities. Nursing has a stronger political influence in the government now than in the past, because some nurses have run for office and have undertaken careers in primary political offices in order to better influence health policy.

ASK YOURSELF   www

Each day our lives is governed by legislative acts that had as their goal our health and safety. Think about the activities of your last 24 hours and try to recount ways that policies have protected or harmed you.

INFORMATION BOX 7-1

Want to know about the American Recovery and Reinvestment Act? Go to the website for the Agency for Healthcare Research and Quality (AHRQ) for a great overview of this legislation: www.ahrq.gov

☐ Professional Organizations

There are hundreds of professional organizations for nurses, including the American Academy of Nursing, the American Nurses Association (see INFORMATION BOX 7-2 for information on how to further explore the ANA's stance on forming policies), the American College of Nurse Practitioners, and other state, national, international, and specialist nursing associations. Any or all of these organizations can be influential in health promotion by lobbying the government or by providing public services. At the annual meetings of nursing associations, many presentations specifically focus on health promotion policy, offering opportunities for association members to become active in developing health policies. Individual organizations may also employ lobbyists or submit opinions to convince legislators to work on specific policy matters of importance to the organization's membership (for example, laws permitting nurse practitioners to prescribe medications in rural states where there are few doctors available). A comprehensive list of nursing organizations with hyperlinks to specific websites is available at http://www.nurse.org/orgs.shtml.

INFORMATION BOX 7-2

Visit the site of the American Nurses Association: www.nursingworld.org. Go to the section called Policy & Advocacy (it is one of the buttons shown across the screen near the top) to review the stance of the ANA on health care reform.

Do you have a special interest in healthcare policy? Here are a few specialty journals about policy: *Health Care Analysis (HCA): Journal of Health Philosophy and Policy; Health Expectations: An International Journal of Public Participation in Health Care and Health Policy*; and *Journal of Health Care Law and Policy*.

☐ Community

You may practice in the community, but you may also live there. You have a personal interest in supporting health promotion activities in your home community. You can shape policy in your community by participating in parent–teacher organizations, chambers of commerce, and civic organizations. Community participation is particularly important if you hope to have a direct effect on local government or workplace policy, as other members of the community are more likely to listen to a person they know to be actively involved in the community's well-being.

These are a few examples of how the nursing spheres of policy influence health promotion. It is important to recognize that despite the fact that each sphere is distinct, they interact with and affect the other spheres. Lack of participation in one sphere may render you less effective in influencing changes in other spheres (Mason et al., 2007).

Incorporating Policies in Health Promotion

You have several roles to play in health promotion policy. On the one hand, when policies are created to promote certain health behaviors, nurses are often the very people who educate the public about the policy and promote it to citizens who may either be unaware of, or skeptical of, the initiative. You also can help in the development of health promotion policies. As a primary point of contact between policy makers and patients, you are in a unique position to understand what health challenges are most important to the public, as well as what practices work for overcoming such challenges.

Nurses as Policy Implementers

You can be influential in promoting new health policies. For example, consider the use of automobile safety seats. Child safety seats were invented in 1962, and car seat use was recommended by the American Academy of Pediatrics in 1974 (Lincoln, 2005), but they did not come into widespread use until the 1980s, when studies began to show that injuries to children could be reduced by placing children in car seats with restraints (Johnston, Rivara, & Soderberg, 1994; Turbell, 1974; Tingvall, 1987).

Research has shown that the greatest factor affecting injury and death among children placed in car seats is incorrect use of the seat (Fuchs, Barthel, Flannery, & Christoffel, 1989; Stalnaker, 1993). This is an area in which you can assist with promoting a health policy (Tessier, 2010).

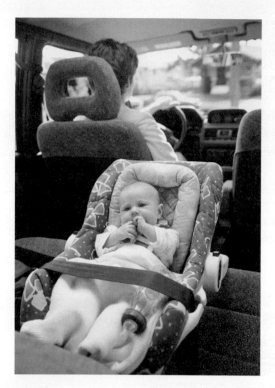

Current recommendations from the American Academy of Pediatrics (2011) direct that infants and toddlers should ride facing the rear of the vehicle until they reach at least 2 years of age and/or weigh at least 30 pounds. Older or larger toddlers and preschoolers ride forward facing in a seat with a harness until they reach the limit of their seat, usually 65–80 pounds. School-aged children need booster seats until adult seat belts fit correctly—usually when the child reaches about 4 feet, 9 inches in height and is between 8 and 12 years of age. All children under 13 should ride in the back seat of the car, properly restrained.

Many parents, particularly new, first-time parents, become overwhelmed when faced with the installation of a car seat. Some pediatric hospitals have nurses in mobile units at specific community centers advocating for the proper use of car seats, and such training outreach is needed because the seats have complex

---

RESEARCH BOX 7-1   School Wellness Policies Change Behavior

» BACKGROUND: In 2006, all local education agencies in the United States participating in federal school meal programs were required to establish school wellness policies. This study documented the strength and comprehensiveness of one state's written district policies using a coding tool, and tested whether these traits predicted school-level implementation and practices.

» METHODS: School wellness policies from 151 Connecticut districts were evaluated based on school principal surveys collected before and after the writing and expected implementation of wellness policies. Changes in school-level policy implementation before and after the federal wellness policy mandate were compared across districts by wellness policy strength, based on district-level demographics.

» RESULTS: Statewide, more complete implementation of nutrition and physical activity policies at the school level was reported after adoption of written policies.

» CONCLUSIONS: Written school wellness policies have the potential to promote significant improvements in the school environment. Future regulation of school wellness policies should focus on the importance of writing strong and comprehensive policies.

Source: Schwartz, M. B., Henderson, K. E., Falbe, J., Novak, S. A., Wharton, C. M., Long, M. W., O'Connell, M. L., & Fiore, S. S. (2012). Strength and Comprehensiveness of District School Wellness Policies Predict Policy Implementation at the School Level. *Journal of School Health, 82*(6), 262–267.

mechanisms to hold the infant and the seat itself in place securely. Hospitals and state police in many states have periodic car seat check programs to assist with this task, but surveys of parents have shown that relatively few (~ 30%) are aware of the programs (Cease, King, & Monroe, 2011). Program staff find many times that car seats are not correctly placed or fastened. Car crashes are a leading cause of death among children age 4 and older (Durbin, 2011), so it is important that parents continue to be educated about the correct use of car seats.

HEALTH PROMOTION CHALLENGE

Did your school district follow the national mandate? If yes, what changes occurred? If not, why not? Make a plan to help your school district follow wellness directives.

You are well situated to provide this education, either in the setting of the maternity ward when an infant goes home with its parents, or in pediatric offices. During routine well-child visits, for example, you can inquire about car seat use and refer parents to a seat check program.

Nurses can also promote health policy by bringing large-scale research findings into the care of individual clients. For example, consider the findings of the Human Genome Project. The **genome** is basically the organism's complete set of DNA. In humans, the genome is arranged into 24 distinct chromosomes.

One goal of the Human Genome Project was to define the sequencing of DNA to aid in biologic research. Doing this has helped researchers identify

RESEARCH BOX 7-2   Preventable Risks For Cancer

The good news is, the major environmental factors that make up nearly 100% of the risk for cancer can be avoided. Here are the statistics.

Proportion of cancer deaths linked to avoidable risk factors (Doll, 1998):

Tobacco	29–31 percent
Diet	20–50 percent
Infections: bacteria, viruses	10–20 percent
Ionizing and UV light	5–7 percent
Occupation	2–4 percent
Pollution: air, water, food	1–5 percent

particular genetic abnormalities. These findings can be used in health promotion by nurses involved in genetic counseling. For example, genetic counseling may be used to determine intrauterine abnormalities during pregnancy or identify risk factors for a variety of specific gene-mediated diseases, such as BRCA-1 breast/ovarian cancer or Huntington's disease. Knowing whether a genetic condition exists offers an opportunity for the client to take prophylactic action.

You, as nurse educator, can provide clients with information about how to stop smoking, change diet, prevent infections, stay away from ionizing UV light, change occupations (if needed), and reduce pollution.

Testing family members of children with type 1 (autoimmune) diabetes may identify a genetic predisposition for the disease and highlight the presence of autoantibodies. Finding these conditions early allows family members to reduce further risk by exercising and staying at the recommended weight. Stay current with advances in gene testing and therapies so you can better advise clients (Loud, 2010; McBride, Wade, & Kaphingst, 2010).

In 2008, President George W. Bush signed the **Genetic Information Nondiscrimination Act (GINA)**, which protects Americans from discrimination based on information found on genetic tests. Specifically, it forbids insurance companies from discriminating through such things as reduced coverage or increased pricing, and it prohibits employers from making employment decisions based on a person's genetic code. Provide this information to clients who are leery of genetic testing.

Nurses as Policy Developers

You can assist in the development of policy. Cohen, March, and Olsen (1972) developed a framework, specifically for nurses, that includes four processes that must be included in activities: buy-in, self-interest, political sophistication, and leadership.

☐ Buy-In

Buy-in is the act of identifying and committing yourself to promoting actions considered to be a priority. This commitment is crucial to convincing others to work on the policy initiative with you. If success in developing the policy does not matter to you on a personal level, then buy-in has not occurred (and it is not likely that the policy initiative will succeed). Buy-in is not strictly formed on the basis of emotions alone. Buy-in can and should be supported by study of the problem to create a strong, convincing case that the action being promoted is the right strategy. The more evidence and data you obtain to bolster the position, the greater your buy-in.

□ Self-Interest

Self-interest is a circumstance that offers a benefit, direct or indirect, if you develop the policy. Self-interest is a key component of developing buy-in, as most people cannot emotionally invest in working hard to promote a policy that will not provide them with a benefit—even if that benefit is simply the satisfaction of feeling that you have helped someone. Where benefits are direct and tangible (e.g., an ICU nurse promoting policies that require specific work-place safety changes to improve hospital working conditions for ICU nurses), self-interest, and by extension buy-in, tends to be high.

□ Political Sophistication

In order to effectively influence the policy-making system, you must become educated in how it works—in other words, must develop political sophistica-tion. This means knowing who the key legislators are and which committees they are on, keeping current on what policy initiatives are being developed in Congress or in a state legislature, and developing systems for collecting data and public input needed to support arguments in favor of (or against) a par-ticular policy decision.

□ Leadership

You become a leader by advocating for a change in current policy. Political sophistication may help in convincing legislators to act, but you have a greater opportunity to make necessary changes in policy if you make an effort to pro-mote these changes *personally*.

Leadership requires you to understand what messages will resonate with lawmakers who are developing health policy, learn how to present public tes-timony in a professional and persuasive manner, and be willing to offer time and energy to the effort of getting a policy enacted. If necessary, run for public office so that you are in a position to influence health policy.

For example, consider the following health topic: the use of helmets by chil-dren whenever they are riding a bicycle. Bicycle riding, even in today's high-tech environment, continues to be a popular recreational sport. The bicycle functions through balance, and therefore a bike and its rider have a chance for falls even without environmental hazards. Although bike paths and bike lanes are becoming more common, it is not unusual for bike riders to have no other recourse but to ride in a street, sharing the road with cars (whose drivers may not always see bike riders or yield to them). Wearing a bicycle helmet is a safety measure that prevents serious brain injuries, yet many children continue to go without them. Even when a child does wear a helmet, it might not fit prop-erly, either not adequately covering the skull or being fitted too loosely. Some

RESEARCH BOX 7-3   Hearing Protection

» BACKGROUND: The Occupational Safety and Health Administration (OSHA) mandated workplace hearing conservation programs for industrial workers in 1983. Thirty million workers in the United States are exposed to harmful noise levels at their place of work. Workers are expected to wear hearing protective devices when noise levels cannot be controlled; however, they do not always take responsibility for using hearing protection devices. Investigators from the University of Michigan conducted a study to test the effectiveness of an individually tailored intervention to increase use of hearing protection devices in a factory setting.

» METHOD: Participants were randomly assigned to one of the following: tailored intervention (computer guided tutorial) ($n = 446$), two other interventions via computer presentation ($n = 447$), or a control group not receiving an intervention ($n = 432$). Follow-up on the groups occurred at 6 months and 18 months. A survey questionnaire that has been used to determine the predictors of hearing protection use by factory workers was administered to participants.

» RESULTS: The study results showed that those with the tailored intervention reported an increased use of hearing protective devices postintervention. This study of health promotion was an attempt to determine the best approach to encourage worker compliance with an OSHA recommendation.

Source: Lusk, S. L., Ronis, D. L., Kazanis, A.S., Eakin, B.L., Hong, O., & Raymond, D.M. (2003). Effectiveness of a tailored intervention to increase factory workers' use of hearing protection. *Nursing Research, 52*(5). 289-295.

helmets may be attractive to look at, but lack sufficient strength to protect the skull against a blow to the head. To promote health in bicyclists, helmets should be worn, they should fit properly, and they should be certified by the United States Consumer Product Safety Commission as being sufficiently strong to withstand the forces involved in a fall or crash.

You may develop buy-in for promoting helmet use after caring for a child with a closed head injury who has sustained the injury while riding on a bicycle without a helmet, or with an inadequate or loose helmet. After the experience, you may not wish to see such an injury again, or perhaps you have children, nieces, or nephews similar in age to the injured child. Such emotional investment in preventing further head injuries is part of your self-interest—the personal stake in the policy.

You may decide to exhibit leadership by volunteering at a grade school and organizing a bike rally with students to educate them about the importance of helmet use. To put on an effective presentation, develop political sophistication by becoming educated in current state laws about the wearing of helmets; this may be taken a step further later on, for instance in identifying local legislators who might be willing to sponsor a bill mandating the use of helmets by cyclists riding in public streets.

Nursing Organizations Involved in Policy

Professional nursing organizations offer support of policy initiatives on many fronts, ranging from developing professional standards to lobbying for broad-scale health reform. One professional organization in nursing is the National League for Nursing (NLN). Currently, the NLN is working on the principle that all individuals must have equitable access to comprehensive healthcare services regardless of the medical condition. The current priorities for the NLN include quality health care for all, ethnic/cultural/gender diversity, nurse workforce development, and the nurse faculty shortages. The NLN organization has information available on its website at http://www.nln.org.

Another nursing organization involved in policy is the American Nurses Association. The ANA advances the nursing profession by fostering high standards of nursing practice, promoting the rights of nurses while in the workplace, public relations of the nursing profession by portraying nursing realistically, and lobbying the Congress and regulatory agencies on healthcare issues affecting nurses and the public. It also has a primary mission statement similar to that of the NLN, which is improving health for all by advancing the nursing profession. The ANA has information available on its website at http://www.nursingworld.org.

Healthcare Policy in the United States

At the heart of most arguments about healthcare policy is one simple question: Who will pay the costs? The traditional model of health care in the United States is that the person receiving the service pays the service provider, either directly or through a third party (an insurance company). This system made complete sense in the era of general practice doctors who made house calls and had few instruments more complicated than a stethoscope, a thermometer, and a tongue depressor. As medicine grew more specialized, more technically complex, and above all more expensive in the post-WWII era, the federal government began to take up a role in providing health services. Initially, this was done by means of legislation such as the Hill-Burton Act of 1946, which offered funding to promote the construction and operation of hospitals throughout the nation. This legislation was intended to make health care more broadly accessible to the public. However, comprehensive health policy identifying the priorities for public health—and figuring out ways to pay for them—did not begin to develop until the 1960s, and is still far from an accomplished feat.

Origins of Health Policy: 1965 Medicare Act

National health policy in the United States truly began the early 1950s, when the census revealed that people were living longer. This meant that new public health concerns related to aging (conditions such as cancers, osteoporosis, and mental deterioration) were becoming more prominent. Then as now, the costs associated with treating such conditions were known to be out of reach for the majority of people.

Partly in response to this development, the **Social Security Act Amendments** statute (also known as the Medicare Act) of 1965 was created and made law under President Lyndon B. Johnson. Although political debate argued that this law was the start of socialized medicine, the **Medicare Act** effectively established a national health insurance program for older adults, financed by a tax on the earnings of employees, matched by contributions of employers. The supplementary medical insurance program resulted in hospital and outpatient insurance for persons aged 65 years of age and older and has proven greatly beneficial (and remarkably popular) over the decades. What was not foreseen by Johnson or subsequent administrations was that the number of people in the aging population would continue to increase, while the population of individuals contributing to the tax pool remained stable or declined.

HOT TOPICS

Here are some topics to explore:
- Policy analysis
- Genetic Information Nondiscrimination Act
- Patient Protection and Affordable Care Act
- Social Security
- Medicare
- International health policy
- WHO and health policy
- Food insecurity

Health Reform in the 1970s and 1980s

The next president to undertake healthcare reform was Richard Nixon, who proposed in 1971 and again in 1974 that a comprehensive national insurance plan be created. Nixon's descriptions of the issues facing American health care resonate eerily when read today (see INFORMATION BOX 7-3), because many of the concerns he raised about health care in his 1974 State of the Union Address are largely unchanged in 2012. His proposals for universal health care were scuttled, ironically, by Democratic legislators such as Ted Kennedy, who wanted a comprehensive national healthcare system but refused to work with Nixon because he felt

INFORMATION BOX 7-3 The More Things Change, the More They Stay the Same: 1974 State President Richard Nixon's of the Union Address

Without adequate health care, no one can make full use of his or her talents and opportunities. It is thus just as important that economic, racial and social barriers not stand in the way of good health care as it is to eliminate those barriers to a good education and a good job …

Today the need [for comprehensive healthcare reform] is even more pressing because of the higher costs of medical care. Efforts to control medical costs … have been met with encouraging success, sharply reducing the rate of inflation for health care. Nevertheless, the overall cost of health care has still risen … so that more and more Americans face staggering bills when they receive medical help today …

For the average family, it is clear that without adequate insurance, even normal care can be a financial burden while a catastrophic illness can mean catastrophic debt.

Beyond the question of the prices of health care, our present system of health care insurance suffers from two major flaws: First, even though more Americans carry health insurance than ever before, the 25 million* Americans who remain uninsured often need it the most and are most unlikely to obtain it. They include many who work in seasonal or transient occupations, high-risk cases, and those who are ineligible for Medicaid despite low incomes.

Second, those Americans who do carry health insurance often lack coverage which is balanced, comprehensive and fully protective … These gaps in health protection can have tragic consequences. They can cause people to delay seeking medical attention until it is too late. Then a medical crisis ensues, followed by huge medical bills—or worse. Delays in treatment can end in death or lifelong disability.

Comprehensive health insurance is an idea whose time has come in America. There has long been a need to assure every American financial access to high quality health care. As medical costs go up, that need grows more pressing.

Now, for the first time, we have not just the need but the will to get this job done. There is widespread support in the Congress and in the Nation for some form of comprehensive health insurance.

Surely if we have the will, 1974 should also be the year that we find the way.

*In 1974, 25 million uninsured persons represented 11.7% of the total population. In 2010, the U.S. Census Bureau estimated the number of uninsured persons at 50.7 million people, or 16.7% of the population.

Source: Nixon, R. 1974. "Address on the State of the Union Delivered before a Joint Session of the Congress." In J.T. Woolley and G. Peters, eds. The American Presidency Project. Santa Barbara: University of California, Santa Barbara. Retrieved from: http://www.presidency.ucsb.edu/ws/index.php?pid=4327#axzz1inX22KFF.

Nixon's proposals did not go far enough (Hall, 2007; Himmelstein & Woolhandler, 2007; Nixon, 1974; Sisk, 2009).

The first significant health policy initiative following these failures was undertaken during the Reagan administration with passage in 1985 of the Consolidated Omnibus Reconciliation Act (COBRA), which sought to address the problems experienced by individuals who were insured through employers. Employees who lost their jobs or who changed jobs were instantly uninsured, whether they could afford to pay for insurance or not. If they had preexisting health conditions, this often meant that they were effectively barred from obtaining new insurance—and it had the unwelcome side effect of locking some employees into a job because they would be unable to sign up for insurance through a new employer if they tried to find a better position. The loss of insurance was particularly harmful for employees who may have been in treatment for a disease such as cancer, where loss of insurance might mean the patient was suddenly faced with a choice between life-saving medication and bankruptcy. COBRA allowed employees to continue their employer-sponsored coverage for a specified length of time so that such preexisting health issues could be treated without interruption.

Many other Congressional and White House healthcare initiatives proposed in the late 1980s, 1990s, and early 2000s fell to partisan bickering. In the 1990s and early 2000s, especially, a variety of healthcare reform schemes were proposed but failed to pass because of opposition from industry and advocacy lobbyists. One that did get enacted into law was the 1997 State Children's Health Insurance Program (SCHIP), which provided health insurance to children in families at or below 200% of the poverty level. Given that the Clinton administration had earmarked health care as a principal issue on its agenda, such limited policy action was disappointing to all concerned.

Modern Healthcare Reform: The Patient Protection and Affordable Care Act of 2010

The most recent and most far-reaching piece of legislation has been the bill referred to, derogatorily and somewhat inaccurately, as "Obamacare"—despite the fact that it was neither created by President Obama nor promoted by him, although he did sign it. The law is properly called the **Patient Protection and Affordable Care Act** (PPACA), with modifications made by the 2010 Reconciliation Act. Some of the basic provisions are:

1. Prohibits insurance discrimination based on employee's wages
2. Permits insurance rating variability on age, family composition, geographic location, and tobacco use, but not on health or gender

3. Provides Medicaid to all individuals under age 65 who are at or below 133% of the federal poverty level

4. Established new program to support school-based health centers and nurse-managed health centers

5. Creates essential benefits package that provides comprehensive set of services

6. Creates an essential benefits package with a comprehensive set of mental health services

7. Supports development of training programs that focus on primary care models that integrate physical and mental health services

Effects of the 2010 Patient Protection and Affordable Care Act on Nurses

The PPACA includes many key provisions related to nursing. As the American Nurses Association states, registered nurses are fundamental to the shift needed in health care, specifically the need to transform the services from a care-of-the-sick system to healthcare system based on prevention.

The Patient Protection and Affordable Care Act has a subcomponent of **Nursing Workforce Development programs** that recruit new nurses into the profession, promote career advancement within nursing, and improve patient care delivery. Some of the provisions include:

- Training and career advancement
- Support for public health nursing
- Support for home health care
- Incentives to address provider shortages

☐ Training and Career Advancement

The bill expanded the Nurse Loan Repayment and Scholarship program to provide loan repayment for students who serve for at least 2 years as a faculty member at an accredited school of nursing. It also authorized grants to accredited nursing schools or health facilities to promote career advancement among nurses, including authorization of the Department of Health and Human Services to award grants to advanced practice nurses who are pursuing a doctorate or other advanced degree in geriatrics—a field in which shortages are predicted in the near future.

☐ Support for Public Health Nursing

To encourage more nurses to go into public health, the bill called for the establishment of a Public Health Workforce Loan Repayment Program to assure an adequate supply of public health professionals to eliminate workforce shortages in public health agencies.

☐ Support for Home Health Care

The bill also coordinated care of Medicaid recipients through a health home for individuals with chronic conditions. The health home provides comprehensive care management, care coordination, and chronic disease management by a provider or a team of professionals.

☐ Incentives to Address Provider Shortages

The bill provided a 10% bonus payment under Medicare for fiscal years 2011 through 2016 to all primary care practitioners, including nurse practitioners and general surgeons, practicing in areas with shortages of healthcare professionals (rural or inner-city zones).

Health Policy in Action: Federal Agencies and the Healthy People Initiative

Health policy is not solely the province of Congress. The executive branch, charged with implementing and enforcing congressional mandates, has considerable leeway in regulating health care and setting public health priorities. Individual agencies have specific programs and agendas intended to promote public health. Providing a comprehensive overview of all federal agencies tasked with promoting health is beyond the scope of this chapter, but we will offer a brief sketch of key executive branch agencies and their mandates and give an in-depth look at one long-term, comprehensive public health policy initiative that is a cornerstone of national health policy planning: the Healthy People initiative.

Agencies Responsible for Healthcare Policy Implementation

The primary federal agency responsible for health in the United States is the Department of Health and Human Services. Within this department are a number of operating divisions with specific mandates (see TABLE 7-1).

Each of these agencies manages distinct, but sometimes overlapping, sectors of public health. However, the primary policy goals of the Department of

Table 7-1 Department of Health and Human Services Operating Divisions and Their Mandates

Administration for Children and Families (ACF)	The ACF is a federal agency funding state, territory, local, and tribal organizations to provide family assistance (welfare), child support, child care, Head Start, child welfare, and other programs relating to children and families. Actual services are provided by state, county, city, and tribal governments, and public and private local agencies. ACF assists these organizations through funding, policy direction, and information services. Some policy areas supervised include adoption and foster care, child neglect and abuse, and temporary assistance for needy families.
Administration for Children, Youth, and Families (ACYF)	The ACYF is a subdivision of the ACF that administers the major federal programs that support the following: social services that promote the positive growth and development of children and youth and their families, protective services and shelter for children and youth in at-risk situations, and adoption for children with special needs. These programs provide financial assistance to states, community-based organizations, and academic institutions to provide services; carry out research and demonstration activities; and undertake training, technical assistance, and information dissemination.
Administration on Aging (AoA)	The mission of AoA is to develop a comprehensive, coordinated, and cost-effective system of home and community-based services that helps elderly individuals maintain their health and independence in their homes and communities.
Agency for Healthcare Research and Quality (AHRQ)	The AHRQ's mission is to improve the quality, safety, efficiency, and effectiveness of health care for all Americans. Information from AHRQ's research helps people make more informed decisions and improve the quality of healthcare services.
Agency for Toxic Substances and Disease Registry (ATSDR)	The ATSDR, based in Atlanta, Georgia, is a federal public health agency of the U.S. Department of Health and Human Services. ATSDR serves the public by using the best science, taking responsive public health actions, and providing trusted health information to prevent harmful exposures and diseases related to toxic substances.
Centers for Disease Control and Prevention (CDC)	The CDC's mission is collaborating to create the expertise, information, and tools that people and communities need to protect their health—through health promotion; prevention of disease, injury and disability; and preparedness for new health threats.
Centers for Medicare and Medicaid Services (CMS)	CMS provides health coverage for 100 million people through Medicare, Medicaid, and the Children's Health Insurance Program. The agency is responsible for managing individual eligibility and provider services.

(continues)

Table 7-1 (Continued)

Food and Drug Administration (FDA)	FDA is responsible for protecting the public health by assuring that foods are safe, wholesome, sanitary, and properly labeled, as well as ensuring human and veterinary drugs, vaccines and other biological products, and medical devices intended for human use are safe and effective. FDA is also charged with advancing the public health by helping to speed product innovations and helping the public get the accurate science-based information they need to use medicines, devices, and foods to improve their health.
Health Resources and Services Administration (HRSA)	HRSA is the primary federal agency for improving access to healthcare services for people who are uninsured, isolated, or medically vulnerable.
Indian Health Service (IHS)	IHS is responsible for providing federal health services to American Indians and Alaska Natives. The provision of health services to members of federally recognized tribes grew out of the special government-to-government relationship between the federal government and Indian tribes. The IHS provides a comprehensive health service delivery system for approximately 1.9 million American Indians and Alaska Natives who belong to 564 federally recognized tribes in 35 states.
National Institutes of Health (NIH)	NIH's mission is to seek fundamental knowledge about the nature and behavior of living systems and the application of that knowledge to enhance health, lengthen life, and reduce the burdens of illness and disability. NIH provides leadership and direction to programs designed to improve the health of the nation by conducting and supporting research.
National Cancer Institute (NCI)	NCI, a subdivision of NIH, is the federal government's principal agency for cancer research and training. The National Cancer Act of 1971 created the National Cancer Program. The National Cancer Institute coordinates the National Cancer Program, which conducts and supports research, training, health information dissemination, and other programs with respect to the cause, diagnosis, prevention, and treatment of cancer; rehabilitation from cancer; and the continuing care of cancer patients and the families of cancer patients.
Office of the Inspector General (OIG)	The inspector general is the senior official responsible for audits, evaluations, investigations, and law enforcement efforts relating to Department of Health and Human Services (DHHS) programs and operations. The OIG manages an independent and objective nationwide organization of over 1,500 professional staff members dedicated to promoting economy, efficiency, and effectiveness in DHHS programs and addressing fraud, waste, and abuse.
Substance Abuse and Mental Health Services Administration (SAMHSA)	SAMHSA's mission is to reduce the impact of substance abuse and mental illness on America's communities. To accomplish its work, SAMHSA administers a combination of competitive, formula, and block grant programs and data collection activities.

Note: Agency descriptions are drawn from each agency's mission statement or "About Us" webpage. See http://www.hhs.gov/open/contacts/index.html to access these pages.

Health and Human Services as a whole are spelled out in the *Healthy People* policy statement. *Healthy People* (see INFORMATION BOX 7-4) has evolved from a brief document to multiple volumes, and now even a large website. One can easily be overwhelmed when approaching any portion of the initiative, with confusing terms such as goals, objectives, leading health indicators, and focus areas. Prior to defining these terms, as well as their specific entities, an overview of the history and process will be covered. This chapter will provide an in-depth description.

INFORMATION BOX 7-4   Healthy People 2020

Healthy People 2020 is based on the accomplishments of four previous Healthy People initiatives:

- 1979 surgeon general's report, *Healthy People: The Surgeon General's Report on Health Promotion and Disease Prevention*
- Healthy People 1990: Promoting Health/Preventing Disease: Objectives for the Nation
- Healthy People 2000: National Health Promotion and Disease Prevention Objectives
- Healthy People 2010: Objectives for Improving Health

Evolution of the Healthy People Initiative

Healthy People is an agenda of prevention for the United States—a tool that identifies what have been found to be the most significant preventable threats to health. It originally grew out of a 1979 surgeon general's report entitled *Healthy People: The Surgeon General's Report on Health Promotion and Disease Prevention*. The findings of this report have been updated in 10-year increments for the past 30 years. Public health threats are identified in such a way as to distinguish how public and private sector focus efforts must be undertaken to address each health concern. The initiative provides information and knowledge on how to improve health for diverse groups in a format that enables them to have the nation work together as a team. Ultimately, *Healthy People* is a very powerful document in that it is based on scientific, evidence-based knowledge and is used for decision making and for planning interventions.

Healthy People 2020

It is worth briefly discussing the definitions in the *Healthy People* document here, as there are certain important distinctions made by this policy. Health is defined as "a condition of wellbeing, free of disease or infirmity, and a basic human right." This definition is based on the definition originating from the

World Health Organization, with an update published in 1998 (p. 11). It is important to recognize that the phrase "a basic human right" is itself a policy statement; that is, it solidifies the idea that the United States' policy regarding health supports health care for *everyone*, whether that person is a citizen of the United States, a resident of the United States, or someone living outside the United States' national borders. Health promotion as defined in *Healthy People 2020* is a process of enabling people to increase control over their health and its determinants and thereby improve their health (again, this is based on the WHO, 1998 definition). Disease prevention, then, is an "approach that covers measures not only to prevent the occurrence of disease, such as risk factor reduction, but also to arrest its progress and reduce its consequences once established" (WHO, 1998, p. 14).

Encompassing all of these concepts are health interventions, which include health promotion, disease prevention, and primary health care. To have a change in health behavior or an activity undertaken by an individual for the purpose of promoting health, an intervention must take place. An intervention, then, is a planned effort designed to produce change in a specific, targeted population (Rossi & Freeman, 1993).

Healthy People establishes national goals, objectives, and priorities. A goal in the health context, as defined by the Centers for Disease Control and Prevention (2007), is a broad, long-term aim that defines a desired result associated with identified strategic issues. The CDC defines objectives as results of specific activities or outcomes to be achieved over a stated period of time. They are specific, measurable, and realistic. Objectives are specific in that they state *who* will experience *what* change or benefit and *how much* change is to occur (CDC, 2007). Finally, priorities are alternatives ranked according to feasibility, value, and/or importance (Green & Kreutner, 1991).

The rationale behind having a 10-year policy for health, with clearly defined objectives that meet specific criteria, is simple: It is to make sure that everyone who works on health policy understands the consensus decision on where the nation's health should be in 10 years. Just as with an individual client or patient, a national health promotion action plan needs to have specific targets to be met in a specified time frame. Particularly given the complexity of the agencies and groups involved in creating policies, setting clear goals and objectives is essential if national health policy is to have positive long-term effects for the health of the nation.

Note that Healthy People 10-year agendas are not always fully reached. Objectives alone cannot guarantee change. Specific actions must be taken for change to occur. For example, only 71% of the Healthy People 2010 objectives were met. On the positive side, deaths from heart disease and strokes declined significantly over the past decade, the nation's overall life expectancy continued to rise, and several objectives related to mental health assessment and treatment met their 2010 targets.

Yet, there is no research to show these changes were due to stating objectives. Wang, Orleans, and Gortmaker (2012) examined the objective for reducing childhood obesity and concluded that aggressive action, not only setting objectives, is needed.

On the downside, disparities in access to health care grew, even though reducing such disparities was an important objective of Healthy People 2010. For an answer to what may be happening in that case, examine the growing loss of the middle class (Boushey, 2011). Obesity, which 2010 objectives had targeted for reduction, grew substantially in all populations, particularly in adolescents age 12–19. Efforts to promote smoking cessation did not work well enough to achieve the target rate of 12% by 2010 (the overall prevalence of smoking was 19.3% in 2010).

HEALTH PROMOTION CHALLENGE

Go on the web and investigate how or if any of the Healthy People objectives were funded for aggressive actions. If not, what can you do about this? Toss around some ideas with several of your classmates and come up with a plan. If possible, implement it.

Health, Policy, and Economics

Earlier, we noted that the question, "Who will pay the costs?", is fundamental to health policy. It would be difficult to understand health promotion without incorporating aspects of economics. In order to understand any economic system, you need to know who the stakeholders are.

Each of the following is a stakeholder in the business of health care in this country:

- The public has the following vested interests: in keeping healthcare costs low and quality high, ensuring that practitioners are qualified and well trained, ensuring that medications and devices are thoroughly tested for safety and efficacy, and ensuring that access to providers and therapies are evenly distributed.
- The insurance industry has a vested interest in keeping healthcare costs and utilization of therapeutic medications/devices low. It also has a vested interest in limiting government regulations that mandate insurance coverage of specific conditions or populations of people and in ensuring that healthcare providers offer appropriate, high-quality care.

- The pharmaceutical industry has a vested interest in keeping drug costs and utilization of drug therapies high, and in increasing access of patients to medical care so they can obtain these drugs and therapies. It also has a vested interest in reducing regulatory hurdles to approval and marketing of its products (e.g., FDA review) as well as the ability to market its products to physicians and consumers. Note the increase in drug commercials on TV that has had an effect on consumers requesting specific drugs and/or buying those available without prescription by making drug-taking socially acceptable (Buczak, Lukasik & Witek, 2010). TV commercials also deploy several linguistic or rhetorical strategies to send a double message for promotional advantage, including syntactic-semantic ambiguity, voice-over risk messages at odds with upbeat visuals, and a vagueness of certain words in particular contexts (Glinert, 2005).

- Physicians, nurses, clinics, and hospitals, represented by their respective associations, have vested interests in ensuring that reimbursements for provider care keeps pace with the cost of providing that care. Physicians have a vested interest in deciding therapy is appropriate without interference from government or insurers. Administrators of hospitals and clinics have a vested interest in paying for their new MRI and other machines by enrolling more consumers in using them. Nurses, physicians, and administrators of hospitals and clinics have a vested interest in believing that therapies offered have been proven safe and effective, even when research provides evidence to the contrary.

- Government agencies represent both public's interest and the interests of various industries, which sometimes leads to conflicts of interest. For example, a pharmaceutical company may have a promising new therapy for congestive heart failure that it urges the FDA to review and approve promptly. Trials of the therapy show that it improves heart function significantly, but there is a slight increase in colon cancer among those who take it—and some physicians' groups argue that the trials were not sufficiently representative of the patient population to be considered adequate. The government's job is to impartially assess the science—not always an easy task—and weigh the interests of the benefits of the drug for patients *plus* the interests of the pharmaceutical company, which wants to take the drug to market, against the interests of prescribing physicians and the patients who could be harmed by the drug. Often, the solution is to find a middle road: for this fictional example, a middle-ground approach might be that the drug is conditionally approved for use in patients at low risk of colon cancer, and colonoscopy screening is required every 2 years in patients taking the drug. The pharmaceutical company may be required to perform additional safety studies before approval for more general use would be granted, and results of these studies will be required to be made public. Even though these steps sound like a solution, they might not solve the underlying problem. Pharmaceutical companies have a vested interest in their drugs having positive effects, providing a perfect setting for the _Rosenthal effect_ to come into play. This effect is the tendency for results to conform to experimenters' expectations unless stringent safeguards are instituted to minimize human bias. The effect was named after Robert Rosenthal, who performed many of the original experiments revealing the problem (Rosenthal, 1963). In addition to bias, fraud and deception have been noted in the FDA's approval of some drugs (Lenzer & Epstein, 2012), while results were fudged for drugs tested ("Drug companies that had medicines tested," 2011), and research results were falsified for over 70 published studies (Gever, 2010).

Taking into consideration all of these factors, the United States healthcare system is, economically speaking, a jumble of competing market forces. Practitioners, hospitals, and research organizations have created a questionable healthcare system, which is more illness-care than health-care, in which public access and funds available to pay for care are unevenly distributed.

HEALTH PROMOTION CHALLENGE

If you were in charge of the healthcare system, what would you do to improve it? Make a list of all the things that would make things better and share your list with at least two other students. Ask for feedback, listen to their list, and provide constructive feedback. If possible, implement a small portion of one of the items on your list.

Basic Healthcare Economics

In health care, patients are the consumers of healthcare services, and doctors, nurses, technicians, and specialists are the providers of those services. In order to provide care, the provider may need to use devices, medications, and therapeutic interventions (surgery, radiation treatments, massage, physiotherapy, etc.), all of which must be paid for. These are the direct costs associated with care. Indirect costs are costs associated with research and development of new therapies or better devices, the cost of training healthcare personnel, and the cost of administering facilities such as hospitals or clinics. Balanced against costs are outcomes—statistics measuring how effective an intervention is at saving (or prolonging) lives, improving health status, improving quality of life, or restoring physical or mental functioning.

Economic Measurements

The role of economic outcomes is important to understand when evaluating health promotion, especially regarding the costs and the benefits. The steps include comparison of the costs to the benefits (cost–benefit analysis), comparison of one intervention to another, and the identification of the stakeholders for analysis purposes (Pender, Murdaugh, & Parsons, 2011).

When analyzing health promotion terms in cost-inclusive evaluations, a few key terms are important to understand. The first is cost, which is the assigned value of the resources consumed to implement the health promotion activity; in most cases, these resources are measured in dollars. Benefits, on the other hand, are the resources produced or saved as a result of the activity, again usually measured monetarily. Effectiveness is the end result of the program implementation and is *not* measured in monetary units. The final term is the cost-effectiveness analysis, defined as the relationship between the value of the resources used in the program implementation and nonmonetary outcomes produced by the program (Yates, 2008). An example of a cost-effective analysis could be evaluating the cost-effectiveness of gastric bypass surgery for weight loss. The method for the analysis may be a decision tree diagram that delineates the progression of morbid obesity, including coexisting disease processes, that can occur. The effectiveness of the bypass was in relation to the weight loss in the quality-adjusted life in years. Direct costs of the treatment of morbid obesity as well as the coexisting diseases are noted in comparison to those who did not have the surgery. The incremental cost-effectiveness ratio may then be calculated for various scenarios. The findings may be then that the incremental cost-effectiveness ratio was higher for the gastric bypass surgery in comparison to those who did not get the surgery.

Cost–benefit and cost-effectiveness analyses are key factors influencing an extremely important facet of American health care: insurance coverage. Very few people could afford to pay all of the direct costs of health care, never mind the indirect costs. One way that this problem is addressed is through the insurance industry.

What Is Health Insurance?

Health insurance is a business model in which the insurer assesses the insured's likely risk of illness and uses that to determine an insurance premium—that is, a monthly payment made in return for coverage of certain health costs. Health insurance is somewhat like a betting system in which the insurer bets that a policyholder will stay well, while the policyholder bets that he or she will get sick. If the insurer is correct, the policyholder will pay premiums but make relatively few claims, which is a win for the insurer financially. If the policyholder is correct, however, then the insurer pays claims for services far in excess of what the policyholder pays in premiums, and the policyholder wins the financial game.

Of course, it is never that simple. Health insurers hedge the bet by selling policies with large deductibles at more attractive prices. The insurer offers the buyer a lower premium payment if the buyer agrees to assume a certain upfront cost. This is one way that insurers lower their risk of having to pay claims. It is almost a side wager that bets that the policyholder will incur only a specific amount of costs and no more than that. For instance, if the policyholder takes a policy with a $1,000 deductible, and incurs only $999.50 in costs in a given year, then the insurer pays nothing toward those costs—the policy holder does, even though the policy holder has paid insurance premiums right along. The insurer makes money and the policyholders pay more than they otherwise would have. If these same policyholders were to have a nasty accident and break multiple bones, needing surgical repair of the bones and extensive physical therapy, then costs could mount into the tens of thousands of dollars. In this case, the insurance policy would prove a good deal for the policy holders.

The nature of the health insurance business is that it tends to be most profitable when consumers who are not likely to get sick believe themselves to be at risk of illness. It is less profitable when consumers who buy policies have a genuine need for health insurance. For this reason, insurers also hedge their bets further by restricting coverage of certain conditions that tend to get expensive, such as cancer, by limiting the total amount they will pay for a service or during a particular time frame, or by excluding certain conditions or circumstances. For example, a favorite method insurers use for limiting risk is to refuse to pay costs associated with preexisting conditions—that is, any health problem that could be shown to exist prior to the purchase of the policy.[1]

Insurers often drop coverage (refuse to renew a policy) for policyholders who develop expensive health conditions, or they may include fine-print exclusions that allow them to evade an obligation to pay a claim. For example, an insurer can include a disclosure clause in the initial insurance contract that voids the obligation to pay claims if the policyholder neglects to give complete and accurate information about all past health conditions. (Very, very few people keep such records, so it is extremely easy for the insurer to look through medical histories and find something to enable an exclusion.)

Consumers obtain health insurance either through an employer, by purchasing the product themselves, or by participating in a government program, such as Medicaid, Medicare, or the Department of Veterans' Affairs medical program.

---

[1] Discriminating against policy holders based on preexisting conditions has been explicitly forbidden by the 2010 PPACA; this clause will go into effect in 2014. Prior to passage of the PPACA, the practice of excluding coverage on the basis of preexisting conditions was illegal only in Maine and Massachusetts.

Real Costs of Healthcare Services

One of the drawbacks of the insurance industry is that once someone has health insurance, that person may be insulated from the costs of each specified healthcare service. The person may pay only small, incremental fees, and at times, none at all. Subsequently, the insured person tends to seek out health care more frequently than those without insurance would—and to have a less realistic idea of what it costs to obtain health care. Moreover, they tend to expect instant gratification. If they feel sick, they want to take a pill or drink a tonic and instantly feel better, usually without considering the costs involved with researching, testing, manufacturing, and marketing that pill or tonic. Because of this nearly universal longing for an instant cure, it may be difficult to empirically determine not only physical benefits, but the cost benefits of health promotion. Medical care has been shown to account for 10–15% of the decline in premature death in the previous century, with the remaining percentage being illness prevention initiatives (Pender et al., 2011).

Many people do not realize that small, simple changes to their own health practices could make a huge difference to the tax structure and economy of the United States. Here is an example: Suppose there's a massive, $30 million public health campaign asking everyone to learn to habitually cover their nose and mouth with their elbows before sneezing or coughing. The goal of the

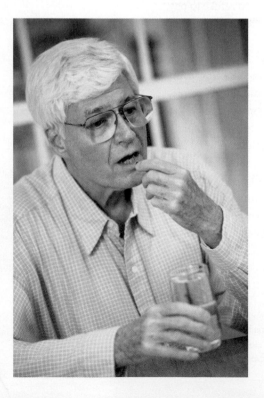

campaign is to lower the rate of viral infections by reducing the transfer of cold viruses and bacteria from the nose and mouth to others either by reducing the presence of droplets carrying these microbes in the air or reducing transfer of germs from hands to doorknobs, light switches, and other people's hands. Would a lot of people consider that a waste of money? Possibly, but let us speculate that it leads to a small reduction of people getting colds—say, 10% of the people who would otherwise have gotten sick do not get sick after this campaign occurs. A 2002 study estimated the economic cost of the common cold at $25 billion (Bramley, Lerner & Sames, 2002), so it is reasonable to assume that the 10% of regained productivity brought about by just 1 person in 10 not getting sick is worth $2.5 billion—almost 85 times what it cost to create the public awareness campaign. Indeed, even at much lower numbers, 1 person in 100, the economic benefit of the campaign still outweighs the cost by more than 8 to 1! Keep in mind, also, that this simple practice would not just affect transfer of common cold viruses, but also influenza, pneumonia, and other communicable respiratory diseases that have profound economic impacts on worker productivity.

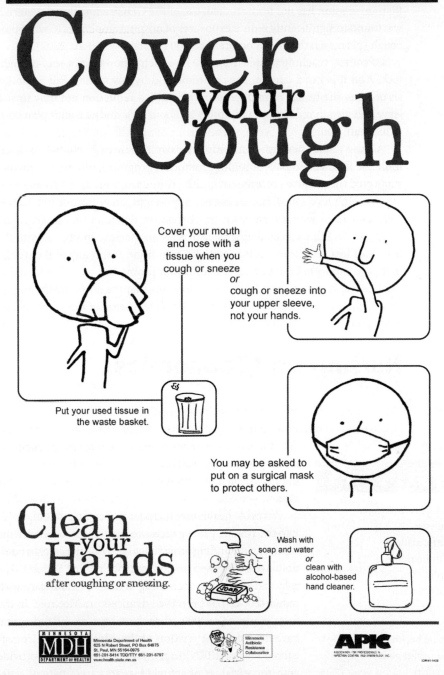

FIGURE 7-3   Cover Your Cough

Source: Centers for Disease Control.

In fact, the CDC has had a cover-your-cough campaign in place for a number of years (see FIGURE 7-3). While its overall effectiveness in preventing cold and flu transmission has not been studied, use of the CDC's educational materials was found to significantly reduce exposures of hospital employees to whooping cough (pertussis) during an outbreak in 2004 (Chatterjee et al., 2007).

Of course, teaching people to sneeze into their elbows is not sexy or high-tech. And it is not a cure for the common cold by any means. But an analysis of work site health promotion programs noted reduction not only in sick leave, but also in reduction in disability by about 25% and of health plan costs (Chapman, 2003).

Aldana (2001) performed a comprehensive review of 72 studies to determine the financial impact of health promotion programs. The review further supported the positive outcomes of health promotion, with the findings showing that high levels of stress, excessive body weight, and multiple risk factors were associated with increased costs. Correlational studies repeatedly found a decrease in illness-related absenteeism with an increase in fitness, with the benefit of less healthcare costs as well. Keep in mind that many of the studies that have supported the cost savings of health promotion were conducted in the 1990s and thus are outdated—which means that the cost–benefit may be even higher, given that the burden of preventable disease in the United States has skyrocketed since 2000.

Nursing and Economics

Nurses are usually employees of healthcare institutions; the demand for their employment is initiated from their employers, who function on a supply-and-demand basis. Currently, there is a decreased demand for inpatient care, yet there is an increase in community nursing needs, such as ambulatory surgery centers and home care.

Access to health care includes three steps: gaining entry into the system, getting access to sites of care to receive the services, and finding providers to provide the care. In addition, access is based on convenience as well as costs. The role that can aid in increasing access to health care with reduced costs has been the advanced practice role. In the first decade of the 2000s, there have been many studies that have described the relation of the advanced practice registered nurse (APRN) to the preventive care they provide with the variables of actual costs incurred, patient satisfaction, hospital recidivism rates, and the actual quality

HOT TOPICS

Here are some topics to explore:
- Policy analysis
- Genetic Information Nondiscrimination Act
- Patient Protection and Affordable Care Act
- Social Security
- Medicare
- International health policy
- WHO and health policy
- Food insecurity

of care delivered. Findings suggest that APRNs can complete a majority of primary care and even preventive care more effectively than the physician providing traditional care (Hoffman, Tasota, Zullo, Scharfenberg, & Donaue, 2005; Steven, 2004). The specific results of the studies have found high satisfaction for the patient and the APRN, as well as direct and comprehensive patient care, support and advocacy, ensuring quality of service, education, research, publication, and leadership (Cumbie, Conley, & Burman, 2004; Mick & Ackerman, 2000). An example may be convenient care clinics, where nurse practitioners manage specific health problems in an accessible place, such as in the local retail pharmacy. Nurse practitioners have also filled the role of primary care provider in rural areas.

APRNs regularly use preventive services through health promotion in primary care to help people achieve and maintain a high quality of life. The APRN uses current evidence-based research to guide these actions. In the relationship that develops between the APRN and the client, counseling can result in primary prevention of:

- postpartum depression by teaching about the effectiveness of more omega-3 fatty acids and counseling
- respiratory infections by helping clients identify and remove sources of second-hand smoke and in-home toxic cleaners and other toxics
- heart disease, cancer of the breast, colon, and rectum; and diabetes mellitus by helping set up a physical activity program (Pruss-Ustum, 2006).

CULTURAL RESEARCH STUDY

A review of: Implications of Food Insecurity on Global Health Policy and Nursing Practice

This literature review examined the concept of food insecurity and its impact on global health policy and nursing. Since the global recession, developing nations have experienced a 17% increase in the prevalence of hunger, mostly occurring in the Middle East and North Africa, sub-Saharan Africa, Asia and the Pacific, and Latin America and the Caribbean. All of these regions are grappling with possible solutions and in many cases are seeking aid.

Implications for nursing in the United States in this review includes participation with other disciplines to assist in education about choosing nutrient-dense foods in cost-effective ways; routine assessment of consumer nutritional status; assessing for adequate macro- and micronutrients; addressing community issues of food storage, transportation, and distribution; and becoming an advocate for adequate nutrition and health promotion on a local level.

Source: Kregg-Byers, C.M., & Schlenk, E. A. (2010). "Implications of Food Insecurity on Global Health Policy and Nursing Practice." *Journal of Nursing Scholarship, 42*(3), 278–285.

Summary

All nursing care is influenced by health policy. Health policy is a decision made to direct the actions of individuals by health promotion. Decisions may be multilevel, and they can be made at a local, state, or federal level, or at all of these.

You can contribute to health policy within the following four spheres of political influence: the workplace, the government, professional organizations, and the community. Workplace-related areas of influence include the policy and procedure manual, occupational and health standards such as those related to needle disposal, biohazard waste, and infectious disease control. In the government realm, you can have influence at all levels. Examples of health promotion laws include those related to tobacco and alcohol and sex education. Professional organization participation may involve supporting recommendations and policies related to such health legislation as seat belt laws, helmet laws, and use of infant car seats. A number of nursing organizations have been instrumental in the promotion of health legislation and recommendations. Within the community setting, areas of participation may include parent–teacher organizations, chambers of commerce, and civic organizations.

A major healthcare reform was the Social Security Act Amendments (also known as the Medicare Act), passed in 1965. This act initiated a plan whereby individuals and employers would pay into a fund throughout an individual's working life and then receive medical coverage at retirement. The 1985 Consolidated Omnibus Reconciliation Act (COBRA) sought to help individuals who were insured through employers to retain insurance coverage even if they lost their jobs. In 1997, the State Children's Health Insurance Program (SCHIP), which provided health insurance to children in families at or below 200% of the poverty level, was enacted.

In 2010, the Patient Protection and Affordable Care Act became law. Major provisions of this include no insurance discrimination based on an employee's wages; insurance rating variability on age, family composition, geographic location, and tobacco use but not on health or gender; Medicaid to all individuals under age 65 who are at or below 133% of the federal poverty level; a new program to support school-based health centers and nurse-managed health centers; a benefits package that provides a comprehensive set of services; a benefits package with a comprehensive set of mental health services; and development of training programs that focus on primary care models that integrate physical and mental health services. Benefits related to health promotion and disease prevention include covering of preventive services as recommended by the U.S. Preventive Services Task Force; variations in insurance rating based on tobacco use; grants to small employers that establish wellness programs for employees; and establishing National Prevention, Health Promotion, and Public Health Council-coordinated federal prevention, wellness, and public health activities. The act also has a subcomponent called the Nursing Work-force Development Program, the purpose of which is to recruit new nurses into the profession, promote career advancement within nursing, and improve patient care delivery. A timeline for the initiation of the various elements of the Patient Protection and Affordable Care Act summarizes components to be phased in each year until 2014.

Health policy mandates passed by Congress are implemented by the Department of Health and Human Services, which has numerous individual agencies. The goals for health policy, however, are identified by 10-year Healthy People plans. Healthy People is an agenda of prevention for the nation. The initiative provides information and knowledge on how to improve health for diverse groups and to encourage the nation to work together as a team. The current plan, Healthy People 2020, was released in 2010, but may require adequate funding to produce expected results.

The ability to evaluate health promotion requires an understanding of economic outcomes, especially information related to costs and benefits. The process involves comparing the costs to the benefits through the effects, comparison of the intervention with another, and identification of stakeholders for analysis purposes. Cost is the assigned value of the resources consumed to implement a project. Benefits are the resources produced or saved as a result of the program implementation. Effectiveness is the end result of the program implementation. Cost-effectiveness analysis is the relationship between the value of the resources used in the program implementation and the nonmonetary outcomes produced by the program. Cost–benefit and cost-effectiveness are used to determine insurance coverage of different therapies. Health insurance is essentially a strategy of balancing the patient's perceived risk of illness against the real likelihood of illness. Along with insurers, economic stakeholders in the business of health care include pharmaceutical companies, providers (including clinics and hospitals as well as individual practitioners), patients, and government bodies.

REVIEW QUESTIONS

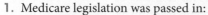

1. Medicare legislation was passed in:
   a. 1941
   b. 1965
   c. 1989
   d. 2000

2. The American Academy of Pediatricians was instrumental in promoting the use of:
   a. Swimming lessons for all children
   b. Bicycle helmets for children when they are riding bicycles
   c. Labeling of food ingredients

3. The Genetic Information Nondiscrimination Act:
   a. Allows insurance companies to insure only those who are low risk
   b. Pays for genetic counseling for all
   c. Prohibits employers from discriminating on the basis of genetic test results

4. Political spheres of influence for the nurse include:
   a. The workplace
   b. The government
   c. Professional organizations
   d. All of the above

5. The Patient Protection and Affordable Care Act includes which of the following provisions?
   a. No insurance discrimination based on employee's wages
   b. Insurance rating not to be based on health and gender
   c. New program to support school-based health centers and nurse-managed health centers
   d. All of the above

EXERCISES

1. Review the various components of the new healthcare legislation that are being phased in each year for the next few years. How will these affect you and your family? Here is one website to use: http://www.nytimes.com/interactive/2010/03/21/us/health-care-reform.html#scenario-1

2. Go to the website for the Food and Drug Administration (http://www.fda.gov/). Find the link for Centers and Offices. Make an outline of the various offices and their responsibilities.

3. Go to the FDA website and find the link for medical devices. Write a brief summary about the ways in which the FDA protects the public through its policies on medical devices.

4. Go to the website for the World Health Organization (http://www.who.int). Summarize its current health policy priorities.

BIBLIOGRAPHY

Barr, D. A. (2007). *Introduction to U.S. health policy: The organization, financing, and delivery of health care in America*. Baltimore, MD: John Hopkins University Press.

Bodenheimer, T., & Grumbach, K. (2008). *Understanding health policy: A clinical approach*. New York, NY: McGraw Hill Medical.

Dove, M. S., Dockery, D. W., Mittleman, M. A., Schwartz, J., Sullivan, E. M., Keithly, L., & Land, T. (2010, September 23). The impact of Massachusetts' smoke-free workplace laws on acute myocardial infarction deaths. *American Journal of Public Health, 100*(11), 2206–2212.

Kogan, M. D., Newacheck, P. W., Blumberg, S. J., Heyman, K. M., Strickland, B. B., Singh, G. K., & Zeni, M. B. (2010). State variation in underinsurance among children with special health care needs in the United States. *Pediatrics, 124*(4), 673–680.

Mackay, D., Haw, S., Ayres, J. G., Fischbacher, C., & Pell, J. P. (2010). Smoke-free legislation and hospitalizations for childhood asthma. *New England Journal of Medicine, 363*(12), 1139–1145.

Mason, D. J., Leavitt, J. K., & Chaffee, M. W. (2011). *Policy and politics in nursing and health care*. Philadelphia, PA: Saunders.

National Vaccine Advisory Committee. (2009). Financing vaccination of children and adolescents: National Vaccine Advisory Committee recommendations. *Pediatrics, 124*, (Suppl. 5), S558–S562.

Patel, K., & Rushefsky, M. E. (2006). *Health care politics and policy in America*. Armonk, NY: M.E. Sharp.

Perrin, J. M. (2010). Treating underinsurance. *New England Journal of Medicine, 363*(9), 881–883.

Prows, C. A., Glass, M., Nicol, M. J., Skirton, H., & Williams, J. (2005). Genomics in nursing education. *Journal of Nursing Scholarship, 37*(3), 196–202.

Schoem, S. R., & Shah, U. K. (2010). Act to keep patients safe: Device-related adverse event reporting. *Otolaryngology Head Neck Surgery, 142*(5), 651–653.

Shi, L., Lebrun, L. A., & Tsai, J. (2010). Access to medical care, dental care, and prescription drugs: The roles of race/ethnicity, health insurance, and income. *Southern Medical Journal, 103*(6), 509–516.

Staff of the *Washington Post*. (2010). *Landmark: The inside story of America's new health care law and what it means for all of us*. Washington, DC: Washington Post.

Tang, N., Stein, J., Hsia, R. Y., Maselli, J. H., & Gonzales, R. (2010). Trends and characteristics of US emergency department visits, 1997–2007. *JAMA, 304*(6), 664–670.

Winickoff, J. P., Gottlieb, M., & Mello, M. M. (2010). Regulation of smoking in public housing. *New England Journal of Medicine, 362*(24), 2319–2325.

REFERENCES

Aldana, S. (2001). Financial impact of health promotion progress: A comprehensive review of the literature. *American Journal of Health Promotion, 15*(5), 296–320.

American Academy of Pediatrics Policy Statement. (2011). Child passenger safety. *Pediatrics, 127,* 788–793.

Boushey, H. (2011). The Endangered Middle Class: Is the American Dream Slipping out of Reach for American Families? Testimony Before the Senate Committee on Health, Education, Labor, and Pensions. Retrieved from http://www.americanprogressaction.org/issues/2011/05/boushey_testimony.html

Bramley, T. J., Lerner, D., & Sames, M. (2002). Productivity losses related to the common cold. *Journal of Occupational and Environmental Medicine, 44*(9), 822–829.

Buczak, A., Lukasik, I. M., Witek A. (2010). Use of painkillers by Polish secondary school students and the influence of TV. *Gesundheitswese, 72*(11), 808–812.

Cease, A. T., King, W. D, & Monroe, K. W. (2011). Analysis of child passenger safety restraint use at a pediatric emergency department. *Pediatric Emergency Care, 27*(2), 102–105.

Centers for Disease Control and Prevention [CDC]. (2007). *National diabetes fact sheet: General information and national estimates on diabetes in the U.S.* Atlanta, GA: U.S. Department of Health and Human Services/CDC.

Chapman, L. (2003). Meta-evaluation of worksite health promotion economic return studies. *Art of Health Promotion Newsletter, 6*(6), 1–16.

Chatterjee, A., Plummer, S., Heybrock, B., Bardon, T., Eischen, K., Hall, M., & Lazoritz, S. (2007). A modified "cover your cough" campaign prevents exposures of employees to pertussis at a children's hospital. *American Journal of Infection Control, 35*(7), 489–491.

Cohen, M., March, J., & Olsen, J. (1972). A garbage can model of organizational choice. *Administrative Scientific Quarterly, 17,* 1–25.

Cumbie, S., Conley, V., & Burman, M. (2004). Advanced practice nursing model for comprehensive care with chronic illness: Model for promoting process engagement. *Advances in Nursing Science, 27*(1), 70–80.

Doll, R. (1998). Avoidable environmental factors. *Recent Results in Cancer Research, 154,* 3–21.

"Drug companies that had medicines tested." (2011). FDA finds U.S. drug research firm faked documents. Retrieved from http://www.reuters.com/article/2011/07/26/us fda cctcro-violation-idUSTRE76P7E320110726

Durbin, D. R., for the Committee on Injury, Violence, and Poison Prevention. (2011). Child passenger safety. *Pediatrics, 127*(4), e1050–e1066.

Fenton, J. J., Foote, S. B., Green, P., & Baldwin, L. M. (2010). Diffusion of computer-aided mammography after mandated Medicare coverage. *Archives of Internal Medicine, 170*(11), 987–990.

Fuchs, S., Barthel, M. J., Flannery, A. M, & Christoffel, K. K. (1989). Cervical spine fractures sustained by young children in forward facing car seats. *Pediatrics, 84*(2), 348–354.

Gever, J. (2010). Research fraud probe leads to criminal charge. Retrieved from http://www.medpagetoday.com/PublicHealthPolicy/Ethics/17985

Glinert, L. H. (2005). TV commercials for prescription drugs: a discourse analytic perspective. *Research in Social and Administrative Pharmacy, 1*(2), 158–184.

Gómez-Cabello, A., Ara, I., González-Agüero, A., Casajús, J. A., & Vicente-Rodríguez, G. (2012). Effects of training on bone mass in older adults: a systematic review. *Sports Medicine 42*(4), 301–325.

Green, L., & Kreutner, M. (1991). *Health promotion planning: An educational and environmental approach* (2nd ed.). Palo Alto, CA: Mayfield Publishing Company.

Hall, K. G. (2007, November 28). *Democrats' health plans echo Nixon's failed GOP proposal*. Washington, DC: McClatchy Washington Bureau. Retrieved from http://www.mcclatchydc.com/2007/11/28/22163/democrats-health-plans-echo-nixons.html

Hoffman, L., Tasota, F., Zullo, T., Scharfenberg, C., & Donaue, M. (2005). Outcomes of care managed by an acute care nurse practitioner/attending physician team in a subacute medical intensive care unit. *American Journal of Critical Care, 14*(2), 121–130.

Irvine, L., Elliott, L., Wallace, H., & Crombie, I. K. (2006). A review of major influences on current public health policy in developed countries in the second half of the 20th century. *Perspectives in Public Health, 126*(2), 73–78.

Johnston, C., Rivara, F. P., & Soderberg, R. (1994). Children in car crashes: Analysis of data for injury and use of restraints. *Pediatrics, 93*(6 Pt. 1), 960–965.

Lenzer, J., & Epstein, K. (2012). The Yas men: Members of FDA panel reviewing the results of popular Bayer contraceptive had industry ties. *Washington Monthly*. Retrieved from http://www.washingtonmonthly.com/ten miles-square/2012/01/the_yaz_men_members_of_fda_pan034651.php

Lincoln, M. (2005). Car seat safety: Literature review. *Neonatal Network, 24*(2), 29–31.

Loud, J. T. (2010). Direct-to-consumer genetic and genomic testing: Preparing nurse practitioners for genomic healthcare. *The Journal for Nurse Practitioners, 6*(8), 585–594.

Mandelblatt, J., Cronin, K., Bailey, S., Berry, D., de Koning, H., Draisma, G.,...Feuer, E. (2009). Effects of mammography screening under different screening schedules: Model estimates of potential benefits and harms. *Annals of Internal Medicine, 151*(10), 738–747.

Mason, D., Leavitt, J., & Chafee, M. (2007). *Policy and politics in nursing and health care* (5th ed.). St. Louis, MO: Saunders.

McBride, C. M., Wade, C. H., & Kaphingst, K. A. (2010). Consumers' views of direct-to-consumer genetic information. *Annual Review of Genomics and Human Genetics, 11*(September 22), 427–446.

Mick, D. J., & Ackerman, M. H. (2000). Advanced practice nursing. Advanced practice nursing role delineation in acute and critical care: application of the strong model of advanced practice. *Heart and Lung: Journal of Acute and Critical Care, 29*(3), 210–221.

National Cancer Institute, (2010). Mammograms: Fact sheet. Retrieved from http://www.cancer.gov/cancertopics/factsheet/detection/mammograms

Nelson, H., Tyne, K., Naik, A., Bougatsos, C., Chan, B., & Humphrey, L. (2009). Screening for breast cancer: An update for the U.S. Preventive Services Task Force. *Annals of Internal Medicine, 151*(1), 727–737, W237–W242.

Nixon, R. (1974). Address on the state of the union delivered before a joint session of the Congress. In J. T. Woolley & G. Peters (Eds.), *The American Presidency Project*. Santa Barbara: University of California, Santa Barbara. Retrieved from http://www. presidency. ucsb. edu/ws/index. php?pid=4327#axzz1inX22KFF

Pender, N., Murdaugh, C., & Parsons, M. (2011). *Health promotion in nursing practice* (6th ed.). Upper Saddle River, NJ: Pearson.

Pruss-Ustun, A. (2006). Executive summary, WHO conference on preventing disease through healthy environments. Retrieved from http://www.who.int/quantifying_ehimpacts/publications/prevdisexecsume.pdf

Rosenthal, R. (1963). On the social psychology of the psychological experiment: The experimenter's hypothesis as unintended determinant of experimental results. *American Scientist, 51*, 268–283.

Rossi, P., & Freeman, H. (1993). *Evaluation: A systematic approach* (5th ed.). Newbury Park, CA: Sage Publications, Inc.

Sisk, R. (2009, August 26). Health care reform was Sen. Ted Kennedy's unfinished life's work. *Daily News (New York)*. Retrieved from http://www.nydailynews.com/news/politics/health-care-reform-sen-ted-kennedy-unfinished-life-work-article-1. 394842

Stalnaker, R. L. (1993). Spinal cord injuries to children in real world accidents. *SAE SP-986* (pp. 173–183). Warrendale, PA: Society of Automotive Engineers (SAE).

Stefanek, M., Gritz, E., & Vernon, S. (2010). Mammography and women under 50: Déjà vu all over again? *Cancer Epidemiology, Biomarkers and Prevention, 19*(3), 639.

Steven, K. (2004). APRN hospitalist: Just a resident replacement? *Journal of Pediatric Health Care, 18*(4), 208–210.

Tessier, K. (2010). Effectiveness of hands-on education for correct child restraint use by parents. *Accident; Analysis and Prevention, 42*(4), 1041–1047.

Tingvall, C. (1987). Children in cars. Some aspects of the safety of children as car passengers on road traffic accidents. *Acta Paediatrica Scandinavica, 339*(Suppl.), 1–35.

Trippel, R. (2011, August 11). U.S. newborn death rate ranked behind 40 other nations. *Health News*. Retrieved from http://www.healthnews.com/en/news/US-Newborn-Death-Rate-Ranked-Behind-40-Other-Nations-/1EQSv5Sff6ovNKSK$bH6TL/

Turbell, T. (1974). *Child restraint systems: Frontal impact performance*. VTI Rapport 36A. Stockholm, Sweden: Swedish Road and Traffic Research Institute (VTI).

Wang, Y. C., Orleans, C. T., & Gortmaker, S. L. (2012). Reaching the healthy people goals for reducing childhood obesity: closing the energy gap. *American Journal of Preventive Medicine, 42*(5), 437–444.

World Health Organization [WHO]. (1998). *Health promotion glossary*. Geneva, Switzerland: Author.

World Health Organization [WHO]. (2012). *Health policy*. Retrieved from http://www.who.int/topics/health_policy/en/

Yamaguchi M. (2012, April 5th). Nutritional factors and bone homeostasis: synergistic effect with zinc and genistein in osteogenesis. *Molecular Cell Biochemistry*. [Epub online before print.] Retrieved from http://www.ncbi.nlm.nih.gov/pubmed/22476903

Yates, B. (2008). Cost-effectiveness and cost-benefit of family involvement initiatives. *The Evaluation Exchange, 14*, 33.

INTERNET RESOURCES

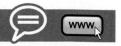

For a full suite of assignments and learning activities, use the access code located in the front of your book to visit this exclusive website: **http://go.jblearning.com/healthpromotion**. If you do not have an access code, you can obtain one at the site.

PART 3

Health Promotion and Evidence-Based Practice

LEARNING OBJECTIVES

Upon completion of this chapter, you will be able to:

1. Describe how qualitative and quantitative research is used in health promotion.

2. Identify three types of quantitative research studies and explain their value to health promotion.

3. Identify three types of qualitative research studies and explain their value to health promotion.

4. Differentiate between independent and dependent variables.

5. Analyze health promotion research studies to determine the strength of the data set and validity of data analysis

6. Critique a health promotion research article.

7. Discuss health promotion nursing research questions.

8. Compare health promotion relationship statements.

KEY TERMS

www

Correlation research

Data analysis

Data collection

Dependent variable

Descriptive research

Ethnographic research

Experiment

Grounded theory

Independent variable

Literature review

Phenomenological research

Problem

Qualitative research

Quantitative research

Quasiexperimental research

Research design

Sample

CHAPTER **8**

Evidence-Based Health Promotion

- Introduction
- Why is Evidence-Based Health Promotion Important?
- Types Of Health Promotion Research
- Steps of Research
- Summary

Introduction

In earlier chapters, we discussed health promotion between you and the client, whether it was an individual, family, or community. In this chapter, we focus on choosing evidence-based health promotion practices that are supported by high-quality data, and when quantitative or qualitative research findings might be more appropriate.

This chapter also provides information necessary to begin generating health promotion nursing questions, suggests some methods that may be most useful in studying health promotion-oriented questions, and suggests some health promotion relationship statements that can be used to test theory and, in eventually, develop research studies (see BOX 8-1).

BOX 8-1   What Are Independent and Dependent Variables?

Variables in research can be independent or dependent. An **independent variable** is a factor that is not affected by or altered by other factors. For example, age, gender, and race are all independent variables. Other factors, such as diet, exercise, and lifestyle, have no effect on any of these independent variables. However, one goal of research is to determine whether the independent variable causes or predicts a change or difference in other factors (**dependent variables**). For example, exercise habits in a group of people might differ substantially depending on age, gender, and possibly even race.

Thus, the independent variable is what the researcher is manipulating, and the dependent variable is the outcome or response that may be affected by altering the independent variable. The relationship between independent and dependent variables, in short, is what the researcher wants to explain.

Why is Evidence-Based Health Promotion Important?

Qualitative and quantitative research are keys to generating evidence that supports nursing goals and practices (Burns & Grove, 2007). Keeping up with the latest health promotion findings is vital whether you work with individual clients, families, or communities. New data may be published tomorrow that can help you with a client. When you start working with a new client, get in the habit of looking up the latest research on that client's goals or issues. Get on the internet and go to www.pubmed.gov and type in the topic in the search box and the latest research on the problem will pop up first.

Types Of Health Promotion Research

Research methods come in two forms, quantitative and qualitative. **Quantitative research** counts or measures phenomena or data points and compares it to other observed phenomena or data points in order to develop ideas about how those phenomena/data relate to one another. Quantitative research is a formal, rigorous process for objectively generating information; it may be used in describing, exploring, or examining new situations, events, or concepts.

Qualitative research is subjective and the information is generated from and is viewed in the context of the experiences of study participants. It is often used to generate hypotheses about a particular phenomena. Quantitative research has been mistakenly labeled as the only true research method. This assumption is incorrect—qualitative research can generate rich data as well, although the process is a bit different and the conclusions reached must be used differently.

Types of Quantitative Research

There are four primary types of quantitative research: descriptive, correlation, quasiexperimental, and experimental. This list is in order of specificity—that is, a descriptive research study is exactly what its name suggests, a study undertaken to describe a poorly known phenomenon or entity, while an experimental research study is a much more concrete examination of how a known entity responds to specific situations.

☐ Descriptive Research

Descriptive research explores and describes a real-life phenomenon in its normal context, thereby depicting accurate accounts of the characteristics of the participants, situations, or even the group as a whole (Kerlinger & Lee, 2000). It seeks to discover how a person or entity behaves in its usual environment.

HEALTH PROMOTION CHALLENGE

Take a look at the descriptive study that follows. How can you use the findings to assist with your health promotion efforts?

RESEARCH BOX 8-1

» OBJECTIVE: To investigate whether the educational initiatives carried out in basic health units in Belo Horizonte, Minas Gerais, Brazil, follow the principles of health promotion.

» METHODS: This descriptive study examined 33 educational health promotion initiatives to determine whether they were guided by five principles, used as categories of analysis: multicausality of the health–disease process, intersectoriality, social engagement, sustainability, and use of dialogic teaching methods (active participation of subjects in the learning process, planning the activity to generate new knowledge, and use of various teaching strategies). Structured observation was used for data collection. The frequency of each category was evaluated in each initiative.

» RESULTS: Multicausality was the most frequent category observed (73.0%), and intersectoriality the least frequent (9.0%). Regarding the use of dialogic methods, 38.0% of the initiatives promoted the active engagement of subjects, 6.0% promoted knowledge generation, and 40.0% employed a variety of teaching strategies.

» CONCLUSIONS: Most educational initiatives were not actively oriented toward health promotion, understood as the strengthening of autonomy and self-management of health processes, social engagement, and employment of dialogic teaching approaches. However, some progress has been made moving away from hegemonic models of education in primary health care.

Source: Carneiro, A. C., Souza, V. D., Godinho, L. K., Faria, I. C., Silva, K. L., & Gazzinelli, M. F. (2012). Health promotion education in the context of primary care. *Revista Panamericana Salud Publica, 31*(2),115–120.

☐ Correlation Research

Correlation research involves more than describing a phenomenon; it usually involves an investigation of the relationship between the study variables (or how they are correlated). An example of correlation research would be to document whether individuals who engage in one behavior (say, twice-yearly dental visits) also engage in another behavior (such as regular flossing). Note that this sort of research cannot say whether either of the correlated behaviors *causes* the other to occur.

An example of how easily correlation research can be misinterpreted is a 2011 study of maternal–child bonding in obese children published in the journal, *Pediatrics* (Anderson, Gooze, Lemeshow, & Whitaker, 2012). The study assessed the relationship between mothers and their children at young ages (15, 24, and 36 months) as recorded in an earlier developmental study, and then returned to the participants when the children were in their teens to see whether there was a correlation between a poor relationship between mother and child and the child's adolescent weight. Having discovered such a correlation, the findings were published under the title, "Quality of Early Maternal–Child Relationship and Risk of Adolescent Obesity." The conclusions of the study were:

> Poor quality of the early maternal-child relationship was associated with a higher prevalence of adolescent obesity. Interventions aimed at improving the quality of maternal-child interactions should consider assessing effects on children's weight and examining potential mechanisms involving stress response and emotion regulation (Anderson, Gooze, Lemeshow, & Whitaker, 2011, p. 132).

The title and the conclusions do not state that the poor relationship between the mother and child causes the child to become obese, but a variety of news outlets interpreted the study that way. "Teenage Obesity Linked to Poor Mother–Child Bond" was the title of a *New York Times* blog on parenting (Dell'Antonia, 2011); "Obesity Linked to Kids Who Have Bad Relationships with Their Mothers," read another parenting blog title (Parenting Source, 2011). As a result of this misunderstanding, popular wisdom came away with the impression that the study showed that bad mothering makes kids grow up to be overweight.

HEALTH PROMOTION CHALLENGE

How can authors of correlation studies ensure this kind of misunderstanding does not happen in the future?

☐ Quasiexperimental Research

A **quasiexperimental research** approach is one step away from being a true *experiment*, with the *quasi* meaning "resembling." A quasiexperiment is not fully experimental because it lacks control by the researcher, specifically over the manipulation of treatment, the setting management, or subject selection (Burns & Grove, 2007).

An example would be a study that randomly tests high school students' blood glucose levels upon entering school to get a sense of how well students eat before going to classes. The results might give a snapshot of the range of blood glucose values among the students on that particular morning, but it likely does not give an accurate perspective on the frequency with which high school students eat breakfast, nor whether they eat healthy breakfasts, nor even whether eating breakfast affects their performance in school. A small subgroup of children who started the day with high-glycemic foods—soda, pastries, or candy, for example—could potentially skew the results higher than reality; alternatively, a small subgroup of children who began the day with a protein shake and a 5-mile jog might skew the results lower. Thus, quasiexperimental studies should be taken with a grain of salt and recognized for what they are—a starting point for further experimental research. For example, this initial quasiexperimental study could be strengthened by selecting a group of 200 students, having them all eat identical breakfasts every day for a set time period, measuring their blood glucose after breakfast each day, and tracking academic performance over time to see if blood glucose and performance correlate.

❑ Experimental Research

Experimental research is highly controlled and has the purpose of identifying a specific relationship in a phenomenon between the independent and dependent variables. The strongest research is a study where subjects are alike or highly similar in certain basic characteristics (e.g., age, gender, and ethnicity) and the variables that are being studied are highly specific (for example, doses of a medication). The goal is to compare like subjects under varying conditions—the apples-to-apples, oranges-to-oranges approach—so that the effects of the variable can be clearly seen. If the subjects are not similar enough, then the dissimilarities can muddy the waters. For instance, a group of male subjects included in a study of muscle strength is only meaningful if the subjects' ages are controlled. A child of 10 cannot reasonably be expected to show the strength level of a 15-year-old adolescent, nor would a 25-year-old man necessarily compare with a 50-year-old man.

HEALTH PROMOTION CHALLENGE

Examine the experimental research health promotion study that appears below. How can you use the findings in the study to help promote health?

Qualitative Research

Qualitative approaches assess the quality of phenomena—a subjective assessment that can be challenging to measure in objective terms. Qualitative research is most appropriate for the discovery of theory and understanding. Its scope is holistic and its methods emphasize interactions of variables. Increasingly, researchers in fields with a traditional quantitative or numbers emphasis, such as psychology, social sociology, and educational research, have shifted to a more qualitative mindset. This shift is in line with a trend toward holistic learning.

Qualitative data are well grounded in real-world observations and contain rich descriptions and explanations of processes, while quantitative data tend

RESEARCH BOX 8-2   A Health-Promoting Lifestyle in University Students

» BACKGROUND: Research has shown that encouraging healthy behaviors, especially among younger people, is an effective way to reduce morbidity and mortality from chronic conditions such as diabetes. This study was conducted in Mexico where diabetes is a major cause of death.

» OBJECTIVES: The aim of this study was to test the efficacy of a brief health-promotion intervention that encouraged a health-promoting lifestyle in university students.

» METHODS: The researchers used a two-group randomized controlled experimental design. Seventy-three freshman Mexican students (31 in the experimental group and 42 in the control group) participated. The experimental group attended a 7-session program, with a duration of 2 hours per session. Lifestyle was measured using the Health-Promoting Lifestyle Profile-II questionnaire. Repeated-measures and factorial analysis of variance were computed.

» RESULTS: There was a significant main effect of the intervention in all dependent health profile variables, $F(2, 138) = 3.46–14.45$, $p < .03$. They also found a significant interaction between group and time for the overall health profile score, $F(2, 138) = 8.73$, $p < .0001$, physical activity, $F(2, 138) = 4.68$, $p = .01$, nutrition, $F(2, 138) = 3.57$, $p = .03$, health responsibility, $F(2, 138) = 5.31$, $p = .006$, and stress management, $F(2, 138) = 8.71$, $p < .0001$.

» DISCUSSION: This interaction indicated that lifestyle differed in the intervention and control groups across the measurements at different times. Students attending the intervention presented a healthier lifestyle than did students in the control group. These results offer interesting experimental evidence to establish guidelines for the design of healthier universities.

Source: Ulla Díez, S. M., Fortis, A. P., & Franco, S. F. (2012). Efficacy of a health-promotion intervention for college students: a randomized controlled trial. *Nursing Research, 61*(2),129–140.

to isolate findings and make analysis difficult when results are unexpected. Qualitative approaches (see INFORMATION BOX 8-1) offer context to phenomena; coupled with quantitative research, they can provide nuances to the data that might otherwise be difficult to interpret.

A prime example of occasions when qualitative data offer superior information may be found in end-of-life care. Quantitative analysis would focus on objective measures of *how long* subjects lived, but might not capture the subjective question of *how well* subjects lived. There is general agreement that taking heroic measures at extending life is not beneficial if the quality of the added days, weeks, or months is low (e.g., a client is unable to speak, move, or interact with others, and/or suffers tremendous pain, confusion, or distress).

Quantitative analysis does not capture such factors well; a person cannot objectively assess another's experience of pain, for example, because each individual responds to and expresses pain and discomfort differently. A person with a low pain threshold may scream or cry out when experiencing pain that

INFORMATION BOX 8-1

Qualitative research uses techniques that are very different from quantitative approaches. There are a number of websites with excellent reviews and guidance about each qualitative approach discussed in this chapter. Here are a few. From North Carolina State University: http://faculty.chass.ncsu.edu/garson/PA765/ethno.htm. This site contains an excellent review of ethnographic research.

Reviews of the grounded theory approaches can be found at http://www.groundedtheoryreview.com/, http://www.scu.edu.au/schools/gcm/ar/arp/grounded.html, and http://www.groundedtheory.com/. An excellent site for information about phenomenology is from the Center for Advanced Research in Phenomenology: http://www.phenomenologycenter.org/phenom.html.

another person, with a higher pain threshold, would simply ignore. Thus, collecting qualitative assessments of distress from the subject (subjective data) is important when attempting to assess quality of life.

See RESEARCH BOX 8-3 that follows. It details a qualitative study of end-of-life care. Notice how themes are identified, which is something impossible to do in a quantitative study. Which of these themes could you use to promote health?

RESEARCH BOX 8-3   Qualitative Study, End-Of-Life Care

» BACKGROUND: The researchers undertook this study of older adults dying from chronic illness in rural areas because they are understudied and have limited access to health services.

» PURPOSE: The purpose of this qualitative descriptive study was to describe the perspectives of primary family caregivers regarding experiences with formal and informal care at the end of life for dying older adults in one rural, agricultural county.

» METHOD: Semi-structured interviews were conducted with 23 caregivers following the death of an older relative.

» FINDINGS: Major themes that emerged from the data were the benefits and challenges associated with care services. Benefits included neighbors, friends, and other volunteers who offered household help and provided respite care. Challenges included limited resources for continuity of care, geographical service boundaries, and lack of knowledge about end-of-life care by paid caregivers.

» IMPLICATIONS FOR FUTURE RESEARCH: Further research that addresses the perspective of rural service providers is needed to better understand the benefits and challenges of end-of-life care in this setting.

Source: Hansen, L., Cartwright, J. C., & Craig, C. E. (2012). End-of-life care for rural-dwelling older adults and their primary family caregivers. *Research in Gerontological Nursing, 5*(1), 6–15.

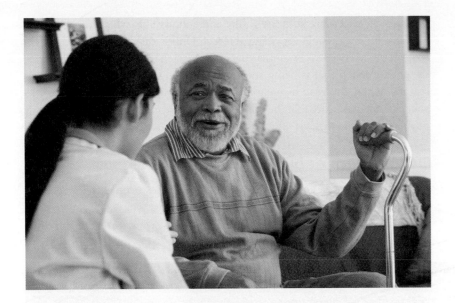

Qualitative approaches include phenomenological research, grounded theory research, ethnographic studies, and historical research.

☐ Phenomenological Research

Phenomenological research captures the lived experience of the participants. This type of research is inductive in nature. If you were doing this kind of study, you would collect observations from a selection of members in a class of people or things and use those observations to generalize about the entire class. The drawback to this is when the class of people or objects is naturally diverse, your findings might not represent the whole class. Another problem with this type of research is that no two observers will describe the same phenomenon in the same way—even if they observed it using the same tools at the same time.

Researchers can limit the range of error of such research by narrowing the subject down to subjects they know to have things in common. They can restrict a study to people of Puerto Rican ethnicity living in New York City, for example. Setting clear limits to establish that the findings of the study apply to one very strictly delimited group can help improve the study's accuracy. Even so, there are still factors that can skew the observations. Imagine for a moment what would happen if four aliens landed on Earth. All of them landed in New York, but one landed at the eastern tip of Long Island on a January morning, a second landed in Central Park on a July afternoon, a third landed in Queens at midnight in October, and a fourth found himself at Rockefeller Plaza on Christmas Eve. If the four then compare notes, they might have very different concepts of what New York looks like and sounds like, what the weather is like, and how its people dress and interact. Unless care is taken to establish congruent observations by similar people subjected to few outside influences, the phenomenon that is being studied can show great variability. For these reasons, when you read a research report and wonder if it would apply to your clients, make sure that the population the researchers used matches your population of clients.

□ Grounded Theory

Grounded theory is an inductive approach that has been developed from sociology—specifically the symbolic interaction theory. The technique involves collecting data and organizing it into categories, which are then used to

---

RESEARCH BOX 8-4   Grounded Theory of Childhood Cancer Decisions

» BACKGROUND: Parents of children diagnosed with cancer must make major treatment decisions with life-altering consequences. The unique experience of these parents is not well represented in the growing literature on cancer treatment decision making (TDM).

» OBJECTIVE: The objective of this study was to describe the process of parents making major treatment decisions for their children with cancer.

» METHODS: The researchers used grounded theory methods and interviewed 15 parents of 13 children with cancer facing major treatment decisions.

» RESULTS: Everything parents encountered and undertook during the TDM process was in the service of making the right decision for their child. All parents expressed conviction that they had made the right decision, but conviction was tempered by doubts triggered by the pervasive uncertainty of the childhood cancer experience. Parents described limited TDM participation by extended family members and the affected children themselves, asserting their primary responsibility to act as their child's surrogate in partnership with the child's medical team.

» CONCLUSIONS: Making the right decision for one's child under challenging conditions is an extension of the parental obligation to act in the child's best interest and a responsibility that parents claim as their own.

» IMPLICATIONS FOR PRACTICE: The findings from this study can serve as the foundation for future studies to refine the conceptualization of TDM in childhood cancer, which will in turn ground the development and evaluation of interventions to support parents in their critical TDM role.

Source: Stewart, J. L., Pyke-Grimm, K. A., & Kelly, K. P. (2012, January 30th). Making the Right Decision for My Child With Cancer: The Parental Imperative. *Cancer Nursing,* 2012 Jan 30. [Epub ahead of print]. Retrieved from http://www. ncbi.nlm.nih.gov/pubmed/22293159

formulate hypotheses or propositions. These hypotheses are then tested and reformulated until a theory is developed. Because there are specific techniques used in grounded theory (and differing methodologies, depending on whether Straussian [Strauss & Corbin, 1990] or Glaserian [Glaser, 1992] methods are chosen), researchers who seek to employ this method should be very clear on the techniques of data collection and organization before beginning a study.

The study that follows shows a summary of grounded theory research.

HEALTH PROMOTION CHALLENGE

Which of the findings in Research Box 8-4 can aid you in your health promotion efforts?

☐ Ethnographic Research

An **ethnographic research** approach involves the collection and analysis of qualitative data in order to learn about cultural phenomena reflecting knowledge and meaning systems for a specific ethnic or cultural group. Data is usually collected via interviews, observation, questionnaires, and so forth.

RESEARCH BOX 8-5   Nursing Practice Values In The NICU And Breastfeeding Promotion

In this ethnographic study, the researcher examined neonatal intensive care unit (NICU) nurses' everyday practice values and explored how breastfeeding promotion fit within this context. The study was conducted over a 14-month period and included participant observation and interviewing of 114 purposively selected nurses in a level-IV NICU in the United States. Uncertainty emerged as a central concern underlying everyday practice values. Three themes described these values: (a) maximizing babies' potentials in the midst of uncertainty; (b) relying on the sisterhood of NICU nurses to deal with uncertainty; and (c) confronting uncertainty through tight control of actions, reliance on technology, and maximal efficiency in use of time. A fourth theme demonstrated how these values were reflected in NICU breastfeeding practices. Although high-control, high-tech, and time-urgent practice values were helpful in confronting uncertainty, these values also posed challenges to ongoing nursing efforts to promote breastfeeding. These values must be addressed for effective breastfeeding promotion.

Source: Cricco-Lizza, R. (2011). Everyday nursing practice values in the NICU and their reflection on breastfeeding promotion. *Qualitative Health Research, 21*(3), 399–409.

Ethnography requires the researcher to have a clear understanding of his or her own cultural biases, and to record behavior and beliefs without judging them.

Read the research summary below and see whether it fits the criteria for an ethnographic approach.

☐ Historical Research

Historical research is just what the term implies—an analysis or narrative of specific events that have already occurred or are retrospective.

CULTURAL RESEARCH STUDY

A review of: Strangers in Strange Lands: A Metasynthesis of Lived Experiences of Immigrant Asian Nurses Working in Western Countries

This study examined the experiences of Asian nurses (the largest group of immigrant nurses in the world) who work in Western countries. The authors found 14 studies in which the lived experiences of this group had been reported. They then conducted a metasynthesis of the studies, utilizing the criteria from Noblit and Hare's 1988 book, *Metaethnography: Synthesizing Qualitative Studies* (Newbury Park, CA: Sage). Metasynthesis involves synthesizing the findings of qualitative studies in order to disclose a grand narrative or interpretation that would be more powerful than any study alone could be. Metasynthesis is an enlargement of interpretation, whereas in the quantitative approach of meta-analysis, the purpose is to reduce findings.

The themes that emerged for the experience of Asian immigrant nurses included: communication as a daunting challenge; differences in nursing practice; marginalization, discrimination, and exploitation; and cultural differences. The authors expanded on implications for nursing knowledge development, policy making, and practice. This study helped to document experience; and knowledge of the experience can help lead to changes in practice.

Source: Xu, Y. (2007). Strangers in strange lands: A metasynthesis of lived experiences of immigrant Asian nurses working in Western countries. *Advances in Nursing Science, 30*(3), 246–265.

HEALTH PROMOTION CHALLENGE

How can these findings help you in your health promotion efforts?

Qualitative Research in Nursing

Nursing exists in the social world, yet nursing research frequently uses quantitative designs. Quantitative research often does not have meaning for the practice world of nursing because researchers reduce variables to a single dimension to look at direct relationships between them. Such an approach overlooks the highly complex and diverse nature of nursing interactions and frequently falls short of providing direction for nursing interventions.

For example, two nursing students searched for correlations between anxiety, loneliness, and grade-point average in their classmates. They did a multiple regression correlation to understand the effects of two or more independent variables on the dependent measure, but there was so much variance unaccounted for that all they were able to conclude was that there was no significant relationship among the three. Such a finding makes no intuitive sense. Emotional considerations affect academic performance in many contexts, so to conclude that nurses are an exception to the general rule defies logic. What if they had gathered some qualitative data such as interviewing a focus sample of students with low or high grade-point averages to find out other variables that the students thought might be involved? Their discussion of findings would have been much richer, and they would have untangled more of the puzzle of the relationship of the variables.

Steps of Research

The quantitative research process involves many steps (TABLE 8-1), with the first leading to the second, and then the third, all the way to the research outcome.

Table 8-1 Steps in Quantitative Research

1. Research problem and purpose
2. Literature review
3. Study framework
4. Research objectives, questions, or hypotheses
5. Study variables
6. Research design
7. Sample
8. Methods of measurement
9. Data collection
10. Data analysis
11. Research outcomes

The initial step is to identify research **problem** and purpose. The problem is the area of focus where there is a gap that will lead to the purpose (the goal or aim) of the study. The next step is the literature review, so the researcher can determine what is currently known or lacking in the research problem. To provide a link to the study, the framework needs to be determined for a theoretical basis for the study. After determining the framework, a "bridge" is needed to link the research problem to the design, and thus the analysis. This bridge consists of the formulation of the research objectives, the questions, and the hypothesis, which is determined by the type of study being conducted. Hypotheses are usually saved for quasiexperimental or experimental types of study.

The **research design**, which many describe as the architectural blueprint for the study, is formulated next. This is when the researcher outlines step by step what the study methods will be and what kind of analysis will be performed on the data. Choosing the sample is next. The **sample** is the part of the population being studied and those who become the study participants. The measurement process, wherein an instrument or instruments are used to measure the study variables, is next, and it is followed by data collection and data analysis. **Data collection** is the gathering of the information, and **data analysis** is the technique that organizes and gives meaning to the data, through the use of statistics (Burns & Grove, 2007). The final step is analyzing the outcomes of the research, which are then used to generate further research.

CASE STUDY   Cognitive Behavioral Group Therapy for Spanish Speaking Women

This case study is a glimpse into the development of a research study. The feasibility research study was conducted by an interdisciplinary team of nurses, counselors, educators, public health educators, social workers, and pastoral care providers. They explored the feasibility of an 8-week cognitive-behavioral group therapy intervention for depressed Spanish-speaking women of Mexican origin, living in an emerging immigrant community in the United States. The study sample number was six.

The literature search for this study would have included searching for information about which of the following?

a.   Latinos in the United States
b.   Immigrant health issues
c.   Cognitive-behavioral therapy
d.   Depression
e.   All of the above

The group decided to use the PRECEDE-PROCEED model for health promotion as its conceptual framework. Health programs and interventions that use this model have a goal of enhancing the quality of life of individuals or populations.

The recruitment of subjects for a study is always an important consideration. In addition, if an intervention is to take place over a long period of time, the issue of retention becomes a concern.

Which of these issues would not be of concern for appropriate subject recruitment?

a.   Assessing presence of depression

b.   Being employed outside the home

c.   Being Spanish speakers

In this study, none of the women were employed outside the home. The tool used to assess for depression was the Spanish version of the Center for Epidemiologic Studies-Depression scale.

Which of the following issues would not be of concern for ensuring participants attended all sessions?

a.   Transportation

b.   Free child care

c.   Small stipend to compensate participants for time commitment

d.   Occupation of spouse

For this study, the investigators ensured that each participant had free childcare and transportation to the sessions. In addition, a $10 gift card was given to participants for attending each session.

This study focused on feasibility issues in order to plan for implementation of this program on a large scale. Issues explored included the logistics of the intervention, retention, transportation, child care, and an evaluation of the reliability and validity of the Center for Epidemiologic Studies-Depression scale, Spanish version. Recommendations of the study included further evaluation of the intervention and of the depression tool through larger samples and controlled, randomized trials.

Source: Shattell, M. M., Quinlan-Colwell, A., Villalba, J., Ivers, N. N, & Mails, M. (2010). A cognitive-behavioral group therapy intervention with depressed Spanish-speaking Mexican women living in an Emerging immigrant community in the United States. *Advances in Nursing Science, 33*(2), 158–169.

HEALTH PROMOTION CHALLENGE

How can these findings help you to promote health?

The qualitative research methodology is different, although it is also successive in nature. The initial step is the selection of participants. The samples in qualitative studies are smaller than those in quantitative studies whereby the total number (N) is determined by a power analysis. In qualitative research, the number is based on the study purpose instead and can be as low as 1 or have an upper limit of thousands, although methodologies will place limits on how many participants there are given that some methods (personal observation of individual behavior, for example) are not always feasible for large numbers of people. Data collection is next; this phase is completed by either observing or interviewing the participants, with the data becoming the written text of these observations or interviews. Therefore, data analysis occurs at the same time as the data collection. Data analysis is a three-stage approach including description, analysis, and interpretation. The techniques involved with this process may include transcribing the interviews, coding the data into categories, and interpreting the themes or the findings. See BOX 8-2.

BOX 8-2   Accessing "Gray Literature"

In addition to published science, medical, and nursing literature, there exists a large body of information that is unpublished. This is often referred to as "gray literature," because while it doesn't exist in black and white (that is, in published form), it often contains valuable information for professionals.

Scientists from around the world have been working steadily to formalize this information. It is not an easy task. Gray literature can consist of e-mails, blog entries, interviews with researchers, notes from phone calls, and even discussions in Wiki. Whatever the source, it must be credible and verified.

Keeping these issues in mind, gray literature offers plenty of potential information and direction for research. Finding it is the main challenge. There is a variety of online databases (CINAHL, EMBASE, EBSCO, OVID, to name a few) that catalogue gray literature resources. Libraries and institutional archives are key sources of gray literature (for example, unpublished doctoral dissertations are usually archived in university libraries). In Europe, a network called GreyNet has attempted to identify, categorize, and catalogue gray literature.

Sources: Pejsova, P., & M. Vaska, for GreyNet, Grey Literature Network Service. (2011). An Analysis of Current Gray Literature Document Typology. *The Grey Journal (TGJ): An International Journal on Gray Literature, 7*(2). Retrieved from http://hdl.handle.net/10068/700013

University of British Columbia/UBC Library. (2011). What Is Grey Literature? Retrieved from http://toby.library.ubc.ca/subjects/subjpage2.cfm?id=878

Literature Review Process

A **literature review** is the process used to acquaint the researcher with the current knowledge of the topic of interest. The result of the literature review is familiarity with the available evidence. The literature used for the review should be primary, meaning it has been written by the person who conducted the research. Secondary sources are a good start for becoming familiar with what is available, but often times the source is not completely objective.

Most research is conducted by searching for references through the use of bibliographic databases, most of which can be readily accessible through a computer. Although Internet search engines such as Google will bring about a lot of information on your subject, most of the information will not be true research literature. You can get somewhat better results by using Google Scholar (www.scholar.google.com), but even so, the organization and quality of the citations you find will vary. There are many commercial vendors available. These include OVID, EBSCOHost, and ProQuest. Whichever one is chosen, it is important to become familiar with the characteristics of the package before

ASK YOURSELF   www

Suppose you have decided to conduct a research study with the purpose of examining the relationship between Alzheimer's disease and caregiver stress. You are not sure what your study design will be or how you will measure stress. You have decided you need to complete a literature search. Devise the plan for your search.

using it. There are some electronic databases that are especially useful for nursing researchers, including Cumulative Index to Nursing and Allied Health Literature (CINAHL), Medical Literature On-Line (MEDLINE), and PubMed (the National Library of Medicine index). The keywords selected are usually the independent and/or dependent variables. Sometimes it requires finding the right way the concept is stated to find the correct literature; for example, instead of searching for "mammograms" you may have better results with the search term "mammography screening." You may also make the search a bit broader by searching for other areas, such as breast cancer screening, women's health, or health promotion.

Assessing Literature

The review starts with the search, but the researcher must also develop skill in critiquing the literature that is found. It is useful to have a literature review protocol that works the best for the reviewer. One approach is the use of 3×5 cards with the sections of the research process outlined on them. Some other approaches include using a binder with individual tabs, or an investigator-generated electronic filing system. These sections could include the following information:

- The citation
- Type of study
- Setting
- Key variables
- Framework/theory
- Design type
- Data sources
- Statistical tests
- Findings
- Recommendations
- An overview of the strengths and weaknesses

It will be tempting to simply use the abstract of the study, but if a researcher is utilizing the aforementioned

HOT TOPICS

Here are some topics to explore:
- Phenomenology
- Grounded theory
- Ethnography
- Literature review
- Meta-analysis
- Correlational research
- PRECEDE-PROCEED model
- Statistical analysis
- Critiquing research

process, many of these items are not readily apparent in the abstract. An abstract is written by the author and may not necessarily accurately reflect the study's quality. Unless you can check the particulars of the methodology, the study's findings may not prove to be statistically powerful enough for your purposes. Cards documenting specific studies can then be sorted into specific themes that may have been found during the research. From those themes, some of the articles may stand out more than the others, and one may even be the landmark study in that area. It is then important to critique those articles more thoroughly.

Critiquing Research

Simply identifying studies is not enough; a researcher must be able to tell whether the study's findings are persuasive. A study may have interesting conclusions, but if the data are weak—either because of methodological errors, small sample size, or incorrectly obtained samples—or the analysis methods are flawed, the conclusions may be inappropriate. Statistical measures are only as powerful as the data used to generate the statistics, which is the basis of the GIGO or "garbage in, garbage out" critique: If the data that go in are garbage, then so, too, are the conclusions that come out. Bailar (2009) identifies the following four key elements to separating good research from bad:

1. Are the data sound?
2. Are key assumptions spelled out?
3. Can results be generalized to other groups or phenomena?
4. Is the study asking appropriate questions?

☐ Are the Data Sound?

Sound or solid data depend on adequacy of sample size, appropriateness of the sample (that is, whether the sample is representative of the total population being studies), and methods used to collect the data. Researchers collecting the data must document what factors influenced their sample selection and why they used the sampling methods they chose. Small sample sizes need not automatically exclude a study's conclusions from being considered strong, but larger samples are usually considered to be more powerful. However, *too* large a sample might run the risk of introducing extra, unrecognized variability into the analysis, unless variations in the population (e.g., age, gender, and ethnicity) can be identified and accounted for.

☐ Are Key Assumptions Spelled Out?

If a research paper does not clearly describe the factors assumed to be true, then there is no way the reviewer can question the base assumptions made by the researcher. Often, assumptions are incorrect. Bailar (2009) cites an example of a dose-response curve generated for carcinogenic chemicals, which for many years were thought to have an effect proportional to the amount of exposure to the carcinogen. In other words, researchers assumed that people exposed to low doses of the chemical had a low likelihood of developing cancer, while those who were exposed to high doses had a high likelihood of developing cancer. Safety recommendations regarding such chemicals often were based on this one-to-one proportionality. When experimental testing of this assumption was finally undertaken, the research showed it to be false. In many cases, cancer risk increased much more rapidly than the increase in exposure, so that even a slight elevation in exposure meant significantly higher rates of cancer.

☐ Can Results Be Generalized to Other Groups or Phenomena?

Some studies use animal subjects because testing a research question in humans would be dangerous or unethical. An example would be studies seeking to determine whether certain food additives pose a health risk in children, who could not be used as test subjects for obvious reasons. Generally, juvenile animals, such as mice, rats, or dogs, are used instead. However, mice, rats, and dogs are not people; while they do respond similarly in many ways, often their responses are not similar enough. A mouse, for example, may respond extremely well to a therapeutic intervention that has no effect in a person, or vice versa. Also, it is important to recognize that the phenomenon under study itself may have variation. For example, studies that examine toxicity of a chemical by feeding it to animals and recording the health effects of this exposure are of little value to someone who is researching the use of that chemical in skin products, because absorption through the gut is not the same type of exposure as absorption through the skin. How well the study results translate into other areas is an important consideration.

☐ Is the Study Asking Appropriate Questions?

Studies that are grounded in faulty assumptions represent one end of the spectrum, but on the other end are studies that take a simplistic approach to a complex problem. For example, a researcher asking the question, "Does air pollution cause asthma?" is asking a question that is both faulty in its base assumption (that asthma has a single cause) and that is overly simplistic (attempts to break down a complicated process into a simple this-causes-that equation). Asthma is a complex disease process with multiple factors; air pollution may be *one of* the causes, but it cannot be considered *the* cause, The interactions between pollutants and specific changes in pulmonary function are not something that occurs on just one exposure. A question such as, "How does incidence of asthma exacerbations relate to air quality measures during the summer?" might be a more appropriate topic for research, or, as Bailar (2009) suggests, a series of research questions might be used to break a complex topic down into simpler, more palatable bites.

There are many critique guides available through any of the research texts (see INFORMATION BOX 8-2). The lists in the next section include a brief idea of what a critique involves.

INFORMATION BOX 8-2

There are a variety of approaches to critiquing nursing research. Here are some sites that offer some guidance: http://www.nursingplanet.com/Nursing_Research/critiquing_nursing_research.html, http://www.sonoma.edu/users/n/nolan/n400/critique.htm, and https://pantherfile.uwm.edu/brodg/www/Handout/critique.htm.

Critique Guidelines

Research Problem and Purpose

- Is the problem concrete as stated?
- Is the problem relevant and significant?
- Does the purpose lead the reader into the aim of the study with the research variables, population, and setting clarified?
- Is the study feasible in terms of the length of study, accessibility of subjects, expertise, and resources available?

Literature Review

- Is the review organized to show progression of the researcher's idea from previous research?
- Is the theoretical base appropriate for the study?
- Does the literature review provide direction for the study?
- Does the synthesis of the literature provide a foundation for the study?

Study Framework

- Is the framework clear?
- Is the framework appropriately linked to the research purpose?
- Is there another framework that may have been better?
- If part of the theory is being tested, can it be clearly linked to the objectives?

Research Objectives, Questions, or Hypotheses

- Are they clear and concise?
- Are they linked to the purpose?
- Are they linked to the framework?

Variables

- Do they reflect the concepts identified in the framework?
- Are they clearly defined based on the literature review?

Design

- Is this the best design to direct the study?
- Is the design able to incorporate the objectives, questions, or hypothesis in the study purpose?
- Are there threats to design validity?
- Is the design logically linked to the sampling method and statistical analysis?
- If an intervention is proposed, is it clearly defined and appropriate for the purpose?

Sample, Population, and Setting

- Is the target population defined?
- Is the sampling method adequate to provide representation?
- Are there possible biases in the sampling method?
- Is the sample size sufficient?
- If more than one group is used, are they equivalent?
- Are the rights of human subjects protected/has there been an institutional review board review done?
- Is the setting typical of clinical settings?

Measurements

- Do the instruments adequately measure the study variables?
- Are the instruments sensitive enough to detect differences between subjects?
- Are the instruments reliable and valid?
- Does the researcher examine reliability and validity?
- If an observation measurement is used, is there interrater and intrarater reliability?
- If a physiologic measure is used, are the accuracy, precision, selectivity, sensitivity, and error of the measure discussed?

Data Collection

- Is the data collection process clear?
- Does the analysis address each objective, question, or hypothesis?
- Is the analysis procedure appropriate?
- Are the results clearly presented?
- Are there tables and figures used to synthesize a large amount of findings?
- Is the analysis interpreted correctly?
- If the results were not significant, was it because there was not a significant sample size?

Interpretation of Findings

- Are the findings discussed in relation to each objective, question, or hypothesis?
- Are both significant and not significant findings explained?
- Were the statistical significant findings also examined for clinical significance?
- Does the interpretation of findings appear biased?
- Are there uncontrolled extraneous variables that may have influenced the findings?
- Do the conclusions fit the results from the analysis?
- Are the conclusions based on statistically and clinically significant results?
- Did the researcher identify important study limitations?
- Are there inconsistencies in the report?

HEALTH PROMOTION CHALLENGE

Find a health promotion study that resonates with you and may help your nursing practice. Ask all the questions above about it and then decide whether the study findings are still relevant.

Not all studies will have satisfactory answers to all of these questions, but a good study should be able to properly answer most of them. In some cases, there may be confounding factors that prevent researchers from addressing particular methodological issues; if these are clearly spelled out by the article's authors, then you can continue to support the study as being fairly strong. If the authors ignore or downplay the issues, it weakens the research findings. One example of methodologically suspect research is retrospective studies of vitamin supplement use based on data collected during qualitative studies of women's health (such as the Women's Health Initiative [WHI] and the Iowa Women's Health Study), where data were collected via questionnaire. Several such analyses have published in reputable medical journals and have received significant media attention (Mursu, Robien, Harnack, Park, & Jacobs, 2011; Neuhouser et al., 2009). In nearly every such study published, the data collected relied on self-reported use of nonstandardized supplements. Qualitative (and potentially unreliable) data from the participants that had no controls for comparability and no way to verify the data's accuracy were analyzed in a quantitative fashion, and the results discussed in quantitative terms—flaws that limit the quality of the study (Huang et al., 2006). For quantitative studies to be strong and useful for drawing conclusions, the data need to be strictly defined, variables limited or controlled, and the parameters of interaction between the dependent and independent variables dictated by the researcher. That is not the case with these multivitamin studies. In order to make these studies valid targets for quantitative analysis, researchers would need to ensure that the study participants used the same supplements (e.g., same dose levels of the same vitamin/mineral combinations) in the same way (daily, twice daily, etc.) for the same length of time, and that all participants were equivalent in terms of their overall health (e.g., roughly the same age, same gender, and either having or lacking specific serious health concerns, such as diabetes or asthma). For still greater strength, the researchers could interview the participants frequently (annually, monthly, or weekly) rather than every 10 years, so that faulty memory does not contribute to poor data quality.

Health Promotion Research Questions

Nursing is focused on the diagnosis and treatment of human responses to health problems (American Nurses Association, 2010). From a wellness and health promotion perspective, examples of the kind of nursing research questions to ask are:

- What is the effect of self-care measures clients use?
- What health promotion measures might reduce destructive personal relationships?
- What health promotion knowledge about their disease risks do clients lack?
- How can health risk knowledge best be provided to clients?
- What knowledge about sexuality do clients lack?
- How can knowledge about sexuality be provided to clients in need?
- What type of activity is best for which types of diagnosed condition?
- What is the type of pain experienced during a sore throat?
- Is imagery or therapeutic touch more useful for this kind of pain?
- What is the effect of confronting irrational beliefs in relationships with others?
- What changes in self-esteem occur when a parent produces an infant with a disability?
- Is value clarification or journal writing a more effective self-care measure for low self-esteem?
- What is the effect of beliefs about the meaningfulness of life on health promotion activities?

Most of these questions are illness oriented, but in health promotion, the goal is to focus on ways to prevent illness and promote wellness. There are a number of ways to turn illness-oriented research questions into wellness and health-promotion ones. One way is to focus on a well population. Although it is possible to use a problem orientation with a well population, it is easier to structure questions to focus on health promotion concerns. For example, one simple research question might be, "What are common determinants of quality of life among a particular population of individuals?" Another way to turn illness-oriented questions into health promotion/wellness ones is to begin to relate problems or human responses to the dimensions of wellness. For example, instead of focusing on the pain or illness experience in otitis media, the focus would be on the prevention and minimization of pain using self-care strategies. Some questions that might be asked are:

- What is the relationship between level of exercise and otitis media?
- What is the relationship between positive expectations about the outcome of otitis media and healing?
- What is the effect of eating additional amounts of high vitamins C, A, and zinc-containing foods on the otitis media process?
- What is the effect of progressive relaxation and healing imagery measures on the otitis media process?
- What is the effect of color, full spectrum light, or noise on the otitis media process?
- What is the effect of peer or family supportive communication on the otitis media process?

Modeling in Health Promotion Research

A variant of this process is to take some of the indicants of whole-person wellness and begin to formulate them into research questions, especially those related to manageability, comprehensibility, and meaningfulness. Antonovsky (1996) developed a model based on the sense of coherence as a determinant of health. His work was relevant for health promotion research because he examined health as a process, not merely as the absence of disease. He also conceives of the process as one of moving toward greater order and meaningfulness. This idea is also relevant for health promotion.

Antonovsky's model is most relevant for the health promotion/wellness dimension of stress but can be expanded to encompass other dimensions. For example, Antonovsky's sense of coherence model was formed from a cluster of attitudes that he calls comprehensibility (perceiving stimuli as making cognitive sense as information, as opposed to finding them unpredictable, random, noisy, and chaotic); manageability (having resources at the client's disposal either directly under the client's control, or having access to resources control by dependable others); and meaningfulness (feeling life makes sense in emotional terms so that some life problems are viewed as worth investing energy in).

Using Antonovsky's concept of coherence, the following wellness/health promotion questions could be formulated:

- What is the relationship between the belief in the ability to influence the level of fitness either already or with the help of others and fitness activities?

- What is the relationship between believing the solution to life problems is worth investing energy in and preventive nutrition?
- What is the relationship between believing the client is able to make sense out of new and risk-requiring situations and attempts to form positive relationships with others?

HEALTH PROMOTION CHALLENGE

Develop at least two other questions from Antonovsky's model.

Mehl's (1981) holistic model may also offer some ideas for research questions. He pointed out the fallacy of thought that underlies the medical model that adverse factors cause an illness or disease. Such a model ignores why one particular, unique human being becomes ill. Until recently, this kind of question was categorized as irrelevant because it is outside the medical model.

Because of the uniqueness of individuals, Mehl (1981) questioned randomization procedures used in quantitative research as valid. If each person has a unique position in time and space, how can randomization of space/time units be appropriate? A holistic model, such as wellness, is based upon the significance of the individual. Theory construction is systematic, based on the assessment of factors affecting individuals and does not require that the same factor affect every individual in exactly the same way to be considered significant.

Using this method, a nurse researcher might begin with a detailed description of the life of individuals with a life problem, such as type 2 diabetes, and consider the following:

- Childhood events
- Stresses pre-illness
- Spiritual beliefs
- Life events
- Emotional changes
- Paralleling changes in their illness and their general world view

HEALTH PROMOTION CHALLENGE

Use Mehl's model to develop at least two research questions.
Share them with your class and ask for feedback.

Only after one individual's pathway to diabetes is understood would the nurse researcher begin to look for similarities and differences among different individual pathways. Theory might be formulated for each individual regarding how diabetes functioned in his or her personal system.

Continuing with the research, it would be important to observe if the course of diabetes changed for each person as life factors changed. Using Mehl's model, an example of a health promotion/wellness-oriented question might be: What are the interactions of exercise on the development of client Jones related to diabetes, spiritual beliefs, life events, emotional changes, paralleling changes in her view of diabetes and her general worldview, stresses and ability to use stress management procedures, positive relationships with others, preventive nutrition, and the amount of full-spectrum light to which she is exposed?

According to Mehl, a holistic approach to research begins with a description of all the possible factors in the life of an individual with a particular disease or condition, leading to an understanding of which combinations of factors affect that particular disease or condition. Only then would other individuals be studied and similarities and differences noted. Theory would then accumulate about the many possible individual pathways of development of the problem. This kind of approach emphasizes the interactive nature of variables rather than the isolation and proof of one effect. It is also congruent with a systems approach that focuses on interactive factors and in which there are many paths to one outcome. In systems terms, this is referred to as equifinality.

Two kinds of approaches are especially suited for studying wellness and health promotion. They both require research procedures that allow the researcher to examine holistic and interactive health promotion processes: qualitative research and action research.

Action Research

Action research is the use of research methodology to solve problems. The underlying assumption of action research is that clients are better able than anyone else to define their problems and propose solutions, because they are best acquainted with their own situations. This assumption implies that it is desirable, and even necessary, for clients to possess decision-making skills—skills that you can teach or support.

In action research, clients are enlisted to define the problem as they see it and then to generate hypotheses. They learn to specify and define terms, decide on how to measure change, determine how changes will be implemented, interpret data to see if it supports or refutes their hunches or hypotheses, and develop generalizations. In action research, hypotheses are ways of stating objectives; they predict the consequences of carrying out actions and move participants towards those actions. An overriding theme is that people are more likely to change if they participate in exploring the reasons for a means of change; the researcher is involved in training the participants in the research process.

Action research tends to enhance the position of the individual and to expand the sources of power. Clients are given freedom, meaningful activity, opportunity to participate, recognition of their worth, needed decision-making and probably some problem-solving skills, and opportunities for growth and security. Each of these aspects seems likely to enhance wellness and promote health; also, the quality of their life is enhanced.

For example, a participant studying the problem of obtaining wellness and health promotion services in the community could be asked to list the subjective barriers. These would be the personal experiences and emotions that prevent the client from obtaining health promotion services. In addition, the objective barriers—that is, organizational and environmental difficulties that interfered with movement toward health—should be considered. The next steps are as follows:

- A 15-minute period for the participants to silently generate ideas.
- A collaborative interaction in which each person shares one problem, which is written on a large pad of paper, organized by number and alternating between subjective and objective columns. No ideas are discussed or critiqued; the participants are encouraged to write new ideas as they are stimulated by others, ideas.
- A 30-minute period allowing participants to discuss, clarify, elaborate, dispute, or add new items; no items are eliminated.
- A 15-minute break.
- The group ranks the priority of items, showing the 10 most critical elements, writing one each on a 3 × 5 card and ranking them in order of importance. A spontaneous discussion follows in which participants can clarify, elaborate, defend, or dispute the preliminary vote. At this point, some problems are redefined.
- The prioritization of items is changed by individuals as they rerank them on their own sheets, assigning a value of 100 to their most important items and values between zero and 100 to the other items.
- The researcher collects the final ratings and reports the votes to the group.
- A 20-minute discussion follows.

HEALTH PROMOTION CHALLENGE

The class chooses a health promotion issue and follows all the steps in the action research process. Pick a leader to keep the group on topic and a recorder to record ideas on the board or somewhere where everyone can see the information. When finished, evaluate your findings and decide whether you want to take action to enhance health promotion.

The nominal group process technique allows for multiple individual inputs simultaneously while keeping participation balance. The method also controls variance (error), which can arise when there is incongruence between the researcher and her practitioner system and the client or user system. The nominal group reduces incongruence. RESEARCH BOX 8-6 reports the use of a nominal group technique for sleep disorders.

RESEARCH BOX 8-6

» BACKGROUND/OBJECTIVES: The International Classification of Functioning, Disability and Health (ICF) provides a comprehensive and universally accepted framework to classify changes in functioning related to health conditions. Comprehensive and brief core sets have been defined for various disorders but not for sleep disorders. Such a core set would greatly enhance the techniques available to describe the impact of sleep disorders on clients. The overarching purpose of this paper is to report on phase 1 of the international and World Health Organization- (WHO-) endorsed consensus process in identifying ICF core sets for sleep disorders.

» METHODS: A formal decision-making and consensus process, which integrated evidence gathered from preparatory studies, was carried out. Relevant ICF categories were selected by a sample of international experts from different backgrounds using the nominal group technique.

» RESULTS: Twenty-six experts from 22 countries and different professional backgrounds attended the consensus conference. Altogether, 120 second- or third-level ICF categories were included in the comprehensive ICF core set with the following ICF component split: 49 categories from body functions, 8 from body structures, 31 from activities and participation, and 32 from environmental factors. The brief ICF core set included a total of 15 second-level categories: 5 body functions (sleep, energy and drive, attention, consciousness, respiration functions); 3 body structures (brain, respiratory system, pharynx); 4 activities and participation (focusing attention, driving, handling stress and other psychological demands, carrying out daily routine); and 3 environmental factors (immediate family; health services, systems, and policies; and health professionals).

» CONCLUSION: A formal consensus process integrating evidence and expert opinion led to the first version of the ICF core sets for persons with sleep disorders. Further validation of the core set is needed.

Source: Gradinger, F., Cieza, A., Stucki, A., Michel, F., Bentley, A., Oksenberg, A., … Partinen, M. (2011). Part 1. International classification of functioning, disability and health (ICF) core sets for persons with sleep disorders: Results of the consensus process integrating evidence from preparatory studies. *Sleep Medicine, 12*(1), 92–96

HEALTH PROMOTION CHALLENGE   www

Make a list of client problems that could benefit from nominal group process. For ideas, visit PubMed (www.pubmed.gov), type "nominal group process" in the search box, and scroll through study titles.

CASE STUDY

Building from Boryc and colleagues' (2010) need assessment of clients with HIV, imagine you are working with clients just diagnosed with HIV. Suppose you plan to administer them a questionnaire that asked questions regarding their demographics, services received, quality of service delivery, and mental health and substance abuse.

Respondents reported further need of referrals to income-generation opportunities, food and nutritional supplement support, and support for children. Boryc and colleagues (2010) also found that 42% of the respondents screened positive for probable depression, and 37% of respondents screened positive for being at risk for a drinking problem.

HEALTH PROMOTION CHALLENGE

What services do you think Boryc and colleagues found to be the most commonly received and requested by respondents with HIV?

Other action research projects might raise some of the following questions:

- How well are we accomplishing our wellness and health promotion goals?
- How might we make our work more expeditious?
- How do we feel about ourselves and what we are accomplishing?
- What should we accomplish in our next health promotion group meeting?
- How can health promotion programs be improved?
- What kind of assistance would help us develop our potential?
- What are the problem areas in health promotion programs that should be changed?
- What is the planning process we used to develop health promotion programs?
- What hypotheses about health promotion can we formulate?
- What is the best way to introduce change to facilitate health promotion behaviors?
- What tools should be used to identify our progress?
- How will our family members react to our health promotion programs?
- What reactions to our health promotion behaviors to our supervisors at work show?

RESEARCH BOX 8-7   Community Consensus Partnered with Participatory Action Research To Establish Self-Directed Medical Mental Health Care

» OBJECTIVE: This article describes a public–academic collaboration between a university research center and the Texas state mental health authority to design and evaluate a unique money-follows-the-person model called self-directed care (SDC). SDC programs give participants control over public funds to purchase services and supports for their own recovery.

» METHOD: Through a participatory action research process, the project combined use of evidence-based practice and community consensus as a tool for system change.

» RESULTS: The story of this effort and the program that resulted are described, along with quantitative and qualitative data from the project's start-up phase.

» CONCLUSIONS: Lessons learned about the importance of community collaboration are discussed in light of the current emphasis on public mental health system transformation through alternative financing mechanisms.

Source: Cook, J. A., Shore, S. E., Burke-Miller, J. K., Jonikas, J. A., Ferrara, M., Colegrove, S., …. Hicks, M. E. (2010). Participatory action research to establish self-directed care for mental health recovery in Texas. *Psychiatric Rehabilitation Journal, 34*(2), 137–144.

HEALTH PROMOTION CHALLENGE   ⭐ (www)

If you were to use Cook and colleagues' action research model, how might you help clients with specific health promotion needs?

Developing Relationship Statements and Testing Theoretical Relationships

According to Chinn and Kramer (2010), theories can only be tested when a translation is made from the theoretical to the concrete. The activity of testing theoretical relationships involves three subcomponents:

1. Formulating the specific statement of relationship, often a hypothesis
2. Determining the operational definitions necessary to validate the statements
3. Validating the statement through systematic methods

Goal indicators must be substituted for abstract concepts. Some possible relationship statements for testing health promotion theory might be:

1. When fitness goals are written, there is a greater likelihood that action toward fitness will follow. When fitness goals are systematically evaluated, there is a greater likelihood that new fitness goals will be set as

previous ones are met. When fitness goals are attained, there is a greater likelihood that movement toward health in other dimensions will occur.

2. When preventive nutrition goals are attained, there is a greater likelihood that movement toward health in other dimensions will occur.

3. There is an inverse relationship between time spent specifying fitness goals and time needed to act upon them. There will be a positive relationship between frequency of health promotion goal facilitation and progress toward goal attainment.

4. The more the nurse serves as a health promotion role model, the more the client will move toward health and health promotion. The more the nurse resolves his or her inconsistent belief systems, the more helpful he or she will be to the client's ability to move toward health and wellness. The greater the movement toward a wellness belief system, the more health behaviors will be exhibited by the client.

5. The more the client participates in self-assessment, the greater the movement toward health and wellness.

HEALTH PROMOTION CHALLENGE

Describe ways to develop health promotion research questions in nursing practice that would work in your clinical area. Discuss ways to develop ways to study health promotion practice. Write a paper on ways you would like to be involved in health promotion research.

Summary

There are two major categories of research studies—quantitative and qualitative. A quantitative research study is a formal and rigorous process for objectively generating information, or describing, exploring, and/or examining new situations, events, or concepts. Qualitative research is subjective and is viewed by the participants' experience, describing the meaning related to an event without generating new ideas, but rather philosophic ideas. The four major types of quantitative research are descriptive, correlational, quasiexperimental, and experimental. Descriptive research is the exploration and description of a phenomenon in a real-life situation, thereby depicting accurate accounts of the characteristics of the participants, situations, or even the group as a whole. Correlational research involves the investigation of the relationship between the study variables. Quasiexperimental research is not experimental because it lacks control by the researcher, specifically over the manipulation of treatment, the setting management, or subject selection. Experimental research is highly controlled and has the purpose of predicting and controlling a phenomenon between the independent and dependent variables. Independent variables are factors that are innate to the study subject and not changeable; dependent variables are factors that are changed or influenced by independent variables.

Qualitative research includes the following types: phenomenological, grounded theory, ethnography, and historical research. Phenomenological research captures the lived experience of the participants; this research is inductive in nature. Grounded theory is an inductive approach that has been developed from sociology—specifically the symbolic interaction theory. The technique involves formulating, testing, and redeveloping propositions until a theory is developed. Ethnographic research involves the collection and analysis of data specifically from a cultural behavior to develop theory. Historical research is an analysis or narrative of specific events that have already occurred or are retrospective. The quantitative research process includes the following steps: identify the research problem and purpose; conduct a literature review; determine the framework; formulate research objectives, questions, and hypotheses; determine research variables; formulate the research design; identify the sample; decide on research instruments or a statistical analysis plan; collect data; analyze data; and examine outcomes and their significance. Qualitative methodology proceeds in this fashion: select participants (usually fewer are needed than in quantitative research), data collection, and analysis (data analysis includes description, analysis, and interpretation). Techniques employed in the process include transcribing the interviews, coding the data into categories, and interpreting the themes or the findings. The literature review is a process used to become acquainted with the current knowledge of the desired topic, which leads to familiarity with available evidence. The literature used should be primary sources, as these are written by the person who conducted the research. Secondary sources can be helpful for becoming familiar with what is available. Bibliographic databases may be used in the search. Electronic databases such as MEDLINE, PubMed, CINAHL, EMBASE, and others are extremely helpful, although the last two mentioned are particularly useful for identifying gray literature sources that do not show up in databases that focus on published articles. The identification of keywords to use in a literature search is an important step. The plan for critique of the literature should involve development of a list of types of information that will be recorded from each article. Some researchers use a 3 × 5 card on which to record such information. Then the cards are sorted into specific themes that are found in the research. Critiquing literature can seem like an overwhelming task but can be less so through the use of a critique guide. A critique guide will usually divide components of an article into sections with a list of questions to be asked with a review of each of these sections. An example of topic division is the following: research problem and purpose; literature review; study framework; research objectives, questions, or hypothesis; variables; design; sample, population, and setting; measurements; data collection; and interpretation of findings.

REVIEW QUESTIONS   `www`

1. Which of the following questions is not part of the interpretation of findings in a research study?
   a. Were the statistically significant findings examined for clinical significance?
   b. Are the findings discussed in relation to each objective, question, or hypothesis?
   c. Is the data collection process clear?

2. Which of the following questions is not part of the assessment of the sample, population, and setting in a research study?
   a. Does the researcher examine reliability and validity?
   b. Are the rights of human subjects protected/has an institutional review board review taken place?
   c. Is the setting typical of clinical settings?

3. The sequential steps in conducting a quantitative research study are:
   a. Identify the research problem and purpose, review the literature, develop hypothesis or research questions, design the study, identify the sample, measure/data collect, analyze data, and interpret finds.
   b. Identify the research problem and purpose, design the study, review the literature, develop a hypothesis or research questions, identify the sample, measure/data collect, analyze data, and interpret findings.
   c. Review the literature, identify the research problem and purpose, design the study, identify the sample, measure/data collect, and interpret findings.

4. Quantitative research is:
   a. A formal and rigorous process for generating information
   b. A method that captures the lived experience of the participant
   c. Subjective research

5. The independent variable is:
   a. The outcome or response that the researcher wants to explain
   b. The analysis or narrative of specific events that have already occurred
   c. What the researcher is manipulating

6. Phenomenological research:
   a. Involves formulation, testing, and redevelopment of propositions until a theory is developed
   b. Captures the lived experience of the participant
   c. Is the collection and analysis of data specifically from a cultural behavior to develop theory

7. Correlation research is:
   a. The exploration of a phenomenon in a real-life situation
   b. An investigation of the relationship between the study variables
   c. Subjective research

8. Data analysis is:
   a. The technique that organizes and gives meaning to the data through the use of statistics
   b. The gathering of information or data
   c. A literature search approach that utilizes citations from relevant studies to track down earlier studies

9. All of the following are types of qualitative research except:
   a. Grounded theory
   b. Quasiexperimental research
   c. Phenomenological research

10. Research design is:
   a. A technique for analyzing data
   b. The process for examining the literature
   c. The architectural blueprint of the study

11. The research problem is:
   a. The area of focus where there is a gap in knowledge that will lead to the purpose or aim of the study
   b. The part of the population being studied
   c. The outcome or response that the researcher wants to explain

12. An **experiment** is/does not:
   a. A highly controlled study
   b. A type of qualitative research
   c. Have the purpose of predicting and controlling a phenomenon between independent and dependent variables

EXERCISES

1. Find two nursing research articles on subjects related to health promotion. Utilize the research critique process presented in this chapter to critique the articles. Write up your findings.

2. Explore the qualitative technique *phenomenology*. Read a couple of research articles that use phenomenology to guide the study. How would you define phenomenology? How would you design such a study? Propose a study you might conduct using this technique.

3. Quantitative research relies on statistical methods for analysis of the study data. Find two studies using quantitative research approaches. Review the statistical methods found in these studies. Did this help you to better understand the results?

4. Find a research study that uses a quantitative approach. Briefly outline each activity of the study that corresponds to the sequence of steps followed in a quantitative study as outlined in this chapter.

BIBLIOGRAPHY

Allen, J. K., & Dennison, C. R. (2010). Randomized trials of nursing interventions for secondary prevention in patients with coronary artery disease and heart failure: Systematic review. *Journal of Cardiovascular Nursing, 25*(3), 207–220.

Anderson, J. M., Reimer, J., Kahn, K. B., Simich, L., Neufeld, A., Stewart, M., & Makwarimba, E. (2010). Narratives of "dissonance" and "repositioning" through the lens of critical humanism: Exploring the influences on immigrants' and refugees' health and well-being. *Advances in Nursing Science, 33*(2), 101–112.

Burns, N., & Grove, S. (2010). *Understanding nursing research: Building an evidence-based practice.* Philadelphia, PA: Saunders.

Conn, V. S., Valentine, J. C., Cooper, H. M., & Rantz, M. J. (2003). Grey literature in meta-analysis. *Nursing Research, 52*(4), 256–261.

Creswell, J. W. (2007). *Qualitative inquiry and research design: Choosing among five approaches.* Thousand Oaks, CA: Sage.

Giorgi, A. (2005). The phenomenological movement and research in the human sciences. *Nursing Science Quarterly, 18*(1), 75–82.

Houser, J. (2007). *Nursing research: Reading, using, and creating evidence.* Sudbury, MA: Jones and Bartlett.

Lafaiver, C. A., Keough, V., Letizia, M., & Lanuza, D. (2007). Using the Roy adaptation model to explore the dynamics of quality of life and the relationship between lung transplant candidates and their caregivers. *Advances in Nursing Science, 30*(3), 266–274.

Mefford, L. C. (2004). A theory of health promotion for preterm infants based on Levine's conservation model of nursing. *Nursing Science Quarterly, 17*(3), 260–266.

Merriam, S. B. (2009). *Qualitative research: Guide to design and implementation.* San Francisco, CA: Jossey-Bass.

Polit, D. F., & Beck, C. T. (2007). *Nursing research: Generating and assessing evidence for nursing practice.* Philadelphia, PA: Lippincott Williams & Wilkins.

Rew, L. (2003). A theory of taking care of oneself grounded in experiences of homeless youth. *Nursing Research, 52*(4), 234–241.

Sandelowski, M., & Barroso, J. (2003). Creating metasummaries of qualitative findings. *Nursing Research, 52*(4), 226–233.

Szanton, S. L., Gill, J. M., & Allen, J. K. (2005). Allostatic load: A mechanism of socioeconomic health disparities. *Biological Research for Nursing, 7*(1), 7–15.

Wallin, L., Estabrooks, C. A., Midodzi, W. K., & Cummings, G. G. (2006). Development and validation of a derived measure of research utilization by nurses. *Nursing Research, 55*(3), 149–160.

Williams, J. K., Barnette, J. J., Reed, D., Sousa, V. D., Schutte, D. L., McGonigal-Kenney, M., … Paulsen, J. S. (2010). Development of the Huntington disease family concerns and strategies survey from focus group data. *Journal of Nursing Measurement, 18*(2), 100–119.

Wuest, J., Hodgins, M. J., Malcolm, J., Merritt-Gray, M., & Seaman, P. (2007). The effects of past relationship and obligation on health and health promotion in women caregivers of adult family members. *Advances in Nursing Science, 30*(3) 206–220.

REFERENCES

American Nurses Association. (2010). *ANA 2010 annual report: Nurses—caring today for a healthier tomorrow.* Silver Spring, MD: Author.

Anderson, S. E., Gooze, R. A., Lemeshow, S., & Whitaker, R. C. (2012). Quality of early maternal–child relationship and risk of adolescent obesity. *Pediatrics, 129*(1), 132–140.

Antonovsky, A. (1996). The salutogenic model as a theory to guide health promotion. *Health Promotion International, 11*(1), 11–18.

Bailar, J. C., III. (2009). Some uses of statistical thinking. In J. C. Bailar, III & D. C. Hoaglin (Eds.), *Medical uses of statistics* (3rd ed., pp. 21–40). Cambridge, MA: Massachusetts Medical Society.

Boryc, K., Anastario, M. P., Dann, G., Chi, B., Cicatelli, B., Steilen, M., … Morris, M. (2010). A needs assessment of clients with HIV in a home-based care program in Guyana. *Public Health Nursing, 27*(6), 482–491.

Burns, N., & Grove, S. (2007). *Understanding nursing research* (4th ed.). St. Louis, MO: Saunders.

Chinn, P. L., & Kramer, M. K. (2010). *Integrated theory and knowledge development in nursing.* St. Louis, MO: Mosby.

Dell'Antonia, K. J. (2011, December 29). Teenage obesity linked to poor mother–child bond. *The New York Times.* Retrieved from http://parenting. blogs. nytimes. com/2011/12/29/teen-obesity-linked-to-poor-mother-child-interaction/

Glaser, B. (1992). *Basics of grounded theory analysis.* Mill Valley, CA: Sociology Press.

Huang, H. Y., Caballero, B., Chang, S., Alberg, A., Semba, R., Schneyer, C., … Bass, E. B. (2006). Multivitamin/mineral supplements and prevention of chronic disease. *Evidence Report/Technology Assessment (Full Report), 139*(May), 1–117.

Kerlinger, F., & Lee, H. (2000). *Foundations of behavioral research* (4th ed.). Holt, NY: Harcourt.

Mehl, L. (1981). *Mind and matter: Foundations for holistic health.* Berkeley, CA: Mindbody Press.

Mursu, J., Robien, K., Harnack, L. J., Park, K., & Jacobs, D. R., Jr. (2011). Dietary supplements and mortality rate in older women: The Iowa women's health study. *Archives of Internal Medicine, 171*(18), 1625–1633.

Neuhouser, M. L., Wassertheil-Smoller, S., Thomson, C., Aragaki, A., Anderson, G., Manson, J. E., … Prentice, R. L. (2009). Multivitamin use and risk of cancer and cardiovascular disease in the women's health initiative cohorts. *Archives of Internal Medicine, 169*(3), 294–304.

Parenting Source: A Blog for Parents. (2011, December 27). Obesity linked to kids who have bad relationships with their mothers [Web log post]. Retrieved from http://parenting-source. com/mommy-tips/obesity-linked-to-kids-who-have-bad-relationships-with-their-mothers/

Strauss A., & Corbin, J. (1990). *Basics of qualitative research: Grounded theory procedures and techniques*. Thousand Oaks, CA: Sage Publications.

INTERNET RESOURCES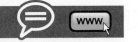

For a full suite of assignments and learning activities, use the access code located in the front of your book to visit this exclusive website: **http://go.jblearning .com/healthpromotion**. If you do not have an access code, you can obtain one at the site.

LEARNING OBJECTIVES

KEY TERMS

Upon completion of this chapter, you will be able to:

1. Discuss the importance of self-management with chronic conditions.
2. Describe natural self-care approaches clients can safely use on their own.
3. Compare the underlying theories that support these approaches.
4. Differentiate specific ways clients can use each approach.
5. Identify rationales for use of these approaches in health promotion.
6. Practice approaches yourself to understand what the client faces.
7. Demonstrate each self-care approach to another student as practice for teaching clients.

Acupressure

Aerobic exercise

Aromatherapy

Centering prayer

Coping skills

Hypnosis

Imagery

Mindfulness meditation

Prana

Qigong

Reflexology

Relaxation procedures

Thought stopping

Transcendental meditation

Yoga

CHAPTER 9

Self-Management and Health Promotion

- Introduction
- Self-Management
- Summary

Introduction

This chapter presents natural, self-care, noninvasive approaches you can teach clients to use to self-manage their health. These approaches are all safe when used as directed and work well as a complement to medicines and surgery or can be used by themselves. They offer something not now available to clients in most hospitals and many other parts of the current healthcare system, which was designed for acute illness (Group Health Research Institute, 2012).

Interventions that encourage clients to acquire self-management skills are essential for chronic conditions. The number of consumers with chronic illness is growing at an astonishing rate because of the rapid aging of the population and the greater longevity of persons with many chronic conditions (Group Health Research Institute, 2012). In this chapter, you will also find theoretical underpinnings and rationales for the use of these self-management approaches.

Natural approaches use therapies that are noninvasive, that utilize no synthetic chemicals or drugs, and that seek to activate the body's innate healing capabilities to resolve or prevent illness. For example, a natural method of reducing high blood pressure might include dietary changes, a daily exercise regimen, affirmations, and stress-reduction techniques. These therapies require that the client be consistent in applying them, and their effects are gradual. Clients may require coaching and encouragement from you to continue their self-care approaches.

Medications that lower blood pressure work much more quickly, but they also are more likely to include unwelcome and/or dangerous side effects ("High blood pressure," 2012; Weber, 2002). Their effectiveness depends on clients being diligent about taking them as prescribed. In many instances, medications are also much more expensive than natural therapies, and some are addictive (LaLie, Rudolph, Luscher & Tan, 2011; Stene, Dyb, Tverdal, Jacobsen & Schei, 2012).

Self-Management

The realization that the needs of clients with chronic conditions are not being met by traditional healthcare approaches is shifting the focus from didactic education to encouragement and support for more effective self-management. Considerable evidence exists that interventions emphasizing client empowerment and the acquisition of self-management skills are effective in managing diabetes, asthma, and other chronic conditions. Most of these interventions are relatively brief. They generally emphasize the client's crucial role in maintaining health and function and the importance of setting goals, establishing action plans, identifying barriers, and solving problems to overcome obstacles (Coleman, Austin, Brach & Wagner, 2009).

You can prepare yourself for this kind of self-management by practicing approaches on yourself and then teaching at least one other student. While demonstrating the intervention, be sure to help your student client set a goal and establish an action plan. Examples include: I will exercise daily for at least 30 minutes. I will say my affirmation 20 times every day. I will eat more vegetables and fruits and limit fries and sodas to once-a-week treats. I will practice foot massage every evening at bedtime. I will do qigong every morning when I get up. I will take a meditation break instead of a coffee break every day. I will put a few drops of lavender under my pillowcase to aid in sleep. I will use positive imagery and coping statements when I'm stressed at work or school. I will take a yoga class to help with my arthritis. I will go to Tai Chi class every week.

Using self-care and self-management modalities calls for you to allow the client to be in charge. This is not always a simple transition. See RESEARCH BOX 9-1 for an example of what obstacles can occur.

Although clients self-manage care, you still provide encouragement (e.g., "You can *do* this.") and self-efficacy promotion (e.g., "That's good, you've mastered the first step; you're well on your way to your goal.")

It is not possible to address every self-care approach in one chapter, but here we will focus on some safe methods that are easy to incorporate into daily living and give pointers for their use in health promotion.

RESEARCH BOX 9-1 Diabetes Management In Primary Care Settings

» BACKGROUND: While the chronic care model has been extensively used for the management of patients with diabetes in primary care settings, it is not clear whether this model can be used effectively in specialty clinics for other chronic disorders.

» METHODS: The chronic care model was introduced to help manage patients with osteoarthritis in an academic rheumatology service with seven pre-specified goals. These goals included measurements of Western Ontario MacMaster (WOMAC) osteoarthritis scores, self-efficacy scores, and exercise time.

» RESULTS: Five a priori goals were achieved in this study: average WOMAC scores less than 1,000 mm as measured on a visual analogue scale, average self-efficacy score of less than 5 mm, average exercise time greater than 90 min, more than 40% of patients exercising at least 60 min per week, and a 20% improvement in self-efficacy scores. The authors were unable to achieve their self-management goal, indicating they had not yet fully implemented the chronic care model into practice.

» CONCLUSIONS: The chronic care model can be effectively introduced into a specialty service and can be used effectively in the management of clients with nondiabetic disorders, in this case osteoarthritis.

Source: Ranatunga, S., Myers, S., Redding, S., Scaife, S. L., Francis, M. D., & Francis, M. L. (2010). Introduction of the chronic care model into an academic rheumatology clinic. *Quality and Safety Health Care, 19*(5), 1–4.

Acupressure

Acupressure is an ancient art that uses the fingers to press key points on the surface of the skin to stimulate the body's natural self-curative abilities. When these points are pressed, they release muscular tension and promote the circulation of blood to aid healing. Such therapies are widely used for self-treatment of tension-related ailments.

A primary advantage of acupressure is that it is safe for clients to do on themselves or others as long as instructions and cautions for the method are followed. Another advantage of acupressure is that because the hands are used, it can be practiced at any time and in any setting. Some of the conditions for which acupressure has been used include ulcer pain, menstrual cramps, backache, constipation, indigestion, anxiety, headaches, head congestion, asthma, fatigue, motion sickness, and insomnia. Acupressure should not be used as the only treatment and acupressure that uses heavy pressure should not be used if the client has a heart condition; just before or within 20 minutes of heavy exercise, a large meal, or taking a bath; if the point in question is under a mole, wart, varicose vein, abrasion, bruise, cut, or any other break in the skin; or when pregnant, especially if more than 3 months along.

☐ Theory Base

Acupressure is based on the theory that a perpetual flow of bioenergy, or life-force, called "chi," "ki," or "qi" flows into the body and along pathways called "meridians," influencing the functioning of all the organs. When healthy, the flow balances internally and externally. When ill, external or internal events disturb the flow. Along the meridians are a large number of pressure points that act as "valves" for the flow of chi. Stimulating acupoints restores balance, relieving symptoms. Try each of the examples in TABLE 9-1 as you read them.

Table 9-1 Acupressure for Headache, Backache, Fatigue, Energizing, Abdominal Pain and Discomfort, Head Congestion

To relieve headache, push hard up and into the skull in the depressions on either side of the cervical vertebrae below the occipital bone. Tenderness in the meridian point is the best indicator the point has been found.

To relieve backache, stimulate the inside of the thigh, just back of the knee cap.

To ease fatigue, press hard in the middle of the eyebrow several times 5 seconds on and 5 seconds off.

To energize, stimulate the point where the big and second toe meet.

To relieve abdominal pain, motion sickness and fatigue, press about 3 inches below the knee.

To relieve congestion in head, sinus infection, colds, pinch skin above nose opposite eyes, push in hard along brow (both sides), right under each eye, alongside nostrils, 5 seconds on, 5 seconds off.

For more assistance, go to http://www.livestrong.com/article/106745-acupressure-instructions/

RESEARCH BOX 9-2   Effect Of Acupressure On Labor

» PURPOSE: To evaluate the effect of acupressure administered during the active phase of labor on nulliparous women's ratings of labor pain.

» DESIGN: Randomized controlled trial.

» SETTING: Public hospital in India.

» SAMPLE: Seventy-one women randomized to receive acupressure at acupuncture point spleen 6 (SP6) on both legs during contractions over a 30-minute period (acupressure group), 71 women to receive light touch at SP6 on both legs during the same period of time (touch group), and 70 women to receive standard care (standard care group).

» METHODS: Experience of in-labor pain was assessed by visual analog scale at baseline before treatment, immediately after treatment, and at 30, 60, and 120 minutes after treatment. Main outcome measure; labor pain intensity at different time intervals after treatment compared with before treatment.

» RESULTS: A reduction of in-labor pain was found in the acupressure group and was most noticeable immediately after treatment (acupressure group vs. standard care group $p < 0.001$; acupressure group vs. touch group $p < 0.001$).

» CONCLUSION: Acupressure reduced pain during the active phase of labor in nulliparous women giving birth in a context in which social support and epidural analgesia were not available. The treatment effect is small, which suggests that acupressure may be most effective during the initial phase of labor.

Source: Hjelmstedt, A., Shenoy, S. T., Stener-Victorin, E., Lekander, M., Bhat, M., Balakumaran, L., & Waldenström, U. (2010). Acupressure to reduce labor pain: a randomized controlled trial. *Acta Obstetricia et Gynecologica Scandinavica, 89*(11), 1453–1459.

Acupressure has been used for many conditions other than those found in Table 9-1. One of them is labor and delivery pain. See RESEARCH BOX 9-2, Effect of Acupressure on Labor, for study specifics.

HEALTH PROMOTION CHALLENGE

Is the sample, size, and research design adequate to determine whether acupressure is effective or not? Justify your response.

There are several kinds of acupressure. One example is high-touch acupressure, which uses gentle pressure to achieve healing. Anyone who can take a pulse can perform the actions. TABLE 9-2 provides some simple actions clients can be taught to do on themselves.

Table 9-2 High-Touch Acupressure Chart for Common Ailments

Directions: Hold index, third, and fourth finger of one hand on any spot on the top side of your other forearm. Hold lightly but tightly enough to feel the pulse in each finger. Experiment until you balance the pulse in all three fingers so they are all pulsating about the same amount. This is the sensation you are aiming for when you do the following actions.

1. *For emotional imbalance or fatigue, weak immune system, can't swallow, or abdominal pain,* hold the middle finger of one hand until balanced, repeat with the other hand.

2. *For tumors,* hold the fingers opposite the tumor; if the tumor is on the right side, hold the left thumb with your three fingers until balanced, then the index finger, then each of the rest of the fingers until they are balanced.

3. *For perspiring when asleep,* hold back of thumb on one hand until balanced, and then the other.

4. *For skin problems, dizziness, sweaty hands and feet, heart racing, or dry tongue,* hold index finger of one hand until balanced, and then the other.

5. *For constipation,* hold index finger of right hand until balanced.

6. *For diarrhea,* hold index finger of left hand until balanced.

7. *For bloated abdomen, craving carbohydrates, food aversions, hair falling out, or perspiring,* hold thumb of one hand until balanced, then other thumb.

8. *For craving sweets, blood pressure problems, dry skin, stumbling over words, fatigued nervous system, intestinal pain, muscle tone, graying hair, hair loss, joint pain/stiffness, or muscle spasms,* hold little finger of one hand until balanced, then the other little finger. (For reproductive organs or fibroid tumors/cysts, treat opposite side.)

9. *For flushed face, feverish palms, excessive thirst, or varicose veins,* hold center of palm of one hand with three fingers until balanced then repeat with other palm.

10. *For osteoporosis, headaches, pain, gas, allergies, muscle or ligament pain, perspiring yet cold, rheumatism, low energy, feeling disconnected or overly attached, cancer, or achy and crusted eyes,* hold ring finger of one hand until balanced, then repeat with other hand.

11. *For dizziness, heart conditions, or back stiffness,* hold ring finger over thumb or vice versa, both hands at once.

12. *For hand ailments,* hold index finger of the same side as ailment, hold under arm pit same side, hold opposite side below head where shoulder meets neck.

Source: Adapted from Betsy Ruth Dayton, M.Ed. (1998). *High Touch Jin Shin Workbook.* 1. Friday Harbor, WA: High Touch Network. For more information, go to www.hightouchnet.com

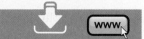

CASE STUDY: Accupressure

Ms. Schroeder, age 28, suffered from insomnia and occasional headaches for many years, as the result of a car accident. Now she's pregnant and tells you, "I feel so tired and weary, nearly all the time. Can you teach me acupressure points to help me now and when I go into labor?"

HEALTH PROMOTION CHALLENGE

Use the information in this section to develop a teaching/learning program in collaboration with Ms. Schroeder.

Affirmations

An affirmation is a thought consciously chosen to produce a desired result. Affirmations can be a useful motivational tool (Martin, Keswick, & Leveck, 2010) and they can also reduce defensiveness (Critcher, Dunning, & Armor, 2010). However, focusing too much on the purpose of an affirmation when teaching clients affirmations can attenuate its effect (Sherman et al., 2009). For anxious clients, affirmations relating to "not being crazy" were reported to be helpful as were affirmations that depression will subside in time for depressed clients. Nurses and clients can benefit from being open to trying innovative self-tailored interventions (Kinnier, Hofsess, Pongratz, & Lambert, 2009).

Stress is implicated in the development and progression of a broad array of mental and physical health disorders. Theory and research suggest that self-affirming activities may buffer these adverse effects (Cresswell et al., 2005). Veterans suffering from posttraumatic stress disorder can benefit from hearing and using positive affirmations about their wartime experiences (Dohrenwend et al., 2004).

☐ Affirmation Examples

It's getting easier and easier to think about stopping smoking (smoking cessation).
Life itself supports me (back pain).
I joyously release the past (hypertension).
I move forward in life with ease and joy (leg and/or feet problems).
It is safe for me to be alive (eating disorders).
I am willing to change and grow (illness).
I love and approve of myself (overweight).

Life supports me in love and peace (osteoporosis).
I see only love and joy (eyes).
I am powerful and desirable (endometriosis).
I am filled with energy (fatigue).
I create only good in my life (tumors and cysts).

☐ Theory Base

Affirmations are based on the theory that both good and disease are the result of mental thought patterns which form life experiences. For every life effect, a thought pattern precedes it. Negative thought patterns produce tension and discomfort. Consistent thought patterns create experiences; by changing thinking patterns, experience can be changed (Hay, 2001).

☐ Guidelines for Affirmation Use

Provide a relaxing, sharing atmosphere. Consider using a relaxation exercise or playing a relaxation tape as a prelude to the affirmation process. Obtain information from the client about health issues and concerns. Dialogue with the client to see whether the affirmation is best stated in the attitude, feeling, or action mode. If affirmations are stated too quickly in the action mode, clients might not be able to benefit from them. To evaluate this, ask the client, "Are you ready to start thinking about changing or are you ready to use affirmations to take action to change?"

Sometimes clients may be unsure of themselves and think they want to change, but may find during the affirmation process that they are not yet ready to change and are really at the contemplation stage. Affirmations are useful for either stage, but should be stated in the appropriate way, e.g., "It's getting easier and easier to smoke 10 cigarettes a day" (behavior mode) vs. "It's getting easier and easier to think about smoking 10 cigarettes a day" (attitude mode).

Assist the client to state the affirmation in his or her own words. Actively listen to the client until it is clear how an affirmation might be stated, but keep checking with the client until the affirmations feels right. For example, "It sounds as if an affirmation for you might be, 'It's getting easier and easier to …' or 'I'm becoming more comfortable with the idea of…'" Once an affirmation has been agreed upon, ask clients to write or say it 10 to 20 times a day while listening to their inner response to hearing it or writing it.

Practice this process with clients at least once. Ask clients to say the affirmation, then ask, "What is your reaction to hearing yourself say that?" Ask clients to repeat the affirmation again, and ask, "How does it sound this time?" Continue working with clients this way. At first, clients may respond with comments such as, "I'll never be able to do it." With repetition, their inner response begins to move toward, "Maybe I can do it."

RESEARCH BOX 9-3   Affirmations and Breastfeeding

» AIMS: To identify strategies used by breastfeeding women to assist them to continue breastfeeding.

» BACKGROUND: These studies were conducted in Australia where breastfeeding initiation is high, but the majority of women wean before the recommended time. The identification of interventions which may increase breastfeeding duration is therefore a research priority.

» DESIGN: The Against All Odds study used a case-controlled design to investigate the characteristics of women who continued to breastfeed in the face of extraordinary difficulties. Phase One of the I Think I Can study employed the Nominal Group Technique to investigate the views of subject matter experts regarding which psychological factors may influence the duration of breastfeeding.

» METHOD: Against All Odds study participants ($n = 40$) undertook a one- to two-hour interview and the transcribed data were analyzed using thematic analysis. Stratified purposeful sampling was employed in the I Think I Can study ($n = 21$), with participants assigned group membership according to their most recent breastfeeding experience. A fourth group was composed of experienced breastfeeding clinicians. The nominal group technique was used to generate group data and segments of the discussion were audiotaped and transcribed for thematic analysis.

» RESULTS: Participants in both the studies identified strategies used to assist them in their efforts to cope with the challenges of breastfeeding and early motherhood. These strategies included increasing breast-feeding knowledge, staying relaxed and 'looking after yourself', the use of positive self-talk (a form of affirmations), challenging unhelpful beliefs, problem solving, goal setting and the practice of mindfulness.

» CONCLUSIONS: Employment of these simple behavioral and cognitive strategies may assist women to cope with the pressures inherent in the experience of early mothering, thereby increasing the duration of breastfeeding.

» RELEVANCE TO CLINICAL PRACTICE: These results provide a 'tool box' of coping strategies for women to use in the postnatal period.

Source: O'Brien, M. L., Buikstra, E., Fallon, T., & Hegney, D. (2009). Strategies for success: a toolbox of coping strategies used by breastfeeding women. *Journal of Clinical Nursing, 18*(11), 1574–1582.

Advise clients to carry their chosen affirmation with them on a 3×5 card and place it in a briefcase, purse, or car dashboard, where it will be read throughout the day. Underscore how hearing themselves on tape, viewing themselves say the affirmation, or writing and reading back the affirmation provides important reinforcing feedback.

Encourage clients to record their affirmations and play them back or look in the mirror and say them, maintaining good eye contact and striving for a relaxed facial expression. Clients can also practice with you or a supportive peer. Provide or ask clients to provide an ongoing reinforcement for continuing the affirmation. Use affirmations to support other medical, nursing, or related therapies clients participate in. Present affirmation as a new method that has proved useful to many clients with many different kinds of problems.

Provide support if clients become frustrated or expect too much, e.g., "This is difficult, but you will get it," "Keep trying, you're making progress," or "Don't expect to change patterns you've taken years to develop overrnight."

For more information on affirmations, go to http://www.vitalaffirmations.com/affirmations.htm

HEALTH PROMOTION CHALLENGE   (www)

Examine the research design in RESEARCH BOX 9-3 and decide whether it is strong enough to support the conclusions drawn. Justify your answer. How can you use the information provided to promote health?

Aromatherapy

Aromatherapy is the use of essential oils via massage or inhalation to improve health. The distillation of oils has a 5,000-year history. Egyptians used the essential oils of myrrh, cedarwood, cinnamon, sandalwood, thyme, and elemi to embalm their dead. Incense was used to help heighten spiritual experiences by deepening meditation and purifying the spirit. The Babylonians, Hindus, Chinese, Japanese, Assyrians, ancient Africans, Greeks, Romans, and Native American shamans all used essential oils. The modern revival began during the 1920s when Gattlefosse, a French chemist and perfumer, coined the term aromatherapy (Stevensen, 1996).

☐ The Theory Behind Aromatherapy

It is believed that the inhalation of essential oils stimulates the part of the brain connected to smell, the olfactory system. A signal is sent to the limbic system of the brain, which controls emotions and retrieves learned memories. This causes chemicals to be released that make the person feel relaxed, calm, or stimulated. If the aromatherapy includes massage, the effect is to further relax the person.

Essential oils are applied topically to activate thermal receptors and destroy microbes and fungi, as well as soothe sore muscles and reduce tension. Internal application may stimulate the immune system, but must only be done under supervision of a certified aromatherapist.

☐ Scientific Basis

The liquid gas chromatograph is used to analyze chemical components of essential oils, which are a mixture of 100 organic compounds. Their therapeutic action include aldehydes (calmants, anti-infectives), esthers (antispasmodics, calmants, antifungicides), ketones (calmants, mucolitics, cicatrisings), coumarins (balancing, calmants), lactones (balancing, calmants), sesquiterpenes (anti-allergics, antihistamines), acids/aromatic aldehydes (immunostimulants, anti-infectives), oxides (expectorants, antiparasitics), C10 terpenes (antiseptics, cortisonelike actions), phenols/C10 alcohols, aromatic aldehydes (antiinfectives, immunostimulatns), C15 and C20 alcohols (estrogenlike actions), and phenyl methyl ethers (anti-infectives, antispasmodics). Some essential oils that have been studied and demonstrate health-promoting qualities include:

1. *Oregano* shows antioxidant and antimicrobial properties (Celik, Nur, Arslan, Zafer & Mercan, 2010).

2. *Bergamot* (*Citrus bergamia*) is a fruit used in aromatherapy to minimize symptoms of stress-induced anxiety, mild mood disorders, and cancer pain by interfering with normal and pathological synaptic plasticity, providing neuroprotection (Bagetta et al., 2010).

3. *Thyme, cinnamon, rose, and lavender* essential oils exhibited the strongest bactericidal activities at a concentration of 0.25% (v/v), and *Propionibacterium acnes* was completely killed after 5 minutes.

4. *Thyme* essential oil exhibited the strongest cytotoxicity towards three human cancer cells. The cytotoxicity of 10 essential oils on human prostate carcinoma cell (PC-3) was significantly stronger than on human lung carcinoma (A549) and human breast cancer (MCF-7) cell lines (Yu et al., 2010).

5. *Clary* oil had the strongest anti-stressor and antidepressive effect, indicating the oil could be used therapeutically for its antidepressant-like effect and may modulate the DAnergic pathway (Seol et al., 2010).

6. *Rosemary and lemon* essential oils in the morning, and *lavender and orange* in the evening, led to significant improvement in personal orientation related to cognitive function for Alzheimer's patients (Jimbo, Kimura, Taniguchi, Inoue, & Urakami, 2009).

7. *Lavandin* (a type of *lavender*) has been shown to reduce pre-operative anxiety (Braden, Reichow, & Halm, 2009).

8. *Lavender and rosemary* oils can reduce anxiety (McCaffrey, Thomas & Kinzelman, 2009).

9. *Bergamot, lavender, and frankincense* (1:1:1), diluted 1.5%, mixed in a carrier oil of 50 ml of sweet almond oil, and used to massage each hand for 5 minutes × 7 days (as opposed to massage with just almond oil) had a significant effect on pain and depression in hospice patients with terminal cancer (Chang, 2008).

10. *Lavender* helps maintain sustained attention during long-term tasks (Shimizu et al., 2008).

11. *Lavender and clary* topical application reduce work-related stress of nurses in an ICU setting (Pemberton & Turpin, 2008).

12. *Lavender bath oil* reduces stress and crying and enhances sleep in very young infants (Field et al., 2008).

13. *Lavender aromatherapy* improves coronary flow velocity reserve in healthy men (Shiina et al., 2008). See RESEARCH BOX 9-4.

RESEARCH BOX 9-4   Essential Oils for Oral Health for Terminal Cancer

» PURPOSE: This study examined the effects of oral care with essential oil in improving the oral health status of hospice patients with terminal cancer.

» SAMPLE: The sample included 43 participants with terminal cancer admitted to K hospital in G city, Korea.

» METHOD: Twenty-two patients were assigned to the experimental group and 21 to the control group. Participants in the experimental group received special mouth care with essential oil (application of essential oil mixture consisting of geranium, lavender, tea tree, and peppermint). The control group received special mouth care with 0.9% saline. The special mouth care was performed twice daily for one week in both groups. The scores for subjective oral comfort, objective oral state, and numbers of colonizing *Candida albicans* were measured before and after the treatment.

» RESULTS: The score for subjective oral comfort and objective oral state were significantly higher in the experimental group compared to the control group. The numbers of colonizing C. albicans significantly decreased in the experimental group compared to the control group.

Source: Kang, H. Y., Na, S. S., & Kim, Y. K. (2010). Effects of oral care with essential oil on improvement in oral health status of hospice patients. *Journal of the Korean Academy of Nursing, 40*(4), 473–481.

Cautions: It is important to follow the product instructions carefully. Concentrated products should be diluted in a carrier oil. Caution clients to wash their hands after handling concentrated essential oil and never touch their eyes before doing so. If clients have any of the following conditions, caution them to be careful using aromatherapy and to follow all directions carefully: allergies, hay fever, asthma, eczema or psoriasis, epilepsy, hypertension, deep vein thrombosis, or if they are breastfeeding or pregnant.

Aromatherapy does sometimes have side effects, but they tend to be very mild and do not last long. These include nausea, headaches, and some allergic reactions.

Essential oils derived from citrus may make the skin more sensitive to ultraviolet light, making the person more susceptible to sunburn. Some oils may change the effectiveness of conventional medicines—if you are not sure, check with a qualified pharmacist or doctor (Nordqvist, 2009).

❑ Methods of Administration

Aromatherapy is generally applied in one of three ways:
- Aerial diffusion includes using diffusers, humidifiers, room sprays, and water bowls. The aim is to give the air a specific fragrance or to disinfect it. A diffuser made especially for essential oils is recommended. It should have a bowl section that is nonporous so it can be wiped clean.
- Direct inhalation. This method is commonly used for respiratory disinfection, decongestion, as well as for psychological benefits. One drop of essential oil is placed in a tissue or handkerchief and sniffed as needed.

A few drops of lavender oil can be placed under the pillowcase to aid in relaxation and sleep.

- Topical applications are applied onto the skin and are commonly used for massage, baths, and therapeutic skin care. Add about seven drops of essential oil in a carrier oil or a small amount of shampoo to an already drawn bath and then mix in by hand to avoid quick evaporation of the oil.

Clients with sensitive skin are advised to do a skin patch test. All you need to do is to mix one drop of the oil you wish to test with a teaspoon (5 ml) of carrier oil, such as sweet almond oil or grapeseed oil. Apply a small amount of this mixed oil to the inside of your wrist or elbow and leave uncovered for 24 hours. This area must not be washed for this period of time. If no sign of itching, redness, or swelling occurs after the 24 hour period, it should be safe for you to use the oil. Consider doing a skin patch test using only the carrier oil. For children between the ages of 4 and 12, as well as for elderly people, only add 4 drops of oil per bath; for children between 1 and 4, as well as for pregnant women, add only 2 drops of oil per bath, and children under 1 year should have no more than 1 drop of oil per bath. After the drops of essential oil are added to the bath water, the bathroom door is closed so vapors do not escape. The client soaks for at least 10 minutes, breathing deeply. For more information, go to: http://www.livestrong.com/article/95458-pure-essential-oil-directions/

Studies that have shown positive effects from using aromatherapy include Ou and colleagues, (2012), for pain relief for dysmenorrhea; Ruepert et al., (2012), for irritable bowel syndrome; and the study that follows.

RESEARCH BOX 9-5 Effect of Aromatherapy Masssage on Menopause Symptoms

- » AIM: This study investigated the effects of aromatherapy massage on menopausal symptoms in Korean climacteric women.

- » METHOD: Kupperman's menopausal index was used to compare an experimental group of 25 climacteric women with a wait-listed control group of 27 climacteric women. Aromatherapy was applied topically to subjects in the experimental group in the form of massage on the abdomen, back, and arms using lavender, rose geranium, rose, and jasmine in almond and primrose oils once a week for 8 weeks (eight times in total).

- » FINDINGS: The experimental group reported a significantly lower total menopausal index than wait-listed controls ($P < 0.05$). There were also significant intergroup differences in subcategories such as vasomotor, melancholia, arthralgia, and myalgia (all $P < 0.05$). These findings suggest that aromatherapy massage may be an effective treatment of menopausal symptoms such as hot flushes, depression, and pain in climacteric women. However, it could not be verified whether the positive effects were from the aromatherapy, the massage, or both. Further rigorous studies should be done with more objective measures.

Source: Hur, M. H., Yang, Y. S., & Lee, M. S. (2008). Aromatherapy massage affects menopausal symptoms in Korean climacteric women: A pilot-controlled clinical trial. *Evidence Based Complementary and Alternative Medicine, 5*(3), 325–328.

HEALTH PROMOTION CHALLENGE

What additional research needs to be done? If you were the researcher, what would be your next step?

Coping Skills

Assisting clients to cope is a major goal for health promotion, so learning coping skills is a natural extension of that idea. **Coping skills** grew out of Meichenbaum and Cameron's (1974) systematic desensitization and relaxation procedures. These activities include replacing defeatist self-talk with stress coping statements and progressive relaxation.

☐ Theory for Coping Skills

Lazarus and Folkman (1984), leaders in the field of coping research, defined coping as "constantly changing cognitive and behavioral efforts to manage specific external and/or internal demands that are appraised as taxing or exceeding the resources of the person" (p. 141). The notion of coping efforts includes the idea that they are constantly changing, which implies it may be necessary for people to learn a variety of possible coping strategies and to assess the situation to determine which strategies might work best.

This theory includes the notion that the issues that give rise to the need for coping may originate outside of the person or from within the person. Improved coping may include examining the appraisal process (the assessment of the demands of the situation), as well as the teaching of coping strategies. Coping is believed to be context specific and coping is a function of the connection between the person and the environment.

☐ Coping Skills Procedures

Coping skills procedures can be used to rehearse for real life events deemed stressful. The procedure is (1) choose a stressful situation, (2) practice progressive relaxation until feeling calm and peaceful, and (3) repeat coping skills statements until the stressful situation can be thoroughly completed in an imaginary rehearsal without feeling stressed. This procedure can effectively reduce anxiety associated with interviews, giving speeches, taking tests, being in social situations, and reducing phobias, especially the fear of heights. According to Davis, McKay, and Eshelman (1995), 89% of hypertense, postcardiac clients who used this approach were able to attain general relaxation, and 79% controlled anxiety and were able to fall into a deep sleep. It can take 1-2 weeks to master progressive relaxation and about 1 week to master the ability to relax the body while picturing the stressful situation.

Coping thoughts can be divided into statements useful for different stages of the stressful situation: preparatory, the situation, and reinforcing success. Examples of statements found effective for each stage follow. Nurses and clients can develop their own list and memorize it and/or carry a copy with them for use in stressful situations.

1. Preparatory Stage:
   - This will get easier if I just start
   - I'll jump in and be fine
   - I can do this
   - No need to worry
   - Soon this will be over

2. The Situation:
   - I'm taking a deep breath and relaxing
   - I won't allow this situation to upset me
   - I can handle this; I'm doing it now
   - I'll just take this step by step
   - It's easy to keep focused on the task
   - I'm not concerned with anyone else, just on doing this
   - I'm deep breathing and it's helping

RESEARCH BOX 9-6   Motivation to Learn Stress Reduction Procedures

» BACKGROUND: Work is often fraught with stress.

» PROBLEM UNDER STUDY: Whether in-person or phone consultations about stress reduction work best.

» METHOD: Support programs for stress reduction were offered independently in two departments (650 employees in total) of an insurance group. Both departments, referred to as comparison group 1 and 2 (CG1 and CG2), offered an Employee Assistance Program (EAP) featuring individual consultations. The employees were addressed through different channels of communication, such as staff meetings, superiors, and email. In CG1, a staff adviser additionally called on all employees at their workplace and showed them a brief relaxing technique in order to raise awareness of stress reduction. Contacting employees personally was also intended to reduce the inhibition threshold for the following individual talks. In CG2, individual talks were done face-to-face, whereas CG1 used telephone counselling.

» RESULTS: By using the new access channel with an additional personal contact at the workplace, an above average percentage of employees in CG1 could be motivated to participate in the following talks. The rate of participants was five times as high as in CG1, with lower costs for the consultation in each case.

Source: Burnus, M., Benner, V., Kirchner, D., Drabik, A., & Stock, S. (2012). Comparison of two access portals of an employee assistance program at an insurance corporation targeted to reduce stress levels of employees. *Versicherungsmedizin, 64*(1), 17–22.

3. Reinforcing Success
   - I did it!
   - I did really well
   - I'm proud of myself
   - Situations will not overwhelm me ever again
   - I'm going to tell _____how successful I was

HEALTH PROMOTION CHALLENGE

How could you use the findings in this study to provide a stress reduction program for a client?

Exercise/Movement

Movement is one of the simplest and most effective modes of stress reduction. It also moderates appetite and serves a preventive function against aging and some chronic conditions, including coronary heart disease, obesity, joint and spinal disc disease, fatigue, muscular tension, and depression. When done correctly, movement and exercise can enhance self-image and self-confidence, reduce joint stiffness, increase circulation, improve posture, reduce depression, positively affect work performance, decrease blood pressure, enhance ability to relate to others, enhance sleep, decrease the need for stimulants, and enhance breathing ability (Physical Activity Guidelines Committee, 2008). Locomotor movement crosses the brain and body's midlines to integrate and organize brain hemispheres, increase blood flow to all parts of the brain, and enhance alertness and energetic learning.

Movement, physical activity, and exercise grow new brain cells essential to learning and memory; bring fuel, oxygen, and glucose to the brain faster; help the brain see letters and numbers on a page; and assist in putting patterns into a sequence.

Other movements that can stimulate brain integration include:

- Hold your nose, reach over or under and grab your nose with the other hand. Switch and switch.
- While writing a signature on an imaginary table, rotate the foot in a clockwise fashion.
- Using thumbs and index fingers, gently pull the ears back and unroll them. Begin at the top and gently massage down and around the curve, ending with the bottom lobe. Do this for about 1 minute. Rolling the ears over activates the brain for concentration, short term memory, and listening skills.
- Placing fingers on the jaw where it meets the ears, rub this area while yawning for about 30 seconds; this relieves the stress that tightens the jaw and decreases nerve function. (Boyd, Vidoni, & Wessel, 2010).

□ Some Theoretical Frameworks For Movement

Movement and fitness frameworks especially suited to a wellness and health promotion outlook are Feldenkrais's Theory of Awareness Through Movement and Kurtz and Prestera's Body Message Theory.

Feldenkrais's Awareness Through Movement

Physiologists found that cells in the motor cortex of the brain are arranged in such a way that they, broadly grouped, correspond to different body parts. This representation is called the homunculus, and it resembles the human body. This is the motor or movement basis for self-image. Feldenkrais contends that everyone's self-image is smaller than it might be and that the combinations and patterning of cells may be more important than their number. For example, people who speak two languages make use of both more cells and more combinations of cells. Some people can speak 30 or more languages; this gives a rough idea of the limitlessness of potential for self-image (Feldenkrais, 1977, pp. 12–15).

Everyone has parts of the body for which there is no awareness. For example it is easy for most people to lie on their back and sense their fingertips, but it is probably difficult for many to sense the nape of the neck or the space between the ears. The parts of the body that are easily defined in the awareness are those that serve humans daily, while the parts that are dull or mute in awareness play only an indirect role in life and are almost missing from self-image when people are in action (Feldenkrais, 1979, p. 27).

Learning to move parts of the body with consciousness will enhance the self-image, according to Feldenkrais. The way a person holds their shoulders, head, and stomach, their voice and expression; their stability; and their manner of presenting themself are all based on self-image. Feldenkrais believed that systematic correction of the self-image is quicker and more efficient than correcting single actions and errors by modes of behavior (Feldenkrais, 1979, p. 23). TABLE 9-3 provides important postulates of Feldenkrais's theory.

Table 9-3 Feldenkrais Theory Postulates

Some important postulates of Feldenkrais (1979, pp. 33–62) theory are:

1. Awareness and self-image are based on movement.
2. Breathing and movement must be coordinated if movement is to be effective.
3. Movement of the eyes organizes movement of the body.
4. When actions are performed correctly, refreshment and relaxation result; when movements are performed too quickly and without attention to breathing, fatigue may result.
5. The body is constantly fighting against the force of gravity unless it is well organized; without appropriate organization, gravity can pull or push the body and affect movement in a negative manner.
6. Individuals can learn to organize their bodies more effectively by practicing slow, gradual movements while breathing correctly and learning to experience the body sensations associated with effective movement.

Kurtz and Prestera's Body Message Theory

Fixed muscular patterns in the body are central to a person's way of being in the world. They form in response to family and early environment. Every emotional feeling is also expressed physically and becomes a way of holding oneself, a fixed muscular pattern and a set attitude toward life. These attitudes and fixed muscular patterns reflect, enhance, and sustain one another (Kurtz & Prestera, 1984, pp. 2–3).

These characteristic patterns inhibit individuals from attaining well-being. When well, the body is capable of allowing the free flowing of feeling. It is efficient and graceful in its movements, and aware and responsive to real needs. Such a body has bright eyes, breathes freely, is smooth skinned, and has an elastic muscle tone. It is well-proportioned, and the various segments coordinate well with each other. The neck is pliable and the head moves easily. The pelvis swings freely. The entire body is lined up efficiently with respect to gravity; in a standing position, there is no struggle with gravity's downward pull.

Pleasure and well-being are characteristic feelings. A person with such a body is emotionally flexible and his or her feelings are spontaneous (Kurtz & Prestera, 1984, p. 3) When there is a wholeness to the body/mind/spirit, expression of feelings flows easily; wholeness is disrupted when the flow of energy in the body is disrupted. When an individual experiences anger, but does not express it directly, breaks in the normally smooth curves of the body can be observed.

HEALTH PROMOTION CHALLENGE   ⭐   (www)

Look at your body right now in the mirror and see if your scapulas are flat and equally so; if not, there is a break in the smooth curve of your back. Likewise, if you look at the front of your body in a mirror, you may see that the right or left side of your chest is more forward, more to the back, wider, longer, or whatever. Any of these will look like breaks in the smooth curve of your body. Everyone has some breaks; the difference in magnitude and quantity differentiates all individuals along a continuum from no movement and energy blocks to effective movement and energy flow. Once you're finished, evaluate at least two other students. Compare and contrast your findings.

Feelings can intersect with the body. In the case of the individual who does not express anger, that unexpressed feeling may be "locked" in a body part. Some individuals may lock it in the arms (instead of striking out); others may hold their anger in their abdominal area, leading to digestive upsets and a tight, tense abdomen that may be excessively held in.

Similarly, an infant whose mother constantly grabbed his arm whenever he reached out to explore his environment may turn into an adult with lifeless arms that hang drooping from narrow shoulders. Here, there is no indication of reaching out to life; instead, the infant waits passively for things to come to him.

Infants are born with the capacity for wholeness, but fear can produce blocks. For example, "in blocking the expression of sadness, we tense the jaw, chest, stomach, diaphragm, and some muscles of the throat and face—all the areas which move spontaneously when the feeling is allowed its natural outlets" (Kurtz & Prestera, 1984, pp. 8–9).

Blocks impede the normal flow of energy as muscles tense, circulation is constricted, and skin tone and temperature change. The holding in of feeling is manifested as rings of muscle and fascia tension or breaks in the areas between the major segments of the body, including the neck and upper shoulders, the diaphragm, the lower back between the abdomen and pelvis, the groin, the knees, and the ankles; feet and eyes can also be held.

FIGURE 9-1 shows body areas where holding is common. Gross changes in function, form, color, and development can occur. Hands and feet may be small and cold. The head may be large or the abdomen blown up while the chest is collapsed. As blood supply is reduced due to increased muscular tension, there is a collection of tissue wastes, setting up a mechanism of toxic spasm and stasis. The nervous system responds by firing more signals, leading to the pain-spasm-pain-spasm of a headache, backache, or heartache. If this occurs chronically, the tissues harden to splint the area against further attack and structural block develops.

According to Kurtz and Prestera, a backache may be the product of a slipped disc, but the original insult may result in an attempt to hold oneself up or back. A heart attack may be the end result of blocked impulses to love or be loved that become a block in energy flow, a decrease in circulation, a pooling and thickening of blood, and eventually a physiological blockage.

Harmony with gravity aids in reaching up and out in the world. Disharmony leads to attempts by the body to compensate. If the chest is going in and down, the belly may go out and up. "The ideal axis for obtaining the greatest balances is that which connects points at the top of the head, middle of the ear, middle of the shoulder, midpoint of the hip joint, center of the knee joint, and center of the ankle joint" (Kurtz & Prestera, 1984, p. 2).

Individuals who are out of balance can express it bodily and emotionally; bodies that are bent forward often express feelings of being over-burdened; those bending backward experience life as an unending struggle.

Tension and stiffness in the lower half of the body, especially legs and feet, makes balancing difficult; it is as if the person is bracing against a fall. Tightening up may be to protect against being a "pushover," or of falling down on the job.

Feet can reveal how reality is dealt with by the way the ground is contacted. If one foot goes one way and the other another way, this may indicate confusion. Feet rotated outward put added stress on the ankle and knee joints. Feet facing forward reduce this stress, allowing more effective weight transfer through the

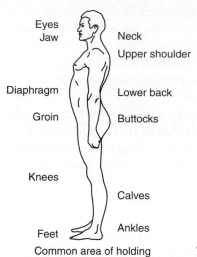

Eyes
Jaw

Neck
Upper shoulder

Diaphragm

Lower back

Groin

Buttocks

Knees

Calves

Feet

Ankles

Common area of holding

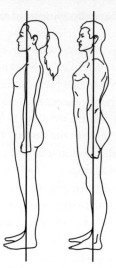

The lateral line and compensated balance

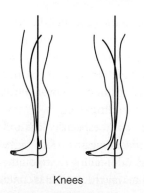

An overburdened individual

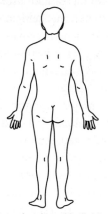

Knees

Bowing backward and forward

FIGURE 9-1   Areas of holding.
© Carolyn Chambers Clark, 2010.

center of the foot. Locking of the knees could indicate an attempt to hold on, hold oneself up, or stand ground (Kurtz & Prestera, 1984. pp. 10–20.)

□ Assessing Fitness

The traditional view of fitness focuses on cardiac fitness, while a wellness/health promotion view holds that fitness is more comprehensive. The deaths of world-class athletes who were apparently "cardiac fit" provides empirical evidence that a more extensive framework is needed to assess fitness, including flexibility.

Flexibility Assessments

There are several ways to assess flexibility. You could also ask clients which areas of the body "feel" tight or stiff, or ask them to complete range of motion or extension exercises. You can also observe the client in action and see whether the body moves as a solid, shuffling block, or if it gives the impression of a spring in the step, a lightness and gracefulness, or something in between. Other questions to ask include: Are body movements well defined with arms swinging in opposition to leg movement, knees bending, hips moving with legs, neck and chest moveable, or does the body move as a whole, or something in between? Is there a difference in the walk when observed from the front and the back in terms of movements, or do both give similar impressions? Does the head slouch forward or is it held back behind the center of gravity? Is the body lifted in an exaggerated manner to move forward? (Key indicators of this problem are shoulders hunched up, walking on the balls of the foot, and lack of thrusting forward of the hip.) Do the feet face straight ahead? Does the client favor one leg? (A thump-thump sound indicates favoring.) Does the client shuffle or scrape the feet?

Try these questions on yourself first. Ask a friend or classmate to film you walking toward and away from the video or phone. A "yes" answer to any of the above indicates a loss of flexibility and could indicate a need for stretching or Feldenkrais interventions.

Look at the foot: high arch indicates tight heel cord and tight joints; average arch indicates average flexibility; flat foot indicates loose joints and extreme flexibility. Loose-jointed clients are best suited for endurance activities and patterned movements such as dancing, gymnastics, cycling, swimming, or running. They are prone to ligament problems, partial dislocations, and knee problems. Tight-jointed clients are best at explosive activities such as basketball, hockey, tennis, racquetball, and sprinting. These clients are most prone to muscle pulls and tears, torn ligaments and cartilage, lower back pain, tendonitis of the shoulder or elbow, and pinched nerves. Remember which activities are most suited to you and your client and suggest the ones less likely to produce injury.

Aerobic Assessments

Aerobic exercise involves sustained, rhythmic activity of the large muscle groups. Aerobic exercise uses large amounts of oxygen, causing an increase in heart rate, stroke volume, respiratory rate, and a relaxation of the small blood vessels, leading to increased oxygenation. The goal of aerobic exercise is to strengthen the cardiovascular system and increase stamina. Approximately 20 minutes of activity at the appropriate heart rate for each age range produces a training effect without straining the heart unduly.

Aerobic exercise not only conditions the cardiovascular system but can also reduce the amount of body fat. Percentage of body fat can be calculated most easily by pinching the back of the back of the upper middle arm; less than 0.25 inch indicates a below average amount of body fat; 0.25–0.75 inches indicate an average amount of body fat. More than 0.75 inches indicates a high percentage of body fat. For men, 12% of body weight as fat is desirable; for women, 18%. Other methods of determining body fat are use of calipers and water displacement. When using calipers, the skin fold sites commonly used are: triceps, sub-scapula, suprailiac, and thigh (Arena, Myers & Guazzi, 2010).

For other measures of body fat go to http://www.1is2fat.com/charts_and_ calculators.htm

☐ Calculating a Safe Range for Aerobic Exercise

Target heart range is the safest range of heartbeats per minute during exercise. Clients can calculate target heart range by subtracting their age from 220 for women (226 for men) and multiplying the answer by both 0.6 and 0.8. The lower number suggests a safe rate for beginners, while the higher number would be the goal as fitness level improves.

For example, a 43-year-old woman subtracts her age from 220 to arrive at 177. Multiplying this number by 0.6% tells her that her safe rate is 106 beats per minute, while her goal would be to bring the rate up to 80%, or 141 beats per minute, as her fitness level improves.

A simple measure for whether a walking or jogging rate is if conversation between the client and an exercise partner can occur.

☐ Movement Interventions

Crawling and creeping are especially helpful in integrating the two hemispheres of the brain (Mills & Cohen, 1979, p. xiv). Crawling on hands and knees for 10-minutes in the morning can also relax painful backs and spines.

Feldenkrais Interventions

Specific Feldenkrais interventions demonstrate the ease and power of his technique. See TABLE 9-4 for the interventions to use for difficulty rising from a

Table 9-4 Feldenkrais Interventions

Intervention No. 1: Standing while Sitting. Sit in a chair and pay attention to how you stand up, note which part of the body moves first and which other parts follow and with what degree of difficulty, tension, effort. Write down what happened prior to continuing.

Now sit on the edge of a chair and let your body rock forward and backward without any sudden increase in effort. Make no attempt to get up. As you continue the movement, grasp the hair at the top of your head so any tensing of the cervical spine can be felt. When tension in the cervical area exists, increase the movement of the head forward and upward by moving the hip joints until the buttocks rise from the chair. Note the difference in effort in rising when the chest muscles, ribs, and chest are relaxed. Repeat the second part of the exercise, making sure to breathe during it. Summarize your findings. This exercise is useful for clients who have difficulty rising from a chair or bed.

Intervention No. 2: Increasing Range of Motion in the Neck. Sit comfortably in a chair. Turn the head slowly and easily to the left as far as is comfortable. Note a spot on the wall or ceiling that marks that spot, then return the head to face front. Remember to keep breathing during the exercise. Next, turn the head slowly and easily to the left while keeping the eyes looking forward. Return the head to facing front. Now turn the eyes and head slowly and easily to the left again. Note how far the head turned this time and compare it with the first time the head turned to the left. Almost everyone reports an increase in range of neck motion as a result of this simple exercise. It supports Feldenkrais's (1977) theory: use small, slow movements; breathe and concentrate on the movement and its results; break the movement into its component parts; and then reconstruct it to attain more efficient movement. This exercise will reduce neck, shoulder, and back pain.

Intervention No. 3: Using Imagery and Movement. Sit comfortably in the chair, breathing in the lower abdomen. When ready, keep the head facing forward, but picture your head turning slowly and comfortably as far as possible to the left and then returning to the front-facing position. Breathe comfortably and slowly turn the head to the left as far as comfortable. Note the spot on the wall or ceiling and compare it with previous efforts. Results from this intervention are frequently astounding. Nearly everyone greatly increased their range of motion with this series. This supports Feldenkrais' theory that imagery alone can affect movement in a positive manner.

Intervention No.4: Improving Movements of the Lower Back. This intervention is effective for tightness or pain in the lower back, tension, and improving efficient use of the lower back. Lie on the floor with knees bent and feet flat on the floor. Cross the right leg over the left knee as if sitting in a chair with the legs crossed. Extend arms out at shoulder level and let them relax into the floor. Continue breathing easily while very slowly and smoothly letting the legs drop to the left toward the floor as far as is comfortable. Continue breathing and using one slow, continuous movement, return the legs to center and let them drop to the right towards the floor. Continue breathing and repeat the exercise, allowing the legs to move slowly to the right side of the floor and then to the left side of the floor. With legs facing front, slowly stretch them out and observe the sensations in the lower back, pelvis, and legs. Lie still, breathing and noting changes and sensations.

Table 9-4 Feldenkrais Interventions (Continued)

Intervention No. 5: Increasing Movement in the Shoulders and Upper Back. This exercise is especially useful for people who sit reading or writing for long periods of time or for those who carry their tension in their chest or back. Complete all parts of the exercise in slow motion, breathing comfortably and easily throughout. Sit in a straight chair or sit up in bed. Cradle one arm in the other arm and gently move that arm as far as possible to the left, then back to center and to the right. Raise the arms slowly above the head while cradled. As you feel the muscles relax, enjoy the sense of relaxation. Place the left palm on the front of the right shoulder and gradually and firmly push the shoulder back as far as is comfortable while breathing deeply in and out. Hold in the extended position and picture tiny lungs breathing in and out at the point of pressure. Relax and note body sensations. Repeat with that arm several times and then repeat with the other shoulder (Feldenkrais, 1977, pp. 139–160).

chair; to reduce neck, shoulder and back pain; to use imagery to improve movement; to improve movement of the lower back and reduce tension; and to increase movement in shoulders and upper back.

❑ Deciding on an Appropriate Aerobic Exercise Regime

Although running and jogging are efficient, inexpensive approaches to increasing cardiovascular fitness and can be begun in stages at any age and by those who have been ill and require rehabilitation, injuries of the ankle, knee, and lower back are common. Some can be prevented by improving posture, using appropriate shoes, and strengthening the abdominal muscles. It might also be wise to consider another form of aerobic exercise if low back pain, previous injury, or poor jogging posture already exists. Swimming is an excellent conditioner if bearing weight on the lower joints is contraindicated. Feldenkrais exercises can help no matter what the chosen exercise to enhance movement.

Besides choosing an aerobic workout that is useful, it is also wise to choose one that is fun, or it will not be continued on a lifelong basis. At least 30 minutes of moderately intense physical activity is recommended on all or most days of the week. Examples of moderate activity include brisk walking, cycling, swimming, or doing home repairs or yard work. All 30 minutes need not be completed at once. Aim for shorter bouts of activity (at least 10 minutes) that add up to a half hour per day. Ask clients who sit at a computer or table all day to set an timer to get up, stretch, move around the room, and maybe do a Feldenkrais stretching exercise every 20 minutes.

Instead of thinking in terms of a specific exercise program, work toward permanently changing the lifestyle to incorporate more activity. Muscles used in any activity, any time of day, contribute to fitness. Some ways to increase movement/exercise to share with clients include: Take the stairs instead of the elevator. Park at the far end of a parking lot and walk to the office or store. Get off public transportation a few blocks before your stop. Get up from your desk during the day to stretch and walk around. Take a brisk walk when you get the urge to snack. Increase your pace when working in the house or yard. Mow your own lawn and rake your own leaves. Carry your own groceries.

Encourage clients to set a reasonable goal for movement/exercise and how to gradually increase expectations. Encourage clients to check with their health care practitioner prior to starting a movement/exercise program.

Here are some tips to help clients make exercise a habit: Choose an activity you enjoy. Tailor your program to your own fitness level. Set realistic goals. Choose an exercise that fits your lifestyle. Give your body a chance to adjust to your new routine. Don't get discouraged if you don't see immediate results. When you do see results, congratulate and reward yourself with a new pair of walking shoes or new workout clothes. Don't give up if you miss a day; just get back on track the next day. Find a partner for a little motivation and socialization. Build some rest days into your exercise schedule. Listen to your body. If you have difficulty breathing or experience faintness or prolonged weakness during or after exercise, consult your physician.

It's a good idea to suggest clients choose more than one type of exercise to give the body a thorough workout and to prevent boredom. For example, you could garden on Monday, walk on Tuesday, dance on Wednesday, Tai Chi on Thursday, swim on Friday, bike on Saturday, and weights on Sunday. Counsel them to choose one indoor exercise and one outdoor activity to allow for changes in their schedule or for inclement weather. Very few people live in a temperate climate year-round. Weather extremes do not have to interfere with an exercise routine if clients make some minor adjustments.

When it is hot or humid: Exercise during cooler and/or less humid times of day, such as early morning or evening. Drink plenty of fluids, especially water. Avoid alcohol, which encourages dehydration. Wear light, loose-fitting clothing. Stop at the first sign of muscle cramping or dizziness.

When it is cold: Dress in layers. Wear gloves or mittens to protect your hands. Wear a hat or cap, as up to 40% of body heat is lost through your neck and head. Adjust the size of your shoes if you need to wear thicker socks. Warm up slowly. Drink plenty of fluids; you can get dehydrated in the winter, too. Stop if you experience shivering, drowsiness or disorientation. You may need help for hypothermia.

Year-round safety: Let someone know where you are going and when you are returning. Carry identification when exercising outside the home. Exercise indoors or try mall-walking when the weather is stormy. Build in warm-up and cool-down periods to decrease risk of injury. Avoid strenuous exercise for 1 to 2 hours after eating. Wear sturdy, well-fitting shoes appropriate for the activity. Wear brightly colored clothing when exercising outdoors. Add lights and reflector tape to body or bike when exercising after dark. Wear helmets and safety pads appropriate for the activity. Move against traffic if you must run or walk on the road. Do not wear headphones, since they can distract from observing traffic and safety concerns. Respect pollution alerts and exercise indoors when warnings are posted, especially if diagnosed with heart or lung disease. Avoid areas where traffic is heavy. Clients who are diabetic or have vascular disease must take special care of their feet, changing socks and shoes after exercising and keeping the feet warm and clean (President's Council on Physical Fitness, 2010).

☐ Diet and Action—the Fitness Combo

Clients need to burn off 3,500 calories more than they take in to lose just one pound. When overweight, eating the usual amount of calories while increasing activity is good, but eating fewer calories and being more active is even better. The following is a list of calories used per hour in common activities. Calories burned vary in proportion to body weight, but are approximately 240 per hour for bicycling 6 mph, 410 per hour for bicycling at 12 mph, 740 per hour for jogging at 5.5 mph, 920 for jogging at 7 mph, 650 for running in place for an hour, 1280 for running for an hour, 750 for jumping rope for an hour, 700 for an hour of cross-country skiing, 275 for swimming 25 yards/minute, 500 for swimming 50 yards/minute, 400 for playing tennis singles for an hour, 240 for walking 2.0 miles per hour, 440 for walking 4.0 miles per hour (American Heart Association, 2012).

Before clients make any major dietary changes, counsel them to check with their healthcare practitioner. However, there are plenty of small changes clients can make on their own, such as avoiding sweets and salty foods and cutting down on fat in their diet, especially saturated fat found in cheese, burgers, and anything fried.

☐ Using Exercise for Depression

Exercise has been used to reduce depression (Murphy et al., 2012). Some tips that can help reduce depression by exercising appear in TABLE 9-5.

☐ Exercise for Special Populations

Probably the best exercise for clients of all ages and conditions is walking. Exercises for bedridden clients are presented in TABLE 9-6.

Additional resource for exercise:
Using Pilates to reduce neck and back pain http://www.youtube.com /watch?v=vYpetZ9aQA8

Table 9-5 Tips for Reducing Depression By Exercising

When using exercise for depression, keep the following considerations in mind:

1. Use a slow, graduated exercise program. It fosters a sense of mastery, a positive self-image, and cathartic relief.
2. Walk with a companion who walks at about the same speed and is not competitive. (An indication of noncompetitiveness is the ability to make complimentary comments regardless of fitness level.)
3. Keep moving even if fatigue necessitates a slow walk.
4. Keep a log of activity for self-motivation, reinforcement of the activity, and to chronicle progress.
5. Make a contract with a peer or practitioner providing a substantial bonus for success and a meaningful penalty for failure.
6. Synchronize breathing with movement; Feldenkrais and yoga are possible interventions to combine with an exercise program to help with synchronization.
7. Provide more extrinsic rewards for novice exercisers until they build their own, intrinsic rewards.

HEALTH PROMOTION CHALLENGE

Try each of the interventions in Table 9-4. Record your results and share them with at least two other students. Decide how you might use this information with clients to promote health.

Table 9-6 Exercises for Bedridden Clients

NOTE: Ask client to breathe throughout all exercises.

1. Raise the head from the pillow as far as possible; add one raise of the head a week to a maximum of 10 repetitions.
2. Turn the head slowly to the left and then to the right; add one turn of the head per week to a maximum of 10 repetitions.
3. Shrug the shoulders up and back toward the ears as far as possible; add one repetition per week to a total of 10 repetitions.
4. Rotate the shoulders clockwise and then counterclockwise, five times in each direction.
5. Bring the right arm (fully extended) over the head, left arm at side; bring down right arm to the side of the body and bring the left arm (fully extended) over the head. Work up to a maximum of 10 repetitions.
6. Cross the wrists at the abdomen and circle both arms at the same time, first clockwise and then counterclockwise; work up to 10 repetitions.
7. Clench the fists tightly and hold for several seconds, then extend the fingers and reach up as far as possible; work up to 10 repetitions.
8. Extend the arms forward and spread the fingers as far as possible; work up to 10 repetitions.
9. Make a fist and rotate the thumbs clockwise and then counterclockwise; work up to 10 repetitions.
10. Raise the right leg up as far as possible and return it to the bed, keeping the leg as straight as possible without straining the lower back; work up to 10 repetitions each leg.
11. Grasp the right knee with both hands and very slowly pull it toward the chest while slowly moving the head toward the knee; work up to 5 repetitions with each knee.
12. Grasp both knees with both hands and very slowly pull them toward the chest while slowly moving the head toward the knees; work up to 10 repetitions.
13. With arms at sides of the body, slowly raise the head, shoulders, and legs several inches; hold, then return to lie flat; work up to 3 repetitions.
14. Extend both ankles toward the bottom of the bed; hold, then flex them toward the shins, hold, then relax. Work up to 10 repetitions.
15. Bicycle both legs slowly, completing up to 10 circles.
16. Lie on the stomach with chin resting on hands. Put heels apart and big toes together; squeeze the buttocks together as though trying to prevent a bowel movement; while squeezing, bring the heels slowly together and hold for 2–3 seconds, then relax on the bed. Work up to 5 repetitions.
17. Lie on the left side in a straight line and raise the left leg as high as possible over the other leg; hold, then return it to the bed. Work up to 10 repetitions. Turn on right side and raise left leg up to 10 repetitions.
18. Raise hips 5"6" off the bed, keeping arms at sides; hold several seconds, then relax into the bed. Work up to 5 repetitions.

HEALTH PROMOTION CHALLENGE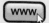

Develop a protocol for using the exercises for bedridden clients information in Table 9-6 and plan a date and place to implement it.

RESEARCH BOX 9-7   Physical Activity and Arthritis

» BACKGROUND: Most women with arthritis are insufficiently active, despite the health benefits derived from participation in moderate physical activity (MPA). Understanding perceived barriers that make it difficult for women with arthritis to be active is needed to inform interventions. Barriers are often assessed through investigator-provided lists, containing mainly general, personal, and situational barriers, common across populations (e.g., lack of time). Identifying an encompassing range of problematic barriers that challenge women's activity participation is needed. Such barriers may be general or arthritis specific (e.g., pain). Problematic barriers may be best identified through assessment of whether individuals actually experience these barriers (i.e., are present) and, for present barriers, their extent of limitation on activity.

» PURPOSE: The primary study purpose was to examine whether the presence of general and arthritis-specific barrier categories and the limitation of these overall categories were significant predictors of participation in MPA among women with arthritis (n = 248).

» METHODS: On-line measures of barriers and MPA were completed.

» FINDINGS: A multiple regression model predicting activity was significant (r(2)(adjusted) = .22; p < .01). Both arthritis-specific and general barrier limitation were the strongest predictors of activity. Arthritis-specific personal barriers were reported as being present most often (e.g., pain).

» CONCLUSION: Interventions should identify problematic barriers, taking into account the extent to which both general and disease-specific barriers limit activity, and then target their alleviation through the use of coping strategies as a way to improve activity adherence and health among women with arthritis.

Source: Brittain, D. R., Gyurcsik, N. C., McElroy, M., & Hillard, S. A. (2010). General and arthritis-specific barriers to moderate physical activity in women with arthritis. *Womens Health Issues, 21*(1), 57–63.

HEALTH PROMOTION CHALLENGE

What coping strategies would you teach women with arthritis who are resistive to exercise?

Imagery

Imagery has been mentioned throughout most of recorded history. Hippocrates, the father of medicine, used it. Aristotle believed that images could change body function, create illness, and assist healing. Freud believed that bringing images to consciousness was a basic growth process, and Jung was also convinced of the power of images (Epstein, 2004).

Imagery is a process that involves the use of symbols to imagine the changes the individual desires taking place. This may include imagining that their problem is like many other familiar situations that are curable like cuts, bruises, a sore throat, and other conditions.

The body has its own healing system and imagery helps clients tap into it. Everyone has had experiences with self-generated images, from dreams and daydreams to fantasies. These images are generated by the right side of the brain.

While visualization has been used for many centuries, it gained a lot of attention in the early 1970s when clients diagnosed with cancer were encouraged to use imagery to fight cancer cells in their bodies. Since then, clients have been encouraged by nurses and other healthcare practitioners to imagine the cells of their immune system attacking the cancer cells and watching the cancer cells being subdued. Scientific research has looked into guided imagery and found that the nervous system can alter cancer metastasis and tumor growth (Ondicova & Mravec, 2010).

☐ Theoretical Model for Imagery

Orenstein's (1972) model postulates that imagery allows direct access to the subconscious and autonomic nervous system function. It bypasses the left brain, which has a tendency to try to solve problems in a logical manner. Although useful in many situations, when the logical approach goes awry, rumination and repetitive worrying occur, raising stress and anxiety. Imagery can bypass rumination to the essential core of the problem.

Rossman (1993) also adds to the theoretical and conceptual basis for imagery. According to him, the mind does not differentiate between the image of a situation and the actual experience. Practicing imagery in a relaxing, safe environment provides experience that can be used in a stressful, real-life situation. Positron emission tomography (PET) has demonstrated that the same parts of the cerebral cortex are activated whether imagining a situation or actually experiencing it (Rossman, 1993).

☐ Uses for Imagery

There are four basic ways to use guided imagery:

1. *Decreasing negative feelings.* When using guided imagery in this mode, help clients identify feelings, dissatisfactions, tensions, and images that are affecting body functioning and change them to helpful elements. Ask clients to get into a relaxed position and state and then ask them to picture the negative feelings, picture a container to hold them, put the feelings inside the container, put a tight lid on it, and lock it tightly so they no longer exert any influence.

2. *Healing.* When you use guided imagery for healing, you help clients erase bacteria or viruses; build new cells to replace damaged ones; make rough areas smooth, hot areas cool, sore areas comfortable, or tense areas relaxed; drain swollen areas, release pressure from tight areas, bring blood

to areas that need nutrients or cleansing, make moist areas dry or dry areas moist, bring energy to fatigued areas, and enhance general wellness.

Ask the client what needs healing and to "go inside yourself and describe what you see in that area." If clients don't provide much description, ask, "What color is the area?" and "What temperature is the area?" Once a color and temperature have been identified, ask the client to "Make that dark area lights" or "Make that red area a cool, soothing color," or "Make that gray, cold area pink and warm." A general rule is to prescribe picturing the opposite of what the client describes or to "picture the area that needs healing so it looks like a healthy area."

3. *Problem solving.* Used this way, clients learn to consult their intuitive sources of wisdom in a structured way or break down barriers to clear thinking. Help the client to get into a relaxed position and state, then ask, "Tell me in three or four words what the problem is." Once you have a clear idea, ask, "Are you ready to solve this problem?" If the answer is "yes," proceed to the next step. Otherwise, select another problem. Ask the client to picture a clearly defined problem in a bordered frame. Ask the client to "See the solution to the problem in another frame, using a different color to create a border around the solution." If the client cannot complete the task, ask them to spend time practicing the exercise until they are successful.

4. *Preparing for upcoming situations.* By working back and forth between feeling relaxed and picturing a feared upcoming situation, clients can teach their bodies to stay relaxed in future situations. Ask clients to choose an upcoming, anxiety-provoking situation for practice. Assist clients to close their eyes, attain a relaxed state, and signal you by raising the index finger of their left hand when they feel relaxed and comfortable. Ask the client to "Imagine yourself as the director of a movie that you are going to run in your mind's eye. As director, you can stop or start the movie at any point that discomfort occurs. Picture everything about the situation, what is said, what you feel, what the other people say or do, smells, sounds, sensations. When you notice yourself becoming uncomfortable, stop the movie in your mind and go back to focusing on relaxing your body. When you've relaxed again, begin the movie a second before you became anxious. Work back and forth between relaxing and running your movie until you complete the whole scene and feel satisfied and relaxed."

❑ Deciding When to Use Imagery

When descriptions by clients are vivid enough that a picture can be formed, guided imagery may be the approach of choice. It is a versatile modality that is often combined with relaxation therapy, music therapy, and self-hypnosis.

If clients are wary of the procedure or have difficulty obtaining a clear image, it may be useful to have them touch an object, then close their eyes and picture it. Another way to enhance imaging skill is to ask the client to view a movie, then close the eyes and picture a critical scene.

HEALTH PROMOTION CHALLENGE

How can you use the information in RESEARCH BOX 9-8 to use guided imagery with clients? Share your ideas with at least two other students and ask for feedback.

RESEARCH BOX 9-8   Self-Management for Osteoarthritis

» BACKGROUND/AIM: Supporting safe self-management interventions for symptoms of osteoarthritis (OA) may reduce the personal and societal burden of this increasing health concern. Self-management interventions might be even more beneficial if symptom control were accompanied by decreased medication use, reducing cost and potential side effects. Guided imagery with relaxation (GIR) created especially for OA may be a useful self-management intervention, reducing both symptoms and medication use.

» DESIGN: A longitudinal randomized assignment experimental design was used to study the efficacy of GIR in reducing pain, improving mobility, and reducing medication use. Thirty older adults were randomly assigned to participate in the 4-month trial by using either GIR or a sham intervention, planned relaxation. Repeated-measures analysis of variance revealed that, compared with those who used the sham intervention, participants who used GIR had a significant reduction in pain from baseline to month 4 and significant improvement in mobility from baseline to month 2.

» FINDINGS: Poisson technique indicated that, compared with those who used the sham intervention, participants who used GIR had a significant reduction in over-the-counter (OTC) medication use from baseline to month 4, prescribed analgesic use from baseline to month 4, and total medication (OTC, prescribed analgesic, and prescribed arthritis medication) use from baseline to month 2 and month 4. Results of this study support the efficacy of GIR in reducing symptoms, as well as in reducing medication use.

» RELEVANCE TO CLINICAL PRACTICE: Guided imagery with relaxation may be useful in the regimen of pain management.

Source: Baird, C. L., Murawski, M. M., & Wu, J. (2010). Efficacy of guided imagery with relaxation for osteoarthritis symptoms and medication intake. *Pain Management Nursing,* *11*(1), 56–65.

Journal Writing

A journal is a book of dated writings. It can contain the day's events, or the writer's feelings, dreams, dialogues, or fantasies. The journal is a tool for recording the process of a life, but the entries also integrate musculoskeletal processes with memory and sensory systems to promote harmony and wholeness (Snyder, 1998).

Journaling is a teaching technique that provides the opportunity for learners to reflect on and analyze their life experiences (Mayo, 1996). Through the journaling process, clients can learn to identify thoughts, feelings, and behavior patterns, as well as solve problems. Because the record is permanent, clients can return to passages again and again to glean new responses to a pattern. While thought patterns often become repetitive and memory fades, a journal preserves the essence of an experience. Working with a journal can also assist clients to think logically and in a goal-oriented manner. Although writing in a journal or talking to a good listener produce comparable effects, it is not always easy to find a suitable ear (Segal & Murray, 1994).

Progoff (1975) developed an Intensive Journal method for helping individuals move through uncertain times of transition. This method helps participants to identify stoppages, readjustments, or difficult decisions and restructure life goals. Some of the areas Progoff used are Steppingstone Periods, Intersections, Roads Taken and Not Taken, Reconstructing an Autobiography, Dialogue with Persons, Dialogue with Works, Dialogue with Body, Dialogue with Events, and Situations and Circumstances.

The main attribute of a journal process is to promote self-understanding. Often, clients have a clear sense that something is wrong in their lives, but are unable to identify what that something is. Journal writing can help to focus on a portion of life experience and uncover major concerns.

☐ Theoretical Underpinnings

Writing requires the client to simultaneously represent ideas in all three of Jerome Bruner's modes of representation—enactive, ikonic, and symbolic—forcing a degree of thought integration not found in other modes of expression. Feedback and opportunity for reflection are also cited as powerful writing features that support learning (Bruner, 1990).

☐ Research Base for Journal Writing

Several studies (Davison, 1999; Johnson & Kelly, 1990; Pennebaker, 1997; Pennebaker & Bell, 1986; Petrie et al., 1995; Spera et al., 1994) used writing as a healing tool. This work is based on research showing that inhibiting strong feelings gradually undermines the body's defenses. Like other stressors, it can inhibit the immune, cardiovascular, and nervous systems. Confession in writing can neutralize the effect of inhibition. (Epstein, Sloan, & Marx, 2005; Kearns, Edward, Calhoun, & Gidycz, 2010).

☐ Uses of Journaling

Disclosure through writing can be used to help clients faced with chronic or life-threatening illnesses process and understand the role of their condition in their lives. This type of writing can also assist clients to develop conceptions of the cause and impact of the condition.

Journaling also provides a context for change. In order for change to occur, clients must prepare interior acceptance for change and provide internal and external suppor systems for making change. Journal work can provide both (Baldwin, 1977).

Specific individuals who may benefit from journal writing include those faced with heart disease, cancer, pain (especially backache and headache), downsizing, childhood asthma, secrets clients fear to disclose, depression, eating disorders, and death or separation from important others. See TABLE 9-7 for specific directions for using journal writing with clients to enhance health.

Table 9-7 Specific Directions for Using Journal Writing with Clients

Ask clients to purchase a journal that has meaning for them. The size, color, number of pages, etc. is dependent on what feels right for the client. Choose a writing implement that allows for free-flowing writing. Sit in a quiet place for a few moments in stillness. Let the breathing become slow and deep. Begin writing by saying to yourself: "I'm thinking about ___ (topic)," remembering that journaling is not writing down facts, but rather allowing deeper thoughts and feelings to rise up from inside. This free-flowing writing pays no attention to the structure of what is written; nothing is censored. Trust the process of resonance that occurs as the flow of energy produces words. Begin a journal entry entitled "Expectations of myself" and use the information to remember how expectations can sabotage growth. Constantly question: What am I leaving out of this entry? Do I forgive myself and others for past experiences? What family myths am I still adhering to that prevent me from being totally honest in my journaling? Always let the original writing stand, but go back frequently to re-read entries and add to them after the original entry, as new ideas and memories surface.

HEALTH PROMOTION CHALLENGE

Based on the results of this study, pair up with another student, who takes the role of client, to plan and implement a program that uses journal writing to reduce anxiety or depression.

RESEARCH BOX 9-9 Effect of Journaling on Anxiety and Depression

» AIM: In this study, researchers investigated the extent to which outpatient psychotherapy clients benefited from Pennebaker's expressive writing protocol adapted for use as a homework intervention.

» DESIGN: Participants were randomly assigned to written emotional disclosure or writing control conditions. Pre- and post-intervention outcome measures were collected for three consecutive therapy sessions.

» FINDINGS: Clients in the written emotional disclosure group showed significantly greater reductions in anxiety and depressive symptoms as well as greater overall progress in psychotherapy in comparison to the writing control group.

» RELEVANCE TO CLINICAL PRACTICE: Results suggest that emotional disclosure writing homework, in conjunction with outpatient psychotherapy, facilitates therapeutic process and outcome.

Source: Graf, M. C., Gaudiano, B. A., & Geller, P. A. (2008). Written emotional disclosure: a controlled study of the benefits of expressive writing homework in outpatient psychotherapy. *Psychotherapy Research, 18*(4), 389–399.

Meditation

Meditation is a self-directed practice that is used to relax the body and calm the mind. During the practice of meditation, the mind settles down into a silent state and the body's internal mechanisms repair the body, providing physiological benefits, including: synchronous alpha, theta, and beta waves as indicated by an electroencephalogram (EEG); light and/or suspended breathing pattern; decreased heart rate; decreased plasma cortisol, TSH, and lactate; increased plasma prolactin and phenylalanine; and redistribution of blood flow away from the abdomen and toward the brain (Peressutti, Martin-Gonzalez, Garcia-Manso, & Mesa, 2009). Meditation has been utilized to reduce stress and anxiety, enhance general well-being, and expand awareness (Yang, 2010). See TABLE 9-8.

☐ Types of Meditation

1. **Transcendental meditation** (TM) is the most well-known type of meditation. Transcendental meditation is the process of focusing on a thought or word, called a *mantra*, until attention transcends its common meaning. As a result of this focus, subtler meanings of thought are perceived. It is believed that **prana**, the cosmic vibratory energy of the universe, connects the individual to a transcendental existence during which slow, rhythmic, nasal and abdominal breathing prevail. Unlike

Table 9-8 Guidelines for Meditation

1. Choose a time to meditate that is at least 2 hours after eating; digestion interferes with meditation.
2. Select a quiet place where you will not be disturbed.
3. Sit in a comfortable position in a chair with a straight back.
4. Close your eyes.
5. Use a relaxation exercise or relaxation tape to prepare for meditation.
6. Focus on your breathing, allowing the breath to go in and out effortlessly.
7. Use your focus word (or symbol) or focus on your chosen object for at least 20–30 minutes for each meditation session.
8. Meditate at least daily, preferably twice a day.
9. Understand it may take 6–7 teaching sessions to learn meditation and about a month of practice may be needed before significant mind–body change occurs.
10. Avoid meditating if any of the following occur; light-headedness, hallucinations, depression, or suicidal thoughts.
11. If taking any medication, discuss the effects of meditation on dosage.(Meditation frequently results in needing a smaller dosage of insulin, sedatives, and cardiovascular medications.)

breathing exercises, in TM, breathing is not guided. There is no attempt to interfere with breathing. It is simply allowed to happen.

2. **Centering prayer** is another kind of meditation, but is more Christian-based. This type of meditation is designed to withdraw attention from the ordinary flow of thoughts by focusing on a sacred word.

3. **Mindfulness meditation** is used to help the client remain a detached observer of internal mental processes. The stream of thoughts, feelings, drives, and images that occur are focused on in turn without being considered an intrusion. The here-and-now becomes the focus for this approach. The client stays in a relaxed, observer role while attending to activities in both inner and outer worlds.

4. Even walking and counting can be considered meditative. Anything that keeps the mind from straying will work.

☐ Research Base

Meditation can reduce stress related to organ transplant (Gross et al., 2010), reduce anxiety and depression (Leite et al., 2010), reduce sleep need (Kurtz, Kaul, Passafiume, Sargent, & O'Hara, 2010), decrease heart rate and blood pressure (Zeidan, Johnson, Gordon, & Goolkasian, 2010), reduce alcohol dependence (Garland, Gaylord, Boettiger, & Howard, 2010), enhance cerebral blood flow (Newberg, Waldman, Amen, Khalsa, & Alavi, 2010), reduce pain (Goyal et al., 2010), and reduce stress and disability in breast and gynecological cancer (Loizzo et al., 2010).

RESEARCH BOX 9-10   Mindfulness Meditation

» OBJECTIVES: This study evaluated whether a mindfulness meditation intervention may be effective in caregivers of close relatives with dementia and helped refine the protocol for future larger trials.

» OBJECTIVES: This study evaluated whether a mindfulness meditation intervention may be effective in caregivers of close relatives with dementia and helped refine the protocol for future larger trials.

» DESIGN: The researchers used a pilot randomized trial to evaluate the effectiveness of a mindfulness meditation intervention adapted from the Mindfulness-Based Cognitive Therapy program in relation to two comparison groups: an education class based on Powerful Tools for Caregivers served as an active control group, and a respite-only group served as a pragmatic control.

» SETTINGS/LOCATION: Data were collected at the Oregon Health & Science University, Portland, OR.

» SAMPLE: The participants included community-dwelling caregivers, aged 45–85 years, of close relatives with dementia.

» INTERVENTIONS: The two active interventions lasted 7 weeks, and consisted of one 90-minute meditation session per week along with at-home implementation of knowledge learned. The respite-only condition provided the same duration of respite care that was needed for the active interventions.

» OUTCOME MEASURES: Participants were assessed prior to randomization and again after completing classes at 8 weeks. The primary outcome measure was a self-rated measure of caregiver stress, the Revised Memory and Behavior Problems Checklist (RMBPC). Secondary outcome measures included mood, fatigue, self-efficacy, mindfulness, salivary cortisols, cytokines, and cognitive function. The researchers also evaluated self-rated stress in the subjects' own environment, expectancy of improvement, and credibility of the interventions.

» RESULTS: There were 31 caregivers randomized and 28 who completed the study. There was an intervention effect on the caregiver self-efficacy measure and on cognitive measures. Although mindfulness was not impacted by the intervention, there were significant correlations between mindfulness and self-rated mood and stress scores.

» CONCLUSIONS: Both mindfulness and education interventions decreased the self-rated caregiver stress compared to the respite-only control.

Source: Oken, B. S., Fonareva, I., Haas, M., Wahbeh, H., Lane, J. B., Zajdel, D., & Amen, A. (2010). Pilot controlled trial of mindfulness meditation and education for dementia caregivers. *Journal of Alternative and Complementary Medicine, 16*(10), 1031–1038.

HEALTH PROMOTION CHALLENGE

How would you change the design of the study to provide you with different information?

Qigong

For thousands of years, the Taoists researched the connection between body and mind. Nine Palaces of **Qigong** is a powerful practice that cleanses and balances the body through a combination of movement, visualization, and specialized breathing. Nine is a sacred number in this system. It is the number of Heaven and signifies the fusion of Yin and Yang.

A big advantage of Qigong is that being healthy or fit is not a pre-requisite to do any of the exercises, yet they tone the muscles of the back, legs, and abdomen while increasing the circulation in the hands, feet, ears, and blood-rich stomach channels. After a few months of practice, digestion, sleep, inflexibility, common colds, and gastric problems can become a thing of the past (Wu, 2006).

☐ Theoretical Background

The nine openings in the body (eyes, ears, nostrils, mouth, urethra, and anus) are related to nine major internal organs. In Chinese Medicine, the kidneys are associated with the ears. The urethra is connected to the bladder and uterus, the and anus connects to the intestines, the mouth to the stomach and spleen.

Qigong helps to protect against toxic substances linked to cancer and other illnesses by increasing the power of the body's own currents. The practice forms a protective sheath around an individual's delicate cellular and neural circuitry, just as a surge protector safeguards a computer during a thunderstorm.

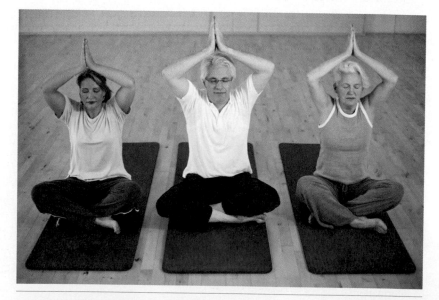

FIGURE 9-2 Qigong Exercises

The steady practice of Qigong can protect the immune system. Combined with specialized stretches that open up the meridian points along the length of the spine, nerve impulses can be sent unobstructed to all body organs, enhancing the body's self-healing properties.

By using controlled breathing, the internal organs are massaged and toned. Qigong also teaches the body to use the skin surface to stimulate and detoxify the organs and circulatory systems (Wu, 2006).

Use TABLE 9-9 to practice Qigong and aid clients in learning movements that can promote health.

Table 9-9 How to Practice Qigong

- Avoid practicing on a carpet.
- Wear flat shoes that enclose the foot securely.
- Wear breathable clothes that do not restrict the waist.
- To attract Qi most similar to your own, wear a color that corresponds to the season of your birth: green for spring, red for summer, yellow or orange for Indian summer, white for fall, and black for winter.
- Whenever possible, practice outside, facing the sun, around trees and plants to surround yourself with Qi that nourishes the body; if unable to be outside in the sun, face south to do the exercises. If that isn't possible, stand in a spot that makes you feel comfortable.
- Avoid practicing near bodies of still water such as swimming pools. Standing by a waterfall or the ocean is purifying. A backyard, park, or balcony will work, although it is always better to have the feet directly on the ground.
- Early in the morning, about 6 a.m., is the best time to practice. If this isn't possible, practice at time when you can be calm and focused. No matter what time you practice, the most important thing is to practice every day.
- Empty your mind and body of all concerns (Wu, 2006).

Try each of these as you read through and jot down the changes in your body.

1. *Nourishing your essence.* Sit upright in a chair, at the edge of the seat so that your back is straight. Put your hands palm up on the knees and press the soles of the feet together for a moment. This will collect your Qi and create a space to practice inside you. Put the feet back on the floor, legs together, but slightly apart. Rest the back of the right hand on the palm of the left hand. With the thumb and first finger of the left hand, encircle the right palm, pressing into the center of the palm with the thumb and the back of the hand with the forefinger. Hold the hands clasped in this position at the level of the genitals, keeping the arms relaxed and the elbows bent. Touch the tip of the tongue to the roof of the mouth behind the front teeth. Close your eyes and hold in the energy behind them. Feel your eyeballs relax and close off your ears from the outside world. Inhale through the nose and exhale through the nose and pores of the skin. If you do only one exercise, do this one.

(continues)

Table 9-9 (Continued)

2. *Awakening the body.* Flick the fingers outward in a burst, striking the fronts of the ears. The ear is a miniature representation of the body, including all the acupuncture points, meridians, and organs. Flicking the ears vigorously activates the entire physical structure. In Chinese medicine, the ears represent the kidneys and even look like kidneys. Flicking the ears also increases the blood circulation and can enhance memory and strengthen the hands. Now flick the fingers from the back of the ears (believed to help regulate blood pressure) nine times, then rub from the back to the front of the ears nine times. For cold, flu, or ear infection symptoms, flick the ears throughout the day. Next, using the thumb and forefinger, gently squeeze the rims of the ear, pinching them nine times from the top to the bottom, ending with a tug on the ear lobes. Place the hands on the ears and create a suction cup, then pull out from the ears nine times; think of it as a plunger unlocking a backed-up toilet, dislodging accumulated debris in the ear ducts and canal. This stimulates the kidneys; reduces motion sickness, dizziness, and problems with plane take offs and landings; and improves hearing.

3. *Beating the Heavenly Drum.* With the hands pressed firmly over the ears and the fingers resting on the back of the head, cross the forefingers over the middle fingers and then flick down with them onto the soft spot at the base of the skull. This is the terminal nerve bundle of the spinal cord (feng fu point). Any tightness or constriction here will restrict blood flow and nerve impulses to and from the brain. Repeat 9 or 13 times to correct blood flow, posture, pain, fatigue, slurred speech, difficulties standing upright, blood pressure, heart problems, and insomnia.

4. *Neck Self-Massage.* Start at the base of the skull and squeeze as much of the width of the back of the neck as much as possible between the heel of the palm and the fingers of the right hand. Work down to slightly below the juncture of the shoulders and neck. For a deeper massage, tilt the head slightly the left and dig into the right side of the spine with the fingertips of the left hand. The main object of Taoist massage is to warm the neck and increase circulation. Once that is accomplished, the muscles relax on their own. Be sure to inhale four beat to one beat for an exhale to allow more Qi to flow into the spine. Neck massage is used to check the buildup of bone spurs and disk erosion; keeping the neck supple is the Taoist route to longevity.

5. *Neck exercises.* Remember to breathe in sync with the heartbeat and stretch the neck out and down as far as it can go, pressing the chin into the chest, opening all the muscles from the back of the neck to the top of the head and back down to the chest. Squeezing firmly into the chest keeps the spine and back muscles aligned and shoots energy into the brain. With practice, you can feel the opening down the back all the way to the heels. If you sit all day, practice this exercise throughout the day to reduce fatigue, as should women who wear high heels. After stretching the neck down, tilt the head back as you stretch upward, lifting the entire neck, not just the chin. Remember to breathe through each exercise. Tilt the head to the right shoulder, then the left, always keeping the shoulders down, following the rhythm of the breath. Neck rolls can coordinate you with the earth's rotation.

Table 9-9 (Continued)

6. *Neck stretch.* Being gentle, place the left hand on top of the head near the hairline and bring the right hand up under the chin, cupping it with the soft mound at the base of the thumb. Keep the jaw relaxed and tug the head down three times toward ear. Switch hands and repeat, sending energy into the brain and never forcing the head. This stretch can prevent TMJ, headache, teeth grinding, and bone spurs in the neck. Repeat nine times.

7. *Neck pinch.* Grasp the soft skin at the base of the neck between the thumb and fingers of the left hand. Pinch the skin and pull it out away from the head. This movement can improve eyesight, glaucoma, and astigmatism; lower eye pressure; and reduce redness, burning, and dark circles under the eyes.

8. *The shoulder twist.* Cross the arms and grasp the shoulders, holding onto the back with your fingers. Keep the chin tucked into the neck at all times as you twist the body as far as you can comfortably go left and then right for nine times. You should feel the spine, waist, hips, and rib cage twist from one side to the other. This twist exercises every segment of the spine and all the internal organs.

9. *For back pain or trauma to internal organs.* Crawl on all fours for 10 minutes every morning to ease the pressure on the viscera and spine. Keep shoulders loose and arms hanging lightly. With a comfortable, balanced spine, it's possible to regain the sensitivity to impending weather changes animals never lost.

10. *Bring Qi to the kidneys.* Reach out and grab the Qi with the thumb, first, and second fingers of both hands. Keeping the legs straight, reach down and rotate your fingers around the knee caps; circle both kneecaps at once in a clockwise direction at least 27 times a day, feeling the knees being nourished. The meridians to the kidney run down the back of the legs, so this exercise can help nourish the kidneys.

11. *Stimulate the brain.* While standing and with hands in front like holding onto a giant beach ball, rock back on the heels then up on the toes. If worried about balance, stand with your back near to a wall. This exercise also strengthens the back and abdominal muscles. Continue rocking until waist is warm and feet are hot. Toxins are being shaken down to the feet. The exercise also balances the kidneys and calms an overactive heart.

12. *For digestion and constipation.* Lean forward a bit to relax abdominal muscles. Using the thumbs, knead down the abdomen to the flesh under the pubic bone, then squeeze and pull out with a quick movement as though allowing built up tension to escape. Repeat twice more. Then do three repetitions with the fingers interlaced and rub down with the fatty part of the heel of the hand. Massaging at the pubic bone may be helpful for menstrual pain, impotence, and premature ejaculation. The full abdominal massage is thought to help with weight loss and digestion.

(continues)

Table 9-9 (Continued)

13. *The Second Heart.* Women put their left hand over the right, men the right over the left, covering the abdomen. Stand straight and kick down the center of the back of the left calf with the edge of the right food straight down to the ankle. Repeat nine times. Then switch and kick down with the edge of the left foot. Heavy toxins in the body tend to settle in this area. The stomach channel and the spleen channel are found on either side of the calf muscle. If there are problems with the heart, this is the area that is treated in Taoist medicine. Kicking is a wonderful self-massage technique and standing on one foot enhances the sense of body alignment and gravity. Standing tall with head straight ahead will help maintain balance. If balance is a problem, use a sturdy chair to hold onto while doing this exercise. Calf-kicking is helpful when fatigued, after a long hike or being on your feet all day, when feeling a tightness over the heart, or when the body feels swollen or tender.

14. *Sending the eyes out.* This exercise clears the eye/liver channel and promotes healing in hepatitis, chronic fatigue, eyestrain, cataracts, and glaucoma. While standing, raise the hands, gently bent and facing the body, at eye level, pinkies aligned with eyebrows. With eyes closed and breathing steady, imagine your eyes opening and looking outward to the centers of the palms. Picture the eyes looking straight through the palms and out into the room. Try to see the room around you up through the ceiling and outside, even high above the city streets, maybe to the ocean, then to distant horizons, through the sky and clouds to outer space. Try to open your third eye between your eyes at brow level, and continue looking out through space. Bring your eyeballs back to your palms and visualize the color green. Feel the warmth from your palms pass down into your liver. Then remove your hands from your eyes and place them on the liver. If you taste a sour flavor like a salted plum in your mouth, you have opened your liver meridian. Practice will help if the taste doesn't happen the first time.

15. *Wake up the kidneys.* Stand with feet 1–2 feet apart; choose the distance that makes it possible to lean over and reach the small of the back above the waist. First, flick the fingertips on one hand against the fingertips of the other hand. Then, flick the hands at the wrists. This will bring energy into the hands. Now, bend over and rub the kidneys.

16. *Stimulate the brain.* Stand with feet 4–5 inches apart. Put the hands out in front as if holding a big beach ball. Rock forward, bringing the heels up off the floor or ground, then rock back onto the heels.

17. *Spin a cocoon.* With legs a few feet apart and knees bent, place a hand on the opposite shoulder and make figure eights back and forth from one side of the body to the other. This loosens the shoulders, neck, hips, and spine.

HEALTH PROMOTION CHALLENGE

Based on what you learned about Qigong, develop a plan to use all or portions of the approach to promote health with clients. Discuss your plan with at least two classmates and ask for feedback.

RESEARCH BOX 9-11   Qigong

» OBJECTIVE: The objective of this study was to explore the feasibility and efficacy of adding integrative Qigong meditation to residential treatment for substance abuse.

» METHODS: Qigong meditation, which blends relaxation, breathing, guided imagery, inward attention, and mindfulness to elicit a tranquil state, was introduced into a short-term residential treatment program. At first clients chose to participate in qigong meditation on a voluntary basis during their evening break. Later they chose to participate in either meditation or Stress Management and Relaxation Training (SMART) twice a day as part of the scheduled treatment. Weekly questionnaires were completed by 248 participants for up to 4 weeks to assess their changes in treatment outcomes. Participants in the meditation group were also assessed for quality of meditation to evaluate the association between quality and treatment outcome.

» RESULTS: Most participants were amenable to meditation as part of the treatment program, and two thirds chose to participate in daily meditation. While both groups reported significant improvement in treatment outcome, the meditation group reported a significantly higher treatment completion rate (92% versus 78%, p < .01) and more reduction in craving than did the SMART group. Participants whose meditation was of acceptable quality reported greater reductions in craving, anxiety, and withdrawal symptoms than did those whose meditation was of low quality. Female meditation participants reported significantly more reduction in anxiety and withdrawal symptoms than did any other group.

» CONCLUSIONS: Qigong meditation appears to contribute positively to addiction treatment outcomes, with results at least as good as those of an established stress management program. Results for those who meditate adequately are especially encouraging. Meditative therapy may be more effective or acceptable for female drug abusers than for males. Further study is needed to assess ways to improve substance abusers' engagement and proficiency in meditation.

Source: Chen, K. W., Comerford, A., Shinnick, P., & Ziedonis, D. M. (2010). Introducing qigong meditation into residential addiction treatment: a pilot study where gender makes a difference. *Alternative and Complementary Medicine, 16*(8), 875–882.

Reflexology

Reflexology is the stimulation of reflex points to enhance the functioning of body organs. Reflex points also influence functional relationships to that organ. For example, stimulating the heart reflex on the foot may help balance energy flow to the heart as well as the rest of the circulatory system (blood vessels, lymphatics, etc.). There are other areas with reflex points (wrist, hand, neck, abdomen, face, head, arms, legs, nose, and iris), but the feet are the most effective because; (1) they link with energy from the Earth and are strong energy poles of the body; (2) working on feet is relatively nonthreatening and noninvasive; (3) feet accumulate deposits of acids and tensions (due to the effects of gravity, pressure, and the normal wear and tear of walking upright), causing tissue degeneration, which can easily be felt, seen, and treated; (4) touching the feet is a soothing gesture that can deeply affect others—for example, agitated children can be calmed by rubbing their feet; (5) clearly charted representations of the body organs on the feet are available; (6) because feet are usually covered with shoes and socks, and because there is less body musculature than in most other parts of the body, they remain tender to the touch and more sensitive than some other reflex points; and (7) feet are a symbolic representation of the infinite energy in the universe. Jesus washed the feet of his disciples, linking, cleaning, protecting, and blessing their whole being (Berkson, 1977).

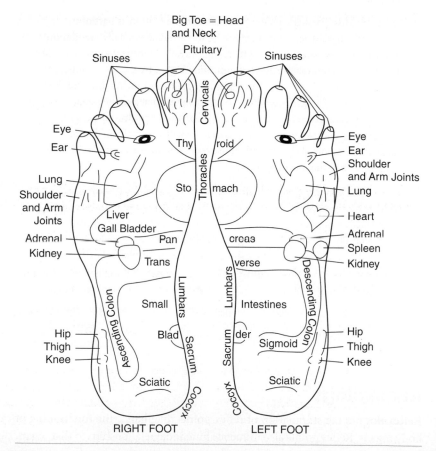

FIGURE 9-3   Foot reflexology points
© Carolyn Chambers Clark, 2010.

☐ Reflexology Assessments

Prior to using reflexology, Berkson (1977) suggested asking the following questions: What does the skin color tell me? Are the heels of the shoes worn evenly? Are the eyes clear? Is the tongue coated? Are the nails strong and hair shiny? What do the client's voice and posture tell me? Which joints rotate easily? Which reflex points are the most tender or the most difficult to relieve? How does bone feel under the skin? How do muscles feel? What temperature differences are there (an even, warm temperature indicates balance)? What differences in texture are there (bunions and calluses can indicate imbalance)? What areas on the foot indicate a hard resistance (indicating tension, deposits, or degeneration, unless a bone, tendon, or ligament resides there)? What areas feel hollow or recessed indicating lack of nutrition and energy imbalance?

☐ Theory of Reflexology

Reflexology is based on the premise that body organs have corresponding reflex points on other parts of the body. The reflex points are believed to be up to 20 times more sensitive than the corresponding organs. The foot is viewed as one of the scanner screens that records body functions. Working the reflexes in the feet helps rebalance organs by releasing blocks that impede the smooth flow of body energy. The thumb and index finger pinch and massage these points. The fingernail can also be used if a point itches. For a very painful spot, go gently and only work on that spot for a few seconds several times a day until the area is not so reactive.

RESEARCH BOX 9-12   Reflexology During Pregnancy

» STUDY PROBLEM: What is the effect of foot massage (reflexology) for decreasing physiological lower leg edema in late pregnancy?

» SAMPLE: The research was conducted between March and August 2007 in Manisa Province Health Ministry Central Primary Health Care Clinic 1, in Manisa, Western Turkey.

» METHOD: Eighty pregnant women were randomly divided into two groups The study group received a 20 minute foot massage daily for 5 days whereas the control group did not receive any intervention beyond standard prenatal care.

» FINDINGS: Compared with the control group, women in the experimental group had a significantly smaller lower leg circumference (right and left ankle, instep, and metatarsal-phalanges joint) after 5 days of massage. The results obtained from our research show that foot massage was found to have a positive effect on decreasing normal physiological lower leg edema in late pregnancy.

Source: Coban, A., & Sirin, A. (2010). Effect of foot massage to decrease physiological lower leg oedema in late pregnancy: a randomized controlled trial in Turkey. *International Journal of Nursing Practice, 16*(5), 454–460.

HEALTH PROMOTION CHALLENGE   www

Using the research design for this study and the foot chart in Figure 9-3, devise a study to test the significance of foot reflexology for clients with a condition other than edema.

Relaxation Procedures

Relaxation procedures have been shown useful for decreasing anxiety and pain (Barsky et al., 2010; Palermo, Eccleston, Lewandowski, Williams, & Morley, 2010).

☐ Theory Base

In 1914, Cannon described the fight or flight response that prepares individuals to fight or run. Physiological changes, include an increase in blood pressure, heart rate, and respiration; peripheral vascular constriction; reduction of testosterone; and release of epinephrine. If stress is chronic, the immune system weakens, transient hypertension can become permanent, stomach upset can turn into colitis or ulcers, and so forth. Stress has been related to many diseases and ailments including headaches, arthritis, colitis, diarrhea, asthma, cardiac arrhythmias, circulatory problems, muscle tension, and cancer. Symptom relief is a powerful motivator for using stress reduction and **relaxation procedures**.

☐ Relaxation Procedures

1. *Breathing.* Breathing is essential for life, yet many of us breathe in the upper part of the chest, not allowing sufficient blood to reach the lungs, brain, and other tissues. Under stress, many people restrict their breathing even further, increasing fatigue, muscular tension, irritability, and anxiety. Breathlessness interventions can help (Howard, Dupont, Haselden, Lynch, & Will, 2010).

   While breathing exercises can be learned readily, it is important to maintain continued practice of them in a nonstressful, relaxing environment to attain full benefits. The first step in enhancing breathing is breathing awareness.

   Steps in enhancing awareness include:
   A. Lie on a rug or blanket on the floor with legs straight and slightly apart; toes pointed comfortably out; arms at sides, not touching the body; palms up; and eyes closed.
   B. Place one hand on the spot that seems to rise and fall during inhalation and exhalation. Place the other hand on the abdomen and think about bringing the breathing to that area. Eventually, breathing will move lower in the body toward the abdomen.

2. *The Relaxation Sigh.* Either sitting or standing, expel a deep sigh upon exhalation. Let a sound of deep relief rush out of the lungs. Allow inhalation to occur naturally. Repeat the procedure as necessary.

3. *Breathing and Imagery.* Breathing can be combined with imagery to provide a powerful healing stimulus. The breath is accomplished in a comfortable position while sitting or lying. The hands are placed on the abdomen. Upon inhalation, energy is pictured rushing into the lungs and moving into the solar plexus for storage. Upon exhalation, energy is pictured flowing to all parts of the body. In the case of an injury or illness, picture energy flowing to the injured or ill part.

4. *Alternate Breath.* The alternate breath has been found useful for general relaxation and to alleviate tension or sinus headache. Directions include:

    1. Sit in a comfortable position using good posture.
    2. Rest the index and second finger of the right hand on the forehead, and the hold the right nostril closed gently with the thumb.
    3. Inhale through the left nostril.
    4. The left nostril is then gently closed with the ring finger, and the right thumb is simultaneously removed from the right nostril.
    5. Air is exhaled slowly and soundlessly through the right nostril.
    6. Continue the cycle of inhaling and exhaling in a slow and even manner.
    7. Five cycles are suggested for beginners, slowly working up to 10 to 25 cycles.

5. *Progressive Relaxation.* Progressive relaxation was developed by Jacobson (1938) and involves tightening and relaxing the muscle groups of the body. See TABLE 9-10 for progressive relaxation directions.

Table 9-10   Directions for Progressive Relaxation

A. Check for relaxation in your arms and legs, the middle of your body, and your head.

B. Agree on a signal, such as raising the index finger of the right hand when relaxation is achieved in a body area.

C. Beginning with your right hand, take 5 to 10 seconds to relax all the muscles in your fingers and palms.

D. Now relax the muscles in lower right arm and upper arm.

E. Relax the muscles in your left hand and arm.

F. Relax the muscles in your right foot and leg.

G. Relax the muscles in your left foot and leg.

H. Relax the muscles in your trunk and all your internal organs.

I. Relax the muscles in your buttocks, lower back, and upper back.

J. Relax the muscles in the neck, back and top of head, jaw, cheeks, eyes, forehead, and ears.

CAUTIONS: Depressed and out of contact clients may withdraw more. Toxic effects of medications may increase as circulation improves. Tightly tensing muscles can increase blood pressure in clients with cardiac conditions; suggest non-tensing relaxation exercises in these cases. For clients who experience heightened pain as a result of focusing their attention on body functions, suggest imagery as the treatment of choice.

Self-Hypnosis

Hypnosis is a wakeful state of deep relaxation that includes an increase in the ability to focus in on a particular situation and being more open to suggestion. Most people have experienced a trance state while concentrating on a book, movie, television program, or work project. All hypnosis is really self-hypnosis because no one will accept suggestion unless ready to do so.

When using self-hypnosis as an intervention, ask the client to listen to a taped relaxation and suggestion session or work with the client directly. With practice, clients can learn to assume a relaxed state rather quickly.

☐ Theory for Hypnosis

A new theory of hypnosis used DNA microarrays to show that hypnosis showed increased brain activity and a reduction in stress and inflammation (Atkinson et al., 2010).

☐ The Importance of Suggestion

Suggestions are used all the time by clients and professionals, e.g., "She'll never recover from this," "It's malignant, the patient doesn't have a chance," "You can't be helped; you'll have to learn to live with your condition." According to hypnosis, people hear and act on suggestions they hear.

☐ Instructions for Self-Hypnosis

1. Prior to practicing self-hypnosis, decide on the suggestions to give while in a highly relaxed and receptive state. Always phrase them in the positive to promote health and confidence, e.g., "I will feel comfortable and confident during the interview tomorrow (as opposed to, "I will not feel tension tomorrow.") Phrase suggestions in a becoming mode, e.g., 'My comfort is gradually increasing," and "I will come out of hypnosis when I'm ready."
2. Sit or lie in a comfortable position.

3. Use a candle, picture, crack in the ceiling, fire in the fireplace, or some other object to encourage eye fixation.
4. While watching the object, suggest your eyes are getting heavier, are beginning to sting, or are starting to flutter (whichever works best) to induce eyelid heaviness.
5. Preselect a word or phrase to use at the moment eyes close. The words, "relax now," or a color or a place that is beautiful and has special meaning to you, can also be used.
6. With eyes closed, begin relaxing all muscles, starting with forearms and biceps; first tighten, then relax them. Move to the face, neck, shoulders, chest, stomach, lower back, buttocks, thighs, calves, and toes.
7. Picture the top of an escalator with the steps moving down in front of you. As you step on, count back slowly from 10 to 0. Repeat counting back slowly for two more floors.
8. Begin to notice a feeling of heaviness in your right arm (if right-handed, or left arm if left-handed). Notice your arm getting lighter and lighter as if balloons are tied to it, lifting it higher and higher. Soon your hand will begin to move, to float, moving closer and closer to you face. When you hand touches your face, you will be in hypnosis. You may feel tingling, warmth, or some other sensations, but whatever you experience will be relaxing.

Smoking Cessation

About 46 million American adults smoke cigarettes, but most smokers are either actively trying to quit or want to quit. Since 1965, more than 49% of all adults who have ever smoked have quit.

☐ American Heart Association Scientific Position

According to the 2004 Surgeon General's Report, *The Health Consequences of Smoking*, eliminating smoking can greatly reduce the occurrence of coronary heart disease and other forms of cardiovascular disease. Smoking cessation is important in the medical management of many contributors to heart attacks, including atherosclerosis (fatty buildups in arteries), thrombosis (blood clots), and coronary artery spasm and cardiac arrhythmia (heart rhythm problems). Quitting smoking also can help manage several other disorders, especially arteriosclerotic peripheral vascular disease (fatty buildups in peripheral arteries) and chronic obstructive pulmonary disease.

According to the Surgeon General, tobacco smoking remains the number one cause of preventable disease and death in the United States. About 23% of adult men and 19% of adult women smoke. This figure is down considerably from 42% in 1965. Changes in smoking habits during the late 1960s, the 1970s, and the 1980s have very likely contributed to the drop in cardiovascular deaths that occurred at the same time.

☐ Why Quit?

After one year off cigarettes, the excess risk of coronary heart disease caused by smoking is reduced by half. After 15 years of abstinence, the risk is similar to that for people who have never smoked. In 5 to 15 years, the risk of stroke for ex-smokers returns to the level of those who have never smoked. Male smokers who quit between ages 35 to 39 add an average of 5 years to their lives, while female quitters in this age group add 3 years. Men and women who quit at ages 65 to 69 increase their life expectancy by 1 year.

More than four in five smokers say they want to quit, and each year about 1.3 million smokers do quit. With good smoking cessation programs, 20–40% of participants are able to quit smoking and stay off cigarettes for at least 1 year. According to the Agency for Healthcare Research and Quality's Treating Tobacco Use and Dependence, new, effective clinical treatments for tobacco dependence have been identified in the past decade. Combining interventions such as physician advice and follow-up with nicotine gum and behavior modification may increase success rates.

HEALTH TIP: Smoking cessation programs seem especially helpful for people who smoke more than 25 cigarettes a day.

☐ American Heart Association Advocacy Position

The American Heart Association advocates for adequate resources for tobacco cessation programs. While prevention programs may be able to prevent new smokers from ever becoming addicted to nicotine, about one-third of tobacco users will die prematurely because of their dependence on tobacco unless treatment efforts are increased. Tobacco-use cessation or treatment programs offer the best hope for helping these people.

☐ Counseling for Smoking Cessation

Self-help materials, the most common type of counseling, were not found to be particularly effective. Both individual counseling and group counseling were found to increase the success rates for cessation of smoking. Proactive

RESEARCH BOX 9-13   Self-Control and Smoking Cessation

» BACKGROUND/HYPOTHESIS: Research has suggested that practicing small acts of self-control can lead to an improvement in self-control performance. Because smoking cessation requires self-control, it was hypothesized that a treatment that builds self-control should help in quitting smoking.

» SAMPLE: A total of 122 smokers were used.

» DESIGN: Participants either practiced small acts of self-control for 2 weeks before quitting smoking or practiced a task that increased their awareness of self-control or feelings of confidence, without exercising self-control. Their smoking status was assessed using daily telephone calls and biochemically verified.

» FINDINGS: Individuals who practiced self-control remained abstinent longer than those who practiced tasks that did not require self-control. Supplemental analyses suggested that the increased survival times were a product of building self-control strength and were not produced by changes in feelings that practicing should help in cessation, effort exerted on the practice task, or thinking more about self-control while practicing.

Source: Muraven, M. (2010). Practicing self-control lowers the risk of smoking lapse. *Psychology of Addictive Behavior, 24*(3), 446–452.

telephone calls are a relatively new form of delivering counseling and are also quite effective. A number of states now have "quit lines" that can provide this kind of proactive counseling to residents at no charge.

Regardless of how counseling is delivered, certain types of information increase the chance of success. A problem-solving approach works well for many smokers. An example of this would be thinking about times of the day one is likely to smoke (e.g., first thing in the morning or after meals) and then planning something to distract oneself when the urge strikes (e.g, leaving the situation or deep breathing). Social support, in the form of encouragement, caring, and concern, clearly increases the success rate of smoking cessation. Social support can come both from healthcare providers (intra-treatment social support) and from family, friends, and other community members (extra-treatment social support) (Jorenby, 2001).

Thought Stopping

Thought stopping is an effective way to reduce and even eliminate negative thoughts that interfere with productive behavior. By interrupting negative and even frightening feelings, stress is reduced.

☐ Theory of Thought Stopping

Thought stopping may work because (a) distraction occurs, (b) the interruption behavior serves as a punishment and what is punished consistently is apt to be inhibited, (c) it is an assertive response and can be followed by reassuring or self-accepting comments, and (d) it interrupts a chain of negative or frightening thoughts leading to negative an frightening feelings, thus reducing stress level (Kenner et al., 2010).

☐ What to Tell Clients about Thought Stopping

1. Choose a problematic thought
2. Bring the nagging thought to attention.
3. Imagine a stressful situation in which the thought is apt to occur.
4. Interrupt the nagging thought with a snap of the fingers, timer, or picturing the word, "STOP."
5. Replace the nagging thought with a positive statement, e.g., "I am confident in my ability to lose weight (exercise, eat well, stop smoking, feel safe, digest my food, etc.)."
6. Practice this sequence for 3 to 7 days for effective mastery.
7. If you cannot totally extinguish the thought, choose a less intrusive thought and success will be easier. After mastering that thought, move to the more intrusive thought; success will be more likely.
8. Intrusive thoughts may recur in the future, especially during stressful times. Repeat the procedure above whenever necessary.

Time Management

Time management can reduce stress at home and at work (Hafner & Stock, 2010). Symptoms of ineffective time management include rushing, fatigue, or listlessness with many slack hours of nonproductive activity, chronic vacillation between unpleasant alternatives, chronic missing of deadlines, insufficient time for rest or personal relationships, and the sense of being overwhelmed by demands and details.

Most methods of time management include three steps: establishing priorities, eliminating low priority tasks, and learning to make decisions.

The first step in time management is exploring how time is currently being spent. An easy way to do this is to divide the day into three segments: waking through lunch, end of lunch through dinner, and end or dinner until bedtime. Carry a small notebook and record the number of minutes for each activity in each time segment. Keep the inventory for 3 days. At the end of the time, note the total amount of time spent in each activity.

Touch

Dr. Dolores Krieger, who developed therapeutic touch, pictures the healer as a person with excess prana, or energy, who has a strong sense of commitment and intention to help clients. The act of healing in therapeutic touch includes the channeling of energy flow by the healer for the well-being of the client. Healers are thought to accelerate the healing process by giving the healee an extra boost to the recuperative system (Krieger, 1979).

☐ Krieger's Theory of Therapeutic Touch

Krieger (1979) theorizes that prana (Sanskrit term for energy) is transferred in the healing act. She draws on Eastern literature, finding apt analogies in Western thought. For example, the source of prana in Eastern thinking is the sun; likewise, the source of energy for photosynthesis is the sun. Eastern thinking follows the idea that well people have an excess of prana. Western physiology texts state there is a great deal of redundancy in the human body.

☐ Research Support for Theory

Studies have shown therapeutic touch is significantly better than usual care for post-surgical pain (Coakley & Duffy, 2010; Monroe, 2009) and anxiety (Gomes, Silva & Araújo, 2008). Nursing leaders have been shown to reduce their stress when using healing touch (Tang, Tegeler, Larrimore, Cowgill, & Kemper, 2010). Even tactile touch has been shown to reduce anxiety and stabilize circulation (Henricson, Ersson, Määttä, Segesten, & Berglund, 2008).

Table 9-11   Therapeutic Touch Directions

Prior to any intervention, close your eyes and center yourself in the now; hold the intention to heal. Unruffling the field is accomplished by placing the hands with palms facing away from the body at the area where pressure is felt and then moving the hands away from the body in a sweeping gesture.

According to Kreiger (1979), energy can also be directed from a higher energy area to a low energy area by moving the hands in the appropriate direction in a brushing movement.

Another use of therapeutic touch is to act as a channel for energy to bring it to the client from a universal energy source. This is particularly helpful if the client is fatigued or needs concentrated energy to heal. With eyes closed, center, protect yourself (e.g., by picturing a protective shield around the body), and picture energy being channeled through the hands to the area in need of healing or energizing (Krieger, 1979).

RESEARCH BOX 9-14   Effects of Therapeutic Touch for Pain after Vascular Surgery

» BACKGROUND: Therapeutic Touch (TT) is a complementary modality that has been demonstrated to reduce psychological distress and help patients to relax. It is unclear if there is an impact of TT on biobehavioral markers such as cortisol and natural killer cells (NKCs). There is some preliminary evidence that suggests relaxation may have positive effects on the immune system.

» PURPOSE: To test the efficacy of TT on pain and biobehavioral markers in patients recovering from vascular surgery.

» FRAMEWORK: The study was grounded in a psychoneuroimmunology framework to address how complementary therapies affect pain and biobehavioral markers associated with recovery in surgical patients.

» DESIGN: This was a between-subjects intervention study.

» SAMPLE: Twenty-one postoperative surgical patients.

» MEASURES: Measures of level of pain and levels of cortisol and NKCs were obtained before and after a TT treatment.

» RESULTS: Compared with those who received usual care, participants who received TT had significantly lower levels of pain, lower cortisol levels, and higher NKC levels.

» CONCLUSIONS AND IMPLICATIONS: Evidence supports TT as a beneficial intervention. Future research on TT is still needed to learn more about how it functions. However, there is evidence to support incorporating TT into nursing practice.

Source: Coakley, A. B., & Duffy, M. E. (2010). The effect of therapeutic touch on postoperative patients. *Journal of Holistic Nursing, 28*(3), 193–200.

Therapeutic Touch Interventions The main therapeutic touch intervention is "unruffling the field." As the nurse sweeps the hands down the client's body, any areas that feel like pressure or congestion are "unruffled."

HEALTH PROMOTION CHALLENGE ☆ [www]

Pretend you are the researcher in the study described in RESEARCH BOX 9-14. What research design would you use to learn how therapeutic touch functions? Share your ideas with at least two other students and obtain feedback.

Yoga

Yoga is not only a set of physical exercises, but an inner spiritual experience as well. Yoga is devoted to balance. All forward bending postures are balanced by a backward bending one. Postures are meant to be performed slowly, almost meditatively, while breathing consciously. Postures should be performed on a cushioned floor, before eating, and while wearing loose clothing. Breathing should be in and out through the nostrils.

HEALTH TIP: Advise clients to breathe through each yoga exercise.

☐ Postures

The Bow. Reported useful for gastrointestinal disorders, constipation, upset stomach, sluggish liver, and abdominal fat. While lying flat on the stomach, grasp ankles, inhale, and lift legs, head, and chest, arching the back into a bow. Hold, then exhale and lie flat. Repeat 3–4 times, resting in between and noting effects.

Cobra. Reported to tone ovaries, uterus, and liver; relieves constipation; limbers spine; and is excellent for slipped discs. WARNING: Not recommended for those with peptic ulcer, hernia, or hyperthyroid. Lie on the stomach, arms at shoulder level. Push the upper body up with the arms, arch the back and look up while inhaling; hold and exhale while lowering the upper body slowly to the floor.

Corpse Pose. Reported to stimulate blood circulation; alleviate fatigue, nervousness, neurasthenia, asthma, constipation (enhance by visualizing increased circulation and movement of material through the intestines), diabetes (enhance by visualizing circulation to and from pancreas), indigestion, insomnia, and lumbago (enhance by visualization enhanced circulation to nourish back muscles); improve concentration; and generally increase relaxation. Lie flat on the back, legs and arms a comfortable distance from the body; allow body to sink into the floor.

During the second and third trimester of pregnancy, lie on the side, using pillows as necessary.

Knee to Chest. Reported to relieve stiffness and soreness of back and extremities, constipation, diabetes, and flatulence. Lie flat on back and bring knees to chest; rock back and forth gently, massaging the spine. Lower the legs one at a time, slowly. Bring one leg to the chest, pulling it in using a controlled stretch, fingers interlocked. Hold the position and breathe. Slowly bring the head toward the knee; hold and exhale. Inhale and bring knee to nose and hold for a count of 10; exhale and repeat 5–10 times. Repeat with other leg. Draw up both legs to knee moves toward the nose; hold while breathing and exhale. Return legs to floor and rest, noting the effect.

Kneeling Pose. Reported to increase circulation to prostate gland and uterus. Sit on heels, keeping back straight. While breathing through nostrils, separate the feet and slowly sink in between, moving buttocks toward the floor. Move gently, avoiding straining knee ligaments. Keep feet facing straight back.

The Lion. Report to relieve sore throat and stimulate circulation to throat and tongue (enhance by visualizing relaxation of throat and improve circulation to the area). Sit on the heels, palms on knees, fingers fanned out. Protrude the tongue as far as possible, open eyes and mouth as far as possible, roll eyeballs upward. Exhale saying "Ahhhh" and feeling the sensation in the back of the throat.

Locust. Reported to relieve problems of abdomen and lower back. WARNING: Not recommended for those with hernia or acute back problems. Lie flat on stomach, head facing forward, chin on the floor; relax and breathe. Keeping arms close to the body, palms up, slowly raise one leg toward the ceiling, using the lower back muscles. Hold briefly and then exhale while lowering the leg to the floor. Rest. Repeat with the other leg. Repeat up to 2–3 times each side, but not to the point of fatigue.

The Mountain. Reported to strengthen lungs, purify blood, improve digestive system, and tone nervous system. Sit cross-legged on the floor; stretch arms up toward the ceiling, fingertips together. Stretch up while breathing slowly and deeply 5–10 times; exhale and lower arms.

Neck and Eye Exercises. Reported to relieve headache and eyestrain, improve eyesight, and relax neck and shoulder tension. Sit cross-legged on the floor, wrists at rest on knees. Nod head forward slowly 3–4 times, then nod toward the left and right shoulder 3–4 times, allowing the mouth to fall open. Inhale and shut the eyes tightly; hold, then exhale, opening eyes wide and blinking rapidly 8–10 times. Hold the eyes open wide while looking around the entire circumference of the eyeballs; reverse the circle. Look diagonally from left upper to right lower and vice versa. Look up and down 10 times. Remember to breathe throughout. Rub palms together, close eyes, and cover them with the palms while completing five slow breaths. Repeat until eyes relax. Visualize energy and brightness moving into the eyes.

Uddiyana. Reported to alleviate constipation, indigestion, gastrointestinal problems, diabetes, and obesity. WARNING: Avoid if pregnant or hypertensive. Stand with feet apart, knees slightly bent; lean forward and arch back. Keep hands on thighs. While exhaling, hunch abdomen toward the spine and hold for several seconds. Relax and repeat on exhalation. Work up to 20 repetitions with one exhalation.

Cat Stretch. Reported useful in relieving back pain of pregnancy and aids in generalized relaxation. While on all fours on the floor, arch back and then concave it.

Spinal Twist. Reported to increase spinal flexibility, aid in the return of the uterus to its nonpregnant size, strengthen oblique abdominals (stretched during pregnancy), and stimulate elimination from the intestines and bladder. Sit on the floor, right knee bent at a 90-degree angle to left leg. Bend the knee and place the left foot in front of the right knee. Place right hand directly behind right hip. Place left hand directly behind right hand. While exhaling, move the left hand in a circle (feel spinal stretch) to rest on the floor behind left hip; hold, then rest. Return the left hand to the position behind the right hand by completing a slow semicircular movement in front of and to the side of the body. Switch legs and repeat, twisting first to the right and then to the left.

Triangle Pose. Reported to prevent degenerative arthritic changes, tone the sides of the body, and maintain joint health in the feet, ankles, knees, and hips. Stand with feet 3–5 feet apart, right foot at a 90-degree angle to left foot. Gradually reach down with right hand to grasp right ankle; hold left arm straight up in the air directly above right arm, eyes watching the left hand while breathing and holding the post. Repeat on left side of the body.

Shoulder Stand. Reported to regulate the thyroid, increase flow of venous blood from the lower extremities to the heart, prevent varicose veins, and reduce gravitation pressure on internal organs. WARNING: Contraindicated in cases of hypertension; neck problems; ear, throat, or eye infection; and obesity. Lie on the back, palms facing the floor; press palms down and lift legs up and over the head, supporting the neck with the hands and resting so the chin is on the chest. Align the chin with navel and big toes. Relax, breathe, enjoy.

Sun Salutation. Reported to invigorate and calm; exercise arms and spinal cord; prevent and relieve stomach ailments; reduce abdominal fat;

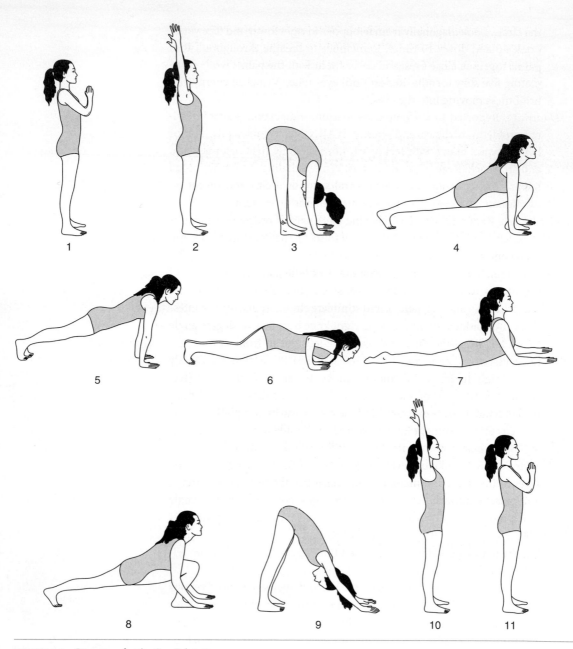

FIGURE 9-4   Directions for the Sun Salutation

© Carolyn Chambers Clark, 2010.

improve digestion and circulation; limber spine; tone abdominal, thigh, and leg muscles; and strengthen nerves and muscles of arms, legs, shoulders, and chest. An all-around preventive posture that should be done at least every day by everyone. See FIGURE 9-4.

RESEARCH BOX 9-15   Yoga for Fibromyalgia

» BACKGROUND: A mounting body of literature recommends that treatment for fibromyalgia (FM) encompass medications, exercise, and improvement of coping skills. However, there is a significant gap in determining an effective counterpart to pharmacotherapy that incorporates both exercise and coping.

» STUDY PROBLEM: The aim of this randomized controlled trial was to evaluate the effects of a comprehensive yoga intervention on FM symptoms and coping.

» SAMPLE: A sample of 53 female FM patients participated in the study.

» RESEARCH DESIGN: Participants were randomized to the 8-week Yoga of Awareness program (gentle poses, meditation, breathing exercises, yoga-based coping instructions, group discussions) or to wait-listed standard care. Data were analyzed by intention to treat.

» FINDINGS: At posttreatment, women assigned to the yoga program showed significantly greater improvements on standardized measures of FM symptoms and functioning, including pain, fatigue, and mood, and in pain catastrophizing, acceptance, and other coping strategies.

» CONCLUSIONS: This pilot study provides promising support for the potential benefits of a yoga program for women with FM.

Source: Carson, J. W., Carson, K. M., Jones, K. D., Bennett, R. M., Wright, C. L., & Mist, S. D. (2010). A pilot randomized controlled trial of the Yoga of Awareness program in the management of fibromyalgia. *Pain, 151*(2), 530–539.

> ## HEALTH PROMOTION CHALLENGE
>
> What is the next research step using yoga to treat women with fibromyalgia? Share your ideas with at least two other students and obtain feedback.

Summary

Considerable evidence exists that interventions emphasizing client empowerment and the acquisition of self-management skills are effective in diabetes, asthma, and other chronic conditions. They generally emphasize the client's crucial role in maintaining health and function and the importance of setting goals, establishing action plans, identifying barriers, and solving problems to overcome obstacles. Health promotion self-care approaches presented include acupressure, aromatherapy, exercise/movement, imagery, journaling, meditation, qigong, reflexology, relaxation procedures, self-hypnosis, smoking cessation, touch and yoga.

REVIEW QUESTIONS

`www.`

1. Which of the following is not true of acupressure?
   a. It is safe to do on yourself.
   b. It can be used to relieve headaches.
   c. It is not appropriate to practice in public.

2. Which of the following statements is true about Qigong?
   a. It draws from martial arts.
   b. It is more challenging than t'ai chi.
   c. It is an excellent exercise for frail, elderly clients.

3. Which of the following statements is not true about affirmations?
   a. They are consciously chosen to produce a desired result.
   b. They can be a useful motivational tool.
   c. Stress is not touched by affirmations.

4. Aerobic exercise not only conditions the cardiovascular system, it
   a. Relaxes large muscles.
   b. Reduces body fat.
   c. Can strain the heart unduly.

5. The following are true about imagery except
   a. It's a fairly new approach.
   b. It helps tap into the body's healing system.
   c. It may help client fight cancer.

6. Yoga postures:
   a. Should be balanced
   b. Should not be practiced by pregnant women
   c. Are relatively easy for someone who is out of shape

7. Which are the most effective reflex points?
   a. Those on the neck
   b. Those on the face
   c. Those on the feet

8. Who developed therapeutic touch?
   a. Aristotle
   b. Sigmund Freud
   c. Dolores Krieger

EXERCISES

1. Attend or observe at least one yoga, t'ai chi, or Qigong class. Interview the instructor and/or a student in the class about his or her beliefs in the therapeutic benefits of the practice as well as his or her level of training in the practice. Write a brief paper outlining your experience in the class and the interviewee's thoughts.

2. Ida Cummings is a client you are assigned. She has a heart condition, diabetes, never has enough time to do what she wants to do, is bothered by nagging guilt feelings, and complains of anxiety, depression, and fatigue. From all the self-management approaches you've learned, which ones would you suggest to Ms. Cummings and why? Share your choices with at least two students and obtain feedback.

3. Try out all the approaches described in this chapter. Keep track of your successes and questions. Discuss your experience with at least two students, ask for feedback, and listen to their experiences.

REFERENCES

American Heart Association. (2012). Get moving. Retrieved from http://www.heart.org/HEARTORG/GettingHealthy/PhysicalActivity/Physical-Activity_UCM_001080_SubHomePage.jsp

Arena, R., Myers, J., & Guazzi, M. (2010). The future of aerobic exercise testing in clinical practice: Is it the ultimate vital sign? *Future Cardiology, 6*(3), 325–342.

Atkinson, D., Iannotti, S., Cozzolino, M., Castiglione, S., Cicatelli, A., Vyas, B., & Rossi, E. (2010). A new bioinformatics paradigm for the theory, research, and practice of therapeutic hypnosis. *The American Journal of Clinical Hypnosis, 53*(1), 27–46.

Bagetta, G., Morrone, L. A., Rombolà, L., Amantea, D., Russo, R., Berliocchi, L., … Corasaniti, M. T. (2010). Neuropharmacology of the essential oil of bergamot. *Fitoterapi, 81*(6), 453–461.

Barsky, A. J., Ahern, D. K., Orav, E. J., Nestoriuc, Y., Liang, M. H., Berman, I.T., … Wilk, K. G. (2010). A randomized trial of three psychosocial treatments for the symptoms of rheumatoid arthritis. *Seminars in Arthritis and Rheumatism, 40*(3), 222–232.

Berkson, D. (1977). *The foot book: Healing the body through reflexology.* New York, NY: Harper and Row.

Boyd, L. A., Vidoni, E. D., & Wessel, B. D. (2010). Motor learning after stroke: is skill acquisition a prerequisite for contralesional neuroplastic change? *Neuroscience Letters, 482*(1), 21–25.

Braden, R., Reichow, S., & Halm, M.A. (2009). The use of the essential oil lavandin to reduce preoperative anxiety in surgical patients. *Journal of Perianesthesia Nursing, 24*(6), 348–55.

Bruner, J. (1990). *Acts of meaning.* Cambridge, MA: Harvard University Press.

Cannon, W. (1914). The emergency function of the medulla in pain and the major emotions. *American Journal of Physiology, 33*, 356–372.

Celik, A., Nur Herken, E., Arslan, I., Zafer Ozel, M., & Mercan, N. (2010). Screening of the constituents, antimicrobial and antioxidant activity of endemic Origanum hypericifolium. *Natural Product Research, 24*(16), 1568–1577.

Chang, S.Y. (2008). Effects of aroma hand massage on pain, state anxiety and depression in hospice patients with terminal cancer. *Taehan Kanho Hakhoe Chi, 38*(4), 493–502.

Coakley, A. B., & Duffy, M. E. (2010). The effect of therapeutic touch on postoperative patients. *Journal of Holistic Nursing, 28*(3), 193–200.

Cohen, M. & Mills. B. B. (1979). *Developmental movement therapy.* Durham, NC: The School for Developmental Movement Therapy.

Creswell, J. D., Welch, W. T., Taylor, S. E., Sherman, D. K., Gruenewald, T. L., & Mann, T. (2005). Affirmation of personal values buffers neuroendocrine and psychological stress responses. *Psychological Science, 16*(11), 846–851.

Critcher, C. R., Dunning, D., & Armor, D. A. (2010). When self-affirmations reduce defensiveness: Timing is key. *Personality and Social Psychology Bulletin, 36*(7), 947–959.

Dohrenwend, B. P., Neria, Y., Turner, J. B., Turse, N., Marshall, R., Lewis-Fernandez, R., & Koenen, K. C. (2004). Positive tertiary appraisals and posttraumatic stress disorder in U.S. male veterans of the war in Vietnam: The roles of positive affirmation, positive reformulation, and defensive denial. *Journal of Consulting and Clinical Psychology, 72*(3), 417–433.

Ellis, A. (2009). *The practice of rational emotive therapy.* New York, NY: Springer Publishing Company.

Epstein, G. (2004). Mental imagery: the language of spirit. *Advances: The Journal of Mind–Body Health, 20*(3), 3–9.

Feldenkrais, M. (1977). *Awareness Through Movement*. New York, NY: Harper and Row.

Field, T., Field, T., Cullen, C., Largie, S., Diego, M., Schanberg, S., & Kuhn, C. (2008). Lavender bath oil reduces stress and crying and enhances sleep in very young infants. *Early Human Development, 84*(6), 399–401.

Garland, E. L., Gaylord, S. A., Boettiger, C.A., & Howard, M. O. (2010). Mindfulness training modifies cognitive, affective, and physiological mechanisms implicated in alcohol dependence: results of a randomized controlled pilot trial. *Journal of Psychoactive Drugs, 42*(2), 177–192.

Gomes, V. M., Silva, M. J., & Araújo, E. A. (2008). Gradual effects of therapeutic touch in reducing anxiety in university students. *Revista Brasileira de Enfermagem, 61*(6), 841–846.

Goyal, M., Haythornthwaite, J., Levine, D., Becker, D., Vaidya, D., Hill-Briggs, F., & Ford, D. (2010). Intensive meditation for refractory pain and symptoms. *Journal of Alternative and Complementary Medicine, 16*(6), 627–631.

Gross, C. R., Kreitzer, M. J., Thomas, W., Reilly-Spong, M., Cramer-Bornemann, M., Nyman, J. A., … Ibrahim, H. N. (2010). Mindfulness-based stress reduction for solid organ transplant recipients: a randomized controlled trial. *Alternative Therapies in Health and Medicine, 16*(5), 30–38.

Group Health Research Institute. (2012). Experience and the chronic health model. Retrieved from http://www.grouphealthresearch.org/maccoll/maccoll_experience.html

Häfner, A, & Stock, A. (2010). Time management training and perceived control of time at work. *Journal of Psychology, 144*(5), 429–447.

Hay, L. L. (2001). *Heal Your Body*. Carlsbad, CA: Hay House, Inc.

Henricson, M., Ersson, A., Määttä, S., Segesten, K., & Berglund, A. L. (2008). The outcome of tactile touch on stress parameters in intensive care: a randomized controlled trial. *Complementary Therapies in Clinical Practice, 14*(4), 244–254.

High blood pressure. (n.d.) *Merck manual home health handbook for patients and caregivers*. Retrieved from http://www.merckmanuals.com/home/heart_and_blood_vessel_disorders/high_blood_pressure/high_blood_pressure.html

Hjelmstedt, A., Shenoy, S. T., Stener-Victorin, E., Lekander, M., Bhat, M., Balakumaran, L., & Waldenström, U. (2010). Acupressure to reduce labor pain: a randomized controlled trial. *Acta Obstetricia et Gynecologica Scandinavica, 89*(11), 1453–1459.

Howard, C., Dupont, S., Haselden, B., Lynch, J., & Wills, P. (2010). The effectiveness of a group cognitive-behavioural breathlessness intervention on health status, mood and hospital admissions in elderly patients with chronic obstructive pulmonary disease. *Psychology, Health and Medicine, 15*(4), 371–385.

Jimbo, D., Kimura, Y., Taniguchi, M., Inoue, M., & Urakami, K. (2009). Effect of aromatherapy on patients with Alzheimer's disease. *Psychogeriatrics, 9*(4), 173–179.

Jorenby, D.E. (2001). Smoking cessation strategies for the 21st century. *Circulation, 104*, e51.

Kang Y. (2010). Mind-body approach in the area of preventive medicine: Focusing on relaxation and meditation for stress management. *Journal of Preventive Medicine & Public Health, 43*(5), 445–450.

Kearns, M. C., Edwards, K. M., Calhoun, K. S., & Gidycz, C. A. (2010). Disclosure of sexual victimization: the effects of Pennebaker's emotional disclosure paradigm on physical and psychological distress. *Journal of Trauma Dissociation, 11*(2), 193–209.

Kinnier, R. T., Hofsess, C., Pongratz, R., & Lambert, C. (2009). Attributions and affirmations for overcoming anxiety and depression. *Psychology and Psychotherapy, 82*(Pt 2),153–169.

Kinzelman, A. O. (2009). The effects of lavender and rosemary essential oils on test-taking anxiety among graduate nursing students. *Holistic Nursing Practice, 23*(2), 88–93.

Kreiger, D. (1979). *The therapeutic touch*. Englewood Cliffs, NJ: Prentice-Hall.

Kurtz, R., Kaul, P., Passafiume, J., Sargent, C.R., & O'Hara, B. F. (2010). Meditation acutely improves psychomotor vigilance, and may decrease sleep need. *Behavioral and Brain Functions, 29*(6), 47.

Lazarus, R. S., & Folkman, S. (1984). *Stress, Appraisal, and Coping*. New York, NY: Springer Publishing Co.

Leite, J. R., Ornellas, F. L., Amemiya, T. M., de Almeida, A. A., Dias, A. A., Afonso, R., ... Kozasa, E. H. (2010). Effect of progressive self-focus meditation on attention, anxiety, and depression scores. *Perceptual and Motor Skills, 110*(3 Pt 1), 840–848.

Loizzo, J. J., Peterson, J. C., Charlson, M. E., Wolf, E. J., Altemus, M., Briggs, W. M., ... & Caputo, T. A. (2010). The effect of a contemplative self-healing program on quality of life in women with breast and gynecologic cancers. *Alternative Therapies in Health and Medicine, 16*(3), 30–37.

Martin, C. T., Keswick, J. L., & Leveck, P. (2010). A welfare-to-wellness-to-work program. *Journal of Community Health Nursing, 27*(3), 146–159.

Mayo, K. (1996). Social responsibility in nursing education. *Journal of Holistic Nursing, 14*, 24–32.

McCaffrey, R., Thomas, D. J., Johnson, J. B., & Kelly, A.W. (1990). A multifaceted rehabilitation program for women with cancer. *Oncology Nursing Forum 17*, 691–695.

Monroe, C. M. (2009). The effects of therapeutic touch on pain. *Journal of Holistic Nursing, 27*(2), 85–92.

Morley, S. (2010). Randomized controlled trials of psychological therapies for management of chronic pain in children and adolescents: an updated meta-analytic review. *Pain, 148*(3), 387–397.

Meichenbaum, D., & Cameron, R. (1974). Modifying what clients say to themselves. In M. Mahoney & R. Cameron (eds.), *Self control: Power to the Person*. Monterey, CA: Brooks/Cole.

Murphy, S. M., Edwards, R.T., Williams, N., Raisanen, L., Moore, G., Linck, P., ... Moore, L. (2012, May 10th). An evaluation of the effectiveness and cost effectiveness of the National Exercise Referral Scheme in Wales, UK: a randomised controlled trial of a public health policy initiative. *Journal of Epidemiology and Community Health*. [Epub ahead of print]. Retrieved from http://www.ncbi.nlm.nih.gov/pubmed/22577180

Newberg, A. B., Wintering, N., Waldman, M. R., Amen, D., Khalsa, D. S., & Alavi, A. (2010). Cerebral blood flow differences between long-term meditators and non-meditators. *Consciousness and Cognition, 19*(4), 899–905.

Nordqvist, C. (2009). What is aromatherapy? Retrieved from http://www.medicalnewstoday.com/articles/10884.php

O'Brien, M. L., Buikstra, E., Fallon, T., & Hegney, D. (2009). Strategies for success: a toolbox of coping strategies used by breastfeeding women. *Journal of Clinical Nursing, 18*(11), 1574–1582.

Ondicova, K., & Mravec, B. (2010). Role of nervous system in cancer aetiopathogenesis. *Lancet Oncology, 11*(6), 596–601.

Ornstein, R. (1972). *The psychology of consciousness*. San Francisco, CA: W.F. Freeman and Company.

Ou, M. C., Hsu, T. F., Lai, A. C., Lin, Y. T., & Lin, C. C. (2012). Pain relief assessment by aromatic essential oil massage on outpatients with primary dysmenorrhea: A randomized, double-blind clinical trial. *Journal of Obstetrics and Gynaecological Research, 38*(5), 817–822.

Palermo, T. M., Eccleston, C., Lewandowski, A. S., & Williams, A. C. (2010). Randomized controlled trials of psychological therapies for management of chronic pain in children and adolescents: an updated meta-analytic review. *Pain, 148*(3), 387–397.

Pemberton, E., & Turpin, P. G. (2008). The effect of essential oils on work-related stress in intensive care unit nurses. *Holistic Nursing Practice, 22*(2), 97–102.

Pennybaker, J. W. (1997). *Opening up, the healing power of expressing emotions.* New York, NY: Guilford Press.

Pennybaker, J. W., & Beall, A. J. (1986). Confronting a traumatic event. Toward an understanding of intuition and disease. *Journal of Abnormal Psychology, 95*, 274–281.

Peressutti, C., Martín-González, J. M., M García-Manso, J., & Mesa, D. (2009). Heart rate dynamics in different levels of Zen meditation. *International Journal of Cardiology, 145*(1), 142–146.

Petrie, K. J., Booth, R. J., Pennebaker, J. W., Davison, K. P., & Thomas, M. (1995). Disclosure of trauma and immune response to Hepatitis B vaccination program. *Journal of Consulting & Clinical Psychology, 63*, 787–792.

Prestera, H. (1984). *The body reveals.* New York, NY: Harper and Row.

Progoff, I. (1975). *At a journal workshop: The basic text and guide for using the intensive journal.* New York, NY: Dialogue House Library.

Rossman, M. (1993). Imagery: Learning to use the mind's eye. In D. Goleman & J. Gurin (Eds.). *Mind/Body Medicine.* Yonkers, NY: Consumers Union.

Ruepert, L., Quartero, A. O., de Wit, N. J., van der Heijden, G. J., Rubin, G., & Muris, J. W. (2012). Bulking agents, antispasmodics and antidepressants for the treatment of irritable bowel syndrome. *Cochrane Database System Review, 8*, CD003460.

Segal, D.L., & Murray, F. J. (1994). Emotional processing in cognitive therapy and vocal expression of feeling. *Journal of Social and Clinical Psychology, 13*, 189–206.

Seol, G. H., Shim, H. S, Kim, P. J., Moon, H. K., Lee, K. H., Shim, I., … Min, S. S. (2010). Antidepressant-like effect of Salvia sclarea is explained by modulation of dopamine activities in rats. *Journal of Ethnopharmacology, 130*(1), 187–190.

Sherman, D. K., Cohen, G. L., Nelson, L. D., Nussbaum, A. D., Bunyan, D. P., & Garcia, O. J. (2009). Affirmed yet unaware: exploring the role of awareness in the process of self-affirmation. *Journal of Personality and Social Psychology, 97*(5), 745–764.

Shiina Y., Funabashi, N., Lee, K., Toyoda, T., Sekine, T., Honjo, S., … Komuro, I. (2008). Relaxation effects of lavender aromatherapy improve coronary flow velocity reserve in healthy men evaluated by transthoracic Doppler echocardiography. *International Journal of Cardiology, 129*(2), 193–197.

Shimizu, K., Gyokusen, M., Kitamura, S., Kawabe, T., Kozaki, T., Ishibashi, K., … Kondo, R. (2008). Essential oil of lavender inhibited the decreased attention during a long-term task in humans. *Bioscience, Biotechnology and Biochemistry, 72*(7), 1944–1947.

Snyder, M., & Lindquist, R. (1998). *Complementary/alternative therapies in nursing.* New York, NY: Springer.

Spera, S. P., Buhrfeind, E. D., & Pennebaker, J. W. (1994). Expressive writing and coping with job loss. *Academy of Management Journal, 37*(3), 722–733.

Stene, L. E., Dyb, G., Tverdal, A., Jacobsen, G. W., & Schei, B. (2012). Intimate partner violence and prescription of potentially addictive drugs: prospective cohort study of women in the Oslo Health Study. *BMJ Open, 2*(2), e000614.

Stevensen, C.J. (1996). Aromatherapy. In Micozzi, M.S. (Ed.), *Fundamentals of complementary and alternative medicine* (pp. 137–148). New York, NY: Churchill Livingston.

Tang, R., Tegeler, C., Larrimore, D., Cowgill, S., & Kemper, K. J. (2010). Improving the well-being of nursing leaders through healing touch training. *Journal of Alternative and Complementary Medicine, 16*(8), 837–841.

U. S. Department of Health and Human Services, Physical Activity Guidelines Committee. (2008). Physical activity guidelines for Americans. Washington, D. C.: Author.

U. S. Department of Health & Human Services. (2008). *Physical activity guidelines for Americans, 2008*. Retrieved from http://www. health. gov/paguidelines/default. aspx

Weber, M. A. (2002). Calcium channel antagonists in the treatment of hypertension. *American Journal of Cardiovascular Drugs, 2*(6), 415–431.

Wu, B. (2006). *Qi Gong for total wellness*. New York, NY: St. Martin's Press.

Yu, H., Liang, L., Fu, Y., Efferth, T., Liu, X., & Wu, N. (2010). Activities of ten essential oils towards Propionibacterium acnes and PC-3, A-549 and MCF-7 cancer cells. *Molecules, 15*(5), 3200–3210.

Zeidan, F., Johnson, S. K., Gordon, N. S., Goolkasian, P. (2010). Effects of brief and sham mindfulness meditation on mood and cardiovascular variables. *Journal of Alternative and Complementary Medicine, 16*(8), 867–873.

INTERNET RESOURCES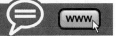

For a full suite of assignments and learning activities, use the access code located in the front of your book to visit this exclusive website: **http://go.jblearning .com/healthpromotion** If you do not have an access code, you can obtain one at the site.

Upon completion of this chapter, you will be able to:

1. Choose effective health promotion programs for clients.

2. Co-facilitate health promotion programs for more than one client with an advanced practice nurse.

3. Refer clients to advanced practice nurses when you are unable to answer client questions.

4. Describe how to measure health promotion programs.

5. Identify ways to evaluate health promotion programs.

6. Delineate how to sustain health promotion programs.

Awareness programs

Behavior change program

Community opinion survey

Evaluation

Lifestyle change programs

Objective evidence

Outcome

Outcome evaluation

Pretesting

Resource inventory

Self-evaluation

Spin-off effects

Supportive environment programs

CHAPTER 10

Health Promotion Programs: Developing, Facilitating, Measuring, and Evaluating

- Introduction
- What are the Steps in Building a Health Promotion Program?
- When the Client is a Community
- Objectives and Work Plan
- Summary

http://go.jblearning.com/healthpromotion

For a full suite of assignments and learning activities, use the access code located in the front of your book to visit the exclusive website: http://go.jblearning.com/healthpromotion. If you do not have an access code, you can obtain one at the site.

Introduction

In this chapter, we outline the steps to take to choose, develop, and facilitate effective health promotion programs. We examine the difference between individual-oriented and community-oriented health promotion, focusing on how to build client investment (whether the client is a person or a group).

What are the Steps in Building a Health Promotion Program?

To create a successful health promotion program, follow four steps. First, assess the need for a program. Obtain client input about health promotion programs as part of the assessment.

Second, formulate health promotion goals based on client input. Goals should be specific, measurable, time limited, and realistic if the client is to succeed. They need to be spelled out in writing, particularly if more than one person is involved.

The third step is to develop a work plan that spells out the goals and describes the steps that the client will take to reach those goals. In developing the plan, build involvement, ownership, and consensus. If the client lacks personal involvement and ownership in the plan, it is unlikely that the plan will be executed well or at all.

The fourth step in the health promotion program is to lay the groundwork for the activity. This includes arranging for facilities, scheduling activities, gathering and providing educational materials or experiences, and facilitating health promotion programs. This may involve something as simple as connecting a client to a group that supports what the client is trying to achieve (for example, a fitness class offered at a nearby YMCA) or as complex as organizing a series of public seminars and luncheons to promote healthy nutrition for pregnant and lactating women at a hospital or birthing center.

Assessing Client Needs

Whether you are working with an individual client, a group, or a community, it is important to assess client needs. During this phase, determine priority health problems, risk factors that contribute to the health problems, and what influences risk factors in the community. Identifying client resources helps determine what additional materials or facilities are necessary. Find out what programs exist and connect clients to them rather than putting time and energy into creating something new. For example, a family seeking help with an alcohol issue can be referred to Alcoholics Anonymous, Al-Anon, Alateen, medical detoxification facilities and care, and individualized or family-centered counseling. Any or all of these resources, individually or in combination, offer effective, comprehensive programs to help families deal with substance abuse issues. In this instance, your role is to act as coordinator of programs for the family, rather than creating or operating a program(s) that will benefit family health.

FIGURE 10-1 provides questions for assessing health and wellness for a client even if the client is a community of people.

Formulating Goal Statements

Goal setting is a key consideration in health promotion. Setting goals establishes commitment—it says, "This is where I want to go," so that you can then decide how to get there. It is not enough to recognize that a health issue exists and needs to be addressed; goals for health promotion must be specific.

For instance, suppose you are working with a family in which every member is overweight or obese. Some members are moderately overweight, while others are seriously obese—and all of them want to lose weight. The weight issue in the family is identified as the health concern to be addressed, but a goal such as "The goal is for everyone in the family to lose weight," is not workable—it is too vague. The nurse needs to sit with the family and identify goals that will enable family members to address the health issue in a way that is concrete, that is challenging but not unreachable, and that gets satisfying results without sacrificing each individual's safety and well-being. For example, a goal of losing five pounds a month might be workable if the family is willing to commit to changing their eating and exercise patterns. Having identified goals and given the individual or family tools to help them reach their goals, you then work with them to make a step-by-step plan for behavioral change. This may require developing a collection of short- and long-term goals that can be prioritized to form an action plan (see BOX 10-1). Assess the clients' motivations for change and help them to learn strategies for increasing motivation on a daily basis, so that the clients, not the nurse, ultimately become the people driving changes.

Follow-Up With the Client

After setting goals and developing a plan for change, check in with the client to make sure all is going according to plan. Even the best-organized clients have trouble implementing changes. Long-standing habits can be hard to break, even in the face of a health crisis. It is essential to keep in contact with the client to provide support for change. Encourage any positive move toward meeting the goal. Comment on small actions such as talking about the change in a positive way or eating one less donut a week to help the client see change is occurring.

If the client proves unable to stick to the plan, a session to assess why the problem exists is necessary. Hidden factors (emotional or mental health issues, for instance) may be interfering with the client's ability to put the plan

1. What is the age and gender of the client(s) and how might that affect health promotion?
2. How is space used by the client?
3. How safe and healthful are work, school, and social environments?
4. What cultural actions does the client follow?
5. How acculturated is the client to his/her community?
6. How able is the client to pay for health promotion activities?
7. What is the level of health information?
8. What is the client's perception of available health information?
9. What health promotion actions is the client already taking?
10. What does the client's occupation tell you about his/her education, health problems, problem-solving patterns, and methods of learning?
11. What client resources are available and where are they? How might the availability of exercise facilities; location, accessibility and number of cigarette machines; and number of grocery stores with a low-fat meat labeling program all influence an individual's behaviors?
12. What other data must be collected to help identify client health problems?
13. Are health promotion needs met or prevented from being met by space, culture, age, gender, family, income, occupational level, or resources?
14. What does the client say about the type of health promotion programs he or she would participate in if available?
15. What specific risk factors exist in the client and how are they being addressed or not?
16. How can family members or friends be considered in planning and implementing health promotion programs?
17. What types of religious, spiritual, or support individuals or groups exist that could support health promotion efforts?
18. What kinds of formal health promotion programs are already being used by the client?
19. How could existing programs or groups be used more effectively?
20. Does the client make decisions before adequate information has been obtained? What possible effects might this have on health promotion programs?
21. Is communication with the client fragmented and inefficient? How might this affect health promotion?
22. Is there a sense of trust between nurse and client?
23. Does the client emit a sense of power and self-control?
24. How will the client be affected if health is promoted?
25. What factors are operating to inhibit change toward health?
26. What information is needed prior to change toward health?
27. What new procedures or experiences will need to be developed prior to change toward health and wellness?
28. How is the client apt to suffer from the change?
29. How aware is the client of the need for change?
30. Is the client sufficiently involved in planning for change?
31. What is the relationship between nurse and client?
32. How open has the client been to change in the past?
33. How can free and open communication, support of and reward for problem-solving efforts, shared decision making, sufficient decision-making time, written statements of what change goals will be, concern for long-term planning, timing, and client confidence in the ability to change be enhanced to lower resistance to change?

FIGURE 10-1 Client Assessment
© 2010, Carolyn Chambers Clark.

into action. If this is the case, you may be able to promote the existing plan by providing additional resources or referrals. If that is unsuccessful, you and the client may need to set new goals and priorities.

Box 10-1 SMART Goal-Setting Techniques

Use the catchphrase **SMART** when setting goals:

Specific
Measurable
Achievable
Relevant
Time-Bound

The best way to help clients to both establish goals and ensure they work toward them is to have the client put health goals and any important related life goals in writing. There are a variety of goal-setting templates available online that you may use to organize your health goals. Some are limited (one template = one goal), and others comprehensive (one template contains goals for multiple areas of life).

When the client has a collection of goals written down, divide them into short- and long-term goals. Work with the client to assess whether each goal meets the SMART criteria, and eliminate or alter any that do not. If there are any goals that are related, highlight them; goals that support other goals may become higher priority. Then, ask the client to prioritize the goals and plan out how to start working on reaching them. The plan should be written down so the client can refer back to it, and you should keep a copy of the plan for the next session. At the follow-up, discuss how well the client was able to follow the plan, and what motivational aspects may or may not need to be improved.

HEALTH PROMOTION CHALLENGE

Using the information provided so far in this chapter, how would you go about developing a health promotion program for Mr. Simmons, diagnosed with diabetes, hypertension, and arthritis?

When the Client Is a Community

When the client is the community, it is vital to involve formal and/or informal community leaders in health promotion programs. They will help you identify problems, resources, and obstacles to change. For example, Birch and Ventura (2010) examined what works to prevent childhood obesity and found most childhood obesity prevention programs have focused on school-aged children and have had little success. The researchers suggested that, given these findings, prevention efforts should be expanded to explore other contexts in which children live as possible settings for intervention efforts, including the family and childcare settings. Given that 25% of preschool children are already overweight, intervening with children before school entry should be a priority. A review of experimental research on developing controls of food intake in infancy and childhood suggests possible intervention strategies, focusing on parenting and aspects of the feeding environment. Epidemiological findings point to even earlier modifiable risk factors, including gestational weight gain, maternal pre-pregnancy weight, and formula feeding.

Building Involvement, Ownership, and Consensus

When working with a family, it is important to involve every member. If one or two members are not involved or disagree with the effort, it is likely that they will consciously or unconsciously undermine the activities of the rest of the family.

Ownership of the health promotion process is all the more important when working with a community. Representation of all major community institutional sectors is important, including commercial, volunteer, political, religious, recreational, medical, public health, and media. For example, a coalition may include representatives from public and private schools and colleges, hospitals/clinics, public health advocates, and government health department officers. There may already be an appropriate interested group in the community. If so, this group may want to expand its responsibilities or be involved in the organization of the coalition in some way. If such a group exists, it is imperative that its leadership is informed/involved in some way to avoid competition and other obstacles that might arise.

Working with the Media to Enhance Interest

To convince community leaders of the need for health promotion, it may be necessary to begin a public awareness campaign. The use of the media throughout this process is critical to the success of the effort. The purpose of this initial campaign is to generate awareness and understanding of the planned effort in the community. It will raise the awareness of local leaders to the issues of health in the community and set the stage for recruiting volunteers for the program.

Prior to working with the media, conduct a community opinion survey and/or community resource inventory. A **community opinion survey** helps determine what are perceived to be the major community health problems, while a **resource inventory** identifies what resources exist in the community to meet health needs. The procedure for both includes interviews with identified community leaders. These interviews are tools for analyzing the community and connecting with community leaders and are two of the first steps in the community organization process. They are also the introduction of the project to important community leaders and begin to build support for later program activities (State of Minnesota, 2010).

Gathering Data and Potential Client Input

The opinion survey and the resource inventory data will provide information on the level of awareness of people in the community, indicate allies, and suggest how to approach the community (State of Minnesota, 2010).

Box 10-2 Community Assessment Questions

Some questions you might wish to ask to assess the community are:
1. Who do you think are leaders in the community?
2. What do you think are the most important health problems in the community for which programs need to be developed?
3. What resources does the community have already that could be enhanced?

The next step is to analyze the collected data. Collect as much community-specific data as possible. Organizing and summarizing data into charts and graphs that are easily viewed and understood by others is important (State of Minnesota, 2010).

Developing focused and relevant health promotion interventions is critical for behavioral change in a low-resource or special population. Established evidence-based interventions may not match the specific population or health concern of interest. The multisource method (MSM), in combination with a workshop format, may be used by health professionals and researchers in health promotion program development. The MSM draws on positive deviance practices and processes, focus groups, community advisors, behavioral change theory, and evidence-based strategies. The MSM may be useful in designing future health programs designed for other special populations for whom existing interventions are unavailable or lack relevance (Walker, Kim, Sterling, & Latimer, 2010).

1. Avoid using tables with lots of numbers. They are fine as a reference tool, but they can be confusing and hard to decipher.
2. Use percent/proportions instead of total numbers when comparing yourself with other populations. Average at least 3 years prior to comparing.
3. Use numbers when estimating how many people will use a particular health promotion program. This will enable you to determine whether the program is cost-effective.
4. Present your data in terms that speak to the community. Use number of events per minute or day.
5. Take percentages/proportions or rates and translate them into a situation that strikes close to home for the community.
6. Proportions represent the percent of the population, not the rate, which is the number of events per multiplier.
7. Use pie charts to demonstrate proportions, e.g., the leading causes of heart disease by percentage.
8. Use line graphs to show change across time, e.g., prevention of smoking among adults.
9. Use bar graphs to show differences among different groups of people, e.g., teen pregnancy by race and ethnicity.

FIGURE 10-2 Tip Sheet for Presenting Data

FIGURE 10-2 provides a tip sheet for presenting data to the community.

Once the community is aware of health promotion needs, you can begin to generate interest and obtain client input. You may also want to consider partnering with segments of the community to obtain information about health promotion needs (Perry & Hoffman, 2010).

Community Goal Setting

If working with a community rather than an individual or family client, you would take a slightly different tack. Instead of giving the client information and expecting the client to take the lead in goal setting, present a selection of data-driven goals, along with the supporting data, to the core group and/or community coalition for further discussion and development. Community awareness and participation are critical to the success of community-based health promotion efforts.

Community organization is the vehicle that informs and involves people in the project. The community is mobilized through ever-increasing involvement of its leaders and citizens (Larsen & Stock, 2011). Discussions need to produce agreement on the health problems or needs of the community and achieve a consensus on the goals and priorities for action (State of Minnesota, 2010).

Schools	Strengthening health education in school curriculum and including parents in related activities
Media	Involving media personnel in local health activities
Grocers	Promoting availability of healthy food choices
Businesses	Fitness, nutrition, and stress management programs for employees

FIGURE 10-3 Examples of Community Programs

Goal setting for a community may be complicated if there are multiple competing goals, or goals that may require many years' work to achieve. Work with community leaders to assemble a core planning group of a local coordinator and at least three people willing to participate in long-term planning. This core group may be assembled before data collection, or it may be assembled after data collection is completed. The core group assists the coordinator in the planning and administration of the project, helps identify resources necessary to accomplish the objectives, and assists in recruiting coalition members.

The coordinator serves as a catalyst in the process of identifying what needs to be done and recruits core group and coalition members to use their collective strength to solve the health problems of the community. The coordinator will be the organizer, the communicator, and the person through whom all paperwork will flow.

Some communities use the core group to collect data and participate in conducting the surveys. This necessitates training core group members, but has the advantages of involving them from the beginning and in sharing the workload. Based on data and the collective wisdom of the core group, target populations and possible interventions are discussed (Marrett, Northrup, Pichora, Spinks, & Rosen, 2010). FIGURE 10-3 shows examples of community programs.

Objectives and Work Plan

Measurable objectives define the work of the coalition, are time limited, specific, and stated in measurable terms. Write objectives using strong, active verbs such as *challenge, solve, question, participate, choose, apply, eliminate, analyze, experiment, organize, ask, demonstrate, practice, identify, explain,* and *evaluate.* Avoid passive, weak verbs or actions that cannot be observed such as *seems* and *understands.* Groene, Brandt, Schmidt, and Moeller (2009) studied the use of a balanced scorecard to develop strategic objectives.

It may be helpful to build a program around an existing conceptual model. For example, nurses in Canada developed their health promotion program around the Ottawa Charter for Health Promotion, which includes:

- Build healthy public policy
- Create supportive environments for health
- Strengthen community action for health
- Develop personal skills
- Reorient health services (Lee, Kim, Ahn, Ko, & Cho, 2010).

You will be most likely to have success if the client participates in designing or choosing the health promotion strategies and offers input regarding potential obstacles and solutions. The client should also be involved in setting a timeline for reaching the objective, but be prepared to counsel the client on whether this timeline is realistic. For example, the overweight family we described earlier might set a goal such as, "All family members will lose 20% of their body weight in the next 3 months," which may not be safe or even possible for family members who are seriously obese (300 lbs. or more). Setting goals that are unreachable for some members of the group is self-defeating. Your job is to guide the client(s) to set goals in a time frame that allows for success.

Once those goals have been achieved, new, more challenging goals can be set. For our overweight family, you might suggest that family members set a 3-month goal that focuses less on number of pounds lost and more on achieving goals of developing better eating habits and reaching a certain level of physical activity per week. Such goals can be worked on by all family members without penalizing those who have greater challenges in terms of absolute weight they need to lose. After the 3 months have passed, you can sit down with the family, find out how they have done in terms of meeting the initial

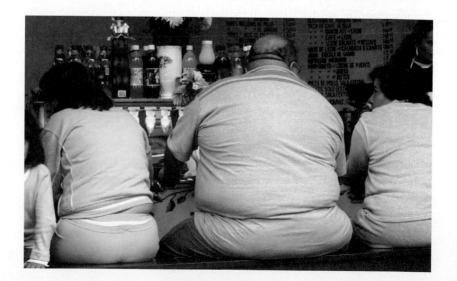

goals, and then perhaps set more challenging goals with the individual family members about losing specific amounts of weight in a set time frame.

How to Recruit Members

To create community ownership, invite leading citizens with a stated interest or known commitment to the project to join the planning group. Ask them to suggest names of others they think might be helpful to the program. These names will probably be similar to those mentioned in the community opinion survey or community resources inventory. Issue invitations to heads of organizations and individuals identified as community leaders.

Recruit representatives from all segments of the community. Beyond that, members must be enthusiastic and excited about the goals and believe that the objectives can and will be accomplished if people work together. It is important to recruit positive thinkers who will look for opportunities, strengths, and are multiple-solution people who enjoy a challenge.

Create a balance of community members who may lend their names and voices to the effort but do not have the time to give active participation, and those members who will be the doers. The core group should discuss whether a formal or informal invitation, phone call, or visit would be most likely to influence each candidate to join. Whichever approach is chosen, provide concise written materials explaining the mission of the coalition and the role each member will be expected to play.

HEALTH PROMOTION TIP

To retain volunteers, be sure to:
- Be flexible and adjust your expectations about completion of tasks
- Get to know each volunteer and learn about each one's special skills and abilities
- Choose worthwhile and varied tasks for each volunteer
- Assign tasks clearly and explain procedures and expectations
- Develop a job description for each volunteer
- Provide training, positive feedback, and appreciation for each task completed

If volunteers understand the mission and their role in it, are trained and actively involved, are recognized for their efforts, and are supported by staff, the turnover problem will be kept to a minimum. Continue to conduct periodic training sessions for coalition members, task force members, and other volunteers. Answer their questions and provide encouragement, pointing out movement toward the goal.

Clarify the Mission

The need for clear roles and expectations for coalition members is paramount to a successful effort. Without a clear mission, people may work at cross-purposes, and when difficulties arise, the differing agendas of these members can become insurmountable obstacles. Coalition members need to see themselves working toward a common goal that they should be able to describe in a few short words.

It is helpful to define individual coalition members' jobs. Job descriptions or agreements include such things as the length of the commitment, training opportunities, support from staff, personal expectations, and financial commitment. Active involvement by coalition members is critical. It may take 6–10 months to build mutual respect and program ownership. Members need training and sufficient time to digest this type of broad public health program. Training about health promotion and project goals will help members feel confident of their participation in decision making. Training may take many forms, such as in-service meetings or weekend seminars with family members invited. Devoting a portion of each meeting to training yields long-term benefits.

Group consensus is the most effective method for decision making. For this to occur, the coalition must take time to resolve member concerns and periodically determine who is not in accord and why. It is important to hear from all members; silence does not necessarily mean assent. Members who may be opposed to an idea, but not skilled at airing their views, can later block implementation. In effective decision making, all members volunteer or are asked to share their views before a decision is made.

Successful community organization efforts offer specific rewards, benefits, and incentives to members. The core group should plan and provide for recognition and incentives for the coalition and task force members. Focusing on early and small successes—which will promote optimism, positivity, and involvement in the community—should be part of the plan of the core group for the coalition and task force members.

The coalition's overall responsibility is to plan and coordinate community-wide program activities. This is a self-directed group, and participants will need to discuss and determine its own methods of accomplishing the goal. The coalition may decide that task forces are needed to concentrate on specific health risk areas such as smoking, nutrition, stress reduction, or exercise. Organizing task forces broadens the base of community support and involvement in the project, but will be dependent on the size of the community and goals of the coalition. A coalition member typically chairs a task force.

Task force members are doers with a strong interest in the specific topic area. It is important to involve members of the target population(s) in the task force. The coalition should provide direction to task forces in the form of written goal statements, measurable objectives, data presentation supporting the goals and objectives, ideas for possible strategies, and clear expectations that results must be measured. Task forces need staff support. The coordinator, or another staff member if the coordinator is not available, should attend every task force meeting and provide positive feedback and encouragement.

Program Design and Implementation

During program design, designers make decisions about the content, level of intensity, and topic areas for the programs. Often, they collaborate with a segment of the community to ensure appropriate interventions are included. For example, Cowart and colleagues (2010) collaborated with a church population to develop an obesity reduction program. Doing so ensured that bonds between participants were already established, which strengthened the buy-in of the individuals to the group's purpose. It also meant that the resources and organizing skills of the church group could be put to use in outreach to the broader community.

RESEARCH BOX 10-1 shows how one type of program design was implemented in a Canadian study.

RESEARCH BOX 10-1 Canadian Program Design Study

» BACKGROUND: Sexually transmitted infections (STIs) are high and rising in British Columbia, Canada, and youth ages 15–24 account for a disproportionate amount of the infections. As a result, new public health interventions have increasingly turned towards media such as the Internet to reach youth populations at risk for STIs/HIV. This study describes youth's perceptions about online sexual health services.

» METHODS: The researchers used in-depth, semi-structured interviews with 38 men and 14 women between the ages of 15 and 24 who discussed online STI/HIV testing, counseling, and education services.

» RESULTS: The researchers found youth were familiar with, receptive to, and had an affinity for online sexual health services. Participants suggested that online STI/HIV risk assessment and testing as well as online counseling and education could enhance opportunities for low-threshold service provision. Online services appealed to youth's needs for convenience, privacy, as well as expedient access to testing and/or counseling. Participants also appear to have relatively low tolerance for technologies that they perceive to be antiquated (e.g., printing lab requisition forms), revealing the challenges of designing online approaches that will not quickly become outdated.

» RECOMMENDATIONS: Globally, pilot programs for Internet-based sexual health services such as online testing and partner notification have shown promising results. As Canadian interventions of this type emerge, research with youth populations can provide relevant insights to help program planners launch effective interventions.

Source: Shoveller, J., Knight, R., Davis, W., Gilbert, M., & Ogilvie, G. (2012). Online sexual health services: examining youth's perspectives. *Canadian Journal of Public Health, 103*(1), 14–8.

Contact Source: School of Population and Public Health, University of British Columbia, Vancouver, BC. jean.shoveller@ubc.ca

□ Determining the Type of Health Promotion Program

The assessment performed at the beginning of the process should offer guidance as to what type of health promotion program is most needed by and beneficial for a client or a community. Health promotion programs generally emphasize one of three types of change: awareness, lifestyle change, or supportive environment. We will discuss programs focused on communities here because they are generally more complex than programs for individuals or families.

Awareness programs typically use newsletters, health fairs, posters, and screening to increase client interest. Awareness programs seek to educate a community about a health issue so that individuals will begin to consider their own behaviors or circumstances. Health promotion campaigns should also consider tapes, video, written information, in-person coaching, and other approaches. The Internet is still a largely untapped area for health promotion (Kaufman, 2010).

Behavior change programs, such as fitness or weight-loss programs, teach skills, require a supportive environment, and usually require 8–12 weeks to see an improvement. **Supportive environment programs** help to alter aspects of community life to help maintain a long-term, sustained, healthy lifestyle. Examples might be working with health food stores and restaurants to offer healthier food selections and to provide recognition for role models as well as rewards and recognition for program participants (State of Minnesota, 2010).

An example of a behavioral change health promotion program is a 2010 study that tested a peer-based, personal risk, network-focused HIV prevention

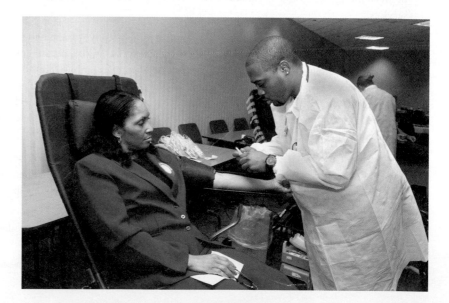

intervention to (1) train injection drug users to reduce injection and sex risk behaviors, (2) conduct outreach to behaviorally risky individuals in their personal social networks (called risk network members [RNMs]), and (3) reduce RNM HIV risk behaviors (Tobin, Kuramoto, Davey-Rothwell, & Latkin, 2010). Researchers used a randomized controlled trial with prospective data collection at 6, 12, and 18 months. Intervention condition consisted of five group sessions, one individual session, and one session with the RNMs. Outcomes included (1) injection risk based on sharing needles, cookers, and cotton for injection and drug splitting; (2) sex risk based on number of sex partners, condom use, and exchanging sex; and (3) index HIV outreach behaviors. At the end of the study, the researchers found a significant intervention effect on increased condom use among female RNMs and concluded that training active intravenous drug users to promote HIV prevention among individuals in their networks who engaged in high-risk behaviors is feasible, efficacious, and sustainable.

Lifestyle change programs undertake behavior change on a grander scale—changing not one, but multiple behaviors so that overall lifestyle is altered toward health. One well-known example of a lifestyle change program is the television show, *The Biggest Loser,* in which show contestants receive all-encompassing coaching on diet, exercise, emotional wellness, and physical health to promote weight loss. Although improvement in overall health is an unstated goal, the nature of the program focuses attention on body mass. The show's producers also seek to engage the audience by offering online programming and incentives to encourage audience members to participate at home. (It is not known how successful this engagement is in promoting weight loss among viewers).

HEALTH PROMOTION TIP: Choosing an Appropriate Health Promotion Program

It is important to pick a health promotion program that meets your criteria. How do you know if the health promotion program is right for you? Consider whether the program:

1. Can be accomplished in the given time period
2. Fits your budget
3. Is attractive to your client(s)
4. Fits health promotion goals
5. Does not duplicate another program
6. Is easy to implement
7. Can be easily incorporated in the client's life or the community
8. Provides incentives to help the client achieve stated goals.
9. Is within the nurse's expertise to facilitate
10. Can be evaluated for program results

The community assessment should help identify the strengths and weaknesses of the community's ability to make these three types of change. The health promotion program can be designed to take advantage of the strengths while addressing the weaknesses. All three are necessary for long-term behavior change to occur.

☐ Determine the Level of Intensity of the Program

The level of intensity of the program determines the degree of success but is affected by the resources, time, and staff available. For instance, awareness levels of people attending a weekend retreat will be greater than the levels of those attending a health fair. Intensity is also determined by the level of support offered in the community, so intensity can be increased by fostering a supportive environment. For example, people who have or are given access to exercise facilities, healthy food choices, and recognition or other incentives for healthy behaviors will have a greater chance of maintaining healthy behaviors than those who do not have such access.

☐ Select Program Areas and Identify Resources Needed to Implement the Proposed Activity

The pros and cons of each possible program area should be thoroughly analyzed. What will be acceptable to the community and special target group? In addition, availability of resources may be a limiting factor when identifying program areas. For each activity, resources such as instructors, facilities, equipment, and materials will need to be determined and the cost of each of these estimated.

Task force members who represent their organizations may be able to bring independent resources to the activity and provide many of the needed program resources. Efforts to identify and find solutions for potential obstacles should be undertaken as early as possible in the planning process.

Here is an example of ways to overcome potential obstacles. A smoking cessation program whose target is high risk pregnant women may have the following potential obstacles and possible solutions:

Potential Obstacles	Possible Solutions
Cost of attending programs may be too high	Scholarships and free babysitting services provided
Last time a smoking cessation program was attempted in the community, it was cancelled due to lack of participants	New and comprehensive promotion campaign incentives offered (e.g., free babysitting)

HEALTH PROMOTION CHALLENGE

Identify a health promotion program you would like to design. List the potential obstacles and brainstorm possible solutions.

Here is an idea to get you started. A study by Patel and colleagues (2009) identified potential obstacles and barriers to helping middle school children lose weight. The researchers used trained observers who visited four Los Angeles Unified School District (LAUSD) middle schools. Observers mapped cafeteria layout; observed food/beverage offerings, student consumption, waste patterns, and duration of cafeteria lines; spoke with school staff and students; and collected relevant documents. Data were examined for common themes and patterns. Results included:

- Food and beverages sold in study schools met LAUSD nutritional guidelines, and nearly all observed students had time to eat most or all of their meal.
- Some LAUSD policies were not implemented, including posting nutritional information for cafeteria food, marketing school meals to improve student participation in the National School Lunch Program, and serving a variety of fruits and vegetables. Cafeteria understaffing and costs were obstacles to policy implementation.

The researchers concluded that site visits were a valuable methodology for evaluating the implementation of school district obesity-related policies and contributed to the development of a community-based participatory research intervention to translate school food policies into practice. Future community-based participatory research studies may consider adding site visits into their toolbox of formative research methods (Patel et al., 2009).

☐ Estimate Total Costs, Develop a Budget, and Consider Funding Options

The funding options depend on the type of program and its focus. Voluntary agencies such as the following may be able to supply materials, training of instructors, or equipment:

- American Heart Association: http://www.americanheart.org
- American Lung Association: http://www.lungusa.org
- American Cancer Society: http://www.cancer.org

Interested organizations can pool resources. Partnerships can be formed with local chambers of commerce and individual businesses. Applications for grants from local, state, federal, or private foundations may be submitted. Program fees can offset a certain amount of costs. If groups use creativity, successful activities are possible without necessarily incurring significant expense.

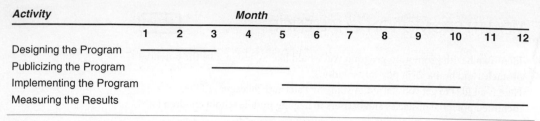

Activity	Month											
	1	2	3	4	5	6	7	8	9	10	11	12
Designing the Program	———————											
Publicizing the Program				———————								
Implementing the Program						———————————————						
Measuring the Results						————————————————————————						

FIGURE 10-4 An example of a timeline.

☐ Set a Timeline

Make a timeline of all the events needed to accomplish each activity and iden-tify who is responsible for each activity. FIGURE 10-4 is an example of a timeline.

☐ Arrange for Facilities and Staff

A wide variety of facilities in the community may be used for health promotion activities. Appropriateness, accessibility, cost, and size should be considered. In some instances, political climate may also need to be pondered.

Staff for health promotion programs may include health educators, phy-sicians, nurses, and interested volunteers. Voluntary agencies have excellent training opportunities for volunteers, or local health professionals may provide needed training. Employer-provided health promotion services can decrease staff dissatisfaction (Wilkins & Shields, 2009).

☐ Schedule Activities

A schedule that is convenient for participants and volunteers is critical to a successful program. The time of year, day of week, time of day, and length of program should all be analyzed to consider the program's target group, its human resources, and the community. Even the best-planned programs may run into scheduling difficulties, so have an alternate plan in mind (Klima, Norr, Vonderheid, & Handler, 2009).

Hildebrand and Neufeld (2009) explored recruitment strategies based on the transtheoretical model (TTM) with older adults living in a naturally occur-ring retirement community (NORC). These naturally occurring communities are found in high-rise, city-based apartment buildings, but also in clusters of suburban-based, single family homes. The researchers sought to encourage enrollment in a physical activity promotion program called Active Living Every Day (ALED). They identified reasons for participation or nonparticipation in the health promotion program. Recruitment strategies were designed to move older adults through the TTM stages of change to enroll in ALED and were built on meetings and resources established by St. Louis NORC's supportive service program. Analysis of interview data identified that scheduling and cost were primary reasons for nonenrollment in ALED. The researchers concluded that using theoretically based recruitment methods for older adults and a neighborhood approach through organizations such as a NORC may result in greater numbers of older adults participating in health promotion programs.

☐ Gather Educational Materials

Successful programs usually provide a variety of educational materials. Materials such as brochures, videos, films, newsletters, and slide tapes are often available either free or at low cost from voluntary agencies. If a program is likely to be repeated on a weekly, monthly, or annual basis, online webinars, chats, and informational pages should be considered as well, as these have the advantage of being relatively low in cost to maintain and are easily updated.

HEALTH PROMOTION TIP: Publicize the Activity

Provide at least 6 weeks of intensive publicity for each program. Promoting the program is crucial to its success. The public awareness campaign will raise general awareness levels but specific publicity for each program or event should be planned. Carefully consider the target group and design media and advertising around their interests.

Many community efforts are turning to environmental, rather than individual or family approaches. RESEARCH BOX 10-2 provides some ideas for developing programs to reduce obesity.

Evaluation

Evaluation is an integral part of the entire process of developing community-based health promotion programs. It is important to determine the extent to which proposed activities have been carried out (process evaluation) and the actual effectiveness of the program, i.e., what impact the program has had on the community's health risks (**outcome**).

Evaluation must be planned during the initial stages of the program so that necessary records, observation, and other data, are collected at the appropriate times. It is not possible to design an effective evaluation at the end of a project. Whenever possible, an evaluation should be based on **objective evidence** rather than observation. This type of evidence may include such things as activity reports, surveys, changes in scores, and measurable changes in health (e.g., decreases in smoking rates or cholesterol levels).

RESEARCH BOX 10-2

» BACKGROUND: Obesity among Americans is a public health threat affecting about one-third of the population. Obesity rates are even higher among racial and ethnic minority populations living in the South. Novel approaches for curtailing obesity disparities are desperately needed. Behavioral change interventions designed to improve individuals' energy balance are necessary, but they may be insufficient for achieving and maintaining the goal of obesity reduction among disparate populations. Environmental interventions focused on improving access to healthy foods are emerging as a complement to individually oriented approaches. The Centers for Disease Control and Prevention (CDC) recently released several state-level indicators focused on promoting public health by increasing the availability of healthy food retail outlets, such as farmers' markets, in communities. Farmers' markets are community health promotion interventions that increase access to fresh fruits and vegetables. As farmers' markets continue to develop, it is important to strategically locate them in settings that are accessible to populations affected by health disparities. One potential setting is a community health center.

» GOAL: The goal of this analysis was to extend existing research on community readiness to identify indicators of preparedness among community health centers for establishing onsite farmers' markets.

» METHOD: The sampling frame for the readiness assessment included all community health centers in South Carolina (N = 20) representing 163 practice sites. Data collection included two brief online surveys, in-depth key informant interviews, and secondary analysis of contextual data.

» FINDINGS: Five themes related to readiness for establishing a farmers market at a community health center were identified: capacity, social capital, awareness of health problems and solutions, logistical factors, and sustainability.

» CONCLUSIONS: Findings from this study provide guidance to researchers and community health center staff as they explore the development of environmental interventions focused on reducing diet-related health conditions by improving access to healthy foods.

Source: Darcy, A., Freedman, D. A., Whiteside, Y. O., Brandt, H. M., Young, V., Friedman, D., & Hebert, J. R. (2012). Assessing Readiness for Establishing a Farmers' Market at a Community Health Center. *Journal of Community Health, 37*(1), 80–88. The entire manuscript for this study is available at http://www.ncbi.nlm.nih.gov/pmc/articles/PMC3208118/?tool=pmcentrez

❑ Types of Evaluation

No matter what kind of evaluation approach you choose, it is important to develop a monitoring system that enables you to have an accurate count of how many clients were served during the year, what services were provided, and clientele characteristics. A monitoring system will provide information about your program's capacity for success.

Outcome evaluation measures consequences attributable to health promotion program activities and can show whether you are attaining your program objectives. Examples of positive outcome measures are:

- Increase in health knowledge
- Change in attitudes to belief in ability
- Increase in healthy behaviors
- Decrease in risk factors
- Decrease in morbidity and premature mortality

Outcomes can be measured in terms of immediate and long-term impact. Many programs offer short-term health promotion but do not follow up in measuring the client's long-term compliance with the processes generated in the activity. To be truly effective, health promotion should make a lasting impact on clients' health, and it is important that plans for measurement of long-term impact be considered. Measures of short-term impact include:

1. Number of health promotion sessions attended
2. Improved knowledge of cancer risk factors
3. Increased belief in the preventability of chronic disease
4. Increased levels of regular exercise
5. Decreased cigarette smoking
6. Reduced consumption of saturated fats
7. Increased consumption of fruits and vegetables

Achieving positive change in these or similar factors is a great short-term impact, but the real measure of success is determining whether the behavior change instilled by the program lasts beyond the duration of the program. If 90% of clients who take part in an 8-week smoking cessation program quit smoking, that program has phenomenal short-term success. If 95% of those clients who quit are smoking again within a year of the program, then overall, only 4.5% of the clients who started the program are free of cigarettes. This kind of finding means very few people have actually seen a health benefit from their participation. The goal of any health promotion program must be geared toward both short- and long-term health impacts.

Consider using other kinds of evaluation goals. Impact evaluation can show spin-off or secondary benefits for participants in the program. Examples of **spin-off effects** would be a reduction in drunk driving incidents, incidence of drinking among adolescents, and alcohol-related domestic violence after a program aimed at reducing alcohol use, or a decrease in emergency department visits related to asthma and chronic obstructive pulmonary disease (COPD) following a public health campaign about the dangers of secondhand smoke.

Self-evaluation measures show clients they are part of the health promotion team and that their input is valued. Simple self-evaluation methods include asking clients to rate their symptoms before and after treatment sessions from 1 (uncomfortable symptoms) to 10 (relief; comfort) (TABLE 10-1), and completing a wellness or feelings diary. A wellness diary (TABLE 10-2) includes a chart of clients' intake, bowel movements, activities, symptoms, and mood changes by time of day. A feelings diary (TABLE 10-3) includes the

Table 10-1   Assessment/Treatment/Evaluation

Date: 8/24 Client: Jason Stimtrex Session No.5

Current Medications: *"The doctor is giving me V antibiotics 6x/week for my sinus infection and asthma. He cut back my medications. Now I only get a sleeping pill, my blood pressure medicine, and Xanax.*

Current Supplements: *Garlic capsules 3x/day, vitamin E 400 IU/day, vitamin C 500 mg 3x/day, calcium/magnesium (1,500/750 mg) a day.*

Current Eating Plan: *Vegetarian: no wheat or white rice. Chicken or fish 3x week. "I like rice pudding—my wife makes it for me."*

Current Exercise Plan: *Walk daily x 40 minutes, yoga class 1x week.*

Current Sources of Support: *Wife and grown daughter, men's church group.*

Other: *Dogs, Charlie & Izzie*

Goal: *"Get rid of sinus infection and diarrhea."*

RATING: MINIMAL. . . . . UNBEARABLE

SYMPTOM 1: *Sinus "headache"*

Rating at beginning of session:	1	2	3	4	5	6	7	8	9	⑩
Rating at end of session:	1	2	③	4	5	6	7	8	9	10

SYMPTOM 2: *"Cold feet" (diabetes)*

Rating at beginning of session	1	2	3	4	5	6	7	8	⑨	10
Rating at end of session:	1	2	3	④	5	6	7	8	9	10

SYMPTOM 3: *"upset stomach and diarrhea"*

Rating at beginning of session:	1	2	3	4	5	6	7	8	9	⑩
Rating at end of session:	1	2	3	4	5	6	⑦	8	9	10

SYMPTOM 4: *"Sore neck and shoulders"*

Rating at beginning of session:	1	2	3	4	5	6	7	8	9	⑩
Rating at end of session:	①	2	3	4	5	6	7	8	9	10

SYMPTOM 5: *"Floaters and sore eyes"*

Rating at beginning of session	1	2	3	4	5	6	7	⑧	9	10
Rating at end of session:	1	2	3	④	5	6	7	8	9	10

TREATMENTS:

Affirmations: *I refuse to let anyone irritate me and breathe in peace and joy.*

It's getting easier and easier to follow a healthy meal plan.

I enjoy the taste of my food and digest it well.

Aromatherapy: *Peppermint oil to sinus area.*

Art/ritual: Start a wellness diary.

Assertiveness: *Discussed trying role playing client–physician interactions during next session*

Breathing: *practiced diaphragmatic breathing in session.*

Coping skills: *I will not allow this situation to upset me.*

Exercise: *Encouraged client to continue exercise program.*

Feng Shui: *Consider having the dogs sleep on the other side of the house from your bedroom*

Table 10-2   One Day of a Wellness Diary

Start Date: *Wednesday*
Stop Date: *Tuesday*

Date	Time	Food/Liquids/ Condiments	Bowel Movements (consistency, gas. bloating)	Activities (with whom for how long)	Symptoms and mood (include changes for 1 hour after eating and at any other time)	Vitamins/ medications (include dosage once, then any changes)
Wed	7:30 a.m	orange juice, coffee	gas, bloating	arguing with son		multi-vitamin vitamin E 400 IU
	8:30 a.m				depressed	
	9:30 a.m			boss gave me a terrible assignment	angry	2 Tylenol
	10 a.m noon	Snickers, burger & fries, Coke		working on new project alone	pain all over, tired, dizzy	
	1 p.m		hard bowel movement			
	3 p.m	2 mints				
	3:30 p.m				tired	
	3:45 p.m	coffee				
	6:30 p.m	broiled chicken, mashed potatoes and gravy, apple		husband came home late	annoyed	
	9. p.m		gas, indigestion		exhausted	Mylanta

date, time, setting, conversations/thoughts, feelings, approaches tried to change feelings, and results.

❑ Designs for Evaluation

When choosing an evaluation design, keep in mind the limitations of the design as well as the practical, ethical, and financial constraints you are under. You may not be able to use a randomized population group because of informed consent issues, the voluntary nature of many health promotion programs, and the difficulty in finding a control group. There are many other kinds of evaluation designs that can provide important evaluation information.

Table 10-3   Feelings Diary

Name						Date:	
Date	Time	Setting	Conversation/Thoughts	Feelings	Approaches Tried to Change Feelings	Results	
10/12	9 a.m	Work	Boss told me I wasn't producing. I think he's a dope.	Rage	Deep breathing Guided imagery	At least I didn't punch him.	
10/12	noon	Cafeteria	Waitress told me there wasn't any fish. She's too lazy to get it.	Real angry	Told myself it was irrational to think there was fish when maybe there wasn't.	I didn't cool down for an hour and that spoiled my lunch hour.	
10/12	5 p.m	Driving	Someone cut me off and I rolled down the window and told him what I thought.	Rage	Picturing him in his underwear	I laughed and realized what a jerk I was being.	

The Inventory Approach To use this method, collect information periodically, at specific intervals, by setting target dates, identifying the expected target levels, and completing surveys or observations of your participants. You may consider this approach if you want to collect data on the decline in absenteeism and hospitalization, weight loss, smoking cessation, or any behavior you wish to examine at entry into the program and after completing the program.

The Comparative Approach If you select this method, you can buy or borrow standardized forms developed by other people or companies. Protocols and comparison data information may be available for smoking cessation and weight loss, among other programs. Large companies such as AT&T or government research organizations, such as the National Health Survey, provide standardized questionnaires, allowing you to compare your data with national or regional data, thus providing a form of control group.

The Controlled Comparison or Quasiexperimental Approach To use this approach, find another hospital or clinic similar to yours that will not participate in your health promotion program; this will be your control group. Both your clinic and the other clinic would then assess specific markers of patient satisfaction so that you can determine how your program compared to a standard approach to the health issue in question.

The Controlled Experimental Approach This is similar to a clinical trial used in pharmaceutical drug research. To use this approach, it must be feasible to deny your health promotion program to half of the population group; that becomes the control group. The group that receives your health promotion program is called the experimental group. Usually, participants are invited to participate. Once they agree, they are randomly assigned to two or more programs; for example, they might be assigned to a self-study group, a lecture group, or an online support group. These experimental groups can then be compared with control groups that do not receive any health promotion program, but which are monitored for major historical events that could affect study outcomes. Often, the control groups are offered the health promotion program after study measurements have been taken.

The Randomized Control Group In this approach, you can flip a coin to see which clients receive which health promotion approach and which receive some other experience. If you are working with the community, entire groups can be randomized to different health promotion programs.

Choose an approach somewhere between the simplicity of an inventory approach and the complexity and time intensity of the randomized control group design. To determine the best design for you, identify the outcomes you want to measure. Then choose a design that provides the data necessary to know whether you are achieving your objectives or not.

☐ Factors That Can Affect Evaluation

A number of problems can affect attempts to evaluate health promotion programs, including the complexity of public health problems that reflect multiple determinants and involve outcomes that may take years to achieve, the decentralized and networked nature of public health program implementation, and the lack of reliable and consistent data sources and other issues related to measurement. All three of these challenges hinder the ability to attribute program results to specific public health program efforts (DeGroff, Schooley, Chapel, & Poister, 2010).

To properly evaluate a program's effectiveness, the following steps must be undertaken:

1. *Summarize why the program was needed.* A program summary states in clear, short, simple terms the rationale for undertaking the program in the first place. This summation need not be more than a few sentences. For example, a program initiated in a school setting to promote helmet use was summarized by Germeni and colleagues as follows:

   The school environment has been often identified as a prosperous venue for public health improvement. This study is a cluster randomized controlled trial evaluating the impact of a school-based helmet promotion program on knowledge, attitudes, and practices of eligible adolescent drivers. (Germeni et al., 2010, p. 895)

2. *Describe the (intervention) program.* If the program is adapted from a field-tested project, identify the key components necessary to carry it out and ensure the integrity of the program. If the program is a community effort, the development of coalitions or task forces to implement community health promotion is an important element to include in the evaluation. Thow and colleagues (2010) demonstrated the importance of coalitions that included governmental policy makers who came on board when they learned the fiscal advantages of such actions.

   Components to discuss include:
   - Data collection through community assessment
   - Levels of support and commitment from community leaders and organizations
   - Types of community participation utilized

3. *State the goals and objectives of the program.* The program's criteria for success must be established in measurable terms. For example, a community's goal may be to reduce premature death due to cardiac arrest in the community. An example of an objective for this goal could be to reduce the percentage of smokers from 22% to 18% in the community by 2014. The balanced scorecard can provide a useful way to break down goals into workable objectives (Groene et al., 2009). Because goals and objectives determine the data that need to be collected to evaluate the program, it is essential that those goals and objectives to be stated in a manner that is clear and measurable. If they are not, the evaluation will be unable to determine whether the data that were gathered actually fulfilled the program's goals and objectives.

4. *Determine whether data collection met the needs of the program.* Data can be considered units of measure—for example, the number of people who quit smoking, the percentage of the population screened for cholesterol or the frequency with which participants attended programs. The value of the data collected is an alternative means of assessing a program's effectiveness. If the data collected cannot be used either to support the program's interventions or to assess the outcomes of those interventions, then they are of little value to the program. It should also be decided whether additional information was needed, would be useful, or would merely be interesting. A program is not effective if it collects more information than is necessary or manageable. There may be data points that offer interesting insights, but if they do not affect outcomes, do not offer any ideas for further interventions, and/ or were more trouble to collect than the information they provide is worth, then they constitute a poor return for the effort. Program designs should always seek to maximize resources; collection of unnecessary data is wasted resources, and a program that wastes resources should be evaluated accordingly.

5. *Develop the evaluation design.* A good evaluation design should include a focused dialogue between program planners and evaluators. Such an approach can result in more rigorously planned programs and the development and implementation of evaluation designs that have greater potential for policy and programmatic influence (Sridharan and Nakaima, 2011). There are many evaluation designs. The following examples illustrate three designs for the same program: introducing a new curriculum into a school health program. They are listed in order of increasing effectiveness, complexity, and cost (State of Minnesota, 2010).

   - *Simple record keeping* is an ongoing system that answers such questions as who, what, where, when, how many, or how much. For example, records are kept on the number of students who attended classes, how many teachers received training in the new curriculum, and what the differences were between the old and new curriculum. Record keeping has limited ability to provide assessment of program effects.
   - *Preimplementation and postimplementation measurement* is a system of collecting before and after information to measure change. In addition to the simple record-keeping data, tests are given to the students before and after the curriculum is taught. The test scores are then measured for differences, although differences cannot necessarily be attributed to the program.
   - *Controlled comparison* is a system of comparing the effects of an intervention in similar, but randomly assigned populations. For example, several school populations are pretested. Half the schools are randomly assigned to receive the new curriculum instruction while the other half does not receive it. Both groups are then tested again, and a comparison is made. Random assignment of the schools to either of the groups helps ensure that the population sample is representative, that the programs results are reproducible and generalizable, and that results are attributable to the program and not some inherent characteristics of the school assigned to either group. Controlled comparisons are highly complex, time consuming, and costly, but the results they generate are accurate representations of the program's effects.

6. *Determine data collection methods.* The evaluation relies on assessing evidence of the program's success or failure. Give some thought to how to best collect the evidence needed for the evaluation. Shoddy data collection yields shoddy results; a highly valuable program can be shot down with a bad evaluation if the evaluator collects evidence in a careless manner. Depending on the activity, any of the following methods may be used:

- Interviews
- Questionnaires
- Counting the number of events that occur
- Focus groups
- Surveys
- Observation

Whatever method is chosen, a collection form, such as a questionnaire or checklist, will be needed so that data are collected in a standard manner and in a common format. A cost–benefit analysis will tell you if the cost provides sufficient health promotion benefit. Costs are assumed to be the cost of implementation and administration of the program, which are usually monetary. Benefits may be somewhat more difficult to assess, as the quality of life improvements among clients cannot be assessed in monetary terms. Reduced usage of healthcare services resulting from improved health can be assigned monetary values, as can hours of worker productivity.

7. *Assess the study population/sample.* Evaluating a program's effects nearly always means making some sort of contact with participants. This contact may be direct, e.g., through the use of follow-up surveys, or indirect, e.g., assessing changes in health markers in the general population where the health program was offered. There are two key factors to assess in evaluating the program's effectiveness. First, did it reach the appropriate clients? Second, can an appropriate subsample of program participants be identified for following up how well the program accomplished its health goals?

Some key methods for assessing study population include:
- Using a census for small populations
- Imitating a sample size of similar studies
- Using published tables
- Applying formulas to calculate a sample size (Israel, 2009)

8. *Develop and pretest forms for data collection.* Many tools already exist for data collection. An existing form can be adapted or a new one can be developed. For questionnaires, careful consideration must be given to the type of questions needed to elicit the proper responses.

9. *Ensure consistency in data collection.* Two considerations that need to be addressed include the consistency of collection methods and the training of those collecting the data. If those collecting data (e.g., administering a phone survey or reading questionnaire responses) do not know how to review and code data, the opportunities for errors to creep into the data set increase. Data collected using inconsistent methods (for instance, by collecting some responses via phone and others via e-mail) introduces the possibility of lack of comparability in the data points—

HEALTH PROMOTION TIP

Pretest the forms that you develop. **Pretesting** is the process of measuring the effectiveness of a tool. It will help identify problems with wording, interpretation, or information gaps. After pretesting, the forms may need to be revised and improved.

the old apples and oranges dilemma, in which the two items being compared are from different populations. All data should be collected using one, consistent method by individuals trained in this method, preferably in a single set of training sessions developed and implemented by a single trainer.

10. *Organize and analyze the data.* Compile and analyze the information you selected and collected, bringing order to the data so that patterns can be identified. If applicable, compare preprogram and postprogram data. Ask whether the program made any difference to participants' health, and if so, how much?

Hazel and colleagues (2010) described how they compared modeled to measured mortality reductions, applying the Lives Saved tool to evaluation data. By examining studies that are similar to programs you plan to set up, you can derive ideas for your evaluation process.

Understand that evaluating the program's effectiveness is at least as important as designing and carrying out the program in the first place. If you do not evaluate the program after it is complete, you have no information as to whether the methods and activities you used are effective—which means you do not have a basis for deciding on whether to use similar methods and activities in the future.

ASK YOURSELF

Why is a program evaluation important?

Modify and Sustain Programs as Needed

Activities that are successful are activities that should be assessed with an eye toward enhancement. If a program obtained improvement among 70% of participants, then consider how the program might be changed to obtain improvement among 80% or 90% of participants. Eliminate or improve activities that were not successful.

Once programs have been evaluated and deemed successful, maintaining that success takes continued systematic planning, periodic review, and active community support. The goal now is to integrate the programs into the community to ensure the maintenance of good health in the present and the future.

In working with communities, develop oral and written progress reports and present them to the coalition, task forces, and the involved community organizations. Remember that communities are not static. New leaders will need to be identified and available resources in the community reviewed on a periodic basis (State of Minnesota, 2010).

HEALTH PROMOTION CHALLENGE

Cheryl O., ARNP, developed a physical activity health promotion program for adults and now is planning an evaluation component. Based on the information in this chapter, what advice would you give Cheryl?

RESEARCH BOX 10-2 Physical Activity in Overweight Adults

» BACKGROUND: Physical activity is related to being overweight.

» STUDY QUESTION: How does a health promotion program affect physical activity in overweight adults?

» RESEARCH DESIGN: Data from two randomized clinical trials (RCTs) were used to examine the extent to which a health promotion intervention affected changes in growth trajectories of psychosocial constructs, and if so, whether these constructs in turn explained changes in physical activity (PA).

» SAMPLE: 842 overweight adults in the United States.

» MEASURES: PA and psychosocial measures were collected in two RCTs evaluating Internet-based behavior change interventions with assessments at baseline and at 6 and 12 months. A physical activity latent variable at 12 months was created using indicators of self-reported walking and leisure time activities.

» FINDINGS: Intervention-mediated effects on PA at 12 months were found via latent growth curves representing self-efficacy and behavioral strategies, where increasing growth curves across time were associated with higher PA values at 12 months. These findings provide some evidence that web-based self-help intervention programs worked through targeted behavior change constructs to influence physical activity levels in overweight adults.

Source: Roesch, S. C., Norman, G. J., Villodas, F., Sallis, J. F., Patrick, K. (2010). Intervention-mediated effects for adult physical activity: A latent growth curve analysis. *Social Science and Medicine, 71*(3), 494–501.

Summary

Awareness programs typically use newsletters, health fairs, posters, and screening to increase client interest. Awareness programs seek to educate a community about a health issue so that individuals will begin to consider their own behaviors or circumstances. Behavior change programs, such as fitness or weight-loss programs, teach skills, require a supportive environment, and usually continue for 8–12 weeks to see an improvement. A community opinion survey helps determine what are perceived to be the major community health problems, while a resource inventory identifies what resources exist in the community to meet health needs. Evaluation is an integral part of the entire process of developing community-based health promotion programs. Evaluation is the process whereby the effects of a health promotion program are measured. Objective evidence may include such things as activity reports, surveys, changes in scores, and measurable changes in health (e.g., decreases in smoking rates or cholesterol levels).

Supportive environment programs help to alter aspects of community life to help maintain a long-term, sustained, healthy lifestyle. Examples might be working with health food stores and restaurants to offer healthier food selections and to provide recognition for role models as well as rewards and recognition for program participants. Lifestyle change programs undertake behavior change on a grander scale—changing not one, but multiple behaviors so that overall lifestyle is altered toward health. Outcome evaluation measures consequences attributable to health promotion program activities can show whether you are attaining your program objectives. Examples of positive outcome measures are increase in health knowledge, change in attitudes to belief in ability, increase in healthy behaviors, decrease in risk factors, and decrease in morbidity and premature mortality. Pretesting is the process of measuring the effectiveness of a survey or other measurement tool. Pretesting will help identify problems with wording, interpretation, or information gaps. Self-evaluation measures show clients they are part of the health promotion team. Their input is valued. Three simple self-evaluation methods include asking clients to rate their symptoms before and after treatment sessions from 1 (uncomfortable symptoms) to 10 (relief; comfort) and completing a wellness or feelings diary. A wellness diary includes a chart of clients' intake, bowel movements, activities, symptoms, and mood changes by time of day, and a feelings diary.

REVIEW QUESTIONS

1. Which of the following is not a good word to use in writing objectives?
    a. Eliminate
    b. Demonstrate
    c. Understand
    d. Identify

2. What is the most effective method for decision making?
    a. Selecting a popular leader
    b. Group consensus
    c. Secret ballots
    d. Doing what worked in the past

3. Why is it important to hear all group members' views before making a decision?
    a. Those who are opposed to a proposed idea might not say so until it is too late
    b. To make everyone happy
    c. Someone might have a better idea
    d. All of the above

4. Which of the following is not an example of an outcome measure?
    a. Change in knowledge
    b. Change in attitudes
    c. Change in behaviors
    d. Change in number of program participants

5. When choosing an evaluation design, what should you consider?
    a. Limitations of the design
    b. Practical, ethical, and financial constraints
    c. Both A and B
    d. None of the above

6. What is the chief significance of evaluating a health promotion program?
    a. To determine whether the methods and activities are effective
    b. To determine whether you can use similar methods in the future
    c. It's a required part of the grant
    d. To understand statistics

EXERCISES

1. Find out what your school or hospital setting is doing to evaluate health promotion programs. Write a 2–4 page paper on your findings.

2. Work with a graduate nursing student to help evaluate a health promotion program.

3. Help the graduate nursing student you are working with to write up the evaluation findings and share what you learned online.

4. Write a short two- to four-page paper on what you learned from working with the graduate nursing student and share it with at least three other students.

5. Check out websites to learn more about developing health promotion programs for individuals and communities. Include http://www.ncbi.nlm.nih.gov/pubmed/ in your search. Write a two- to four-page paper summarizing what you found and including web links. Share your findings with at least two other nursing students.

6. Find out what your school or hospital setting is doing to encourage health promotion in clients and the community. Write up your findings in a two- to four-page paper and share it with at least two other students.

REFERENCES

Birch, L. L., & Ventura, A. K. (2010). Preventing childhood obesity: What works? *International Journal of Obesity (London), 33*(Suppl 1), S74–S81.

Cowart, L. W., Biro, D. J., Wasserman, T., Stein, R. F., Reider, L. R., & Brown, B. (2010). Designing and pilot-testing a church-based community program to reduce obesity among African Americans. *The ABNF Journal, 21*(1), 4–10.

DeGroff, A., Schooley, M., Chapel, T., & Poister, T. H. (2010). Challenges and strategies in applying performance measurement to federal public health programs. *Evaluation and Program Planning, 33*(4), 365–372.

Germeni, E., Lionis, C., Kalampoki, V., Davou, B., Belechri, M., & Petridou, E. (2010). Evaluating the impact of a school-based helmet promotion program on eligible adolescent drivers: Different audiences, different needs? *Health Education Research, 25*(5), 865–876.

Groene, O., Brandt E., Schmidt W., & Moeller, J. (2009). The balanced scorecard of acute settings: Development process, definition of 20 strategic objectives and implementation. *International Journal of Quality Health Care, 21*(4), 259–271.

Hazel, E., Gilroy, K., Friberg, I., Black, R. E., Bryce, J., & Jones, G. (2010). Comparing modelled to measured mortality reductions: Applying the lives saved tool to evaluation data from the Accelerated Child Survival Programme in West Africa. *International Journal of Epidemiology, 39* (Suppl 1), i32–i39.

Hildebrand, M., & Neufeld, P. (2009). Recruiting older adults into a physical activity promotion program: Active living every day offered in a naturally occurring retirement community. *Gerontologist, 49*(5), 702–710.

Israel, G. D. (2009). Determining sample size. Publication No. PEOD6. Jacksonville: University of Florida, FAS Extension. Retrieved from http://edis.ifas.ufl.edu/pd006

Kaufman, N. (2010). Internet and information technology use in treatment of diabetes. *International Journal of Clinical Practice Supplement,* (166), 41–46.

Klima, C., Norr, K., Vonderheid, S., & Handler, A. (2009). Introduction of centering pregnancy in a public health clinic. *Journal of Midwifery and Women's Health, 54*(1), 27–34.

Larsen, E. L., & Stock, C. (2011). Capturing contrasted realities: Integrating multiple perspectives of community life in health promotion. *Health Promotion International, 26*(1),14–22.

Lee, C. Y., Kim, H. S., Ahn, Y. H., Ko, I. S., & Cho, Y. H. (2009). Development of a community health promotion center based on the World Health Organization's Ottawa Charter health promotion strategies. *Japan Journal of Nursing Science, 6*(2), 83–90.

Marrett, L. D., Northrup, D. A., Pichora, E. C., Spinks, M. T., & Rosen, C. F. (2010). The second national sun survey: Overview and methods. *Canadian Journal of Public Health, 101*(4), 110–113.

Perry, C., & Hoffman, B. (2010). Assessing tribal youth physical activity and programming using a community-based participatory research approach. *Public Health Nursing, 27*(2), 104–114.

Sridharan, S., & Nakaima, A. (2011). Ten steps to making evaluation matter. *Evaluation and Program Planning, 34*(2):135–46.

State of Minnesota. (2010). Tip sheets, work sheets, and suggestions for developing health promotion programs. Retrieved from http://www.health.state.mn.us/divs/hpcd/chp/hpkit/text/hcheck_design_main.htm

Thow, A. M., Quested C., Juventin, L., Kun, R., Khan, A. N., & Swinburn, B. (2011). Taxing soft drinks in the Pacific: Implementation lessons for improving health. *Health Promotion International, 26*(1), 55–64.

Tobin, K. E., Kuramoto, S. J., Davey-Rothwell, M. A., & Latkin, C. A. (2011). The STEP into Action study: A peer-based, personal risk network-focused HIV prevention intervention with injection drug users in Baltimore, Maryland. *Addiction, 106*(2), 366–375.

Walker, L. O., Kim, S., Sterling, B. S., & Latimer, L. (2010). Developing health promotion interventions: A multisource method applied to weight loss among low-income postpartum women. *Public Health Nursing, 27*(2), 188–195.

Wilkins, K., & Shields, M. (2009). Employer-provided support services and job dissatisfaction in Canadian registered nurses. *Nursing Research, 58*(4), 255–263.

INTERNET RESOURCES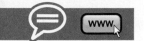

For a full suite of assignments and learning activities, use the access code located in the front of your book to visit this exclusive website: **http://go.jblearning .com/healthpromotion** If you do not have an access code, you can obtain one at the site.

LEARNING OBJECTIVES

Upon completion of this chapter, you will be able to:

1. Define chronic condition
2. Discuss the economic and societal impact of chronic conditions
3. Identify actions clients can take to prevent chronic conditions
4. Discuss the relationship of quality of life to chronic conditions
5. Explain the various elements of the chronic disease self-management model and how they impact on chronic health care

KEY TERMS

Chronic conditions

Chronic disease self-management model

Functional limitations

Health-related quality of life

Quality of life

CHAPTER 11

Prevention and Self-Management of Chronic Conditions: Using the Evidence

http://go.jblearning.com/healthpromotion

For a full suite of assignments and learning activities, use the access code located in the front of your book to visit the exclusive website: http://go.jblearning.com/healthpromotion If you do not have an access code, you can obtain one at the site.

Introduction

Chronic conditions are the United States' greatest healthcare problem. This chapter examines **chronic conditions** and their link to high healthcare costs and low quality of life. We will examine the statistics on chronic conditions and their effect on death and ability to perform activities of daily living (ADLs). We will also provide some insight into the major causes of chronic conditions and how they can be prevented.

The Incidence of Chronic Conditions

In 2005, it was estimated that 133 million people had at least one chronic condition, with a projected 50% of the population being affected by 2020 (Anderson, 2004; Centers for Disease Control and Prevention [CDC], 2009). CDC statistics for 2010 indicate that chronic conditions comprise 10 of the top 15 causes of death and that 70% of all deaths are caused by a chronic disease.

The top four causes of death are all chronic conditions (heart disease, cancer, chronic obstructive pulmonary disease (COPD), asthma, and cerebrovascular diseases) (Murphy, Xu, & Kochanek, 2012). In addition, some individuals, particularly older adults, may have multiple chronic conditions.

Chronic Conditions and Functional Limitations

Individuals with some chronic conditions also have **functional limitations**, defined by one or more of the following factors:

- Limited in performing physical activity, such as difficulty walking, bending, or stooping
- Limited in taking part in normal life activity, such as work, housework, or school
- Requires assistance with ADLs: bathing, eating, dressing, transferring (e.g., from bed to chair), toileting, and walking
- Receives assistance with instrumental ADLs: doing housework, preparing meals, taking medications, shopping, telephoning, and managing money

While only 14% of Americans have both a chronic condition and functional limitations, the healthcare expenses of this group accounts for 46% of all healthcare spending in the United States (Alecxih, Shen, Chan, Taylor, &

Drabek, 2010). It is estimated that 83% of the nation's medical care costs are associated with treating individuals with chronic conditions (Anderson, 2004). Care for chronic conditions has been the most common reason for Americans to seek care for the previous decade, if not longer (CDC, 2002). It is clear that preventing and managing chronic conditions so that individuals experience optimal well-being is an important social and financial priority for the United States.

The Effect of Chronic Conditions on National Healthcare Costs and Treatment

Why have chronic conditions become such a key factor in healthcare spending? One reason is that many diseases that used to be fatal are not anymore. Individuals with HIV/AIDS, type 1 diabetes, cystic fibrosis, hemophilia, lymphoma, and other illnesses now can live longer and healthier lives, depending on how well their condition is managed.

Another reason for the high cost of chronic care is that the American medical care system is fragmented and physicians are primarily prepared to deal with acute conditions. No one specific institution or practice is responsible for managing a client's entire health circumstance, so the need to visit multiple specialists adds to the complexity and cost.

The lack of support for prevention activities is another factor that adds to national healthcare costs. Even though prevention is more cost-effective than treatment, the economic structure of health care rewards treatment, but only rarely supports prevention.

Another reason for the high cost of health care is that our system is set up as to treat the acute illnesses that were more prevalent in the past and is geared towards acute, episodic, and curative care (Holman & Lorig, 2004).

The medical healthcare system has not embraced health promotion and prevention over disease diagnosis and treatment. That perspective must change to reduce the development of chronic conditions and reduce the burden of healthcare costs.

HEALTH PROMOTION CHALLENGE

If prevention is more cost-effective than treatment, why isn't prevention driving the healthcare system? Come up with evidence to back up your answer and share your findings with at least two classmates.

Nurse practitioners, not physicians, are in the forefront of providing prevention and wellness services. One example is a nurse-run clinic in Sheridan, Colorado, that offers health education programs, prevention services, and integrated providers. Nurse-managed clinics have "emphasized the importance of a holistic approach to overcome social and environmental barriers to health, instead of merely treating disease." (Domrose, 2012, p. 11.)

Ever since Lillian Wald established the Henry Street Settlement in 1893 to provide health and education to the poor of New York, over 250 nurse-managed clinics operate nationwide. One of these clinics serves a large homeless population, as well as poor, working adults in San Francisco's Tenderloin neighborhood, and operates in the same building as Glide Memorial Methodist Church, which runs a free meals program. The wellness center offers education, complementary healing, and movement classes such as tai chi. Clients can see a mental health provider, an addiction counselor, and/or take a yoga or meditation class. The center also offers a healthy eating and cooking class, stress reduction training, smoking cessation support, and information on domestic violence (Domrose, 2012).

HEALTH PROMOTION CHALLENGE

If you could develop a nurse-managed prevention clinic, what would you include? Share your ideas with at least two classmates and ask for feedback.

Four Major Causes of Chronic Conditions

We already know the four modifiable health risk behaviors responsible for the suffering and early death due to chronic conditions. According to the Center for Disease Control and Prevention (2010), these four modifiable health risk behaviors are:

1. lack of physical activity,
2. poor nutrition,
3. tobacco use, and
4. excessive alcohol consumption.
- More than one-third of all adults do not meet recommendations for aerobic physical activity based on the 2008 Physical Activity Guidelines for Americans, and 23% report no leisure-time physical activity at all in the preceding month.

- In 2007, less than 22% of high school students and only 24% of adults reported eating 5 or more servings of fruits and vegetables per day.
- More than 43 million American adults (approximately 1 in 5) smoke.
- In 2007, 20% of high school students in the United States were current cigarette smokers.
- Lung cancer is the leading cause of cancer death, and cigarette smoking causes almost all cases. Compared to nonsmokers, men who smoke are about 23 times more likely to develop lung cancer and women who smoke are about 13 times more likely. Smoking causes about 90% of lung cancer deaths in men and almost 80% in women. Smoking also causes cancer of the voicebox (larynx), mouth and throat, esophagus, bladder, kidney, pancreas, cervix, and stomach, and causes acute myeloid leukemia.
- Nearly 45% of high school students report consuming alcohol in the past 30 days, and over 60% of those who drink report binge drinking (consuming 5 or more drinks on an occasion) within the past 30 days.
- Drinking alcohol is a risk factor for primary liver cancer, and more than 100 studies have found an increased risk of breast cancer with increasing alcohol intake. The link between alcohol consumption and colorectal (colon) cancer has been reported in more than 50 studies (Center for Disease Control and Prevention, 2010).

HEALTH PROMOTION CHALLENGE

Choose one of the four modifiable health risk behaviors for death due to chronic conditions and develop a health promotion program in your school to reduce that risk. You can use a newsletter, website, lunchtime lecture/discussion, or any other method you're comfortable with to provide information and change behavior.

Preventing Heart Conditions

Clients can make simple changes in their daily lives to reduce or eliminate risk for heart attack and related conditions. Some of these changes include eliminating added sugars, maintaining a healthy weight, not smoking or being around others who do, exercising for 30 minutes a day, and eating healthy foods.

Welsh and colleagues (2010) found that eating sugars can lead to dyslipidemia, a lipid profile known to increase cardiovascular disease. They found a statistically significant correlation between dietary added sugars and blood lipid levels among U. S. adults. Many Americans consume 22–46 teaspoons of sugar daily in processed or prepared foods, energy drinks, sodas, cookies, candy, pies, cakes, etc. The best remedy is to eat whole foods, such as 5 to 10 servings of fruits and vegetables a day; whole grains; low-fat dairy products; beans; and low-fat sources of protein, including certain types of fish. Salmon and mackerel are good sources of omega-3 fatty acids that protect against irregular heartbeats and lower blood pressure. Limiting saturated fats (red meat, dairy products, coconut and palm oils) and trans fats (deep-fried fast foods, bakery products, packaged snack foods, margarine, and crackers) is important because saturated fats increase the risk of coronary artery disease by raising cholesterol levels.

Following a heart-healthy regime means drinking alcohol only in moderation—no more than two drinks a day for men, and one a day for women. More than that becomes a health hazard. Women with a history of breast cancer may not want to drink at all.

Eating too much and not exercising enough can lead to weight gain, and the excess weight can lead to increased chance of heart disease, high blood pressure, high cholesterol, and diabetes.

Waist circumference is a simple way to measure abdominal fat. Men are overweight if their waist is greater than 40 inches, women if theirs is greater than 35 inches. Even a small weight loss of 10% is beneficial because that decrease can lower blood pressure and blood cholesterol levels and reduce risk of diabetes (Mayo Clinic Staff, 2012b). For specific, evidence-based preventive and health promotive actions, see the Appendix.

Cancer Prevention

Despite widespread availability of cancer prevention programs, policies, and guidelines, evidence-based interventions (EBIs) are not broadly implemented (Sanchez et al., 2012). With the increase of sedentary lifestyle and overweight, many chronic diseases have also increased, including cancer (Inumara, 2012). Besides overweight/obesity, other known causes of cancer that can be prevented include elimination of tobacco use and reduction in exposure to environmental carcinogens (Kripke, 2012).

The American Institute for Cancer Research (2012) provided additional information for preventing cancer:

1. Be as lean as possible without becoming underweight. Staying slim also protects against diabetes and heart disease. Carrying excess fat around the waist can be particularly harmful. This weight acts like a "hormone pump" releasing estrogen into the bloodstream as well as raising levels

of other hormones in the body that are strongly linked to colon cancer and probably to cancers of the pancreas and endometrium (lining of the uterus), as well as breast cancer (in postmenopausal women).

2. Be physically active for at least 30 minutes every day, but 60 minutes is better. Studies show that regular activity can help to keep hormone levels healthy, which is important because having high levels of some hormones can increase cancer risk. Physical activity may also strengthen the immune system, help keep our digestive system healthy, and allow clients to consume more food and more cancer-protective nutrients— without gaining weight. Shorter bouts of activity are just as beneficial; it's the total time that is important. Caution clients to start with brisk walking or anything that gets their heart beating a bit faster and makes them breathe more deeply.

3. Avoid sugary drinks. Limit consumption of energy-dense foods that are processed and contain added sugar, e.g., chocolate. Eating an apple is a better choice; for example, 3.5 oz. of chocolate contains 10 times more calories than the same amount of apple: 3.5 oz of milk chocolate = 520 calories, 3.5 oz. of apple = 52 calories. By choosing a diet based on low-energy-dense foods, such as fruits and vegetables, you can actually eat more food but consume fewer calories.

4. Make your diet plant-based. Eat a variety of vegetables, fruits, whole grains, and legumes such as beans. When preparing a meal, aim to fill at least two-thirds of your plate with vegetables, fruits, whole grains, and beans. Research shows that vegetables and fruits protect against a range of cancers, including mouth, pharynx, larynx, esophagus, stomach, lung, pancreas, and prostate. As well as containing vitamins and minerals, which help keep the body healthy and strengthen the immune system, plant-based foods are also good sources of substances like phytochemicals, which can help to protect cells in the body from damage that can lead to cancer. Foods containing fiber are also linked to a reduced risk of cancer. These foods include whole-grain bread and pasta, oats, and vegetables and fruits. Fiber is thought to have many benefits, including helping to speed up "gut transit time," or how long it takes food to move through the digestive system. Plant foods can also help maintain a healthy weight because many of them are lower in energy density (calories).

5. Limit consumption of red meats (such as beef, pork, and lamb) and avoid processed meats (ham, bacon, pastrami, salami, hot dogs, and sausages). The evidence that red meat is a cause of colorectal cancer is convincing: heme iron in red meats has been shown to damage the lining of the colon. Research on processed meats shows the cancer risk increases with each portion. Meat that is preserved by smoking, curing,

or salting, or by the addition of preservatives, can form substances that damage cells in the body and lead to the development of cancer.

6. After treatment, cancer survivors should follow these recommendations for cancer prevention.

Preventing COPD/Asthma and Promoting Health for Clients Diagnosed with COPD/Asthma

According to the Mayo Clinic Staff (2012a), the controllable risk factors for COPD/asthma are:

- Being overweight
- Being a smoker
- Exposure to secondhand smoke
- Exposure to exhaust fumes or other types of pollution
- Exposure to occupational triggers, such as chemicals used in farming, hairdressing and manufacturing.

The American Academy of Allergy, Asthma, and Immunology (2012) provides additional suggestions for preventing asthma, including breastfeeding, how and when to introduce solid foods, and environmental factors that can be controlled.

Breastmilk is the least likely to trigger an allergic reaction, strengthens an infant's immune system, and protects a baby from lung infections and asthma. Experts recommend exclusive breastfeeding for the first 4 to 6 months.

For infants at risk for food allergy who are not exclusively breast fed, the use of hydrolyzed infant formulas instead of cow's milk formula may be considered as a preventive strategy.

After 4 to 6 months, single-ingredient infant foods including fruits, vegetables, and cereal grains can be introduced one at a time. This slow process gives parents or caregivers a chance to identify and eliminate any food that causes an allergic reaction. The introduction of solid foods, even potential allergens, should not be delayed beyond 4 to 6 months of age.

There are also environmental actions that can prevent asthma. One of them is controlling dust mites, airborne substances that can trigger allergy or asthma symptoms. Reducing contact with these substances early in life may delay or prevent allergy or asthma symptoms. Using zippered, "allergen-impermeable" covers on pillows and mattresses and washing bedding in hot water weekly can be beneficial. Also, indoor humidity should be kept below 50%. If possible, carpets and upholstered furniture should be removed from an infant's bedroom.

Early exposure to animals (cats and dogs in particular) may protect children from developing allergic responses. Newer research suggests children raised on farms develop fewer allergies and asthma.

Exposure to tobacco smoke before or after birth increases the chance of a child wheezing during infancy. Exposing children to secondhand smoke has also been shown to increase the development of asthma and other chronic respiratory illnesses.

Exercise is also important as a prevention strategy. Movement helps stretch the lungs and bronchial tubes, which in turn can reduce the resistance to breathing. There has obviously been a tremendous change in children's lifestyles, from being active and exercise-based to sedentary and technology-based. This lack of exercise, and the possible obesity associated with it, may in fact play a role in the increasing burden of asthma. "For those who already have developed asthma, aerobic exercise might trigger attacks, but these can easily be prevented by using an inhaler (such as albuterol) before the activity. asthma that is triggered by exercise should certainly not prevent a person from having an active lifestyle or participating in sports" (Szeftel, 2007).

As well as dealing with the above risk factors, exercise is an important component in promoting health in clients already diagnosed with COPD/ Asthma. Some of the types of exercise that proved beneficial were aerobic training (walking a 6-minute mile), resistance training (such as weight lifting), balance training, or a combination of all three (Reid et al., 2012). Nutrition and weight management are also important interventions with these clients (Evans, 2012).

Preventing Strokes

Controllable factors that stress carotid arteries and increase the risk of injury, buildup of plaques, and stroke include:

- *High blood pressure.* Excess pressure on the walls of the carotid arteries can weaken them and leave them more vulnerable to damage. Losing weight and learning stress reduction measures can help lower blood pressure. See Appendix for other suggestions.
- *Smoking.* Nicotine can irritate the inner lining of the arteries. It also increases heart rate and blood pressure.
- *Abnormal blood-fat levels.* High levels of low-density lipoprotein (LDL) cholesterol, the "bad" cholesterol, and high levels of triglycerides, a blood fat, encourage the accumulation of plaques. Some of these changes can be prevented by eating a healthy diet that includes 10 servings of fruits

and vegetables a day, salmon or mackerel, and other whole foods, while limiting sugar and saturated and trans fats.

- *Obesity.* Carrying excess pounds increases chances of high blood pressure, atherosclerosis, and diabetes.
- *Physical inactivity.* Lack of exercise contributes to a number of conditions, including high blood pressure, diabetes, and obesity (Silver, 2012; Li & Siegrest, 2012).

HEALTH PROMOTION CHALLENGE

Based on information in this chapter, devise a heart disease, cancer, COPD/asthma, or stroke prevention program. Share your program with at least two classmates and ask for feedback.

Obesity and Its Effect on Other Chronic Conditions

While our healthcare system is good at treating short-term problems, such as broken bones and infections, obesity is reaching epidemic proportions. Obesity increases the risk of developing other chronic conditions, such as diabetes and heart disease. The rate of obesity in adults has doubled in the last 20 years, has almost tripled in children ages 2–11, and has more than tripled in children ages 12–19.

Obesity can harm the cardiovascular system and being overweight during childhood can accelerate the development of heart disease. The processes that lead to a heart attack or stroke start in childhood and often take decades to progress to the point of overt disease. Obesity in childhood, adolescence, and young adulthood may accelerate these processes. Other obesity-related disorders—metabolic, digestive, respiratory, skeletal, and psychosocial—are appearing in children either for the first time or with greater severity or prevalence.

HEALTH PROMOTION CHALLENGE

How should obesity prevention components be embedded within health, education, and care systems to attain long term impact? Draw up a plan to embed obesity prevention components in one school or care system. Share your ideas with at least two other students and seek feedback. If possible, work with a more seasoned nurse researcher to test out your ideas.

Examples include high blood pressure, early symptoms of hardening of the arteries, type 2 diabetes, nonalcoholic fatty liver disease, polycystic ovary disorder, and disordered breathing during sleep.

The increasing prevalence and severity of childhood obesity may reverse the modern era's steady increase in life expectancy, with today's youth on average living less healthy and ultimately shorter lives than their parents. Should this happen, this will be the first such reversal in lifespan in modern history. Such a possibility makes obesity in children an issue of utmost public health concern (Daniels, 2006).

See RESEARCH BOX 11-1 for a study on how to prevent childhood obesity.

RESEARCH BOX 11-1 Prevention of Childhood Obesity

» BACKGROUND: Prevention of childhood obesity is an international public health priority given the significant impact of obesity on acute and chronic diseases, general health, development, and well-being. The international evidence base for strategies that governments, communities, and families can implement to prevent obesity, and promote health, has been accumulating but remains unclear.

» OBJECTIVES: This review of research aimed to update the previous Cochrane review on prevention of childhood obesity and determine the effectiveness of evaluated interventions intended to prevent obesity in children, assessed by change in Body Mass Index (BMI). Secondary aims were to examine the characteristics of the programs and strategies to answer the questions "What works for whom, why, and for what cost?"

» SEARCH METHODS: The researcher searched relevant websites including CENTRAL, MEDLINE, EMBASE, PsychINFO and CINAHL in March 2010. Non-English language papers were included and experts were contacted.

» SELECTION CRITERIA: The review includes data from childhood obesity prevention studies that used a controlled study design (with or without randomization). Studies were included if they evaluated interventions, policies, or programs in place for 12 weeks or more. If studies were randomized at a cluster level, six clusters were required.

» DATA COLLECTION AND ANALYSIS: Two review authors independently extracted data and assessed the risk of bias of included studies. Data were extracted on intervention implementation, cost, equity, and outcomes. Outcome measures were grouped according to whether they measured adiposity, physical activity (PA)-related behaviors, or diet-related behaviors. Adverse outcomes were recorded. A meta-analysis was conducted using available BMI or standardized BMI (zBMI) score data with subgroup

(continues)

analysis by age group (0–5, 6–12, 13–18 years, corresponding to stages of developmental and childhood settings).

» RESULTS: The majority of studies targeted children aged 6–12 years. The meta-analysis included 37 studies of 27,946 children and demonstrated that programs were effective at reducing adiposity, although not all individual interventions were effective, and there was a high level of observed heterogeneity ($I(2)=82\%$). Overall, children in the intervention group had a standardized mean difference in adiposity (measured as BMI or zBMI) of $-0.15\text{kg/m}(2)$ (95% confidence interval (CI): -0.21 to -0.09). Only eight studies reported on adverse effects and no evidence of adverse outcomes such as unhealthy dieting practices, increased prevalence of underweight, or body image sensitivities was found. Interventions did not appear to increase health inequalities although this was examined in fewer studies.

» CONCLUSIONS: The researchers found strong evidence to support beneficial effects of child obesity prevention programs on BMI, particularly for programs targeted to children aged 6 to 12 years. A synthesis of findings indicated the following to be promising policies and strategies: school curriculum that includes healthy eating, physical activity, and body image; increased sessions for physical activity and the development of fundamental movement skills throughout the school week; improvements in nutritional quality of the food supply in schools; environments and cultural practices that support children eating healthier foods and being active throughout each day; support for teachers and other staff to implement health promotion strategies and activities (e.g. professional development, capacity building activities); and parent support and home activities that encourage children to be more active, eat more nutritious foods, and spend less time in screen based activities. Childhood obesity prevention research must now move towards identifying how effective intervention components can be embedded within health, education, and care systems and achieve long term sustainable impacts.

Source: Waters, E., de Silva-Sanigorski, A., Hall, B. J., Brown, T., Campbell, K. J., Gao, Y., . . . Summerbell, C. D. (2011). Interventions for preventing obesity in children. *Cochrane Data Base System Reviews* Published online, December 7(12), CD001871.

High Blood Pressure

Older adults are the most rapidly growing population group in the world. Hypertension increases with age. The risk of many other chronic conditions including coronary artery disease, stroke, congestive heart disease, chronic kidney insufficiency, and dementia is also increased as blood pressure rises (Lionakis, Mendrinos, Sanidas, Favatas, & Georgopoulou, 2012). RESEARCH BOX 11-2 provides some ideas for lowering blood pressure without using pharmacological approaches.

RESEARCH BOX 11-2 Effects of Exercise and Relaxation on Blood Pressure.

» OBJECTIVE: To study the aftereffects of exercise and relaxation, performed alone and in combination, on blood pressure (BP) measured at baseline and during stressful conditions.

» DESIGN: The researchers conducted a clinical trial with comparison groups and repeated measures in each group.

» PARTICIPANTS: Fourteen normotensive (NT) and 16 essential hypertensive (HT) participants in the exercise laboratory at the University of Sao Paulo, Brazil.

» INTERVENTIONS: The researchers conducted four random experimental sessions: relaxation (RX-20 min); exercise (EX-cycle for 50 min); exercise plus relaxation (EX+RX); and control (C-73 min rest). Measures were taken before and after interventions at baseline and during a Stroop color test.

» MEASURES: Auscultatory and plesthysmographic BPs.

» RESULTS: The decreases in both BPs were significantly greater after the EX+RX session, and were also greater in the HT EX+RX session. During mental stress, systolic BP increased significantly and similarly after all the experimental sessions. Diastolic BP also increased significantly during stress, but the increase was significantly greater after the RX session. At the end of the mental stress, diastolic BP was significantly lower after the EX and EX+RX sessions than after the C and RX sessions.

» CONCLUSIONS: In NT and HT subjects, a single bout of exercise or relaxation has hypotensive effects, further enhanced by their combination, and greater in the HT. Moreover, exercise performed alone or in combination with relaxation decreases systolic and diastolic BPs during mental stress.

Source: Santaella, D. F., Araújo, E. A., Ortega, K. C., Tinucci, T., Mion, D. Jr., Negrão, C. E., & de Moraes Forjaz, C. L. (2006). Aftereffects of exercise and relaxation on blood pressure. *Clinical Journal of Sports Medicine, 16*(4), 341–347.

Chronic Conditions and Quality of Life

Pain, stress, lack of mobility, and more can affect the **quality of life** of a client with a chronic condition. Since the early 1980s, researchers have worked to define the concept of **health-related quality of life** (HRQoL) and describe how to measure it. The CDC (2012) has defined HRQoL as "an individual's or group's perceived physical and mental health over time" (Lubkin & Larsen, 2006).

One of the most widely used and adapted tools for measuring HRQoL is a questionnaire called the "short form 36" or SF-36 questionnaire (Hickey, Barker, McGee, & O'Boyle, 2005; McHorney, Ware, Lu, & Sherbourne, 1994). This questionnaire was developed as part of the RAND Corporation's Medical Outcomes Study in 1992. SF-36 focuses on eight scaled scores, which are the weighted sums of all questions in each section. Each scale is directly transformed into a 0–100 scale on the assumption that each question carries equal weight.

The factors scored are:

- Vitality
- Physical functioning
- Bodily pain
- General health perceptions
- Physical role functioning
- Emotional role functioning
- Social role functioning
- Mental health

While the SF-36 has been found to be useful for getting a general sense of quality of life, many researchers looking at people with specific disease states (for instance, HIV) found that it was not specific enough for their purposes. The solution for many researchers is to alter or adapt the SF-36 questionnaire to meet their need. This solution has been met with mixed results; in some instances, the adapted questionnaires still do not address important considerations in particular populations (children and adolescents, for example) (Coons, Rao, Keininger, & Hays, 2000; Ravens-Sieberer et al., 2006). In other instances, even adapted questionnaires failed to adequately capture key aspects of specific disease states (Reaney, Martin, & Speight, 2008).

These problems have led researchers to develop more specific tools for assessing HRQoL. For example, quality of life in people with morbid obesity may be measured using the Laval Questionnaire, developed by a bariatric surgery clinic at Laval Hospital in Canada (Therrien et al., 2011).

INFORMATION BOX 11-1

The Partnership for Solutions is an initiative led by Johns Hopkins University and the Robert Wood Johnson Foundation to improve the care and quality of life for Americans with chronic health conditions. The group is engaged in the following three major activities: (1) conducting original research and identifying existing research that clarifies the nature of the problem; (2) communicating these research findings to policy makers, business leaders, health professionals, advocates, and others; and (3) working to identify promising solutions to the problems faced by people with chronic health conditions. Its website contains research articles and links to governmental groups and health organizations that are involved with chronic disease work. Go to http://www.partnershipforsolutions.org/ for more information.

A tool called the PedsQL (Pediatric Quality of Life Inventory) has been developed to measure HRQoL in children age 2–18 (Varni, Seid, & Kurtin, 2001). HIV clients' quality of life is measured using a tool called FAHI (Functional Assessment of HIV Infection) (Feinberg et al., 2011). In short, there are a multitude of specific measurement instruments for HRQoL that are both generic and disease and population specific. To assess client quality of life, make use of both types by utilizing the SF-36 in addition to more specific questionnaires, depending on what the most recent research data show about the utility of different tools.

Chronic Pain as a Quality of Life Indicator

One key factor in assessing quality of life is the level of pain experienced by a client. Health and function issues include such things as how a person perceives his or her health, how he or she is able to complete the activities of quality of life independently, and if there are any pain experiences.

Pain is especially a priority in that it can easily disrupt a person's quality of life with a chronic condition. Chronic pain, if left untreated or treated inadequately, can also lead to depression, anxiety, fatigue, and sleep disturbance, further disrupting a client's well-being. Thus, some healthcare providers include an assessment of a client's pain experiences at every encounter. Pain levels are now regarded as a fifth vital sign needed to assess health by many health practitioners.

The fact that healthcare providers have developed an awareness of the importance of pain does not mean that pain is well managed, particularly chronic pain. A study by the Veterans Administration found that on the contrary, efforts to highlight pain as the fifth vital sign failed to improve pain management (Mularski et al., 2006). Healthcare providers are often hesitant to treat chronic pain because they fear the potential for addiction, the physiologic response of physical dependence that a person exhibits if he or she has been on medication for a long period of time. Even when addiction does not occur, drug tolerance may occur, which requires higher doses of administration—doses with which the healthcare provider may not be comfortable because of concerns about harmful side effects (e.g., liver damage).

In order to support good quality of life, interventions for pain focus on using the nursing process of assessing, diagnosing, planning, intervening, and evaluating. Nonpharmacologic interventions that do not damage the liver or any other body part can be integrated into the plan of care. Possible interventions include yoga, guided

HOT TOPICS

Here are some topics to explore:
- Chronic disease self-management model
- Quality of life
- Self-management behaviors scale
- Chronic pain
- Yoga
- Guided imagery
- Tai Chi

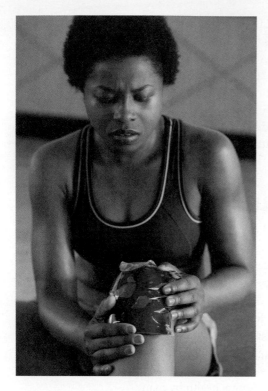

imagery, the local application of heat and cold, and biofeedback. See Appendix for suggestions for use.

Positive Outcomes for Health Promotion in Chronic Disease

What constitutes a positive outcome for a health promotion activity undertaken with a client or family coping with a chronic condition? There are a number of factors that could be considered positive outcomes; these will be discussed in the following sections.

☐ Relief of Symptoms or Reduction of Disease Impact

In some clients, learning to manage the chronic condition is a way to reduce the experience of symptoms or adverse events. For example, persons with allergic asthma might learn strategies for identify triggers so they can take steps to avoid them, resulting in fewer acute asthma exacerbations (Göksel et al., 2009). Individuals with rheumatoid arthritis or fibromyalgia might learn mind-body techniques for reducing pain (Shariff et al., 2009), or a person with irritable bowel syndrome might undertake lifestyle modifications to decrease gastrointestinal symptoms (Kang et al., 2011). Reduction in disease symptoms is often a first step toward improving quality of life. See Appendix for specific approaches that support health and wellness and can reduce symptoms.

There are some chronic conditions that lack overt unpleasant symptoms, but which have effects on daily life, that can be mitigated by a successful health promotion program. For example, osteoporosis is a "silent" disease in that individuals with very low bone density may be unaware of the disease until they either receive a diagnosis based on a screening test (e.g., DEXA) or break a bone from a low-impact fall. Knowledge of (and fear related to) the high risk of fracture can affect the individual's quality of life and emotional well-being. A health promotion program aimed at fall prevention by improving balance via a tai chi class, or educating the client about ways to reduce the risk of falling in the home, such as removing throw rugs, modifying bath tubs to include grab bars, and installing adequate lighting, can promote health.

Preventive actions include asking adults to mark their height (or have a family member or friend help) by placing a pencil line on the wall every year, which can provide information about how the body is getting smaller as bone

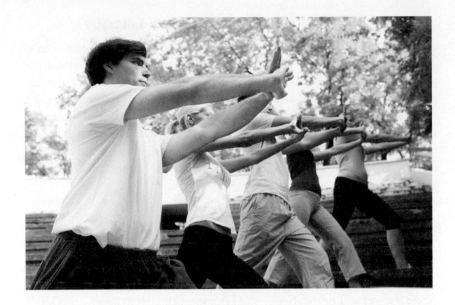

mass recedes. Engaging in bone strengthening activities such as a daily walk and making sure to eat calcium- and magnesium-rich foods are preventive measures to discuss with clients no matter what their chronic condition.

☐ Development of Skill Sets for Self-Management of a Chronic Condition

Clients with specific conditions may require a health promotion intervention that teaches them certain skills. An example would be a person who is diagnosed with type 1 (insulin-dependent) diabetes, who must develop the capacity to manage blood glucose levels with insulin in order to live and be healthy. To be effective, management of this lifelong chronic illness involves learning all of the following techniques:

- How and when to calculate and inject insulin doses in order to maintain appropriate blood glucose levels.
- How to recognize and correct blood glucose levels that are too high or too low.
- How to project the effects of different foods on blood sugar so that insulin doses can be adjusted accordingly.
- How to evaluate the effects that other factors have on blood sugar levels, such as exercise, weather, sleep, stress, and infectious illness.
- Steps to take to prevent development of secondary complications, such as diabetic ketoacidosis, neuropathy, or kidney dysfunction.

A client who learns these necessary skills and is able to effectively manage his or her condition so that he or she remains relatively healthy and functional (in the context of the disease) can be considered a health promotion success.

☐ Independence and Perceived Self-Efficacy

Another measure of how effective a health promotion program has been is the extent to which it increases the client confidence and ability to manage the chronic condition independently. Particularly in children who have grown up with a chronic condition, or in older adults living alone, merely developing a skill set may not be enough to assure independence. Health promotion activities may also entail developing a mindset that supports the idea that the client can and will manage the disease effectively. This factor is referred to in the literature as perceived self-efficacy—the confidence one has about doing things.

☐ General Improvement to Quality of Life

Living with a chronic condition can be frustrating, tiresome, and difficult. The added stresses and demands of managing a condition can decrease quality of life, sometimes to as great or greater an extent than the physical problems involved with the disease do. Interventions that either directly reduce some of these stresses and/or reduce physical symptoms enough to lower stress levels promote increased quality of life, which in turn can help to improve physical wellness (Gellis et al., 2012). For examples of evidence-based stress reduction measures, see Appendix for each chronic condition.

A Model of Chronic Disease Management

Health promotion in chronic disease settings has sparked a great deal of research. Models of how to manage chronic disease have developed as researchers examine commonalities among clients living with chronic illness.

The Chronic Disease Self-Management Model

The **chronic disease self-management model** was developed by Dr. Kate Lorig at Stanford University School of Medicine, who researched, developed, and evaluated it through a randomized, controlled trial. The content used for the trial was developed as a result of focus groups with people with chronic diseases who discussed what content area was most important to them. To use this model for promoting chronic disease self-management, a program leader teaches the program's curriculum to lay leaders at community sites, with 10–15 participants per class. A pair of leaders who have received 20 hours of training teach the chronic disease self-management model, using a detailed, scripted manual. Leaders can also be laypersons with chronic diseases.

ASK YOURSELF

www

Suppose you have decided to develop a program for chronic disease self-management similar to the program at Stanford, for clients with heart failure. Should this be a multidisciplinary program? What professionals should be involved? What content would you include?

The program content has been published in *Living a Healthy Life with Chronic Conditions* (Lorig et al., 2007), which will be given to each participant. The program incorporates modeling and social strategies that enhance self-efficacy, including guided mastery of skills through weekly action plans and feedback of progress; modeling of self-management behaviors and problem-solving strategies; reinterpretation of symptoms; social persuasion through group support; and guidance for individuals' self-management skills.

INFORMATION BOX 11-2

Would you like to know more about the Stanford chronic disease self-management program? Go to the website http://patienteducation.stanford.edu/programs/cdsmp.html You will find detailed information about the program, leader manual information in multiple languages, information on training to become a program leader, and information about research tools developed or adapted for use by Stanford.

The program is provided in six weekly sessions of 2.5 hours duration. Content includes adoption of exercise programs; use of cognitive symptoms management techniques; nutritional change; fatigue and sleep management; use of medication and community resources; managing emotions; training in communication with healthcare providers and others; health-related problem solving; and decision making.

CULTURAL RESEARCH STUDY

» BACKGROUND: Despite the recognized importance of patient involvement in primary care interactions, little information describing women's needs and expectations for these interactions is available.

» CONCEPTUAL FRAMEWORK: This participatory action study was based in Critical Action Theory.

(continues)

» PURPOSE: To describe any emancipatory interests that surfaced when eight ethnically diverse women examined their interactions with primary care nurse practitioners (PCNPs) over the course of five successive focus group meetings.

» DATA SOURCES: Focus group meeting transcripts, field notes, interaction notations, seating maps, and first impression summaries.

» CONCLUSIONS: Participants wanted to learn how to "stand up" for themselves in primary care interactions. They believed this could be accomplished by developing a positive sense of self-esteem. Ultimately, they identified the right way to "talk back" to clinicians and created a method for regaining control of their own health care and maintaining equality in interactions with primary care clinicians.

» IMPLICATIONS FOR PRACTICE: Nurses and nurse practitioners working in the primary setting are especially well situated to support self-management and foster patient participation by women as they live with chronic disease, engage in health promotion activities, and deal with common symptomatic problems for themselves and their families.

Source: Alexander, I. M. (2010). Emancipatory actions displayed by multi-ethnic women: Regaining control of my health care. *Journal of the American Academy of Nurse Practitioners,* *22*(11), 602–611.

Contact Source: Yale University School of Nursing, 100 Church Street South, New Haven, Connecticut 06536-0740, U.S.A. ivy.alexander@yale.edu

HEALTH PROMOTION CHALLENGE

Using the format and findings of the emancipatory actions study above in the Cultural Research Study, develop a format to elicit health promotion needs from multi-ethnic women with chronic conditions. Share your findings with at least two classmates.

Summary

There are a great many interventions to help clients prevent chronic conditions or enhance their health if they have already been diagnosed. Chronic conditions are not circumscribed; they can continue on for life. Some individuals with chronic conditions also have functional limitations such as difficulty walking, bending, or stooping; limited ability to take part in normal life activities; or need assistance with ADLs. Even though prevention is more cost-effective, physicians are trained to function in acute conditions. Nurse practitioners are in the forefront of providing preventive and wellness services for community residents with chronic conditions.

Four causes of chronic conditions are lack of physical activity, poor nutrition, tobacco use, and excessive alcohol consumption. Clients can prevent heart disease by eliminating added sugars, maintaining a healthy weight, not smoking or being around others who smoke, exercising 30 minutes a day, and eating healthily. Cancer prevention activities include keeping lean, being physically active, avoiding sugary drinks, following a plant-based diet, limiting consumption of red meats and avoiding processed meats. To prevent COPD/asthma, clients can lose weight if men have a waist bigger than 40 inches or women have one bigger than 35 inches; stop smoking; and avoid exposure to secondhand smoke other sources of pollution, and occupational triggers. Parents can also take steps to help prevent COPD/asthma in their children. Strokes can be prevented by lowering blood pressure, losing weight, eating healthily, avoiding smoke and smoking, and increasing physical activity. Prevention of childhood obesity is an international public health priority. Factors that affect quality of life for clients with a chronic condition include pain, stress, and lack of mobility. A measure of an effective health promotion program is the extent to which it increases a client's confidence and ability to manage a chronic condition. A self-management model can be used to help clients develop a program for chronic condition management.

REVIEW QUESTIONS

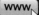

1. An acute disease:
   a. Lasts a short period of time and will end with recovery or death
   b. Is an irreversible process that requires supportive care and self-care for continued function and prevention of further disability
   c. Is a condition that relates to a specific pathophysiologic process
   d. Is the experience of symptoms and suffering and how the individual lives with and responds to these symptoms

2. A chronic disease:
   a. Lasts a short period of time and will end with recovery or death
   b. Is an irreversible process that requires supportive care and self-care for continued function and prevention of further disability
   c. Is a condition that relates to a specific pathophysiologic process
   d. Is the experience of symptoms and suffering and how the individual lives with and responds to these symptoms

3. The chronic disease self-management model:
   a. Is a program developed by Dr. Kate Lorig for clients with chronic diseases
   b. Incorporates modeling and social strategies that enhance self-efficacy, guided mastery of skills with action plans, and feedback
   c. Includes program evaluation that incorporates the areas of health status, health behaviors, perceived self-efficacy, and health services utilization
   d. Meets all of the above descriptions

4. Health-related quality of life includes:
   a. Health and physical function
   b. Emotional well-being
   c. Roles and social function
   d. All of the above

5. The four major causes of death are:
   a. Heart disease, cancer, suicide, and cerebrovascular disease
   b. Cancer, suicide, cerebrovascular disease, and domestic violence
   c. Heart disease, cancer, COPD/asthma, and cerebrovascular disease
   d. Suicide, cerebrovascular disease, cancer, and heart disease

6. The most cost-effective treatment is:
   a. Prevention
   b. Acute care
   c. Chronic care
   d. Health promotion

7. Clients can help prevent heart disease by:
   a. Eliminating added sugars
   b. Exercising 15 minutes a day
   c. Limiting consumption of processed meats
   d. Avoiding exposure to pollution

8. Clients can help prevent strokes by doing all but:
   a. Losing weight
   b. Lowering blood pressure
   c. Losing weight
   d. Resting their bodies

9. A health promotion program is effective if it:
   a. Reduces bothersome symptoms and unnecessary pain
   b. Reduces significant pain and increases mobility
   c. Increases client confidence to manage the condition
   d. Meets the client's goals for pain and decreased stress

EXERCISES

[www]

1. Do some research on the chronic condition self-management model. Construct a condition-specific curriculum using the model.

2. Complete a literature search on a chronic condition of interest. Obtain the articles and make an annotated bibliography (summarize each article briefly) to share with your fellow students.

3. Make a list of factors that may be considered perceived barriers to preventive behaviors.

4. Select an ethnic group to research. Investigate factors for this group that would increase health prevention behaviors and those that would be perceived barriers.

5. Select a chronic condition of interest and find information related to it in the Healthy People 2010 data.

REFERENCES

Alecxih, L., Shen, S., Chan, I., Taylor, D., & Drabek, J. (2010). *Individuals living in the community with chronic conditions and functional limitations: A closer look.* A report for the Office of the Assistant Secretary for Planning & Evaluation, US Department of Health & Human Services. Retrieved from http://aspe.hhs.gov/daltcp/reports/2010/closerlook.pdf

American Academy of Allergy, Asthma & Immunology. (2012). Prevention of allergies and asthma in children: Tips to remember. Retrieved from http://www.aaaai.org/conditions-and-treatments/library/at-a-glance/prevention-of-allergies-and-asthma-in-children.aspx

American Institute for Cancer Prevention. (2012). Recommendations for cancer prevention. Retrieved from http://www.aicr.org/reduce-your-cancer-risk/recommendations-for-cancer-prevention/

Anderson, G. (2004). *Chronic conditions: Making the case for ongoing care.* Retrieved from http://www.partnershipforsolution.partnership.org/DMS/files/chronicbook2004.pdf

Andrén S., & Elmståhl, S. (2005). Family caregivers' subjective experiences of satisfaction in dementia care: Aspects of burden, subjective health and sense of coherence. *Scandinavian Journal of Caring Sciences, 19*(2), 157–168.

Centers for Disease Control and Prevention [CDC]. (2009). *The power of prevention: Chronic disease . . . the public health challenge of the 21st century.* Retrieved from http://www.cdc.gov/chronicdisease/pdf/2009-Power-of-Prevention.pdf

Centers for Disease Control and Prevention [CDC]. (2010). Chronic diseases and health promotion. Retrieved from http://www.cdc.gov/chronicdisease/overview/index.htm

Centers for Disease Control and Prevention [CDC]. (2012). *Health related quality of life (HRQOL): How can HRQoL be measured?* Retrieved from http://www.cdc.gov/hrqol/concept.htm#3

Daniels, S.R. (2006). The consequences of childhood overweight and obesity. *Future Child, 16*(1), 47–67.

Domrose, C. (2012). Top-notch care around the corner: APN-run clinics are gems to neighborhood residents. *Nurse.com/Advanced Practice* (Special issue, May 21st).

Downie, W., Latham, P., Rhind, V., Wright, V., Branco, J., & Anderson, J. (1978). Studies with pain rating scales. *Annals of the Rheumatic Diseases, 37*(4), 378–381.

Evans, A. (2012). Nutrition screening in patients with COPD. *Nursing Times, 108*(11), 12–14.

Feinberg, J., Saag, M., Squires, K., Currier, J., Ryan, R., Coate, B., & Mrus, J. (2011). Health-related quality of life in the gender, race, and clinical experience trial. *AIDS Research and Treatment,* 349165.

Gellis, Z. D., Kenaley, B., McGinty, J., Bardelli, E., Davitt, J., & Ten Have, T. (2012). Outcomes of a telehealth intervention for homebound older adults with heart or chronic respiratory failure: A randomized controlled trial. *Gerontologist.* Advance online publication.

Göksel, O., Celik, G. E., Erkekol, F. O., Güllü, E., Mungan, D., & Misirligil, Z. (2009). Triggers in adult asthma: Are patients aware of triggers and doing right? *Allergologia et Immunopathologia (Madr), 37*(3), 122–128.

Hickey, A., Barker, M., McGee, H., & O'Boyle, C. (2005). Measuring health-related quality of life in older patient populations: A review of current approaches. *Pharmacoeconomics, 23*(10), 971–993.

Holman, H., & Lorig, K. (2004). Patient self-management: A key to effectiveness and efficiency in care of chronic disease. *Public Health Reports, 19,* 239–243.

Inumaru, L. E., Inineu, G. D., Quintanilha, M., Aparecida da Silveira, E., & Velosi Naves, M. M. (2012). Risk and protective factors for breast cancer in midwest of Brazil. *Environment and Public Health* 2012: 356851.

Kang, S. H., Choi, S. W., Lee, S. J., Chung, W. S., Lee, H. R., Chung, K. Y., . . . Jeong, H. Y. (2011). The effects of lifestyle modification on symptoms and quality of life in patients with irritable bowel syndrome: A prospective observational study. *Gut and Liver, 5*(4), 472–477.

Kripe, M. L. (2012). Reducing death from cancer: what will it take? *Tumour Biology.* Retrieved from http://www.ncbi.nlm.nih.gov/pubmed/2266494

Lionakis, N., Mendrinos, D., Sanidas, E., Favatas, G., Georgopoulou, M. (2012). Hypertension in the elderly. *World Journal of Cardiology, 4*(5), 135–147.

Lorig, K., Holman, H., Sobel, D., Laurent, D., Gonzalez, V., & Minor, M. (2007). *Living a healthy life with chronic conditions* (3rd ed.). Boulder, CO: Bull Publishing Company.

Lorig, K., Stewart, A., Ritter, P., Gonzalez, V., Laurent, D., & Lynch, J. (1996). *Outcome measures for health education and other healthcare intervention.* Thousand Oaks, CA: Sage.

Lubkin, I., & Larsen, P. (2006). *Chronic illness: Impact and interventions* (6th ed.). Sudbury, MA: Jones and Bartlett.

Mayo Clinic Staff. (2012a). Asthma. Retrieved from http://www.mayoclinic.com/health/asthma/DS00021/DSECTION=risk-factors

Mayo Clinic Staff. (2012b). Five medication-free strategies to help prevent heart disease. Retrieved from http://www.mayoclinic.com/health/heart-disease-prevention/WO00041

Meier, C., Bodenmann, G., Mörgeli, H., & Jenewein, J. (2011). Dyadic coping, quality of life, and psychological distress among chronic obstructive pulmonary disease patients and their partners. *International Journal of Chronic Obstructive Pulmonary Disease, 6,* 583–596.

Mularski, R. A., White-Chu, F., Overbay, D., Miller, L., Asch, S. M., & Ganzini, L. (2006). Measuring pain as the 5th vital sign does not improve quality of pain management. *Journal of General Internal Medicine, 21*(6), 607–612.

Murphy, S. L., Xu, J., & Kochanek, K. D., for the CDC Division of Vital Statistics. (2012). Deaths: Preliminary data for 2010. *National Vital Statistics Report, 60*(4), 1–68. Retrieved from http://www.cdc.gov/nchs/data/nvsr/nvsr60/nvsr60_04.pdf

O'Donnell, M.J., Xavier, D., Liu, L. (2010). Risk factors for ischaemic and intracerebral haemorrhagic stroke in 22 countries (the INTERSTROKE study): a case-control study. *Lancet, 376,*112–123.

Ravens-Sieberer, U., Erhart, M., Wille, N., Wetzel, R., Nickel, J., & Bullinger, M. (2006). Generic health-related quality-of-life assessment in children and adolescents: Methodological considerations. *Pharmacoeconomics, 24*(12), 1199–1220.

Reaney, M. D., Martin, C., & Speight, J. (2008). Understanding and assessing the impact of alcoholism on quality of life: A systematic review of the content validity of instruments used to assess health-related quality of life in alcoholism. *Patient, 1*(3), 151–163.

Reid, W. D., Yamabayashi, C., Goodridge, D., Chung, F., Hunt, M. A., Marciniuk, D. D., . . . Camp, P. G. (2012). Exercise prescription for hospitalized people with chronic obstructive pulmonary disease and comorbidities: a synthesis of systematic reviews. *International Journal of Chronic and Obstructive Pulmonary Disease, 7,* 297–320.

Ritter, P., Gonzalez, V., Laurent, D., & Lorig, K. (2006). Measurement of pain using the visual numeric scale. *Journal of Rheumatology, 33*(3), 574–580.

Sanchez, M.A., Vinson, C.A., Porta, M. L., Viswanath, K., Kerner, J. F., & Glasgow, R. E. (2012). Evolution of Cancer Control P.L.A.N.E.T.: moving research into practice. *Cancer Causes Control, 23*(7), 1205–1212.

Shariff, F., Carter, J., Dow, C., Polley, M., Salinas, M., & Ridge, D. (2009). Mind and body management strategies for chronic pain and rheumatoid arthritis. *Qualitative Health Research, 19*(8), 1037–1049.

Siegrist, J., & Li, J. (2012). Physical activity and risk of cardiovascular disease—a meta-analysis of prospective cohort studies. *International Journal of Environmental Research in Public Health* (2), 391–407.

Silver, B. (2012). An evidence-based approach to stroke prevention: Important Advances in the last decade Retrieved from www.rimed.org/medhealthri/2012-03/2012-03-77.pdf

Szeftel, A. (2012). Exercise preventing asthma? MedicineNet.com. Retrieved from http://www.medicinenet.com/script/main/art.asp?articlekey=16696

Therrien, F., Marceau, P., Turgeon, N., Biron, S., Richard, D., & Lacasse, Y. (2011). The Laval questionnaire: A new instrument to measure quality of life in morbid obesity. *Health and Quality of Life Outcomes, 9*, 66.

Varni, J. W., Seid, M., & Kurtin, P. S. (2001). PedsQL 4.0: Reliability and validity of the Pediatric Quality of Life Inventory version 4.0 generic core scales in healthy and patient populations. *Medical Care, 39*(8), 800–812.

Welsh, J. A., Sharma, A. S., Abramson, J. L, Vaccarino, V., Gillespie, C., & Vos, M. B. (2010). Caloric sweetener consumption and dyslipidemia among U. S. adults. *Journal of the American Medical Association, 303*(15), 1490–1497.

INTERNET RESOURCES

For a full suite of assignments and learning activities, use the access code located in the front of your book to visit this exclusive website: **http://go.jblearning.com/healthpromotion** If you do not have an access code, you can obtain one at the site.

PART **4**

Appendix

Index of Evidence-Based Self-Management
Interventions for Chronic Conditions

APPENDIX

Index of Evidence-Based Self-Management Interventions for Chronic Conditions

- Using Health Promotion Evidence
- Alzheimer's Disease, Dementia, and Memory Loss
- Anxiety
- Bladder Conditions (Cystitis)
- Blood Pressure/Hypertension
- Breast Cancer
- Cervical Cancer
- Colon and Rectal Cancer
- Depression
- Digestion (Constipation, Crohn's Disease, Diarrhea, Gastroesophageal Reflux Disease, Irritable Bowel Syndrome)
- Endometrial Cancer
- Falls
- Fatigue
- Fibroids
- Gastric Cancer
- Heart/Blood Vessels
- Incontinence
- Insomnia
- Kidneys
- Liver
- Lung Conditions
- Menopause
- Migraines
- Osteoporosis/Osteopenia
- Ovarian Cancer
- Overweight/Obesity
- Pain
- Pancreatic Cancer
- Premenstrual Syndrome
- Polycystic Ovary Syndrome
- Pregnancy/Labor/Delivery
- Prostate Cancer
- Stroke

http://go.jblearning.com/healthpromotion   www

For a full suite of assignments and learning activities, use the access code located in the front of your book to visit the exclusive website: http://go.jblearning.com/healthpromotion If you do not have an access code, you can obtain one at the site.

Using Health Promotion Evidence

This appendix presents evidence-based approaches for 32 conditions. When available, environmental actions, exercise/movement therapies, touch and herbal approaches, and stress management interventions are described, and research references are provided for these interventions.

Levels of Evidence

Rich (2005) identified the following three levels of evidence:

- Level A (the best) = Well-conducted randomized controlled trials
- Level B (next best) = Well-conducted case-control studies, poorly controlled or semicontrolled (with one or more major or three or more minor method flaws) trials, observational studies with high potential for bias (case series with comparison to historical controls), case series or case reports, conflicting evidence with more support
- Level C = Expert opinion

Some additional terms may help you evaluate the usefulness of clinical studies to your practice.

Systematic review occurs when a group of reviewers search the available literature via bibliographic databases. When a systematic review is undertaken, it is usually restricted to randomized controlled trials. The reviewers critically evaluate the method and content of all related studies. The final product is a synthesis of the properly completed and meaningful research into information that is relevant to practicing clinicians. The Cochrane Database of Systematic Reviews is one example. You can find relevant systematic reviews for specific conditions at http://www.cochrane.org/

Meta-analysis is a subset of systematic reviews that uses statistical methods to combine and analyze multiple investigations.

Randomized controlled trials are studies that select participants via a randomization procedure; that is, participants in the study are randomly allocated to each group included in the study. Each participant has an equal chance of being assigned to an intervention group, a control group, a placebo group, or a sham treatment group. This eliminates the overrepresentation of any one characteristic to one group. If the randomization is correctly performed, each group should be similar with respect to baseline characteristics. Randomization also eliminates any bias in the assignments of individuals to groups. Without this method, it is possible for a researcher to knowingly or unknowingly assign the less involved clients in the intervention group and the more involved clients in the control group. Randomized controlled trials are known to be the gold standard for establishing the effects of a treatment.

Cohort studies are also called prospective studies and longitudinal studies. A cohort study involves the selection of a large population of people who have the same condition and/or receive a specific intervention and are followed over time and compared to a group not affected by the condition. This study employs observation as the research method. The interventions are not manipulated.

A *matched case-controlled study* is a design that involves choosing two clients, or two groups of clients, who were exposed to two different interventions. The investigator retrospectively looks back to which group or client achieved a better outcome.

Outcomes research is a research design requiring larger groups of individuals to receive the same interventions. The participants are evaluated retrospectively for outcomes.

Case series are reports on a series of clients with the same preidentified problem.

A *case report* is a report on the intervention and outcome for a single client (Rich, 2005).

Other Factors to Consider When Evaluating Evidence

Research neither proves nor disproves a hypothesis; it only provides evidence for or against it. A large study that includes a control group (that does not receive the treatment) and selects clients for treatment or not by using a random method provides more evidence than findings from an interview or questionnaire method/design. Several studies provide more information than one study; a meta-analysis (review of studies) provides even more evidence.

Bear in mind that large studies using randomization are costly; while pharmaceutical companies can generally afford such research, the makers of herbal and nutraceutical products do not have the funds available to complete such studies. Lack of available funding is an important reason that there is often a dearth of evidence for many supplements or health promotion approaches. These approaches may be valid, but little evidence exists to show that they work. Because of this issue, the studies in this appendix provide primarily level B evidence. None are based on level C evidence. Few, if any, are level A studies.

Even when large, randomized studies are completed, they can be biased, especially when the studies are funded by industry sources with an economic stake in the study's findings. For example, a review of six pesticide studies using human subjects found that the studies were flawed by conflict of interest, failure to meet ethical standards, unacceptable informed consent procedures, inadequate statistical power, and inappropriate test methods and end points. All of the studies were funded by pesticide manufacturers, and all ethics committees responsible for approving the study protocols were part of the contract research organizations paid by the company to conduct the studies. Importantly, such biases could result in higher allowable exposures for both children and adults, which would be to the financial benefit of the studies' funders but could potentially cause harm to the health of participants, and ultimately to citizens, who would be exposed to higher levels of chemicals (Lockwood, 2004). For findings to be trustworthy (reliable and valid) studies must include disclaimers or conflict of interest statements explaining whether the authors of the study have ties to industry that could pose a source of bias.

The placebo effect can bias results also. When you read the results of a study, it is not uncommon to see that the placebo group did as well as the treatment group. This response could be due to the placebo effect—the mind's ability to stimulate a response in the body simply on the basis of expectation. The more participants believe they will benefit from a treatment, the more likely it is they will experience a benefit.

Also keep in mind that even a randomized, double blinded, placebo-controlled study may be flawed, in that there are no substances that can be considered to have no effect on the body. To judge what possible effect a placebo has, researchers should identify what exactly was in the placebo.

Among the uncommon cases where placebo composition has been noted, there are documented instances in which the placebo composition apparently produced spurious effects. Two studies used corn oil and olive oil placebos for cholesterol-lowering drugs: one noted that the "unexpectedly" low rate of heart attacks in the control group may have contributed to failure to see a benefit from the cholesterol drug. Another study noted "unexpected" benefit of a drug to gastrointestinal symptoms in cancer patients. But cancer patients bear increased likelihood of lactose intolerance—and the placebo was lactose, a "sugar pill." When the term "placebo" substitutes for actual ingredients, any thinking about how the composition of the control agent may have influenced the study is circumvented. A different dece(i)bo problem beset Ted Kaptchuk's recent Harvard study in which researchers Another explanation consistent with these results is specific physiological benefit. The study used a nonabsorbed fiber—microcrystalline cellulose—as the "Placebo" that subjects were told would be effective. The authors are applauded for disclosing its composition. But other nonabsorbed fibers benefit both constipation and diarrhea—symptoms of irritable bowel—and are prescribed for that purpose; psyllium is an example. Thus, specific physiological benefit of the "Placebo" to symptoms cannot be excluded.

Thus, rather than facilitating sound reasoning, evidence suggests that in many cases, including high stakes settings in which inferences may propagate to medical practice, substitution of a term—here, "placebo," "placebo effect"—for the concepts they are intended to convey, may actually thwart or bypass critical thinking about key issues, with implications to fundamental concerns for us all. (Golomb, 2012, p. 1)

Cautions

Whenever possible, avoid recommending supplements (especially for pregnant or lactating women, babies, children, and older frail adults) and recommend the appropriate foods instead. When recommending herbs or essential oils, always consult with an expert in the method prior to making a recommendation. Certain methods (e.g., yoga) should be undertaken with the assistance of a licensed, trained professional who can ensure that the technique is used safely and correctly.

Read the studies referred to in this book and search for updated information on any approach at PubMed (http://www.ncbi.nlm.nih.gov/pubmed/) prior to using it with clients, always keeping in mind the possible flaws in the research. It is also beneficial to use the method yourself whenever possible prior to recommending it to clients. Not only will you be a better role model, but you can also anticipate client questions and recommend how to use the approach for best results.

When you are unsure of how to proceed, refer the client to an advanced nurse practitioner or health promotion expert on the approach who possesses a doctorate and at least several years of experience with clients using the method.

REFERENCES

Golumb, B. (2012). The Dece(i)bo Effect. Accessed from http://edge.org/response-detail/1664/what-scientific-concept-would-improve-everybodys-cognitive-toolkit

Hadorn, D. C., Baker, D., Hodges, J. S., & Hicks, N. (1996). Rating the quality of evidence for clinical practice guidelines. *Journal of Clinical Epidemiology 49*, 749–754.

Lockwood, A. H. (2004). Human testing of pesticides: Ethical and scientific considerations. *American Journal of Public Health, 94*(11), 1908–1916.

Rich, N. (2005). Levels of evidence. *Journal of Women's Health Physical Therapy, 29*(2), 19–20.

Alzheimer's Disease, Dementia, and Memory Loss

Environment

Environmental approaches for Alzheimer's disease and memory loss include teaching clients how to:

1. *Avoid being exposed to aluminum.* This includes antacids, buffered aspirin, aluminum cookware, and underarm antiperspirants, which have been shown to cause the same pathological changes in brain tissue that are found in those diagnosed with Alzheimer's disease (Shcherbatykh & Carpenter, 2007).

2. *Avoid brain toxins from prescribed and over-the-counter medications.* Brain toxins can interfere with clear thinking and memory (Fogari & Zoppi, 2004; Hale, 1995; Kerr, Powell, & Hindmarch, 1996; Knegtering, Eijck, & Huijsman, 1994; Nye, Clinard, & Barnes, 2010; Puustinen et al., 2007; Van Putten & Marder, 1987).

3. *Use a medication/memory loss diary.* A diary helps to identify which drugs most affect memory. For a list of prescribed and over-the-counter medications found related to memory loss, go to: www.worstpills .org/results.cfm?drug_id=0&drugfamily_id=0&disease_id=0& druginduced_id=97&keyword_id=0.

4. *Avoid fluoridated water in combination with aluminum.* Aluminum has been shown to cause the same pathological changes in the brain tissue that are found in people diagnosed with Alzheimer's disease (de Wolff, 1999; Rondeau, Commenges, Jacqmin-Gadda, & Dartigues, 2000; Shcherbatykh & Carpenter, 2007; Van der Voet, Schijns, & de Wolff, 1999). Drinking distilled water daily and limiting intake of products listed in No. 1 is recommended.

5. *Use a fish aquarium.* Women diagnosed with Alzheimer's disease who had fish aquariums in their dining room and were asked to look at the fish and speak about what they saw showed increased nutritional intake and weight, decreased physical aggression, and decreased need for nutritional supplementation (Edwards & Beck, 2002).

6. *Keep well hydrated.* Low hydration status is related to impaired cognitive functioning, including slowed psychomotor processing speed and poor attention/memory performance in older adults (Suhr, Hall, Patterson, & Niinistro, 2004). Drinking 8–10 glasses of distilled water a day is recommended because much drinking water contains toxic substances (Sedman et al., 2006).

7. *Use a mirror.* When clients diagnosed with Alzheimer's disease use a mirror, it can raise awareness to needed self-care and can increase communication with caregivers. Nurses and caregivers can encourage clients to look at themselves in a mirror and, if they like, to speak about what they see (Tabak, Bergman, & Alpert, 1996).

8. *Listen to music.* Twenty-minute sessions of listening to classical or ballroom dance music and/or familiar songs from a pleasant situation may be best. Such sessions have been shown to aid memory, movement, balance, calmness, anxiety, depression, and fear, as well as increase appetite. Memory retention can increase to 75% when the client is asked to sing, hum, or keep time to the beat. Those diagnosed with Alzheimer's disease who do not talk or interact may sing or dance when music is played (Narme, Tonini, Khatir, Schiaratura, Clement, & Samson, 2012; Oluboyede, & House, 2009; Prickett & Moore, 1991; Ragneskog, Brane, Kihlgren, Karlsson, & Norberg, 1996).

9. *Reduce noise and increase lighting to enhance food intake.* Noise and lighting conditions can affect food intake at mealtimes (McDaniell, Hunt, Hackes, & Pope, 2001).

10. *Avoid power-frequency fields and wireless communications.* Neurological effects and neurodegenerative diseases, such as Alzheimer's disease, are associated with modified brain activity due to electromagnetic energy fields (EEFs). Scientific evidence raises concerns about the health impacts of mobile or cell phone radiation, power lines, interior wiring, and grounding of buildings and appliances such as microwaves, wireless technologies, and electric blankets (Hardell & Sage, 2008).

11. *Use red or blue dishes.* Using high-contrast red or high-contrast blue tableware (as opposed to white tableware) at each meal may increase food intake by as much as 35% and liquid intake by as much as 84% (Dunne, Neargarder, Cipolloni, & Cronin-Golumb, 2004).

12. *Use Snoezelen: A multisensory intervention.* Statistically significant calming and relaxing of agitation is consistent with 30 to 40 minutes of Snoezelen, a pleasant alternative to seclusion or restraints. This multisensory environment includes music, lights of fiber optic strands, calming image projections, vibrations of bubble tubes, and soothing smells. The experience provides a feeling of dignity, initiative, and freedom of choice (Chistsey, Haight, & Jones, 2002; Teitelbaum et al., 2007).

Exercise/Movement

Exercise/movement evidence-based practice for Alzheimer's disease includes teaching clients and caregivers about rocking in a rocking chair and walking or other strenuous activity.

1. *Rocking in a rocking chair.* Thirty to ninety minutes of rocking a day decreases agitation, anxiety, tension, and depression; it also reduces hyperresponsiveness stress and indirectly decreases detrimental cortisol levels. It can decrease vocalization/moaning, pacing, and walking. It may release pain-relieving brain endorphins, thus increasing quality of life. It can decrease requests for pain medication by 1–3 fewer requests per week. Balance can also improve. **Caution:** Use only a platform-style rocking chair with a super-stable, immobile base that moves back and forth easily. Suggest that family members or friends rock together (Watson et al., 1998).

2. *Walking or other strenuous activity.* Exercise can lower the odds of cognitive decline by 13% (for every 10 blocks walked by women 65 years or older) (Yaffe, Barnes, & Nevitt, 2001). For new walkers, start with one block or fewer and walk at a rate where easy conversation can be held. Suggest caregivers walk with the women if possible, pointing out the sights and observing safety rules. Participating in walking, hiking, bicycling, swimming, weight training, or other strenuous activities for at least 15 minutes 3 times/week can improve cerebral blood flow and cut dementia risk by one-third (Larsson et al., 2006). Moderate exercise is best (Geda et al., 2010).

Herbs/Essential Oils

Evidence-based approaches for Alzheimer's disease include the use herbs.

1. *Gingko biloba* may work for some clients, but not for others (Birks & Grimley, 2009). According to a review of studies, gingko is more effective than placebo (Weinmann et al., 2010), and a randomised, placebo-controlled trial confirmed the efficacy, safety, and increase in quality of life for clients and caregivers of a daily dose of 240 mg (Herrschaft et al., 2012).

   When it is effective, it can speed up working memory and information processing, improve social functioning, and improve blood flow to the brain. It has been shown to be equally effective as cholinesterase inhibitors in the treatment of mild to moderate Alzheimer's dementia (LeBars, Katz, & Berman, 1997; Wettstein, 2000). Routes/dosages /frequencies: 24% standardized extract/capsules of 60–80 mg taken one to three times a day, following dosage on bottle.

   Cautions: Gingko must be carefully coordinated with medications because it can interact with aspirin and antiplatelet drugs, increasing clotting time. Avoid using concurrently with anticonvulsants, buspirone, trazodone, St. John's wort, MAOIs, or fluoexetine, and never exceed suggested dosage. Not to be used with coagulation or platelet disorders, hemophilia, seizures, or hypersensitivity to this herb. Adverse reactions could include transient headache, anxiety, restlessness, vomiting, lack of appetite, diarrhea, flatulence, or rash, but a meta-analysis of unconfounded, randomized, double-blind controlled studies found no significant differences between ginkgo and placebo in the percentage of participants experiencing adverse effects (Skidmore-Roth, 2006).

   Other considerations: Discuss use with a certified or expert herbologist for best results. Gingko may take from 1 to 6 months to achieve full effectiveness (Birks & Grimley, 2009).

2. *Lemon balm* may enhance memory, calm, and improve cognitive performance (Kennedy et al., 2003). Routes/dosages/frequencies: Advise clients to steep lemon balm in boiling water for 10 minutes and drink as a tea, starting with 1 cup a day and working up to no more than 3 cups a day. To keep the tea for up to 1 year, it should be stored in a sealed container away from heat and moisture. Lemon balm can also be taken as a standardized extract (1:1) 60 drops/day.

   Cautions: The herb is not to be used by anyone diagnosed with hypothyroidism or by those hypersensitive to it. Adverse reactions may include nausea, anorexia, and hypersensitivity reactions. Lemon balm may potentiate the sedative effects of barbiturates and central nervous system depressants and may decrease the absorption of iron salts, so separate them by 2 hours. For standardized extract, advise clients to follow directions on the bottle. When in doubt, discuss use with a qualitifed herbalist.

3. *Sage* extracts possess antioxidant, estrogenic, and anti-inflammatory properties, and specifically inhibit butyryl- and acetyl-cholinesterase. Acute administration has also been found to reliably improve mnemonic performance in healthy young and elderly cohorts, whilst a chronic regime has been shown to attenuate cognitive declines in sufferers from Alzheimer's disease (Kennedy & Scholey, 2006).

   Sage leaves or bags can be made into a tea or 1–4 ml (1:1) dilution in 45% alcohol can be taken as an extract tid.

   Cautions: Do not use if hypersensitive to the herb. Clients with diabetes or seizure disorders should be monitored closely. Sage may decrease the action of anticonvulsants; avoid concurrent use. Sage may also increase the action of hypoglycemic herbs, sedating herbs, and central nervous system depressants (Skidmore-Roth, 2006).

Nutrition

1. *Apples/apple juice.* Both can improve memory and learning and may protect against Alzheimer's disease by increasing the production in the brain of the essential neurotransmitter acetylcholine, which can slow mental decline in women already diagnosed with the condition. Two

8-ounce glasses of apple juice or 2–3 apples a day is recommended (Chan, Groves, & Shea, 2006; Tchantchoa, Graves, Ortiz, Rogers, & Shea, 2004). Counsel clients to choose juice that includes apple skins but without added sugar; choose organic apples when possible to eliminate toxic effects of spraying.

2. *Blueberries, strawberries, walnuts, and Concord grape juice.* These protect against age-related oxidative stress and improve learning, balance, memory, and coordination. Recommend 1 cup of fresh or frozen berries daily (Goyarzu et al., 2003; Joseph, 1999; Joseph, Shukitt-Hale, & Willis, 2009; Spangler et al., 2003).

3. *Curry.* In a 2006 study, older women (ages 60–93) who consumed curry occasionally, often, or very often had significantly better scores on the Mini-Mental State Examination (MMSE) than those who never or rarely consumed curry. Curcumin, from the curry spice turmeric, possesses potent antioxidant and anti-inflammatory properties and reduces B-amyloid and plaque burden in the brain (Ng et al., 2006). **Cautions:** The herb is safe in food doses and up to 12 grams a day. In large quantities it can have strong activity in the common bile duct that might aggravate the passage of gallstones in women currently suffering from the condition (Anand, Kunnumakkara, Newman, & Aggarwal, 2007).

4. *Fish oil.* Deficiency in essential, mainly omega-3 and omega-6 long chain polyunsaturated fatty acids (LC-PUFA), which are found in fish oil, results in visual and cognitive impairment and disturbances in mental functions in animals and humans (American Academy of Neurology, 2007; Morris, Puskas, & Kitajka, 2006; Morris, 2009). Advise clients to eat fish 3–4 times per week or take oil caplets (available at health food stores) and to follow the directions on the bottle. Clients should keep oil caplets in the refrigerator so they do not become rancid.

5. *Flavonoids in fruits and vegetables.* The intake of antioxidant flavonoids in tea, fruits, and vegetables is inversely related to the risk of dementia. Apples, bananas, and oranges protect against neurodegenerative diseases including Alzheimer's disease (Englehart et al., 2002; Heo et al., 2008; Hughes et al., 2009). Serve 5–10 half cups daily. Fresh or frozen fruits and vegetables contain the most nutrients and the least salt and sugar.

6. *Garlic.* Oxidative damage is a major factor in dementia. Aged garlic extract (AGE) has been shown to prevent Alzheimer's disease progression by scavenging oxidants; increasing superoxide dismutase, catalase, glutathione peroxidase, and glutathione levels; and inhibiting lipid peroxidation and inflammatory prostaglandins (Borek, 2006; Chauhan & Sandoval, 2007). Routes/dosages/frequency: two capsules with meals twice a day. **Caution:** AGE may interact with antiplatelet or anticoagulant drugs, but appears safe for warfarin therapy (Macan et al., 2006).

7. *Green and black tea.* Two to three cups of tea a day protects against the buildup of plaque from myeloid deposits associated with an increase in brain cell damage and death from oxidative stress. Green tea polyphenols might explain the observed association with improved cognitive function. In a 2005 study, women who drank more than 2 cups of green tea a day had a 50% lower chance of having cognitive impairment, compared to those who drank fewer than 3 cups a week (Rezai-Zadeh et al., 2005). Black tea can also protect against the buildup of amyloid proteins (Bastinetto, Brouillette, & Quirion, 2007). **Cautions:** Caffeine may increase restlessness and talkativeness; decaffeinated green or black tea is preferable.

   Advise clients to steep tea bags in boiling water for 10 minutes, let cool, and drink.

8. *High-fat diet.* A high-fat diet may increase risk of Alzheimer's disease, especially in those with the APOE e4 allele marker. In one study, women who consumed the highest fat diets had a sevenfold higher risk of developing Alzheimer's disease than those who ate lower fat diets. Participants aged 20–39 who carried the genetic marker and ate a diet in which more than 40% of calories were from fat had an almost 23-fold higher risk of Alzheimer's disease than those who did not carry the marker and followed high-fat diets (these control subjects also ate more dietary antioxidants via fruits and vegetables) (Petot, 2000). Advise clients to minimize fat intake, especially saturated animal fats (meats, dairy products) and recommend eating 5–10 servings of fruits and vegetables daily (Gustaw-Rothenberg, 2009).

9. *Onion.* Enhanced memory is due to antioxidant effect of onions (Nishimura et al., 2006). If onion breath is a problem, advise clients to cook the onions rather than eating them raw in salads or sandwiches.

10. *Sugary sodas.* Five (and possibly fewer) cans of sugary beverages like soda a day may increase the risk of Alzheimer's disease. Suggest clients replace soda with green tea, filtered water with lemon or frozen berries, or diluted apple juice. Clients can wean themselves off of soda by drinking half soda and half replacement beverage the first day and gradually reducing the amount of soda over a week to 10 days. High sugar intake is also associated with higher cholesterol levels, insulin resistance, learning deficits, and memory loss. Mice fed on a sugar diet had twice as many amyloid plaque deposits, an anatomical hallmark of Alzheimer's disease (American Society for Biochemistry and Molecular Biology, 2007).

11. *Vitamin B₃.* Also known as niacin, vitamin B_3 may restore memory loss associated with Alzheimer's disease (Morris et al., 2004). Foods containing niacin should be eaten daily. Excellent sources of vitamin B_3 (niacin) include crimini mushrooms and tuna. Very good sources include salmon, chicken breast, asparagus, halibut, and venison.

12. *Thiamine.* A significant percentage of women diagnosed with Alzheimer's disease have a thiamine deficiency, which may have an impact on cognitive function (Gold, Chen, & Johnson, 1995), while thiamine levels are low in the brains of both men and women diagnosed with Alzheimer's disease (Lu'o'ng & Nguyen, 2011). Eating thiamine-rich foods (sunflower seeds, wheat germ, soy milk, and baked or black beans) may help improve cognitive function.

13. *Vitamin B_{12} and folate.* Clients with low levels of B_{12} or folate may have twice the risk of developing Alzheimer's disease as do those with higher levels of these two nutrients (Luchsinger, Tang, Miller, Green, & Mayeux, 2007). Taking folic acid and vitamin B_{12} can reduce homocysteine blood levels; homocysteine compromises brain function by damaging the lining of blood vessels in the brain (Kruman et al., 2002; Seshadri et al., 2002). Drinking five or more cups of coffee a day raises homocysteine significantly and should be avoided (Herrmann, 2006). Vegetarians and vegans (who avoid fish, dairy products, and eggs) are especially at risk for folate deficiency. Undigested folic acid accelerates cognitive decline in older adults with low vitamin B_{12} status. Good sources of folate include leafy green vegetables (like spinach and turnip greens), fruits (like citrus fruits and juices), and dried beans and peas (Pettit, 2002). **Cautions:** Advise clients to avoid foods fortified with folic acid and eat foods high in folate instead (Wright, Dainty, & Fingles, 2007). Calcium supplementation can improve B_{12} absorption. The following medications can lead to B_{12} deficiencies and a need for more foods high in folate: H2 blockers (such as ranitidine), proton pump inhibitors (e.g., omeprazole), colchicines, zicovudine, nitrous oxide anesthesia, metformin, phenformin, and potassium supplements.

14. *Lecithin.* Lecithin increases acetylcholine at receptor sites in the nervous system, improving memory. One of the chemical components of lecithin is phosphatidylcholine, a precursor to acetylcholine. Memory may increase significantly after taking lecithin for 4–6 weeks. Use lecithin capsules at 20–45 grams a day, starting at the lower dosage and increase gradually as needed (Higgins & Flicker, 2003).

15. *Pycnogenol.* Also called pine bark, pycnogenol protects against senile plaques characteristic of Alzheimer's disease. It can be taken in capsules for a total of 100–150 mg daily (Liu, Lau, Peng, & Shah, 2000; Skidmore-Roth, 2006). Be sure to remind caregivers to consult with their prescribing healthcare practitioner.

16. *Selenium.* Increasing evidence suggests a role for oxidative stress in several neurodegenerative diseases, including Alzheimer's disease, and that a maximum of 400 micrograms per day of selenium compounds may function as protective antioxidants. For more information on where to find selenium in foods, go to http://ods.od.nih.gov/factsheets/selenium.asp.

If a selenium supplement is taken, factor in the intake of foods to keep the dosage of selenium under 400 micrograms (Schrauzer, 2001; Xiong, Markesbery, Shao, & Lovell, 2007). The highest level of selenium is found in Brazil nuts (275 micrograms/3–4 nuts), fish (20–68 micrograms/3 ounces), and whole wheat spaghetti (36 micrograms /cup).

17. *Vitamins C, E, and A.* Evidence shows that vitamin C, which is water soluble, might serve to recharge the antioxidant capacity of vitamin E (Engelhart et al., 2002). Taken together, 2,000 IU of vitamin E and 2,000 mg of vitamin C daily may slow the progression of Alzheimer's disease (Exposito et al. 2002; Sano et al., 1997; Zandi et al., 2004). **Cautions:** No cautions were noted in the study; however, vitamin E is a blood thinner, and vitamin C should be taken with a full glass of water. The client should use Ester C form or calcium ascorbate if ascorbic acid form is irritating to his or her gastrointestinal tract. A better method of providing these antioxidants is through foods. A meta-analysis of these three dietary elements showed they decreased the risk of Alzheimer's disease, with vitamin E foods showing the strongest protection (Li, Shen & Ji, 2012). **Good food sources of vitamin C** include papaya, parsley, pineapple, kale, spinach, broccoli, red bell peppers, snow peas, tomato juice, kiwi, mango, orange, grapefruit juice, and strawberries. **Good food sources of vitamin A** include mango, broccoli, butternut squash, carrots, tomato juice, sweet potatoes, pumpkin, and beef liver. **Good food sources of vitamin E** include sunflower seeds, almonds, spinach, Swiss chard, turnip greens, papaya, mustard greens, collard greens, asparagus, bell pepper, olive oil, wheat germ, sunflower seeds, avocado, sweet potatoes, shrimp, and cod.

18. *Vitamins and trace elements.* Cognitive functions improve after supplementation with modest amounts of vitamins and trace elements, such as a daily multivitamin pill taken with a meal (Chandra, 2001). Examine multivitamin information on the bottle to make sure there are no fillers, dyes, starches, or other unnecessary substances contained in the tablets or capsules.

19. *Western diet.* Excessive dietary intake of sugar, refined carbohydrates, and animal products (traditional Western diet) is linked with Alzheimer's disease (Berrino, 2002; Whittmer, Gunderson, Barrett-Connor, Quesenberry, & Yaffe, 2005), and recent research suggests that Alzheimer's disease may reflect insulin resistance in the neurons of the brain—something which most likely stems from a diet high in refined carbohydrates (Kim & Feldman, 2012). Avoiding meat, dairy products, sugar, and refined carbohydrates (cakes, pies, candy, etc.) and increasing fish and/or fish oils, vegetables, whole grain cereals, legumes, and soy products can reduce Alzheimer's disease symptoms. For menus to share

with caregivers, go to: http://www.prevention.com/cda/categorypage .do?channel=nutrition.recipes&category=recipes.

Weight Loss

Excessive weight loss is a predictive factor of mortality and decreases quality of life for both clients and their caregivers. A nutrition education program can prevent weight loss and have a significant effect on cognitive function. One approach that has proved successful is the Mediterranean diet, which includes a high intake of vegetables, legumes, fruits, whole grain cereals, fish, and unsaturated fatty acids such as olive oil; a low intake of saturated fatty acids, dairy products, meat, and poultry; and low to moderate intake of alcohol. For more information, go to http://www.mayoclinic.com/health /mediteraneandiet/MY01725. Hispanic women may be more likely to adhere to the Mediterranean food plan than African Americans and may show a 20–40% reduction in risk of Alzheimer's disease after being on the food plan (Riviere et al., 2001; Scarmeas, Stern, Mayeux, & Luchsinger, 2006).

Stress Management

Stress management approaches for Alzheimer's disease include having clients do the following:

1. *Play bingo.* Compared to engaging in physical activity, playing bingo significantly enhanced performance on the Boston Naming Test and a Word list Recognition task in a study by Sobel (2001). Past research has shown that pharmacological measures can enhance functional capacities for those with Alzheimer's disease but may result in unacceptable side effects, while bingo has none.

2. *Incorporate daily mental exercise.* Mental excrcise could be anything, including from reading and solving crossword puzzles, working on the computer, playing musical instruments and board games, visiting museums, or even dancing. Frequent participation in any of these activities can reduce the risk of Alzheimer's disease and memory impairment (Jak, 2012; Geda et al., 2012).

3. *Talk.* Spending 10 minutes a day talking to another person can improve memory and performance. Talking about a social issue can be as effective as engaging in intellectual activities such as doing crossword puzzles (University of Michigan, 2007).

4. *Use imagery.* Having clients repeatedly picture themselves completing a cognitive task is as effective as practicing the task. Coach clients to use imagery up to 45 minutes a day. Ask them to make a vivid mental image of what they want to remember. Teach caregivers how to use imagery

and that daily practice improves results (Wright & Smith, 2007). For more information on using imagery to improve memory, go to: http://www.helpguide.org/life/improving_memory.htm

5. *Practice meditation.* Meditation decreases the chronic stress that can lead to Alzheimer's disease and especially memory loss. Women with memory loss reported their thinking was clearer and their memory better after meditating for 12 minutes a day (Khalsa, 2007; Peavy et al., 2007). Use simple meditation approaches like focusing on breathing in and out or counting 1, 2 while walking. For more ideas on simple meditation procedures, go to http://www.imcleveland.org/meditation/ Teach caregivers how to do meditation if possible.

6. *Get foot acupressure and massage.* Foot acupressure and massage for 10–15 minutes a day decreases agitation and a hyperresponsiveness to stress, which indirectly decreases detrimental cortisol levels. Acupressure can decrease yelling, pacing, and walking and improve quiet time, pulse, respiration, and sleep quality (Sutherland, Peakes, & Bridges, 1999; Yang, Wu, Lin, & Lin, 2007). Contraindications may include venous stasis, phlebitis, and traumatic and deep tissue injuries. Specific acupressure points to use include (1) the middle of the bottom of the feet, about two inches from the toes; (2) around the ankles; and (3) the front webbing about one inch back between the first and second toes. Caregivers can be taught how to do foot massage. For more information on foot massage, go to www.eclecticenergies.com

7. *Undergo hand aromatherapy and massage.* Hand aromatherapy and massage with lavender essential oil daily for 2 weeks decreases negative emotion and agitation significantly (Lee, 2005). Place a few drops of lavender oil in an ounce or two of jojoba or almond oil and then mix. Practice this sequence on yourself first. Place a few drops of mixed oil in the palm of the client's left hand and hold that hand in yours. Massage the client's palm with your thumb, working out in circles. Work down each finger and use the thumbnail to stimulate the ends of the client's fingers. Work up and down the thumb (correlates to the head of the client) with the pad of the thumb, using a very firm stroke. Stroke down the hand and up the forearm using your thumb and fingers. Compare the two hands for tone, color, and temperature. Repeat with the other hand. For more massage specifics go to www.coolnurse.com/massage.htm

8. *Receive therapeutic touch.* Therapeutic touch (TT) twice a day for 5–7 minutes may decrease agitation, loud or irritating vocalizations, pacing, hyperresponsiveness to stress, and detrimental cortisol levels (Woods& Dimond, 2002). **Caution:** The aged, extremely ill, or dying should be given a gentle treatment by an experienced practitioner. Center and calm yourself by closing your eyes and focusing on breathing in your

abdomen. When you are relaxed, rub your hands together and feel the tingling sensation as you slowly pull your hands apart. When you are able to feel the energies balancing between your hands, hold the intent to balance the other person's energy. Start above the client's head and keep an inch or so away from the body, bring your hands slowly down, sweeping down the body slowly, ending a few inches past the feet.

ALZHEIMER'S DISEASE CASE STUDY

Mr. Tom Arnoldson, age 66, has been experiencing loss of memory for several years. His wife is concerned that his confusion is increasing. He left the oven on recently and locked himself out of his home on several occasions. Sometimes he mistakes his wife for his daughter and sometimes sits in a chair for hours, staring off into space. His physician has diagnosed him with Alzheimer's disease and has asked the family to keep Mr. Arnoldson oriented to person, time, and place.

HEALTH PROMOTION CHALLENGE

Read the Alzheimer's disease case study and then go to PubMed (http://www.ncbi.nlm.nih.gov/pubmed/), type "Alzheimer's home care" in the search box at the top of the page, and click on the Search button. Choose three relevant abstracts and tell how the findings could help you teach the family how to help Mr. Arnoldson if he were your client.

REFERENCES

Anand, P., Kunnumakkara, A. B., Newman, R. A., & Aggarwal, B. B. (2007). Bioavailability of curcumin: Problems and promises. *Molecular Pharmacology, 4*(6), 807–818.

American Academy of Neurology. (2007). Eating fish, omega-3 oils, fruits and veggies lowers Risk of Memory Problems. *ScienceDaily*, November 13. Retrieved from http://www.sciencedaily.com/releases/2007/11/071112163630.htm

American Society for Biochemistry and Molecular Biology. (2007). Sugary beverages may increase Alzheimer's risk. *ScienceDaily*, December 10. Retrieved from http://www.sciencedaily.com/releases/2007/12/071208142559.htm

Bastinetto, S., Brouillette, J., & Quirion, R. (2007). Neuroprotective effects of natural products: Interaction with intracellular, amyloid peptides and a possible role for transthyretin. *Neurochemical Research, 32*(10), 1720–1725.

Birks, J., & Grimley, E. J. (2009). Ginkgo biloba for cognitive impairment and dementia. *Cochrane Database System of Reviews, 21*(1), CD003120.

Borek, C. (2006). Garlic reduces dementia and heart-disease risk. *Journal of Nutrition, 136*(3 Suppl.), 810S–812S.

Davinelli, S., Sapere, N., Zella, D., Bracale, R., Intrieri, M., & Scapagnini, G. (2012). Pleiotropic protective effects of phytochemicals in Alzheimer's disease. *Oxidative Medicine and Cell Longevity*, 2012: 386527. Retrieved from http://www.ncbi.nlm.nih.gov/pubmed/22690271

Chan, A., Groves, V., &, Shea, T. B. (2006). Apple juice concentrate maintains acetylcholine levels following dietary compromises. *International Journal of Alzheimer's Disease, 9*(3), 287–291.

Chandra, R. K. (2001). Effect of vitamin and trace-element supplementation on cognitive function in elderly subjects. *Nutrition, 17*(9), 709–712.

Chauhan, N. B., & Sandoval, J. (2007). Amelioration of early cognitive deficits by aged garlic extract in Alzheimer's transgenic mice. *Phytotherapy Research, 21*(7), 629–640.

Chistsey, A., Haight, B. K., & Jones, M. M. (2002). Snoezelen: A multi-sensory environmental intervention. *Journal of Gerontological Nursing, 28*(1), 41–49.

Dunne, T. E., Neargarder, S. A., Cipolloni, P. B., & Cronin-Golumb, A. (2004). Visual contrast enhances food and liquid intake in advanced Alzheimer's disease. *Clinical Nutrition, 23*(4), 533–538.

Edwards, N. E., & Beck, A. M. (2002). Animal-assisted therapy and nutrition in Alzheimer's disease. *Western Journal of Nursing Research, 24*(6), 697–712

Engelhart, M. J., Geerlings, M. I. K., Ruitenberg, A., van Swieten, J. C., Hofman, A., Witteman, J. C., & Breteler, M. M. B. (2002). Dietary intake of antioxidants and risk of Alzheimer's disease. *Journal of American Medical Association, 287*(24), 3223–3229.

Exposito, E., Rotilio, D., DiMatteo, V., DiGiulio, C., Cacchio, M., & Algeri, E. (2002). A review of specific dietary antioxidants and the effects on biochemical mechanisms related to neurodegenerative processes. *Neurobiology and Aging, 23*(5), 719–735.

Fogari, R., & Zoppi, A. (2004). Effect of antihypertensive agents on quality of life in the elderly. *Drugs and Aging, 21*(6), 377–393.

Geda, Y. E., Silber, T. C., Roberts, R. O., Knopman, D. S. Christianson, T. J., Pankratz, V. S., . . . Peterson, R. C. (2012). Computer activities, physical exercise, aging, and mild cognitive impairment: a population-based study. *Mayo Clin Proceedings, 87*(5), 437–442.

Gold, M., Chen M. F., & Johnson, K. (1995). Plasma and red blood cell thiamine deficiency with dementia of the Alzheimer's type. *Archives of Neurology, 51*(11), 1081–1086.

Goyarzu, P., Lau, F. C., Kaufmann, J., Jennings, R., Taglialatela, G., Joseph, J., . . . Malin D. H. (2003). *Age-related increase in brain nf-b is attenuated by blueberry-enriched antioxidant diet*. Program No. 983. [Abstract]. Washington, DC: Society for Neuroscience.

Gustaw-Rothenberg, K. (2009). Dietary patterns associated with Alzheimer's disease: Population based study. *International Journal of Environmental Research and Public Health, 6*(4), 1335–1340.

Hale, A. S. (1995). Critical flicker fusion and threshold and anticholinergic effects of chronic antidepressant treatment in the remitted depressive. *British Journal of Clinical Pharmacology, 42*, 239–241.

Hardell, L., & Sage, C. (2008). Biological effects from electromagnetic field exposure and public exposure standards. *Biomedical Pharmacotherapy, 62*(2), 104–109.

Heo, H. J., Choi S. J., Choi, S-G., Shin, D.-H., Lee, J. M., & Lee, C. Y. (2008). Effects of banana, orange, and apple on oxidative stress-induced neurotoxicity in PC12 cells. *Journal of Food Science, 73*(2), H28–H32.

Herrmann, W. (2006). Significance of hyperhomocysteinemia. *Clinical Laboratory, 52*(7–8), 367–374.

Herrschaft, H., Nacu, A., Likhachev, S., Sholomov, I., Hoerr, R., Schlaefke, S. (2012). Ginkgo biloba extrac EGb 761^R in dementia with neuropsychiatric features: A randomised, placebo-controlled trial to confirm the efficacy and safety of a daily dose of 240 mg. *Journal of Psychiatric Research, 46*(6). 716–723.

Higgins, J. P., & Flicker, L. (2003). Lecithin for dementia and cognitive impairment. *Cochrane Database System of Reviews, 3*: CD001015.

Hughes, T. F., Andel, R., Small, B. J., Borenstein, A. R., Mortimer, J. A., Wolk, A., . . . Gatz, M. (2009). Midlife fruit and vegetable consumption and risk of dementia in later life in Swedish twins. *American Journal of Geriatric Psychiatry*. Retrieved from http://www.ncbi.nlm.nih.gov/pubmed/19910881

Jak, A. J. (2012). The impact aof physical and mental activity on cognitive aging. *Current Topics in Behavioral Neuroscience, 10*, 273–291.

Joseph, J. A. (1999). Reversals of age-related declines in neuronal signal transduction, cognitive, and motor behavioral deficits with blueberry, spinach, or strawberry dietary supplementation. *Journal of Neuroscience, 19*(18), 8114–8121.

Joseph, J. A., Shukitt-Hale, B., & Willis, L. M. (2009). Grape juice, berries, and walnuts affect brain aging and behavior. *Journal of Nutrition, 139*(9), 1813S–1817S.

Kennedy, D. O., Wake, G., Savelev, S., Tildesley, N. T., Perry, E. K., Wesnes, K. A., & Scholey, A. B. (2003). Modulation of mood and cognitive performance following acute administration of single doses of *Melissa officinalis* (lemon balm) with human CNS nicotinic and muscarine receptor-binding properties. *Neuropsychopharmacology, 28*(10), 1871–1881.

Kerr, J. S., Powell, J., & Hindmarch L. (1996). The effects of reboxetine and amitriptyline, with and without alcohol on cognitive function and psychomotor performance. *Journal of Psychopharmacology, 9*(3), 258–266.

Khalsa, D. S. (2007, October). Stress reduction and Alzheimer's prevention: Two studies using SPECT. Presentation at 6th World Congress on Stress, Vienna, Austria.

Kim, B., & Feldman, E. L. (2012, January 13). Insulin resistance in the nervous system. *Trends in Endocrinology and Metabolism, 23*(3), 133–141.

Knegtering, H., Eijck, M., & Huijsman, A. (1994). Effects of antidepressants on cognitive functioning of elderly patients: A review. *Drugs and Aging, 5*(3), 192–199.

Kruman, I. I., Kumaravel, T. S., Lohani, A., Pedersen, W. A., Cutler R. G., Kruman, Y., . . . Mattson, M. P. (2002). Folic acid deficiency and homocysteine impair DNA Repair in hippocampal neurons and sensitize them to amyloid toxicity in experimental models of Alzheimer's disease. *Journal of Neuroscience, 22*(5), 1752–1762.

Larsson, E. G., Wang, L., Bowen, J. D., McCormick, W. C., Teri, L., Crane, P., & Kukull, W. (2006). Exercise is associated with reduced risk for incident dementia among persons 65 years of age and older. *Annals of Internal Medicine, 144*, 73–81.

LeBars, P. L., Katz, M., & Berman, N. (1997). A placebo-controlled, double-blind randomized trial of an extract of gingko biloba for dementia. *Journal of the American Medical Association, 278*, 1327–1332.

Lee, S. Y. (2005). The effect of lavender aromatherapy on cognitive function, emotion and aggressive behavior of elderly with dementia. *Taehan Kanho Hakho Chi, 35*(2), 303–312.

Li, F. J., Shen, L., & Ji, H. F. (2012). Dietary intakes of vitamin E, vitamin C, and B-carotene and risk of Alzheimer's disease: A meta-analysis. *Journal of Alzheimers Disease* [Epub ahead of print]. Retrieved from http://www.ncbi.nlm.nih.gov/pubmed/22543848

Liu, F., Lau, B. H., Peng, Q., & Shah, V. (2000). Pycnogenol protects vascular endothelial cells from beta-amyloid-induced injury. *Biological Pharmaceutical Bulletin, 23*(6), 735–737.

Luchsinger, A., Tang, M.-X., Miller, J., Green, R., & Mayeux, R. (2007). Relation of higher folate intake to lower risk of Alzheimer disease in the elderly. *Archives of Neurology, 64*, 12–14.

Luồng, K. V., & Nguyen, L. T. (2011). Role of thiamine in Alzheimer's disease. *American Journal of Alzheimers Disease and Other Dementias, 26*(8), 588–598

Macan, H., Uykimpang, R., Clconcel, M., Takasu, J., Razon, R., Amagase, H., . . . Niihara, Y. (2006). Aged garlic extract may be safe for patients on warfarin therapy. *Journal of Nutrition, 136*(3 Suppl), 793S–795S.

McDaniel, J. H., Hunt, A., Hackes, B., & Pope, J. F. (2001). Impact of dining room environment on nutritional intake of Alzheimer's residents: A case study. *American Journal of Alzheimer's Disease and other Dementias, 16*(5), 297–302.

Moncrieff, J., & Cohen, D. (2005). Rethinking models of psychotropic drug action. *Psychotherapy and Psychosomatics, 74*, 145–153.

Morris, M. C. (2009). The role of nutrition in Alzheimer's disease: Epidemiological evidence. *European Journal of Neurology, 16*(Suppl 1), 1–7.

Morris, M. C., Evans, D. A., Bienias, J. L., Scherr, P. A., Tangney, C. C., Hebert, L. E., . . . Aggarwal, N. (2004). Dietary niacin and the risk of incident Alzheimer's disease and of cognitive decline. *Journal of Neurology Neurosurgery and Psychiatry, 75*, 1093–1099.

Morris, M. C., Puskas, L. G., & Kitajka, K. (2006). Nutrigenomic approaches to study the effects of N-3 PUFA diet in the central nervous system. *Nutrition and Health, 18*(3), 227–232.

Ng, T. P., Chiam, P. C., Lee, T., Chua, H. C., Lim, L., & Kua, E. H. (2006). Current consumption and cognitive function in the elderly. *American Journal of Epidemiology, 164*(9), 898–906.

Nishimura, H., Higuchi, O., Tateshita, K., Tomobe, K., Okuma, Y., & Nomura, Y. (2006). Antioxidative activity and ameliorative effects of memory impairment of sulfur-containing compounds in allium species. *Biofactors, 26*(2), 135–146.

Nye, A. M., Clinard, V. B., & Barnes, C. L. (2010). Medication nonadherence secondary to drug-induced memory loss. *Consultant Pharmacist, 25*(2), 117–121.

Peavy, G. M., Lange, K. L., Salmon, D. P., Patterson, T. L., Goldman, S., Gamst, A. C., . . . Galasko, D. (2007). The effects of prolonged stress and APOE genotype on memory and cortisol in older adults. *Biological Psychiatry, 62*(5), 472–478.

Petot, G. (2000, July). Alzheimer's disease risk increases with high-fat diet. World Alzheimer's Conference. Washington, DC.

Pettit, J. L. (2002). Vitamin B12. *Clinicians Review, 12*(7), 64, 66.

Prickett, C. A., & Moore, R. S. (1991). The use of music to aid memory of Alzheimer's patients. *Journal of Music Therapy, 28*, 101–110.

Puustinen, J., Nurminen, J., Kukola, M., Vahlberg, T., Laine, K., & Kivela, S. L. (2007). Associations between use of benzodiazepines or related drugs and health, physical abilities and cognitive function. *Drugs and Aging, 24*(12), 1045–1059.

Ragneskog, H., Brane, M., Kihlgren, I., Karlsson, & Norberg, A. (1996). Dinner music for demented patients: Analysis of video-recorded observations. *Clinical Nursing Research, 5*(3), 262–277.

Rezai-Zadeh, K., Shytle, D., Sun, N., Takashi, M., Hou, H., Jeanniton, D., . . . Tan, J. (2005). Green tea epigallocatechin-e-gallate (EGCG) modulates amyloid precursos protein cleavage and reduces cerebral amyloidosis in Alzheimer transgenic mice. *Journal of Neuroscience, 25*(38), 8807–8814.

Riviere, S., Gillette-Guyonnet, S., Voisin, T., Reynish, E., Andrieu, S., Lauque, S., . . . Vellas, B. (2001). A nutritional education program could prevent weight loss and slow cognitive decline in Alzheimer's disease. *Journal of Nutritional Health & Aging, 5*(4), 295–299.

Rondeau, V., Commenges, D., Jacqmin-Gadda, H., & Dartigues, J. F. (2000). Relation between aluminum concentrations in drinking water and Alzheimer's disease: An 8-year follow-up study. *American Journal of Epidemiology, 152*(1), 59–66.

Sano, M., Ernesto, C., Thomas, R., Klauber, M. R., Schafer, K., Grundman, M., . . . Thal, L. J. (1997). A controlled trial of selegiline, alpha-tocopherol, or both as treatment for Alzheimer's disease. *New England Journal of Medicine, 336*(17), 1216–1222.

Scarmeas, N., Stern, Y., Mayeux, R., & Luchsinger, J. A. (2006). Mediterranean diet, Alzheimer's disease and vascular mediation. *Archives of Neurology, 63*, 1709–1717.

Schrauzer, G. N. (2001). Nutritional selenium supplements: Product types, quality and safety. *Journal of American College of Nutrition, 20*(1), 1–4.

Shcherbatykh, I., & Carpenter, D. O. (2007). The role of metals in the etiology of Alzheimer's disease. *Journal of Alzheimers Disease, 11*(2), 191–205.

Sedman, R. M., Beaumont, J., McDonald, T. A., Reynolds, S. Krowech, G., & Howd, R. (2006). Review of the evidence regarding the carcinogenicity of hexavalent chromium in drinking water. *Journal of Environmental Science and Health Part C, 24*(1), 155–182.

Seshadri, S., Beiser, A., Selhub, J., Jacques, P. F., Rosenberg, I. H., D'Agostino, R. B., . . . Wolf, P. A. (2002). Plasma homocysteine as a risk factor for dementia and Alzheimer's disease. *New England Journal of Medicine, 346*, 476–483.

Skidmore-Roth, L. (2006). *Mosby's handbook of herbs & natural supplements*. St. Louis, MO: Mosby.

Sobel, B. P. (2001). Bingo vs. physical intervention in stimulating short-term cognition in Alzheimer's disease patients. *American Journal of Alzheimer's Disease and Other Dementias, 16*(2), 115–120.

Spangler, E. L., K. Duffy, Devan, B., Guo, Z., Bowker, J., Shukitt-Hale, B., Joseph, J. A., & Ingram, D. K. (2003). *Rats fed a blueberry-enriched diet exhibit greater protection against a kainite-induced learning impairment*. Program No. 735.10. [Abstract]. Washington, DC: Society for Neuroscience.

Suhr, J. A., Hall, J., Patterson, S. M., & Niinisto, R. T. (2004). The relation of hydration to cognitive performance in healthy older adults. *International Journal of Psychophysiology, 53*(2), 121–125.

Sutherland, J., Peakes, J., & Bridges, C. (1999). Foot acupressure and massage for patients with Alzheimer's disease and related dementias. *Image, Journal of Nursing Scholarship, 31*(4), 347–348.

Tabak, N., Bergman, R., & Alpert, R. (1996). The mirror as a therapeutic tool for patients with dementia. *International Journal of Nursing Practice, 2*(3), 155–159.

Tchantchoa, F., Graves, M., Ortiz, D., Rogers, E., & Shea, T. B. (2004). Dietary supplementation with apple juice concentrate alleviates the compensatory increase in glutathione synthase transcription and activity that accompanies dietary and genetically induced oxidative stress. *Journal of Nutrition Health and Aging, 8*: 92–97.

Teitelbaum, A., Volpo, S., Paran, R., Zislin, J., Drumer, D., Raskin, S., . . . Durst, R. (2007). Multisensory environmental intervention (Snoezelen) as a preventive alternative to seclusion and restraint closed psychiatric wards. *Harefuah, 146*(1), 79–80.

University of Michigan. (2007, November 1). Ten minutes of talking improves memory and test performance. *ScienceDaily*. Retrieved from http://www.sciencedaily.com/releases/2007/10/071029172856.htm

Van der Voet, G. B., Schijns, O., & de Wolff, F. A. (1999). Fluoride enhances the effect of aluminum concentrations in drinking water and Alzheimer's disease. An 8-year follow-up study. *Archives of Physiological Biochemistry, 107*(1), 15–21.

Van Putten, T., & Marder, S. R. (1987). Behavioral toxicity of antipsychotic drugs. *Journal of Clinical Psychiatry, 48*, 13–19.

Watson, N., Hauptmann, M., Brink, C., Powers, B., Taillie, E. R., Lash, M., & Wells, T. (1998, April). *As elders rock, emotional burden of dementia eases.* Presented to the Eastern Nursing Research Society, Rochester, NY.

Wettstein, A. (2000). Cholinesterase inhibitors and Gingko extracts—are they comparable in the treatment of dementia? Comparison of published placebo-controlled efficacy studies of at least six months' duration. *Phytomedicine, 6*(6), 393–401.

Whitmer, R., Gunderson, E. P., Barrett-Connor, E., Quesenberry, P., Jr., & Yaffe, K. (2005). Obesity in middle age and future risk of dementia: A 27 year longitudinal population based study. *British Medical Journal, 330*, 1360–1364.

Weinmann, S., Roll, S., Schwarzbach, C., Vauth, C., & Willich, S. N. (2010). Effect of ginkgo biloba in dementia: systematic review and meta-analysis. *Biomedcentral Geriatrics, 17*(10), 14.

Woods, D. L., & Dimond, M. (2002). The effect of therapeutic touch on agitated behavior and cortisol in persons with Alzheimer's disease. *Biological Research in Nursing, 4*(2), 104–114.

Wright, C. J., & Smith, D. K. (2007). The effect of a short-term PETTLEP imagery intervention on a cognitive task. *Journal of Imagery Research in Sport and Physical Activity, 2*(1). Retrieved from http://www.bepress.com/jirspa/vol2/iss1/sty1

Wright, J., Dainty, J., & Fingles, P. (2007). Folic acid metabolism in human subjects: Potential implications for proposed mandatory folic acid fortification in the UK. *British Journal of Nutrition, 98*, 667–675.

Xiong, S., Markesbery, W. R., Shao, C., & Lovell, M. A. (2007). Seleno-L-methionine protects against beta-amyloid and iron/hydrogen peroxide-mediated neuron death. *Antioxidants & Redox Signaling, 9*(4), 457–467.

Yaffe, E., Barnes, D., & Nevitt, M. (2001). A prospective study of physical activity and cognitive decline in elderly women: Women who walk. *Archives of Internal Medicine, 161*, 1703–1708.

Yang, M. H., Wu, S. C., Lin, J. G., & Lin, L. C. (2007). The efficacy of acupressure for decreasing agitated behaviour in dementia: A pilot study. *Journal of Clinical Nursing, 16*(2), 308–315.

Zandi, P. P., Anthony, J. C., Khachaturian, A. S., Stone, S. V., Gustafson, D., & Tschanz, J. T. (2004). Reduced risk of Alzheimer's disease in users of antioxidant vitamin supplements. *Archives of Neurology, 61*(1), 82–88.

Anxiety

Environment

Approaches for anxiety include teaching clients environmental techniques.

1. *Music.* Significantly less anxiety may occur in clients who listen to sedative music on CDs, DVDs, or tapes for 30-minute sessions as compared to those who receive either scheduled rest or treatment as usual (Evans, 2002; John Wiley & Sons, Inc., 2007; Voss et al., 2004). Ask the client to assess anxiety from 1 (calm) to 10 (extreme anxiety) before and after listening to calming music. Investigate healing music at www.healing music.org

2. *Smoking cessation.* Panic attacks (a symptom of high anxiety) are strongly associated with both occasional and regular smoking, passive smoking, and nicotine dependence (Isensee, Wittchen, Stein, Hofler, & Lieb, 2003). Investigate smoking cessation programs by visiting http:// www.helpguide.org/mental/quit_smoking_cessation.htm and referring to Chapter 9 in this book. Develop individualized smoking cessation programs for clients based on their lifestyle and input.

Exercise/Movement

Approaches for anxiety include teaching clients about exercise and movement.

1. *Dance.* Modern dance and other dance, for 50–60 minutes a day, as tolerated, can significantly reduce anxiety (Bradt & Dileo, 2009; Leslie & Rust, 1984). Instruct clients to wear appropriate clothes and shoes and only dance on a safe surface. Assess vital signs, balance, and ask clients to consult with primary caregiver prior to undertaking an exercise program. Have clients complete warm-up prior to dancing and cool-down afterwards. For suggestions, go to http://library.thinkquest.org/12819 /text/warmupcooldown.html **Other considerations:** Exercise may be especially useful to decrease pain in joints.

2. *Rocking chair use.* Rocking from 30 minutes to 2½ hours a day decreases agitation, anxiety, tension, and hyperresponsiveness stress, as well as indirectly decreases detrimental cortisol levels. Those who rock the most often improve the most (Pierce, Pecen, & McLeod, 2009; Watson, 1998).

3. *Walking.* As tolerated, walking at the fastest possible pace that still allows for a comfortable conversation significantly lowers anxiety level (Berk, 2007; De Moor, Beem, Stubbe, Boomsma, & De Geus, 2006). **Cautions:** Clear any exercise program with primary care practitioner. Take a baseline measure for agitation and anxiety, and then take a measure after exercise. Ask clients to wear appropriate clothes and shoes and carry sufficient water (preferably distilled or reverse-osmosis filtered) to remain hydrated (1 cup of water every 15 minutes of exercise).

4. *Yoga.* Sixty-minute sessions of yoga can significantly reduce stress (Subramanya & Telles, 2009). For a list of cautions, go to http://yoga.lifetips .com/cat/56770/yoga-cautions/ Because yoga exerts pressure on inter-

nal organs, clients should wait at least 2 hours after a meal and 30 minutes to 1 hour after a snack to practice. For more information on yoga, go to http://www.yogajournal.com/poses/finder/browse_categories /seated_and_twists

Herbs/Essential Oils

Approaches for anxiety include teaching clients about herbs/essential oils.

1. *Lavender and rosemary essential oils.* These oils protect the body from oxidative stress by decreasing the stress hormone, cortisol, when sniffing their aroma for 5 minutes (Atsumi & Tonosaki, 2007). Keep aromatherapy products away from heat and moisture in a sealed container.
2. *Peppermint tea.* Two to three cups of peppermint tea a day produces analgesic and anesthetic effects in the central and peripheral nervous system that may reduce anxiety (McKay & Blumberg, 2006). Remind clients to store peppermint tea in a cool, dry place.

Mind-Set

Approaches for anxiety include teaching clients mind-set techniques.

1. *Affirmations.* Self-affirmation of personal values and beliefs buffers neuroendocrine and psychological stress and anxiety (Kinnier, Hofsess, Pongratz, & Lambert, 2009). The client repeats aloud or writes positive affirmations, such as "I am safe and protected," "I love and approve of myself," or "I trust the process of life, up to 20 times a day." Ensure affirmations are positive and acceptable to the client. Suggest affirmations be written on 3 × 5 cards and placed where they will be read frequently. Find more affirmations information at www.success-consciousness.com/index_00000a.htm
2. *Cognitive-behavioral therapy* (*CBT*). This helps uncover and alter distortions of thought or perception that increase anxiety (Ruwaard et al., 2010). Individuals with persistent panic attacks are encouraged to test out beliefs they have related to an attack, such as specific fears related to bodily sensations, and to develop realistic responses to such beliefs. Clients keep a daily log of thought and perception problems that lead to anxiety. One book to recommend is *How to Stubbornly Refuse to Make Yourself Miserable about Anything* by Albert Ellis. **Cautions:** Clients with acute stress disorder may not find this approach helpful. For more information: visit http://www.mind.org.uk/help/medical_and_alternative_care/ making_sense_of_cognitive_behaviour_therapy

Nutrition

Approaches for anxiety include teaching clients about nutrition.

1. *Vitamin B_6.* Vitamin B_6 deficiency is related to increases in anxiety. Vitamin B_6 is a building block for serotonin; decreased levels of serotonin have been associated with increased stress and anxiety (Mooney, Leuendorf, & Hendrickson, 2009). Food sources of vitamin B_6 include meat, fish, sunflower seeds, bananas, tomatoes, and spinach. For more sources, go to: http://ods.od.nih.gov/factsheets/vitaminb6.asp.

2. *Vitamin C.* Five hundred milligrams a day of vitamin C has been shown to reduce the level of stress hormones circulating in the blood and reduce other typical indicators of physical and emotional stress (Sasazuki et al., 2008). Ester C is less irritating to the stomach and bladder mucosa than other forms of vitamin C. Client recommendations include eating 1 cup of raw red pepper slices (174.80 mg), 1 cup of steamed broccoli (12.40 mg), 2 cups of strawberries (163.30 mg), and 2 kiwi fruit (171 mg) on day one. The next day, eat 1 cup of boiled or steamed cauliflower (54.93 mg), 2 cups of romaine lettuce (26.88 mg), 1½ cups of Brussels sprouts (145.08 mg), 1 grapefruit (46.86 mg), 1 cup of cubed cantaloupe (67.52 mg), 1 orange (69.69 mg), 1 cup of ripe tomatoes (34.38 mg), 1 cup of pineapple (23.87 mg), and 1 cup of raspberries (30.76 mg). Alternatively, suggest clients make fresh juice with oranges, cantaloupe, pineapple, and strawberries. For more food combinations, see http://www.whfoods.com/genpage.php?tname=nutrient&dbid=109. **Cautions:** Counsel clients to avoid taking vitamin C supplements after eating a meal containing fat. Have them drink a full glass of water or juice when taking a vitamin pill. Whenever possible, they should focus instead on eating more vitamin C-rich fruits and vegetables. Remind clients that vitamin C is not stored or manufactured in the body, so a new supply is needed daily.

3. *Coffee/caffeine.* Anxiety attacks, including panic, sweating, and trembling, have been related to consuming large amounts of caffeine daily in the form of coffee, tea, chocolate, sodas, over-the-counter pain medications (such as Anacin, Excedrin, Midol) and alertness aids (NoDoz). Caffeine inhibits the absorption of adenosine—a body hormone that is calming. This can lead to sleep problems. Depending on the person, one or more cups of coffee or caffeinated foods and beverages, or pain medications, can increase anxiety symptoms or set off panic attacks (Nardi et al., 2009). Dehydration is one of the main concerns and along with it, the loss of calcium that can accelerate bone loss and lead to muscle spasms.

Stress Management

Approaches for anxiety include teaching clients stress management.

1. *Autogenic training.* Autogenic training is a relaxation technique consisting of six mental exercises and is aimed at relieving tension, anger, and

stress. Ninety-second sessions five to eight times a day, either sitting or lying down, have been shown to produce a statistically significantly greater reduction in both state (temporary) and trait (long-term) anxiety than laughter therapy or a control group receiving no intervention (Kanji, White, & Ernst, 2006). It may take up to 10 months to master the series (Sakai, 1997). **Cautions:** The solar plexus theme is not used for clients with ulcers, diabetes, or any condition involving bleeding from the abdominal region. **Other considerations:** For more information on the procedure, go to http://www.guidetopsychology.com/autogen.htm

2. *Breathing retraining.* With or without physical exercise, 30 minutes of breathing retraining a day can retrain shallow and rapid breathing, which are frequent causes of anxiety (Han, Stegen, De Valck, Clement, & Van de Woestijne, 1996; Kim & Kim, 2005). For more information go to http://www.citytech.cuny.edu/files/students/counseling/stresshb.pdf

3. *Mindfulness meditation.* In a 2010 study, participants showed statistically significant improvements in anxiety after a 4-day stress reduction intervention (Zeidan, Johnson, Diamond, David, & Goolkasian, 2010). For more information, go to http://www.stjohn.org/innerpage.aspx?PageID=1779 **Other considerations:** Other websites that may be useful are http://www.mindfulnessmeditationcentre.org/breathingGathas.htm and http://www.meditationcenter.com

4. *Relaxation therapy.* Clients may produce a calming effect by stilling the body and relaxation therapy is now supported by strong evidence for the treatment of anxiety. Participation for 20 minutes a day is recommended (Ernst, Pittler, Wider, & Boddy, 2007). **Cautions:** In a relaxed state, lower levels of medication, especially insulin, may be needed. Complete relaxation may result in a hypotensive state. Clients must avoid holding their breath and should picture breathing in and out of the abdomen. For more information go to www.webmd.com/migraines-headaches/guide/relaxation-techniques **Other considerations:** Taking the client's blood pressure at the conclusion of a relaxation training session may help identify individuals prone to hypotensive state.

Supplements

Approaches for anxiety include teaching clients about supplements that may be helpful.

Vitamin D deficiency is associated with anxiety, while sufficient vitamin D is associated with calm (Armstrong, Meenagh, Bickle, Lee, Curran, & Finch, 2007). Vitamin D$_3$ is produced in Caucasians by 4–10 minutes of exposure of face, arms, or back to the noon sun, and by 60–80 minutes of exposure for darker skinned individuals. Individuals living at latitudes north of 35°, who may not receive exposure to the sun, or who are older than 49 years may need to take a tablespoon of cod liver oil daily. Food sources of vitamin D include egg yolks, fish liver oil, dandelion greens, sweet potatoes, and salmon. **Other considerations:** Clients using corticosteroids may require additional vitamin D.

Touch

Approaches for anxiety include teaching clients about forms of touch that may be helpful.

1. *Acupressure.* Applying pressure at specific relaxation points has been shown to be an effective treatment for anxiety (Meeks, Wetherell, Irwin, Redwine, & Jeste, 2007). Acupressure should be applied for 10–15 minutes daily on the foot about one-third of the way down the sole, behind the second and third toes (solar plexus); right below the ankle bone on the outside of the foot; and on top of the foot between the tendons of the big toe and second toe about an inch from the toes. Hand acupressure should be applied on the center of the palm where the middle finger touches the palm when it is gently bent forward; another location is in the middle of the wrist crease between the tendons on the inside of the arm, level with the little finger (for palpitations and irritability). Use the tip of your thumb to press and knead points for 1–2 minutes. Practice these movements on yourself to find the points and the amount of pressure that is healing and does not tickle or is too painful. **Cautions:** Foot acupressure should not be applied to individuals with venous stasis, phlebitis, and traumatic and deep tissue injuries. Acupressure of any kind is not advised for premature infants who can withstand only limited physical contact. **Other considerations:** Find more specific directions and photographs of foot massage at www.chinese-holistic-health-exercises.com/foot-massage-techniques.html

2. *Massage with aromatherapy.* Massage using lavender, chamomile, rosemary, and lemon exerts significant positive effects on anxiety when used for 20-minute sessions 3 times a week for at least 6 weeks (Rho, Han, Kim, & Lee, 2006). **Cautions:** The aged, extremely ill, or dying individuals may require a gentle massage. The head is also a sensitive area, and only gentle sweeping motions are used and energy is not concentrated in that area. For more information, go to http://www.ehow.com/how_12801_aromatherapy-with-bodywork.html **Other considerations:** Avoid concentrating energy in any area where cancer may reside.

3. *Reflexology.* Women who used self foot reflexology daily for 15–60 minutes for 6 weeks often reduced their stress responses (Lee, 2006). **Cautions:** Pregnant women should avoid foot reflexology because certain manipulations can lead to premature labor. Those with foot problems, gout, arthritis, and vascular conditions such as varicose

veins should be careful using this procedure. For foot charts and related information go to: http://groups.msn.com/AlternativesToPain andDisease/reflexologyinstructionspg1.msnw and http://groups.msn .com/AlternativesToPainandDisease/reflexologyinstructionspg2.msnw.

4. *Therapeutic touch.* Therapeutic touch may help reduce anxiety (Jain & Mills, 2010). **Tips for use:** The techniques of therapeutic touch can be learned in a short period of time, perhaps hours, but knowing when and how to use the techniques requires practice. For information, go to http://www.therapeutictouchontario.org/index.php /newsletter/articles-therapeutictouch/whatistherapeutictouch or for work with animals, go to http://www.barbarajanelle.com/kktt/29-A _VERY_SHORTCOURSE_ON_TT_FOR_ANIMAL_OWNERS.htm

ANXIETY CASE STUDY

Ms. Leah Martinez, age 25, comes in for her routine medical examination. She reports that she has been experiencing increased anxiety over the past 6 months. Most of her day is consumed with excessive concern over a variety of issues. She does not like her job, her boyfriend is pressuring her into a long-term relationship, and she has trouble with bills that she cannot pay. Most recently, she has been having difficulty with sleeping through the night. She reports that she wakes up multiple times and has trouble going back to sleep because she worries about what the next day will bring. She is concerned that her anxiety is getting worse and affecting her relationship with her boyfriend and her ability to function at work.

This case study and health promotion challenge were developed by Carolyn T. Martin, RN, CFNP, PhD Graduate Coordinator, California State University, Stanislaus, Department of Nursing.

HEALTH PROMOTION CHALLENGE

Read the anxiety case study and then go to PubMed (http://www.ncbi.nlm.nih. gov/pubmed/), type "anxiety" in the search box at the top of the page, and click on the Search button. Choose three relevant abstracts and tell how the findings could help you teach Ms. Martinez to manage her anxiety.

REFERENCES

Armstrong, D. J., Meenagh, G. K., Bickle, I., Lee, A. S., Curran, E. S., & Finch, M. B. (2007). Vitamin D deficiency is associated with anxiety and depression in fibromyalgia. *Clinical Rheumatology, 26*(4), 551–554.

Atsumi, T., & Tonosaki, K. (2007). Smelling lavender and rosemary increases free radical scavenging activity and decreases cortisol level in saliva. *Psychiatry Research, 150*(1), 89–96.

Berk, M. (2007). Should we be targeting exercise as a routine mental health intervention. *Acta Neuropsychiatrica, 19*(3), 217–218.

Bradt, J., & Dileo, C. (2009), Music for stress and anxiety reduction in coronary heart disease patients. *Cochrane Database System of Reviews*, 2:CD006577.

De Moor, M. H. M., Beem, A. L., Stubbe, J. H., Boomsma, D. I., & De Geus, E. J. (2006). Regular exercise, anxiety, depression & personality: A population based study. *Preventive Medicine, 42*(4), 273–279.

Ernst, E., Pittler, M. H., Wider, B., & Boddy, K. (2007). Mind-body therapies: are the trial data getting stronger. *Alternative Therapies in Health and Medicine, 13*(5), 62–64.

Evans, D. (2002). The effectiveness of music as an intervention for hospital patients: A systematic review. *Journal of Advanced Nursing, 37*, 8–18.

Han, J. N., Stegen, K., De Valck, C., Clement, J., & Van de Woestijne, K. P. (1996). Influence of breathing therapy on complaints, anxiety and breathing pattern in patients with hyperventilation syndrome and anxiety disorders. *Journal of Psychosomatic Research, 41*(5), 481–493.

Isensee, B., Wittchen, H. U., Stein, M. B., Hofler, M., & Lieb, R. (2003). Smoking increases the risk of panic: Findings from a prospective community. *Archives of General Psychiatry, 60*(7), 692–700.

Jain, S., Mills, P. J. (2010). Biofield therapies: Helpful or full of hype? A best evidence synthesis. *International Journal of Behavioral Medicine, 17*(1), 1–16.

John Wiley & Sons, Inc. (2007, July 18). Colposcopy: Playing music helps women relax. Retrieved from http://www.sciencedaily.com/releases/2007/07/070718002440.htm

Kanji, N., White, A., & Ernst, E. (2006). Autogenic training to reduce anxiety in nursing students: Randomized controlled trial. *Journal of Advanced Nursing, 53*(6), 729–735.

Kim, S., & Kim, H. A. (2005). Effects of relaxation breathing exercises on anxiety, depression, and leukocytes in hemopoietic stem cell transplantation patients. *Cancer Nursing, 28*(1), 79–83.

Kinnier, R. T., Hofsess, C., Pongratz, R., & Lambert, C. (2009). Attributions and affirmations for overcoming anxiety and depression. *Psychology and Psychotherapy, 82*(Pt 2), 153–169.

Lee, Y. M. (2006). Effect of self-foot reflexology massage on depression, stress response, and immune functions of middle aged women. *Taehan Kanho Hakkoe Chi, 36*(1), 179–188.

Leslie, A., & Rust, J. (1984). Effects of dance on anxiety. *Perceptual Motor Skills, 58*(3), 767–772.

McKay, D. L., & Blumberg, J. B. (2006). A review of the bioactivity and potential health benefits of peppermint tea. *Phytotherapy Research, 20*(8), 619–633.

Meeks, T. W., Wetherell, J. L., Irwin, M. R., Redwine, L. S., & Jeste, D. V. (2007). Complementary and alternative treatments for late-life depression, anxiety, and sleep disturbance: A review of randomized controlled trials. *Journal of Clinical Psychiatry, 68*(10), 1461–1471.

of contraception, regular douching, deodorant sanitary napkins or tampons, and frequent or vigorous sexual activity while using a condom are predisposing factors.

Exercise/Movement

Approaches for cystitis include teaching clients about exercise/movement.

1. *Exercises that avoid excessive motion in the lower abdomen.* Sixty-minute sessions of swimming, walking in water, or upper and lower body aerobics performed while sitting or standing in place are best because they do not use excessive abdominal motion. Have the client wait at least 1 hour after a meal and 30 minutes after a snack to exercise and to stop any time bladder discomfort occurs (Karper, 2004).

2. *Hatha yoga.* Participation in a yoga class or using a yoga recording for 30–60-minute sessions may reduce pain of interstitial cystitis (Ripoll & Mahowald, 2002). **Cautions:** Go to http://yoga .lifetips.com/cat/56770/yoga-cautions/ Because yoga exerts pressure on internal organs, clients should wait at least 2 hours after a meal and 30 minutes to 1 hour after a snack to practice. For more information about yoga, go to http://www.yogajournal.com/poses/finder /browse_categories/seated_and_twists

Herbs/Essential Oils

Approaches for cystitis include teaching clients about essential oils.

Peppermint, menthol, rosemary, and clove essential oils all have antimicrobial actions (Fu et al., 2007; Luqman, Dwivedi, Darokar, Kalra, & Khanuja, 2007). Ask clients to fill a bathtub until their hips are covered. Instruct the client to place 5–10 drops of either peppermint, menthol, rosemary, or clove essential oil in the water and swirl it around to disperse it, then soak for 15–20 minutes. **Caution:** Advise clients to avoid using essential oils anywhere near the eyes.

Nutrition

Approaches for cystitis include teaching clients about nutrition.

1. *Berry juices.* Fresh juices, especially unsweetened cranberry and blueberry juice, are associated with a decreased risk of recurrence of urinary track infections. Fresh juice may more effective at eliminating existing infections than warding off new ones for some women and vice versa for others (Kontiokari, 2003; University of Michigan Health System, 2007).

Mooney, S., Leuendorf, J-E, & Hendrickson, C. (2009). Vitamin B6: A long known compound of surprising complexity. *Molecules, 14*(1), 329–351.

Nardi, A., Lopes, F., Freire, R., Veras, A., Nascimento, I., Valença, A., . . . Zin, W. A. (2009). Panic disorder and social anxiety disorder subtypes in a caffeine challenge test. *Psychiatry Research, 169*(2), 149–153.

Pierce, C., Pecen, J., & McLeod, K. J. (2009). Influence of seated rocking on blood pressure in the elderly: A pilot clinical study. *Biolgical Research for Nursing, 11*(2), 144–151.

Rho, K. H., Han, S. H., Kim, K. S., & Lee, M. S. (2006). Effects of aromatherapy massage on anxiety and self-esteem in Korean elderly women: A pilot study. *International Journal of Neuroscience, 116*(12), 1447–1555.

Ruwaard, J., Broeksteeg, J., Schrieken, B., Emmelkamp, P., & Lange, A. (2010). Web-based therapist-assisted cognitive behavioral treatment of panic symptoms: A randomized controlled trial with a three-year follow-up. *Journal of Anxiety Disorders, 24*(4), 387–396.

Sakai, M. (1997). Application of autogenic training for anxiety disorders: A clinical study in a psychiatric setting. *Fukuoka Igaku Zasshi, 88*(3), 56–64.

Sasazuki, S., Hayashi, T., Nakachi, K., Sasaki, S., Tsubono, Y., Okubo, S., . . . Tsugane, S. (2008). Protective effect of vitamin C on oxidative stress: a randomized controlled trial. *International Journal of Vitamin and Nutrition Research, 78*(3), 121–128.

Subramanya, P., & Telles, S. (2009). Effect of two yoga-based relaxation techniques on memory scores and state anxiety. *Biopsychosocial Medicine, 13*(3), 8.

Voss, J., Good, M., Yates, B., Baun, M., Thompson, A., & Hertzog, M. (2004). Sedative music reduces anxiety and pain during chair rest after open-heart surgery. *Pain, 112*(1–2), 197–203.

Watson, N. (1998). Rocking chair therapy for dementia patients: Its effect on psychosocial well-being and balance. *American Journal of Alzheimer's Disease, 13*(6), 296–308.

Zeidan, F., Johnson, S. K., Diamond, B. J., David, Z., & Goolkasian, P. (2010). Mindfulness meditation improves cognition: Evidence of brief mental training. *Consciousness and Cognition 9*(2), 597–605.

Bladder Conditions (Cystitis)

Environment

Approaches for cystitis include teaching clients environmental techniques.

Good bladder hygiene that could reduce or eliminate symptoms includes soaking in a warm tub, wiping from front to back, wearing a diaphragm that is not too large, using nonallergenic menstrual pads, changing tampons at each urination, drinking 6–8 glasses of fluid a day, urinating prior to and after intercourse, washing genitals prior to and after intercourse, voiding after intercourse, and making sure the angle of the penis matches the angle of the vagina so abrasions do not occur (Amiri, Rooshan, Ahmady, & Soliamani, 2009; Foxman, Geiger, Palin, Gillespie, & Koopman, 1995; Hooten et al., 2000; Khalsa, 2006). **Cautions:** Chemical contamination from spermicidal barrier methods

Other considerations: Use only 100% natural fruit juice. Corn syrup is correlated with high blood sugar, the buildup of fat cells, and obesity.

2. *Fermented milk products.* Fermented milk products containing probiotic bacteria are associated with a decreased risk of recurrence of urinary tract infections. Ingest acidophilus-soured milk, berry and fruit cultured milk, kefir, or yogurt, three times per week (Kontiokari et al., 2003; Zarate & Nader-Macias 2006). Not all yogurts contain live organisms, so it is important to read labels prior to buying a product.

3. *Tea and garlic.* In a 2003 study, tea and garlic were shown to have strong antibactericidal activity on a broad spectrum of pathogens, including resistant strains such as methicillin- and ciprofloxacin-resistant staphylococci, vancomycin-resistant enterococci, and ciprofloxacin-resistant *Pseudomonas aeruginosa* (Lee, Cesario, Wang, Shanbrom & Thrupp, 2003). **Cautions:** Garlic may interact with some antiplatelet medications but may be safe while taking warfarin (Macan et al., 2006). Tea can be sipped throughout the day and used in sitz baths. Garlic juice can be added to cooked foods.

4. *Triggering foods.* Advise clients to avoid triggering foods including alcohol, apples, artificial sweeteners, avocado, bananas, beans (fava and lima), brewer's yeast, canned figs, cantaloupes, carbonated drinks, cheese (aged), citrus, chocolate, chicken livers, corned beef, grapes, guavas, hot peppers, mayonnaise, nuts, onions, peaches, pickled herring, pineapple, plums, prunes, raisins, rye bread, soy sauce, spicy foods, sour cream, strawberries, tomatoes, vinegar, vitamins buffered with aspartate, and caffeine. These are considered bladder irritants (Shorter, Lesser, Moldwin, & Kushner, 2007). Not all individuals react to all bladder irritants. The best action is to ask clients to complete a food diary and then eliminate possible irritants for several weeks, and especially 2 hours prior to sleep. Once potential irritants have been eliminated, clients can slowly add back the foods one at a time over several weeks until bladder irritants are identified. Irritating symptoms can often be relieved by drinking a glass of water with 1 teaspoon of baking soda stirred in.

Stress Management

Approaches for cystitis include teaching clients stress management techniques.

Relaxation therapy for 20 minutes a day may produce a calming effect by stilling the body and enhancing circulation (Ernst, Pittler, Wider & Boddy, 2007). Ask clients to avoid holding their breath and to let their breathing slowly move toward the center of their abdomen.

Supplements

Approaches for cystitis include teaching clients about supplements.

Vitamins A, B_6, B_{12}, C, D, E; folic acid; and trace elements of iron, zinc, copper, and selenium work in synergy to contribute to the body's natural defense, cellular immunity, and antibody production. Inadequate intake and status of these vitamins and trace elements may lead to suppressed immunity, which predisposes to infections (Maggini, Wintergerst, Beveridge & Hornig, 2007). **Cautions:** Advise clients to follow suggested dosage on bottles and stop taking if a negative reaction occurs.

Touch

Approaches for cystitis include teaching clients about touch.

A meta-analysis of studies on foot reflexology concluded that foot reflexology for 45–60 minutes enhances urination and bladder tonus (Wang, Tsai. Lee, Chang, & Yang, 2008). **Cautions:** Pregnant women should avoid foot reflexology because certain manipulations can lead to premature labor. Those with foot problems, gout, arthritis, and vascular conditions such as varicose veins should be careful using this procedure. Focus on massaging bladder and kidney areas. For foot charts, see http://groups.msn.com/AlternativesToPainandDisease /reflexologyinstructionspg1.msnw.

BLADDER CASE STUDY

Ms. Ronnie Stuart, age 50, has been experiencing frequent bladder infections and increased burning and urgency. During a physical exam, she reported that she is recently divorced and has been having sexual relations with a man she met several months ago. Her favorite foods include chocolate, apples, cheese (aged), pickled herring, pineapple, sour cream, soy sauce, spicy foods, tomatoes, and yogurt.

HEALTH PROMOTION CHALLENGE

Read the bladder case study and then go to PubMed (http://www.ncbi.nlm.nih. gov/pubmed/), type "Cystitis" in the Search box at the top of the page, and click on the Search button. Choose three relevant abstracts and tell how the findings could help you help Ms. Stuart if she were your client.

REFERENCES

Amiri, F. N., Rooshan, M. H., Ahmady, M. H., & Soliamani, M. J. (2009). Hygiene practices and sexual activity associated with urinary tract infection in pregnant women. *East Mediterranean Health Journal, 15*(1), 104–110.

Ernst, E., Pittler, M. H., Wider, B., & Boddy, K. (2007). Mind-body therapies: Are the trial data getting stronger? *Alternative Therapies in Health and Medicine, 13*(5), 62–64.

Foxman, B., Geiger, A. M., Palin, K., Gillespie, B., & Koopman, J. S. (1995). First-time urinary tract infection and sexual behavior. *Epidemiology, 6*(2), 162–168.

Fu, Y., Zu, Y., Chen, L., Shi, W., Wang, Z., Sun, S., . . . Efferth, T. (2007). Antimicrobial activity of clove and rosemary essential oils alone and in combination. *Phytotherapy Research, 21*(10), 989–994.

Hooten, T. M., Scholes, D., Stapleton, A. E., Roberts, P. I., Winter, C., Gupta, K., . . . Stamm, W. E. (2000). A prospective study of asymptomatic bacteriuria in sexually active young women. *The New England Journal of Medicine, 343*(14), 992–997.

Karper, W. B. (2004). Exercise effects on interstitial cystitis: Two case reports. *Urologic Nursing, 24*(3), 202–204.

Khalsa, S. (2006). Living without cystitis. *Health Counselor, 6*(2), 15–17.

Kontiokari, T., Laitinen, J., Jarvi, L., Pokka, T., Sundqvist, K., & Uhari, M. (2003). Dietary factors protecting women from urinary tract infections. *American Journal of Clinical Nutrition, 77*(3), 600–604.

Lee, Y. L., Cesario, T., Wang, Y., Shanbrom, E., & Thrupp, L. (2003). Antibacterial activity of vegetables and juices. *Nutrition, 19*(11–12), 904–906.

Luqman, S., Dwivedi, G. R., Darokar, M. P., Kalra, A., & Khanuja, S. P. (2007). Potential of rosemary oil to be used in drug-resistant infections. *Alternative Therapies in Health and Medicine, 13*(5), 54–59.

Macan, H., Uykimpang, R., Clconcel, M., Takasu, J., Razon, R., Amagase, H., & Niihara, Y. (2006) Aged garlic extract may be safe for patients on warfarin therapy. *Journal of Nutrition, 136*(3 Suppl), 793S–795S.

Maggini, S., Wintergerst, E. S., Beveridge, S., & Hornig, D. H. (2007). Selected vitamins and trace elements support immune function by strengthening epithelial barriers and cellular and humoral immune responses. *British Journal of Nutrition Supplement, 1,* S29–S35.

Ripoll, E., & Mahowald, D. (2002). Hatha yoga therapy management of urological disorders. *World Journal of Urology, 20*(5), 306–309.

Shorter, B., Lesser, M., Moldwin, R. M., & Kushner, L. (2007). Effect of comestibles on symptoms of interstitial cystitis. *Journal of Urology, 178*(1), 145–152.

University of Michigan Health System. (2007, September 6). The power of fruit juice. *ScienceDaily.* Retrieved from http://www.sciencedaily.com/releases/2007/09/070905175237.htm

Wang, M. Y., Tsai, P. S., Lee, P. H., Chang, W. Y., & Yang, C. M. (2008). The efficacy of reflexology: Systematic review. *Journal of Advanced Nursing, 62*(5), 512–520.

Zarate, G., & Nader-Macias, M. E. (2006). Influence of probiotic vaginal lactobacilli on in vitro adhesion of urogenital pathogens to vaginal epithelial cells. *Letters in Applied Microbiology, 43*(2), 174–180.

Blood Pressure/Hypertension

Environment

Approaches for hypertension include teaching clients environmental techniques.

1. *Alcohol and smoking.* Alcohol and smoking both increase diastolic blood pressure. Controlling one or both could result in reduced hypertension (Houston, 2010). For information on tobacco and alcohol cessation, go to http://www.cdc.gov/tobacco/quit_smoking/index.htm and http://www.eckerd.edu/health/links/index.php
2. *Drug links.* A number of prescription and nonprescription drugs can cause transient or sustained increase in blood pressure, including NSAIDS (COX-1 and COX-2), amphetamines, decongestants, anorectics, oral contraceptives, adrenal steroid hormones, cyclosporine and tacrolimus, erythropoietin, licorice, chewing tobacco, ephedra, ma huang, and bitter orange (Chobanian, Bakris, Black, 2003).
3. *Music.* Self-selected music can lower blood pressure (Zanini et al., 2009).

Exercise

Approaches for hypertension include teaching clients exercise techniques.

1. *T'ai chi.* T'ai chi may lower blood pressure nearly as much as moderate-intensity aerobic exercise (Yeh, Wang, Wayne, & Phillips, 2009).
2. *Walking, jogging, ergometric cycling, or swimming.* Even a modest amount of weekly exercise (61–90 minutes a week) can significantly improve blood pressure levels in hypertensive clients (British Medical Journal, 2007; Ishikawa-Takata, Ohta, & Tanaka, 2003; Mayo Clinic, 2007).

Herbs/Essential Oils

Approaches for hypertension include teaching clients about herbs/essential oils, including aromatherapy.

A once-a-day inhaled blend of lavender, ylang-ylang, and bergamot essential oils for 4 weeks significantly reduced blood pressure in clients with essential hypertension, as compared to a placebo group and a control group in a study by Hwang (2006). Either of the following methods can be used: (1) Have clients add 20 drops of blended oil to a half-ounce carrier oil (peanut, castor, olive) and mix well; place three drops in their palm, rub their hands together and inhale for 1 minute; or (2) Have clients place two to three drops under their pillow for night inhalation. **Cautions:** Essential oils are for external use only unless supervised by a qualified aromatherapist. Keep out of reach of children.

Pregnant women should avoid them. Do not expose to mucous membranes or eyes.

Mind-Set

Approaches for hypertension include teaching clients mind-set techniques.

1. *Affirmations.* Self-affirmation of personal values and beliefs buffers neuroendocrine and psychological stress that can raise blood pressure (Kolea & van Knippenberg, 2006; Mann, 2005). Self-affirmations that may be helpful can be repeated aloud or written up to 20 times a day. Examples include: "I am at peace. I joyously release the past" (Creswell et al., 2000). Asking clients for input into writing affirmations can reduce resistance to using the procedure. **Other considerations:** See affirmations information at www.successconsciousness. com/index_00000a.htm

2. *Cognitive-behavioral therapy.* Daily to weekly cognitive-behavioral therapy includes homework. Clients are asked to examine how their thoughts set off negative feelings that raise blood pressure. They learn how to reduce exaggeration and generalization of negative thinking that may raise blood pressure. Indications for use are hyperreactivity to stress, high levels of occupational stress, and difficulty tolerating or complying with antihypertensive drugs (Granath, Ingvarsson, von Thiele, & Lundberg, 2006). For more information, see http://www.mind.org.uk/help/medical_and_alternative_care/making_sense_of_cognitive_behaviour_therapy

Nutrition

Approaches for hypertension include teaching clients about nutrition.

1. *Apples, berries, and onions.* These foods contain quercetin, an antioxidant flavonol associated with reduced blood pressure (Edwards et al., 2007). Suggest clients also eat the skins of apples; they contain the most antioxidants.

2. *Beet juice.* One glass of beet juice a day can significantly reduce blood pressure. Suggest clients combine 1 cup of beetroot juice with a half cup of juice from green, leafy vegetables for an added decrease in blood pressure (Queen Mary, 2008). Juicers are available at health food stores and online.

3. *Calcium.* Calcium (1,200–1,500 mg a day) reduces the risk of high blood pressure in men (Reid et al., 2010) and reduces the risk of both high blood pressure and preeclampsia in pregnant women (Bucher et al., 1996). For information on dairy and nondairy sources of calcium, go to www.health.gov/dietaryguidelines/dga2005/document/html/appendixB.htm Calcium from nondairy sources is more readily absorbed. A high-protein and high-phosphorus diet that includes soda

and milk makes calcium absorption more difficult. Vitamin D is needed for calcium to be absorbed.

4. *Cola beverages.* Consumption of sugared or diet cola is associated with an increased risk of hypertension and rises with number of cans consumed daily (Winkelmayer, Stampfer, Willett, & Curhan, 2005).

5. *Coenzyme Q10.* CoQ10 is an endogenous cofactor required for mitochondrial energy production and has been shown to lower systolic blood pressure by up to 17 mmHg and diastolic blood pressure by up to 10 mmHg (Rosenfeldt et al., 2007; Sha et al., 2007). Food sources of CoQ10 include mackerel, salmon, sardines, organ meats, boiled peanuts, and raw spinach. Teach clients to use only Spanish mackerel and Alaskan salmon for best results and least contamination. CoQ10 is also available as a capsule if additional amounts of the cofactor are required.

6. *Coffee.* Consumption of coffee is associated with increased blood pressure and plasma homocysteine. Cutting out coffee without slowly reducing its effects can result in a withdrawal syndrome. Encourage clients to dilute coffee with a half cup of decaffeinated beverage and slowly eliminate the caffeinated portion over a week's time. Older clients may be more vulnerable to the adverse effects of caffeine (Higdon & Frei, 2006).

7. *The DASH diet.* Especially when combined with exercise, the DASH diet can significantly reduce blood pressure. The DASH diet consists of daily meals high in fruits, vegetables (total of 10 servings or a half cup daily of each), low-fat dairy products, whole grains, poultry, fish, and nuts and reduced in fat, red meat, and refined sugars. It has been shown to lower blood pressure (Blumenthal et al., 2010).

   Encourage clients to begin to switch meal plans away from fat, red meat, and refined sugars and to the DASH diet by increasing the use of chicken and fish and eating more fresh fruit. Simple diet advice from healthcare practitioners can have a positive influence on motivation to make a lifestyle change (Bhatt, Luqman-Arafath, & Guleria, 2007).

8. *Dietary fiber.* Fiber can lower blood pressure according to a review of available studies (Anderson et al., 2009), but fewer than half of Americans eat sufficient fiber. Eating a bowl of steel-cut oatmeal (not instant, which is highly processed); at least four pieces of whole grain bread a day (if tolerated well; dried beans such as black, pinto, or kidney); and four to six fresh fruits and vegetables per day can help lower blood pressure. Advise clients to drink sufficient water (8–10 glasses a day) to process the fiber.

9. *Fish.* Salmon, sardines, and tuna are rich sources of omega-3 fatty acids used to treat hypertension (Mori, 2010). The American Heart Association recommends consumption of two servings of fish per week and foods high in alpha-linolenic acid (tofu and other forms of soybeans;

canola oil, and walnuts, and flaxseed and their oils, which can be converted to omega-3 in the body) for clients with no history of coronary heart disease and more for those with known coronary heart disease. Advise clients to use chunk white tuna and salmon caught off the coast of the United States (to reduce chances of mercury exposure from other fish, including farm-fed types), and to eat a cup of soybeans, a handful of raw walnuts, and flaxseed oil capsules at least several times a week (Norwegian School of Veterinary Science, 2008).

10. *Folate.* Folate has important beneficial effects on endothelial function and risk of incident hypertension, particularly in younger women. Because national surveys revealed most people did not consume adequate folate, a grain fortification program is in place. A large salad of leafy green vegetables (like spinach and turnip greens), fruits (citrus fruits and juices), and a serving of either dried beans or peas, all natural sources of folate, can help meet the suggested amount of 1,000 micrograms a day (Office of Dietary Supplements, 2005). Some clients may not receive sufficient amounts of the nutrient and may need additional amounts. This includes people on diets who do not eat breads, cereals, or pasta; who abuse alcohol; who are pregnant or breastfeeding; who have malabsorption issues; who undergo kidney dialysis; who have liver disease and certain anemias; or who take medications that interfere with folate absorption (anticonvulsant medications, metformin, sulfasalazine, triamterene, methotrexate, or barbiturates). Research has provided evidence that the introduction of flour fortified with folic acid into common foods has been linked to colon cancer, which them a poor source of this nutrient (Blackwell Publishing Ltd., 2007).

    Exceeding 1,000 micrograms per day of folate may trigger vitamin B_{12} deficiency. To compensate, women can take a multivitamin that contains B_{12} or eat at least one food daily that contains B_{12}, such as nutritional yeast (unless susceptible to *Candida*), clams, eggs, herring, kidney, liver, mackerel, seafood, milk, or dairy products (Office of Dietary Supplements, 2005).

11. *Garlic.* Garlic has antioxidant properties that can help lower systolic blood pressure (Reinhart, Coleman, Teevan, Vachhani, & White, 2008) and may be safe while taking warfarin (Macan et al., 2006).

12. *Green tea.* Hypertension decreased by 35% in women who drank 1–2 cups of green tea and was further reduced by 65% for those who drank 3 cups or more (Yang, Lu, Wu, Wu, & Cheng, 2004). Due to the caffeine, high doses of green tea can result in palpitations and irregular heartbeat, anxiety, nervousness, insomnia, nausea, heartburn, and increased stomach acid. The decaffeinated form may be a better choice for these reasons.

13. *Magnesium.* Clients who eat foods containing magnesium are least likely to have hypertension (Song et al., 2006). **Cautions:** Magnesium absorption can be reduced by diuretics, antibiotics, and antineoplastic medications. Substituting alcohol for food, having poorly controlled diabetes or malabsorptive problems, and being older increase risk for magnesium deficiency. To reduce risk of hypertension, advise clients to eat green leafy vegetables, nuts, whole grains (breads, cereals, pastas, and rice) daily.

14. *Salt.* A meta-analysis of available studies led to the conclusion that restricting sodium intake to levels below 6 grams (1 teaspoon) per day clearly reduces blood pressure and may reduce the need for antihypertensives by as much as 30%. Most international guidelines such as those of the U.S. Dietary Guideline Committee and the Scientific Advisory Committee on Nutrition recommend the 6-gram maximum (Walter, Mackenzie, & Dunning, 2007.) It is not necessary to totally restrict salty foods, but it is important to reduce their use.

15. *Sesame oil.* When the light form of sesame oil is used as the sole cooking oil, it can reduce blood pressure to normal in hypertensive women (with a blood pressure reading of 166/101 on the average) who are already taking the calcium channel blocker nifedipine (Pugalendi, Sambandam, & Rao, 2003).

16. *Soy nuts.* To lower blood pressure, substitute soy nuts for other protein sources in a healthy diet at the rate of a half cup of unsalted soy nuts daily (JAMA and Archives Journals, 2007).

Stress Management

Approaches for hypertension include teaching clients stress management procedures.

1. *Autogenic training.* Autogenic training is a relaxation technique consisting of six mental exercises and is aimed at relieving tension, anger, and stress and reducing blood pressure (Watanabe et al., 2003). For more information go to http://www.guidetopsychology.com/autogen.htm

2. *Transcendental meditation.* A meta-analysis of studies showed that transcendental meditation produces a statistically significant reduction in high blood pressure that is at least as great as the changes found with major changes in diet or exercise. The changes due to 1 hour of daily meditation are associated with at least a 15% reduction in rates of heart attack and stroke (University of Kentucky, 2007). It is not necessary or advisable to meditate on an empty stomach. It is permissible to eat lightly prior to meditating. For information on specific kinds of meditation go to http://www.project-meditation.org/htm/meditation_instructions.html

3. *Yoga.* Women who practice yoga for 1 hour for at least 10 weeks may show significant improvement in blood pressure (Sivasan-karan et al., 2006; Zarich, 2006). **Cautions:** Go to http://yoga.lifetips .com/cat/56770/yoga-cautions/ for information on potential areas of concern. For more information on various asanas (yoga postures), go to www.yogajournal.com/poses/

Supplements

Approaches for hypertension include teaching clients about supplements.

1. *Potassium.* Potassium supplementation can significantly reduce blood pressure (Kapoor & Kapoor, 2009). Clients without salt-related hypertension may achieve similar results from eating potassium-rich foods, especially papayas, lima beans, plantains, Jerusalem artichokes, bananas, oat bran, tomatoes, cucumbers, cantaloupe, pears, and mangoes.

2. *Vitamins C and E.* The enhancement of antioxidant status by vitamins C and E supplementation in essential hypertensive clients is associated with lower blood pressure; 1,000 mg vitamin C and 400 IU vitamin E a day were shown to reduce blood pressure significantly (Rodrigo, Prat, Passalacqua, Araya, & Bachler, 2008). **Cautions:** Vitamin E is a blood thinner and can reduce the amount of prescribed blood thinners needed.

Touch

Approaches for hypertension include teaching clients about touch treatments.

1. *Acupuncture.* Acupuncture proved effective and safe for the treatment of mild to moderate hypertension in a randomized, single-blind clinical trial, using 22 sessions of 30 minutes for a period of 6 weeks (Li, Longhurst, & Dodge, 2007).

2. *Foot reflexology.* Performed twice a week, for 4–6 weeks, foot reflexology significantly decreased systolic blood pressure; self-foot reflexology proved just as good for decreasing diastolic blood pressure (Park, & Cho, 2004). **Cautions:** See www.wikihow.com/Give-a-Foot-Massage for more information on possible concerns regarding this treatment.

3. *Massage therapy.* Massage therapy, with or without aromatherapy (using lavender, rose germanium, rose, and jasmine essential oils) is associated with significant reductions in systolic and diastolic blood pressure (Hur et al., 2007; Sharpe, Williams, Granner, & Hussey, 2007). For information on aromatherapy massage, go to http://www.ehow.com /how_12801_aromatherapy-with-bodywork.html

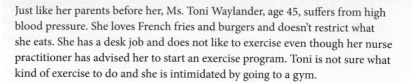

HYPERTENSION CASE STUDY

Just like her parents before her, Ms. Toni Waylander, age 45, suffers from high blood pressure. She loves French fries and burgers and doesn't restrict what she eats. She has a desk job and does not like to exercise even though her nurse practitioner has advised her to start an exercise program. Toni is not sure what kind of exercise to do and she is intimidated by going to a gym.

HEALTH PROMOTION CHALLENGE

Suppose Toni is your client. Go to PubMed (http://www.ncbi.nlm.nih.gov/pubmed/) and search for "hypertension and diet" and for "hypertension and exercise" to see what you might advise for Toni.

REFERENCES

Anderson, J. W., Baird, P., Davis, R. H., Jr., Ferreri, S., Knudtson, M., Koraym, A., . . . Williams, C. L. (2009). Health benefits of dietary fiber. *Nutrition Reviews, 67*(4), 188–205.

Bhatt, S. P., Luqman-Arafath, T. K., & Guleria, R. (2007). Non-pharmacological management of hypertension. *Indian Journal of Medical Science, 61*(11), 616–624.

Blackwell Publishing Ltd. (2007, November 5). Folic acid linked to increased cancer rate, historical review suggests. Retrieved from http://www.sciencedaily.com/releases/2007/11/071102111956.htm

Blumenthal, J. A., Babyak, M. A., Hinderliter, A., Watkins, L. L., Craighead, L., Lin, P. H., . . . Sherwood, A. (2010). Effects of the DASH diet alone and in combination with exercise and weight loss on blood pressure and cardiovascular biomarkers in men and women with high blood pressure: The ENCORE study. *Archives of Internal Medicine, 170*(2), 126–135.

British Medical Journal. (2007, August 20). Even low levels of weekly exercise drive down blood pressure. Retrieved from http://www.sciencedaily.com/releases/2007/08/070813192701.htm

Bucher, H. C., Gayatt, G. H., Cook., R. J., Hotala, R., Cook, D. J., Lang, J. D., & Hunt, D. (1996). Effect of calcium supplementation on pregnancy-induced hypertension and preeclampsia—a meta-analysis of randomized controlled trials. *Journal of the American Medical Association, 275*(13), 1113–1117.

Chobanian, A. V., Bakris, G. L., & Black, H. R. (2003). The seventh report of the Joint Committee on the Prevention, Detection, Evaluation and Treatment of High Blood Pressure: The JNC 7 report. *Journal of the American Medical Association, 289*, 2560–2572.

Creswell, J. D., Welch, W. T., Taylor, S. E., Sherman, D. R., Gruenwald, T. L., & Hay, L. (2000). *Heal your body*. Carlsbad, CA: Hay House.

Edwards, R. L., Lyon, T., Litwin, S. E., Rabovsky, A., Symons, J. D., & Jalili, T. (2007). Quercetin reduces blood pressure in hypertensive subjects. *The Journal of Nutrition, 137*(11), 2405–2411.

Granath, J., Ingvarsson, S., von Thiele, U., & Lundberg, U. (2006). Stress management: A randomized study of cognitive behavioural therapy and yoga. *Cognitive Behavioural Therapy, 35*(1), 3–10.

Han, S. H., Hur, M. H., Buckle, J., Choi, J., & Lee, M. S. (2006). Effect of aromatherapy on symptoms of dysmenorrheal in college students. *Journal of Alternative and Complementary Medicine, 12*(6), 535–54l.

Higdon, J. V., & Frei, B. (2006). Coffee and health: a review of recent human research. *Critical Reviews of Food Science and Nutrition, 46*(2), 101–123.

Houston, M. C. (2010). The role of cellular micronutrient analysis, nutraceuticals, vitamins, antioxidants and minerals in the prevention and treatment of hypertension and cardiovascular disease. *Therapeutic Advances in Cardiovascular Disease, 4*(3):165–83

Hur, M. H., Oh, H., Lee, M. S., Kim, C., Choi, A. N., & Shin, G. R. (2007). Effects of aromatherapy massage on blood pressure and lipid profile in Korean climacteric women. *International Journal of Neuroscience, 117*(9), 1281–1287.

Hwang, J. H. (2006). The effects of the inhalation method using essential oils on blood pressure and stress responses of women with essential hypertension. *Taehan Kanho Hakhoe Chi, 36*(7), 1123–1124.

Ishikawa-Takata, K., Ohta, F., & Tanaka, H. (2003). Just one hour of weekly exercise may lower BP. *American Journal of Hypertension, 16,* 629–633.

JAMA and Archives Journals. (2007, May 29). Soy nuts may improve blood pressure in postmenopausal women. Retrieved from http://www.fda.gov/downloads/ScienceResearch /SpecialTopics/WomensHealthResearch/UCM247900.pdf

Kapoor, R., & Kapoor, J. R. (2009). Blood pressure reduction with potassium supplementation. *Journal of the American College of Cardiology, 53*(13), 1164.

Kolea, S. L., & van Knippenberg, A. (2006). Controlling your mind without ironic consequences: Self-affirmation eliminates rebound effects after thought suppression. *Journal of Experimental Social Psychology, 43*(4), 671–677.

Li, P., Longhurst, J., & Dodge, L. K. (2007, November). *Acupuncture works in lowering blood pressure in hypertensive patients.* Presented at the Society for Neuroscience conference, San Diego, CA. Monday, November 5th.

Macan, H., Uykimpang, R., Clconcel, M., Takasu, J., Razon, R., Amagase, H. . . . Niihara, Y. (2006). Aged garlic extract may be safe for patients on warfarin therapy. *Journal of Nutrition, 136*(3 Suppl), 793S–795S.

Mann, T. (2005). Affirmation of personal values buffers neuroendocrine and psychological stress responses. *Psychological Science, 16,* 846–851.

Mayo Clinic. (2007, July 13). When it comes to walking, it's all good, says Mayo Clinic researcher. *Science Daily.* Retrieved from http://www.sciencedaily.com /releases/2007/07/070711134426.htm

Mori, T. A. (2010). Omega-3 fatty acids and blood pressure. *Cellular and Molecular Biology (Noisy-le-Grand, France), 56*(1), 83–92.

Norwegian School of Veterinary Science. (2008, February 28). Farmed fish fed cheap food may be less nutritious for humans. *ScienceDaily.* Retrieved from http://www.science daily.com/releases/2008/02/080226164105.htm

Office of Dietary Supplements. (2005). *Dietary supplement fact sheet: Folate.* Bethesda, MD: NIH Clinical Center. National Institutes of Health. Retrieved from http://ods.od.nih .gov/factsheets/Folate_pf.asp

Park, H. S., & Cho, G. Y. (2004). Effects of foot reflexology on essential hypertension patients. *Taehan Kanho Hakkoe Chi, 34*(5), 739–750.

Pugalendi, K. V., Sambandam, G., & Rao, M. R. (2003, April). *Sesame oil helps reduce blood pressure-lowering medicine.* Presented to the 15th Scientific Meeting of the Inter-American Society of Hypertension, San Antonio, TX.

Queen Mary, University of London. (2008, February 6). Daily glass of beet juice can beat high blood pressure, study shows. *ScienceDaily.* Retrieved from http://www.sciencedaily .com/releases/2008/02/080205123825.htm

Reid, I. R., Ames, R., Mason, B., Bolland, M. J., Bacon, C. J., Reid, H. E., . . . Horne, A. (2010). Effects of calcium supplementation on lipids, blood pressure, and body composition in healthy older men: A randomized controlled trial. *American Journal of Clinical Nutrition, 91*(1), 131–139.

Reinhart, K. M., Coleman, C. I., Teevan, C., Vachhani, P., & White, C. M. (2008). Effects of garlic on blood pressure in patients with and without systolic hypertension: A meta-analysis. *Annals of Pharmacotherapy, 42*(12), 1766–1771.

Rodrigo, R., Prat, H., Passalacqua, W., Araya, J., & Bachler, J. P. (2008). Diminution of oxidative stress through vitamins C and E supplementation associates with blood pressure reduction in essential hypertension. *Clinical Science (London, England), 114*(10), 625–634.

Rosenfeldt, F. L., Has, S. J., Krum H., Hadj, A., Ng, K., Leong, J. Y., & Watts, G. F. (2007). Coenzyme Q10 in the treatment of hypertension: A meta-analysis of the clinical trials. *Journal of Human Hypertension, 21*(4), 297–306.

Sha, S. A., Sander, S., Cios, D., Lipeika, J., Kluger, J., & White, C. M. (2007). Electrocardiographic and hemodynamic effects of coenzyme Q10 in healthy individuals: A double-blind, randomized controlled trial. *Annals of Pharmacotherapy, 41*(3), 420–425.

Sharpe, P. A., Williams, H. G., Granner, M. I., & Hussey, J. R. (2007). A randomized study of the effects of massage therapy compared to guided relaxation on well-being and stress perception among older adults. *Complementary Therapies in Medicine, 15*(3), 157–163.

Sivasankaran, S., Pollard-Quintner, S., Sachdeva, R., Pugeda, J., Hoq, S. W., Granath, J., . . . Lundberg, U. (2006). Stress management: A randomized study of cognitive behavioural therapy and yoga. *Cognitive Behavioural Therapy, 35*(1), 3–10.

Song, Y., Sesso, H. D., Manson, J. E., Cook, N. R., Buring, J. E., & Liu, S. (2006). Dietary magnesium intake and risk of incident hypertension among middle-aged and older US women in a 10-year follow-up study. *American Journal of a Cardiology, 98*(12), 1616–1621.

University of Kentucky. (2007, December 5). Transcendental meditation effective in reducing high blood pressure, study shows. Retrieved from http://www.eurekalert.org/pub _releases/2007-12/uok-tme120407.php

Walter, J., Mackenzie, A. D., & Dunning, J. (2007). Does reducing your salt intake make you live longer? *Interactions in Cardiovascular Thoracic Surgery, 6*(6), 793–798.

Watanabe, Y., Cornélissen, G., Watanabe, M., Watanabe, F., Otsuka, K., Ohkawa, S., . . . Halberg, F. (2003). Effects of autogenic training and antihypertensive agents on circadian and circaseptan variation of blood pressure. *Clinical and Experimental Hypertension, 25*(7), 405–412.

Winkelmayer, W. C., Stampfer, M. J., Willett, W. C., & Curhan, G. C. (2005). Sodas increase risk of hypertension. *JAMA, 294*(18), 2330–2335.

Yang, Y. C., Lu, F. H., Wu, J. S., Wu, C. H., & Cheng, C. J. (2004). The protective effect of habitual tea consumption on hypertension. *Archives of Internal Medicine, 164*(14), 1534–1540.

Yeh, G. Y., Wang, C., Wayne, P. M., & Phillips, R. (2009). Tai chi exercise for patients with cardiovascular conditions and risk factors: A systematic review. *Journal of Cardiopulmonary Rehabilitation and Prevention, 29*(3), 152–160.

Zanini, C. R., Jardim, P. C., Salgado, C. M., Nunes, M. C., de Urzêda, F. L., Carvalho, M. V., . . . de Souza, W. K. (2009). Music therapy effects on the quality of life and the blood pressure of hypertensive patients. *Arquivos Brasileiros de Cardiologia, 93*(5), 534–540.

Zarich, S. W. (2006). The effect of a six-week program of yoga and meditation on brachial artery reactivity: Do psychosocial interventions affect vascular tone? *Clinical Cardiology, 29*(9), 393–339.

Breast Cancer

Environment

Environmental evidence-based practice for breast cancer includes teaching clients about the following:

1. *Acrylamide.* Acrylamide, a carcinogen linked to breast cancer in humans, is formed when frying, baking or grilling carbohydrate-rich foods at temperatures above 120ºC, including bread, French fries, and biscuits. The longer the cooking time and the lower the water content, the higher the acrylamide content in the heat-processed food. Adding rosemary to dough prior to baking a portion of wheat buns at 225ºC reduced the acrylamide content by up to 60%. Even rosemary in small quantities in 1% of the dough was enough to reduce the acrylamide content significantly. Flavonoids in vegetables, unsweetened chocolate, and tea, especially green tea, considerably reduce the acrylamide content (Linos & Willett, 2007).

2. *Alcohol.* Two drinks a day of beer, wine, or liquor can increase the risk of breast cancer by 10%; three of more drinks increases risk by 30% and is equal to smoking a pack of cigarettes a day. Binge drinking can increase risk by 55%. Although not drinking is preferable, sufficient folate intake can mitigate this excess risk. (See the "Nutrition" section in "Alzheimer's Disease," No. 13 for more information). Risk of breast cancer is strongest among women who drink and take postmenopausal hormones (Zhang et al., 2007).

3. *Aluminum in breast tissue.* Research has linked breast cancer with the use of aluminum-based underarm antiperspirants. The known, but unaccounted for, higher incidence of tumors in the upper outer quadrant of the breast seems to support this theory. **Cautions:** Continuing to use underarm antiperspirants may increase risk for breast cancer. Recommend using deodorants that do not contain aluminum salts. Aluminum is a metalloestrogen; it is genotoxic, is bound by DNA, and has been shown to be carcinogenic (Keele University, 2007).

4. *Cooked meat carcinogens.* During the cooking of meat, mutagenic and carcinogenic heterocyclic amines are formed, the most abundant of which, 2-amino-1-methyl-6-phenylimidazo[4-5-b]pyridine (PhIP), induces mammary gland tumors. PhIP acts as a tumor initiator and promoter, and dietary exposure could contribute to carcinogenesis in breast tissue. PhIP can activate estrogen receptor-mediated signaling pathways following consumption of a cooked meat meal (Creton, Zhu & Gooderham, 2007). Advise clients to gradually replace all cooked meat with other, safer sources of protein, such as fish, soy, beans, rice, and chicken.

5. *Catfish caught in polluted waters.* Exposing estrogen-sensitive breast cancer cells to extracts of channel catfish caught in areas with heavy sewer and industrial waste causes the cells to multiply. Eating any fish caught from polluted waters may expose women to risk of breast cancer. **Cautions:** Researchers at the University of Pittsburgh found vast quantities of pharmaceutical and xeno-estrogenic waste in outflows from sewage treatment plants and from sewer overflows that end up concentrated and magnified in channel catfish (University of Pittsburgh School of the Health Sciences, 2007). Suggest clients eat only fish not caught in areas heavily polluted by industrial and municipal wastes.

6. *Dioxins.* A known human carcinogen and hormone mimicker, dioxin is ubiquitous and is found in the body fat of every human being, including every newborn. It is formed by the incineration of products containing polyvinylchloride (PVC), PCBs, and other chlorinated compounds. Dioxin also comes from industrial processes that use chlorine and combustion of diesel and gasoline containing chlorinated additives. **Cautions:** Clients are exposed to dioxin primarily through consumption of animal products. Sources of dioxin include meat, poultry, dairy products, and human breastmilk. Dioxin enters the food chain when vehicle exhaust or soot from incinerated chlorinated compounds falls on field crops later eaten by farm animals. Exposure to dioxin can be reduced by limiting or eliminating intake of meat, poultry, and dairy products and living far from incineration plants and highways. **Other considerations:** Intrauterine exposure to dioxin can disrupt the development of mammary glands that can predispose offspring to breast cancer (International Agency for Research on Cancer, 1997; Warner et al., 2002; World Health Organization, 2007).

7. *Electromagnetic fields.* Extremely low-intensity electromagnetic field exposure is correlated with breast cancer. **Cautions:** Advise clients to use a headset and carry wireless phones away from the body, limit the duration and number of cell phone calls, and unplug or disconnect the microwave from electrical power before reaching inside. Use cell phones only for emergencies, not for chatting. The World Health Orga-

nization (2011) cautions that cell phones may be carcinogenic. Follow safe use for microwave ovens. If clients purchase or rent a house, suggest they opt for housing far away from cell phone antennas and new, high-tension or upgraded power lines (Hardell & Sage, 2007).

8. *Preventive mastectomy.* Research has failed to show a survival benefit with the second mastectomy. The risk of cancer spread from the original breast to the other body sites during surgery often exceeds the risk of getting cancer in the second breast. A study of 296 women who opted for preventive mastectomy revealed the following regrets: poor cosmetic result (39%), diminished sexuality (22%), lack of education regarding alternative measures (22%), and other reasons (17%). Counsel women not to overestimate the risk for cancer in the healthy breast and convey information about the study of regrets after preventive mastectomy (Montgomery ct al., 1999). **Other considerations:** Counsel women to increase their vitamin D intake to keep their healthy breast and rest of body healthy. See vitamin D deficiency in No. 11.

9. *Pesticides.* Lawn and garden pesticide use is associated with breast cancer risk. There is no known safe level (Teitelbaum et al., 2007). **Cautions:** Advise clients to stay away from lawns and gardens where pesticides are used and to employ xeriscaping and natural pesticides instead. For more information, go to http://www.beyondpesticides.org /lawn/factsheets/. **Other considerations:** Little or no association was found for nuisance/pest pesticides, insect repellants, or products used to control lice, fleas, and ticks on pets.

10. *Sexual assault.* Sexual assault has been associated with an increased risk of breast cancer. Multiple episodes of sexual assault carry a two-to-threefold greater risk of breast cancer compared with a single episode. Every woman should be asked about being sexually assaulted as part of the history and intake process. For more information on sexual assault and how to introduce the topic, go to http://www.justyellfire .com/?gclid=CJ3h6vjt5rACFUJo4AodnV9Ezw or http://www.rainn .org/get-information/sexual-assault-prevention

There is a definitive link between sexual and emotional abuse and breast cancer (Goldsmith et al., 2010), and women or men who have been assaulted should be referred for counseling to help prevent the development of breast cancer in the future (Stein & Barrett-Connor, 2000).

11. *Vitamin D deficiency.* Vitamin D deficiency may precipitate or exacerbate breast cancer or may be a sign of the disease processes. Recommend daily sensible sun exposure (4–10 minutes with face and arms exposed for light-skinned women and 60–80 minutes for dark skin). Longer exposure can increase the risk of skin cancer. Vitamin D supplements are not recommended as they can increase disease in already

ill clients (Autoimmunity Research Foundation, 2008). Sun exposure should be at solar noon when UVB rays are most directly penetrating. Women residing at latitudes north of 35° have a higher incidence of breast cancer. They may need to take a tablespoon of cod liver oil daily, eat fatty fish several times a week, eat eggs several times a week (the yolks are the portion that contain vitamin D), and/or take fish oil supplements.

12. *X-rays, including mammograms.* Low-dose medical radiation exposure, particularly exposures during childhood, increases breast cancer risk. Elevated risks for breast cancer include multiple chest X-rays, seven or more mammograms, CT scans, and women who received dental X-rays without lead apron protection before age 20 years (Brenner & Hall, 2007). Accuracy of X-rays varies by practitioner, so it is not always possible to know the level of exposure (Ma, Hill, Bernstein, & Ursin, 2007). Weigh the dangers of X-rays versus the need for diagnostic information, including whether other, safer methods of diagnosis are available. **Other considerations:** X-rays and Y-rays have been added to the national list of carcinogens. Good alternatives are the AMAS test (AMAS test, 2007) and using a plastic syringe to extract a small amount of breast fluid, a test developed by Dr. Chandice Covington, RN ("*Breast Fluid a Better Option,*" 2003).

13. *Workplace chemical exposure.* Research provides evidence that workplace chemicals increase breast cancer risk among women. **Cautions:** Advise clients to reduce the risk of environmental toxins from exposure to organic solvents, metals, acid mists, sterilizing agents, some pesticides, light during night shifts, and tobacco smoke. Animal cancer bioassays conducted by the National Toxicology Program indicate more than 40 chemicals can induce mammary tumors, and most of these are still in production. People in a variety of occupations worldwide, including healthcare providers and metal, textile, dye, rubber, and plastic manufacturing workers, have been identified as having some evidence of higher breast cancer risk (Snedeker, 2006).

Exercise/Movement

Exercise/movement evidence-based practice for breast cancer includes teaching clients about walking, jogging, running, playing tennis, bicycling, swimming, and aerobic dance.

Giving a breast cancer survivor an exercise workbook or step pedometer can improve her quality of life and fatigue level (University of Alberta, 2007). Women who exercised more than 7 hours per week lowered their risk for breast cancer by 20% more than those women who exercised less than 1 hour per week. In lean, regular-exercising premenopausal women, the risk for breast cancer was reduced by 72%. Previously sedentary postmenopausal women can adhere to a moderate- to vigorous-intensity exercise program that results in changes in estradiol and SHBG concentrations that are consistent with a lower risk for postmenopausal breast cancer (Friedenreich et al., 2010). Exercise can also lower estrogen levels; high levels of estrogen contribute to an increased risk of breast cancer (American Association for Cancer Research, 2008). **Cautions:** Counsel women to start slowly with exercise and inform their healthcare practitioners of plans if they are over 35 years old and have chest pain or shortness of breath, have leg pain when walking, have ankles that swell regularly, or have been told they have heart disease. **Tips for use:** Advise clients to use appropriate clothes and shoes and stop exercising if any untoward signs occur. Women should be able to exercise and carry on a conversation without becoming short of breath.

Herbs/Essential Oils

Herbal evidence-based practice for breast cancer includes teaching clients about:

1. *Astragalus.* A weak immune system is one of the major factors that promote cancer metastases after an operation, chemotherapy, or radiation therapy. Astragalus enhances immune response, stimulates the production of interferon, and protects against mammary tumors. This herb can be taken by mouth as a tincture, decoction, fluid extract, or in capsule form. **Cautions:** Avoid using astragalus during a fever, infection, or inflammation; pregnancy or lactation; or taking concurrently with antihypertensives, cyclophosphamide, immunosuppressants, interleukin-2, or interferon. This herb is generally safe (Deng & Chen, 2009; Nagasawa, Watanabe, Yoshida & Inatomi, 2001).

2. *Curcumin (turmeric).* Curcumin has antiproliferative and antiangiogenic activities that make it therapeutically efficacious for cancer at 400–600 mg three times a day standardized to curcumin content or tincture, 10 ml at 1:5 dilution (Anand, Kunnumakkara, Newman & Aggarwal, 2007; Corona-Rivera et al., 2007). **Cautions:** Pregnant and lactating women or women with bile duct obstruction, peptic ulcer, hyperacidity, gallstones, bleeding disorders, or hypersensitivity to the herb should not use curcumin. Women who take the following drugs should also not use curcumin: anticoagulants, immunosuppressants, or NSAIDs. Advise clients to store curcumin in a cool, dry place and not to take it on an empty stomach. Turmeric/curcumin can be safely sprinkled on food as a spice (Skidmore-Roth, 2006d).

3. *Licorice (Glycyrrhiza uralensis).* Chinese licorice has anticancer effects

against human breast cancer cells (Dong, Inoue, Zhu, Tanji & Kiyama 2007; Jo et al., 2005; Ye, Gho, Chan, Chen, & Leung, 2009). Have the client simmer 1 teaspoon of the cut and sifted root in a cup of boiling water, allow to simmer for 5 minutes, cool, and drink once a day. **Cautions:** Advise clients to avoid licorice when they are pregnant or lactating; during hepatic or liver disease; during a state of hypokalemia if they have hypertension, arrhythmia, or congestive heart failure; if they have a hypersensitivity to the herb; or when taking aloe, buckthorn, cascara, Chinese rhubarb, grapefruit, or diuretics. Drugs that may interact with this herb are cardiac glycosides, antihypertensives, antiarrhythmics, azole antifungals, cytochrome P450, and corticosteroids. Advise clients to keep licorice in a cool, dry place and try to avoid using this herb for longer than 6 weeks or increase potassium intake if taking longer (Skidmore-Roth, 2006e).

4. *Milk thistle.* Silymarin, the active substance in milk thistle, stimulates detoxification pathways, inhibits the growth of certain cancer cell lines, exerts direct cytotoxic activity toward certain cancer cell lines, and may increase the efficacy of certain chemotherapy agents. Milk thistle also protects the liver from drug or alcohol-related injury. Silibinin, a compound of milk thistle, may even prevent the development of liver cancer at 200 to 400 mg per day (Bokemeyer, Fells & Dunn 1996; Cheung Gibbons, Johnson, & Nicol, 2010). **Cautions:** Milk thistle is considered safe and well-tolerated with gastrointestinal upset, a mild laxative effect, and rare allergic reaction being the only adverse events reported when taken within the recommended dose range. Counsel pregnant and lactating women or those who are hypersensitive (have a known sensitivity to ragweed, marigolds, or chrysanthemums) not to use milk thistle. Advise clients to avoid taking milk thistle concurrently with antipsychotics, phenytoin, and halothane. Milk thistle may protect against liver damage from antipsychotics, acetaminophen, phenytoin, and halothane. Preliminary research suggests that silybin may enhance the tumor-fighting effects of cisplatin and doxorubicin.

5. *Rosemary.* Constituents in rosemary have shown a variety of pharmacologic activities for breast cancer prevention when used as a spice in cooking or drunk as a tea (Cheung & Tai, 2007).

Mind-Set

Mind-set evidence-based practice for insomnia in women with breast cancer includes cognitive behavioral therapy.

Cognitive behavioral therapy is a validated, cost-effective intervention for persistent insomnia and can produce a significant reduction in daytime fatigue (Espie et al., 2008).

Nutrition

Evidence-based nutrition approaches for breast cancer include the following:

1. *Berries.* Black raspberry and strawberry extracts showed the most significant ability to inhibit breast cancer cell growth (Seeram et al., 2006). Encourage clients to eat raspberries and/or strawberries at least several times a week.

2. *Curcumin.* A spice also known as turmeric, curcumin can prevent and treat cancer by inhibiting breast cancer cell invasion (Kim et al., 2012). Encourage clients to use curcumin liberally in cooking every day. Caution clients not to use at the same time as anticoagulants, immunosuppressants, or NSAIDs (Skidmore-Roth, 2006d).

3. *Flaxseed.* Flaxseed reduced the growth and metastasis of established ER-human breast cancer, in part due to its lignan and oil components (Chen, Saggar, Corey, & Thompson, 2009; Wang, Chen, & Thompson, 2005). Amount: 2½ teaspoons of ground seeds twice or three times a day in salad, soup, other foods, or water. **Cautions:** Until more research is available, pregnant and lactating women should not use flaxseeds nor give them to children. Women with bowel obstruction, dehydration, or sensitivity to flaxseed should avoid using it. Flax can decrease the absorption of other medications, so advise clients to separate them by several hours. Keep flaxseeds in the refrigerator to prevent fatty acid breakdown. Adequate levels of zinc and acidophilus are needed to metabolize flax. **Other considerations:** Flax may increase the risk of bleeding if taken with anticoagulants/antiplatelets and antidiabetes agents (Skidmore-Roth, 2006b).

4. *Green tea.* Two to five cups of green tea a day is protective against breast cancer before disease occurs and after onset, possibly by creating a detoxifying effect (American Association for Cancer Research, 2007). **Cautions:** Green tea may decrease iron absorption, so advise clients to separate iron-rich foods or iron pills by at least 2 hours from green tea ingestion. Caffeinated green tea can interact with MAOIs and lead to a hypertensive crisis. Counsel clients not to take green tea with anticoagulants/antiplatelets (may increase risk of bleeding), beta-adrenergic blockers (can lead to increased inotropic effects), or benzodiazepines (may increase sedation). Dairy products may decrease the therapeutic effects of green tea, so separate their intake by several hours. Digestive process affects anticancer activity of tea; add citrus (such as lemon juice) or take ascorbic acid (vitamin C) to protect the catechins in green tea from digestive degradation (Skidmore-Roth, 2006c; Espie, 2008).

5. *Mediterranean diet.* The Mediterranean diet is linked with prevention of breast cancer. High daily intake of vegetables, legumes, and fruits that are high in protective fiber is associated with a 40% reduced risk

in developing breast cancer (Do, Lee, Kim, Jung, & Lee, 2007; Fields, Soprano, & Soprano, 2007; Liu, Liu, & Chen, 2005; Mitrou et al., 2007; Taylor, Burley & Cade, 2007). For more information on the diet, go to: http://www.mayoclinic.com/health/mediteraneandiet/CL00011.

6. *Probiotics.* Probiotics (lactic acid bacteria/LAB) are present in many foods such as yogurt. They increase immune cell activity and may suppress the growth of bacteria that convert procarcinogens into carcinogens (Matar & Perdigon, 2007).

7. *Soy.* Soyasaponins have been shown to inhibit the proliferation of cancer cells (Xiao, Huang, & Zhang, 2007). A meta-analysis of the eight studies conducted in high-soy-consuming Asians show a significant trend of decreasing risk with increasing soy food intake (Wu, Yu, Tseng, & Pike, 2008). Eating soy foods in puberty can protect against breast cancer (Georgetown University Medical Center, 2008). **Cautions:** Nonfermented forms of soy foods may reduce assimilation of calcium, magnesium, copper, iron, and zinc due to their high levels of phytic acid. The best soy sources are fermented, including tempeh and miso.

Stress Management

Stress management evidence-based practice for breast cancer includes teaching clients about:

1. *Autogenic training.* Women who participated in autogenic training showed significant reductions in anxiety and depression and increased immune responses (Hidderley & Holt, 2004).

2. *Journaling.* Women who write for at least four sessions about their deepest thoughts and feelings, positive thoughts and feelings, or about their treatment have significantly fewer appointments for cancer-related morbidities (Stanton ct al., 2002).

3. *Mindfulness-based stress reduction program (MBSR).* MBSR is an 8-week program that incorporates relaxation, meditation, gentle yoga, and daily home practice. MBSR is associated with enhanced quality of life and decreased stress symptoms in women with breast cancer (Carlson, Speca, Patel, & Goodey, 2004). For more information, go to http://www.stjohn.org/innerpage.aspx?PageID=1779, http://www.mindfulnessmeditationcentre.org/breathingGathas.htm, or http://www.meditationcenter.com

4. *Yoga* practiced for 1 hour a week reduces perceived stress in women diagnosed with breast cancer, as measured by the Hospital Anxiety and Depression Scale (HADS) and Perceived Stress Scale (PSS). Compared to control groups in two studies, among women not receiving chemo-

therapy, yoga appeared to enhance emotional well-being and mood and might have served to buffer deterioration in both overall and specific domains of quality of life (Banerjee et al., 2007; Moadel et al., 2007). **Cautions:** Go to http://yoga.lifetips.com/cat/56770/yoga-cautions/

Supplements

Supplement evidence-based practice for breast cancer includes teaching clients about:

1. *Coenzyme Q10/riboflavin/niacin.* Coenzyme Q10/riboflavin/niacin, in combination (100 mg/10 mg/ 50 mg daily), suggests a good prognosis and a significant reduction in cytokine levels, and it might even offer protection from metastases and recurrence of cancer (Premkumar, Yuvaraj, Vijayasarathy, Gangadaran, & Sachdanandam, 2007). **Cautions:** Until more research is available, these supplements should not be used by pregnant or lactating women or by those with hypersensitivity to the combination. CoQ10 can interact with anticoagulants, antidiabetes agents, beta-blockers, HMG-CoA reductase inhibitors, phenothiazines, tricyclic antidepressants, or l-carnitine. Clients should avoid use of coenzyme Q10 with phenothiazines, tricyclics, beta-blockers, and cholesterol-lowering agents (Skidmore-Roth, 2006a).

2. *Grape seed extract (GSPE).* Grape seed extract taken at 150–300 mg/day for 21 days, then 50–80 mg/day maintenance, inhibits the growth of breast cancer cells (Agarwall, Sharma, Zhao, & Agarwall, 2000). **Cautions:** Grape seed extract should not be used during pregnancy or lactation or given to children. Assess clients for hepatoxicity; also assess the client's use of anticoagulants and antiplatelets, which could increase the risk of bleeding if taken concurrently.

3. *Maitake extract.* This mushroom exerts an antitumor effect by enhancing the immune system through activation of macrophages and may have the potential to decrease the size of breast tumors (Kodama, Komuta, & Nanba, 2003).

4. *Milk thistle (silymarin).* Milk thistle exerts anticarcinogenic effects, including inhibition of cancer cell growth in human breast cells. The herb protects liver and kidney from toxic effects of drugs, including chemotherapy. **Cautions:** Milk thistle is considered safe and is well tolerated with gastrointestinal upset, a mild laxative effect, and rare allergic reactions being the only adverse events reported when taken in the recommended dose range of 200–400 mg tincture PO, t.i.d. (Post-White, Ladas, & Kelly, 2007).

5. *Pycnogenol.* An extract from the bark of pine trees, pycnogenol selectively induces death in human mammary cancer cells (MCF-7) but not

in normal human mammary tissue (MCF-10) at a dosage of 100 mg/day (Huynh & Teel, 2000).

6. *Selenium* has been associated with decreased risk of cancer at a dose of 300 micrograms/day only (Rayn-Haren et al., 2007). **Other considerations:** Selenium-enriched yeast and selenium-enriched milk are also available. For information on food sources of selenium, go to http://ods.od.nih.gov/factsheets/selenium.asp.

7. *Vitamins A, B, C, D, and E.* Vitamins A, B, C, D, and E can confer protection against breast cancer among women who have low intake of these vitamins (Dorjgochoo et al., 2007). Routes/dosages/frequency: PO daily intake of 10,000 IU vitamin A, 1 B-50 capsule, up to 10 grams of vitamin C, and between 400 and 600 IU of vitamins D and E. **Other considerations:** Women who eat a combined amount of 8–10 servings (half cup) a day of fresh fruits (especially citrus and berries), vegetables (especially leafy greens), legumes (dried beans and peas), and whole grain cereals may be receiving sufficient levels of vitamins necessary to provide protection.

Touch

Touch evidence-based practice for breast cancer includes:

1. *Acupressure.* Acupressure can relieve nausea, vomiting, and retching associated with chemotherapy (Dribble et al., 2007). For information on using acupressure, go to http://www.eclecticenergies.com/acupressure/howto.php

2. *Massage therapy.* Women diagnosed with breast cancer reported being less depressed and angry and having more vigor after receiving 30-minute sessions 3 times per week for 5 weeks of massage therapy. Urine tests showed increased dopamine levels, natural killer cells, and lymphocytes as well (Hernandez-Reif et al., 2005). Aromatherapy massage has been shown to reduce anxiety in women with breast cancer (Imanishi et al., 2009). For massage techniques, to to http://www.wikihow.com/Give-a-Foot-Massage

3. *Foot reflexology.* Foot reflexology significantly reduced nausea, vomiting, and fatigue in women with breast cancer undergoing chemotherapy and significantly improved life satisfaction, the most important predictor of survival for women with advanced cancer (Fox Chase Cancer Center, 2007; Yang, 2005). Self-foot reflexology also enhances natural killer cells and IgG, strengthening the immune system against cancer and possibly preventing tumor development. For more on foot reflexology, go to http://www.how-to-do-reflexology.com/foot reflexology.html

BREAST CANCER CASE STUDY www

Marie Anderson, a breast cancer survivor, age 55, was diagnosed with stage 2 breast cancer 1 year ago, and has just completed treatment of a lumpectomy followed by chemotherapy and radiation. Since her treatments, she has been experiencing some distressing physical symptoms. She has been an active woman who has worked as a nurse, but now has problems with her job because she has been experiencing fatigue, depression, and anorexia. She would like to avoid taking medications related to these symptoms because they may interfere with current medications. She is very interested in complementary and alternative therapies to help with the fatigue.

HEALTH PROMOTION CHALLENGE www

Read the breast cancer case study and then go to PubMed (http://www.ncbi .nlm.nih.gov/pubmed/), type "complementary alternative therapies for breast cancer fatigue" in the Search box at the top of the page, and click on the Search button. Choose three relevant abstracts and tell how the findings can help you teach a client such as Ms. Anderson about the use of complementary and alternative therapies.

This case study and health promotion challenge were written by Cecile A. Lengacher RN, PhD, Professor and Director of the BS-PhD Program, University of South Florida, College of Nursing Tampa, Florida.

REFERENCES

Agarwall, C., Sharma, Y., Zhao, J, & Agarwall, R. (2000). A polyphenolic fraction from grape seeds causes irreversible growth inhibition of breast carcinoma MDA-MB468 cells by inhibiting mitogen-activated protein kinases activation and inducing G1 arrest and differentiation. *Clinical Cancer Research, 6,* 2921–2930.

AMAS test measures lethal replikin gene activity in lung and other cancers. (2007). Retrieved from http://www.reuters.com/article/pressRelease/idUS248597+06-Dec-2007+PRN20071206

American Association for Cancer Research. (2007). Green tea boosts production of detox enzymes, rendering cancerous chemicals harmless. Retrieved from http://www.science-daily.com/releases/2007/08/070810194923.htm

American Association for Cancer Research (2008, March 6). High levels of estrogen associated with breast cancer recurrence. *ScienceDaily.* Retrieved from http://www.sciencedaily .com/releases/2008/03/080306075218.htm

Anand, P., Kunnumakkara, A. B., Newman, R. A., & Aggarwal, B. B. (2007). Bioavailability of curcumin: Problems and promises. *Molecular Pharmacology, 4*(6), 807–818.

Autoimmunity Research Foundation. (2008, January 27). Vitamin D deficiency study raises new questions about disease and supplements. *ScienceDaily*. Retrieved from http://www.sciencedaily.com/releases/2008/01/080125223302.htm

Banerjee, B., Vadiraj, H. S., Ram, A., Rao, R., Jayapal, M., Gopinath, K. S., . . . Prakash Hande, M. (2007). Effects of an integrated yoga program in modulating psychological stress and radiation-induced genotoxic stress in breast cancer patients undergoing radiotherapy. *Integrative Cancer Therapies, 6*(3), 242–250.

Bokemeyer, C., Fells, L. M., & Dunn, T. (1996). Silibinin protects against cisplatin-induced nephrotoxicity without compromising cisplatin on ifosfamide anti-tumor activity. *British Journal of Cancer, 74*, 2036–2041.

Breast fluid a better option for detecting cancer. (2003, July 9). Retrieved from http://www.medicalnewstoday.com/articles/3920.php

Brenner, D., & Hall, E. J. (2007). Computed tomography, an increasing source radiation exposure. *New England Journal of Medicine, 357*(22), 2277–2284.

Carlson, L. E., Speca, M., Patel, K. D., & Goodey, E. (2004). Mindfulness-based stress reduction in relation to quality of life, mood, symptoms of stress and levels of cortisol, dehydroepiandrosterone sulfate (DHEAS) and melatonin in breast and prostate cancer outpatients. *Psychoneuroendocrinology, 29*(4), 448–474.

Chen, J., Saggar J. K., Corey, P., & Thompson, L. U. (2009). Flaxseed and pure secoisolariciresinol diglucoside, but not flaxseed hull, reduce human breast tumor growth (MCF-7) in athymic mice. *Journal of Nutrition, 139*(11), 2061–2066.

Cheung, S., & Tai, J. (2007). Anti-proliferative and antioxidant properties of rosemary. *Oncology Reports, 17*(6), 1525–1531.

Cheung, C. W., Gibbons, N., Johnson, D. W., & Nicol, D. L. (2010). Silibinin—a promising new treatment for cancer. *Anticancer Agents in Medicinal Chemistry, 10*(3), 186–195.

Corona-Rivera, A., Urbina-Cano, P., Bobadilla-Moralies, L., Vargas-Lares, J., Ramirez-Herrera, M. A., Mendoza-Magaua, M. L. . . . Corona-Rivera, J. R. (2007). Protective in vivo effect of curcumin on copper genotoxicity evaluated by comet and micronucleus assays. *Journal of Applied Genetics, 48*(4), 389–396.

Creton, S. K., Zhu, H., & Gooderham, N. J. (2007). The cooked meat carcinogen 2-amino-1-methyl-t-phenylimidazo[4-5-b]pyridine activates the extracellular signal regulared kinase mitogen-activated protein kinase pathway. *Cancer Research, 67*(23), 11455–11462.

Deng, Y., & Chen, H. F. (2009). Effects of Astragalus injection and its ingredients on proliferation and Akt phosphorylation of breast cancer cell lines. *Zhong Xi Yi Jic He Xue Bao, 7*(12), 1174–1180.

Do, M. H., Lee, S. S., Kim, J. Y., Jung, P. H., & Lee, M. H. (2007). Fruits, vegetables, soy foods and breast cancer in pre- and postmenopausal Koren women: A case-control study. *International Journal of Vitamin and Nutrition Research, 77*(2), 130–141.

Dong, S., Inoue, A., Zhu, Y., Tanji, M., & Kiyama, R. (2007). Activation of rapid signaling pathways and the subsequent transcriptional regulation for the proliferation of breast cancer. *Food and Chemical Toxicology, 45*(12), 2470–2478.

Dorjgochoo, T., Shrubsole, M. J., Shu, X. O., Lu, W., Ruan, Z., Zheng, Y., . . . Zheng, W. (2007). Vitamin supplement use and risk for breast cancer: The Shanghai Breast Cancer Study. *Breast Cancer Research and Treatment, 111*(2), 269–278.

Dribble, S. L., Luce, J., Cooper, B. A., Israel, J., Cohen, M., Nussey, B., & Rugo, H. (2007). Acupressure for chemotherapy-induced nausea and vomiting: A randomized clinical trial. *Oncology Nursing Forum, 34*(4), 813–820.

Espie, C. A., Fleming, L., Cassidy, J., Samuel, L., Taylor, L. M., White, C. A., . . . Paul, J. (2008). Randomized controlled clinical effectiveness trial of cognitive behavior therapy compared with treatment as usual for persistent insomnia in patients with cancer. *Journal of Clinical Oncology, 26*(28), 4651–4658.

Fields, A. L., Soprano, D. R., & Soprano, K. J. (2007). Retinoids in biological control and cancer. *Journal of Cell Biochemistry, 10*(4), 886–898.

Fox Chase Cancer Center. (2007, November 1). Quality of life is the most important predictor of survival for advanced cancer patients. *ScienceDaily*. Retrieved from http://www.sciencedaily.com/releases/2007/10/071030170208.htm

Friedenreich, C. M., Woolcott, C. G., McTiernan, A., Ballard-Barbash, R., Brant, R. F., Stanczyk, F. Z., . . . Courneya, K. S. (2010) Alberta physical activity and breast cancer prevention trial: Sex hormone changes in a year-long exercise intervention among postmenopausal women. *Journal of Clinical Oncology, 28*(9), 1458–1466.

Georgetown University Medical Center. (2008, April 9). Eating soy foods in puberty protects against breast cancer, evidence now suggests. *ScienceDaily*. Retrieved from http://www.sciencedaily.com/releases/2008/04/080409091727.htm

Goldsmith, R. E., Jandorf, L., Valdimarsdottir, H., Amend, K. L., Stoudt, B. G., Rini, C. et al. (2010). Traumatic stress symptoms and breast cancer: the role of childhood abuse. *Child Abuse and Neglect, 34*(6), 465–470.

Hardell, L., & Sage, C. (2007). Biological effects from electromagnetic field exposure and public exposure standards. *Biomedicine & Pharmacotherapy, 62*(2), 104–109.

Hernandez-Reif, M., Field, T., Ironson, G., Beutler, J., Vera, Y., Hurley, J., . . . Fraser, M. (2005). Natural killer cells and lymphocytes increase in women with breast cancer following massage therapy. *International Journal of Neuroscience, 115*, 495–510.

Hidderley, M., & Holt, M. (2004). A pilot randomized trial assessing the effects of autogenic training in early stage cancer patients in relation to psychological status and immune response. *European Journal of Oncology Nursing, 8*(1), 61–65.

Huynh, H. T., & Teel, R. W. (2000). Selective induction of apoptosis in human mammary cancer cells (MCF-7) by pycnogenol. *Anticancer Research, 20*(4), 2417–2420.

Imanishi, J., Kuriyama, H., Shigemori, I., Watanabe, S., Aihara, Y., Kita, M., . . . Fukui, K. (2009). Anxiolytic effect of aromatherapy massage in patients with breast cancer. *Evidence-Based Complementary and Alternative Medicine, 6* (1), 123–128.

International Agency for Research on Cancer. (1997). *IARC monographs on the evaluation of carcinogenic risks to humans. Volume 69: Polychlorinated dibenzodioxins and polychlorinated dibenzofurans.* Lyon, France: IARC.

Jo, E. H., Kim, S. H., Ra, J. C., Kim, S. R., Cho, S. D., Jung, J. W., . . . Kang, K. S. (2005). Chemopreventive properties of the ethanol extract of Chinese licorice (*Glycyrrhiza uralensis*) root: Induction of apoptosis and GI cell cycle arrest in MCF-7 human breast cancer cells. *Cancer Letters, 230*(2), 239–247.

Keele University. (2007, September 2). Aluminum in breast tissue: A possible factor in the cause of breast cancer. *ScienceDaily*. Retrieved from http://www.sciencedaily.com/releases/2007/08/070831210302.htm

Kim, S. R., Park, H. J., Bae, Y. H., Ahn, S. C., Wee, H. J., . . . Bae, S. K. (2012). Curcumin down-regulates visfatin expression and inhibits breast cancer cell invasion. *Endocrinology, 153*(2), 554–563.

Kodama, N., Komuta, K., & Nanba, H. (2003). Effect of maitake (*Grifola frondosa*) D-Fraction on the activation of NK cells in patients. *Journal of Medicinal Food, 6*(4), 371–377.

Linos, E., & Willett, W. C. (2007). Diet and breast cancer risk reduction. *Journal of National Comprehensive Cancer Network, 5*(8), 711–718.

Liu, R. H., Liu, J., & Chen, B. (2005). Apples prevent mammary tumors in rats. *Journal of Agricultural and Food Chemistry, 53*(6), 2341–2343.

Ma, H., Hill, C. K., Bernstein, L., & Ursin, G. (2007). Low-dose medical radiation exposure and breast cancer risk in women under age 50 years overall and by estrogen and progesterone receptor status: Results from a case-control and case-case comparison. *Breast Cancer Research, 109*(1), 77–90.

Matar, C., & Perdigon, G. (2007). The application of probiotics in cancer. *British Journal of Nutrition, 98*(Suppl. 1), S105–S110.

Mitrou, P. N., Kipnis, V., Thiebaut, A. C., Reedy, J., Subar, A. F., Wirfalt, E., . . . Schatzkin, A. (2007). Mediterranean dietary pattern and prediction of all-cause mortality in a US population: Results from the NIH-AARP Diet and Health Study. *Archives of Internal Medicine, 167*(22), 2461–2468.

Moadel, A. B., Shah, C., Wylie-Rosett, J., Harris, M. S., Patel, S. R., Hall, C. B., & Sparano, J. A. (2007). Randomized controlled trial of yoga among a multiethnic sample of breast cancer patients: Effects on quality of life. *Journal of Clinical Oncology, 25*(28), 4387–4395.

Montgomery, L. L., Tran, K. N., Heelan, M. C., Van Zee, K. J., Massie, M. J., Payne, D. K., & Borgen, P. I. (1999). Issues of regret in women with contralateral prophylactic mastectomies. *Journal of Surgical Oncology, 6*(6), 546–552.

Nagasawa, H., Watanabe, K., Yoshida, M., & Inatomi, H. (2001). Effects of gold banded lily (*Lillium auratum Lindl*) or Chinese milk vetch (*Astragalus sinicus L*) on spontaneous mammary tumourigenesis in SHN mice. *Anticancer Research, 21*(4A), 2323–2328.

Pari, L., Tewas, D., & Eckel. J. Role of curcumin in health and disease. *Archives of Physiological Biochemistry, 114*(2), 127–149.

Post-White, J., Ladas, E. J., Kelly, K. M. (2007). Advances in the use of milk thistle. *Integrative Cancer Therapies, 6*(2), 104–109.

Premkumar, V. G., Yuvaraj, S., Vijayasarathy, K., Gangadaran, S. G., & Sachdanandam, P. (2007). Serum cytokine levels of interleukin-1beta, -6,-8, a tumour necrosis factor-alpha and vascular endothelial growth factor in breast cancer patients treated with tamoxifen and supplemented with co-enzyme Q(10), riboflavin, and niacin. *Basic Clinical Pharmacology Toxicology, 100*(6), 387–391.

Rayn-Haren, G., Bugel, S., Krath, B. N., Hoac, R., Stagsted, J., Jorgensen, K., . . . Dragsted, L. O. (2007). A short-term intervention trial with selenate, selenium-enriched yeast and selenium-enriched milk: Effects on oxidative defence regulation. *British Journal of Nutrition, 21*, 1–10.

Seeram, N. P., Adams, L. S., Zhang, Y., Lee, R., Sand, D., Scheuller, H. S., & Heber, D. (2006). Blackberry, black raspberry, blueberry, cranberry, red raspberry, and strawberry extract inhibit growth and stimulate apoptosis of human cancer cells in vitro. *Journal of Agricultural and Food Chemistry, 54*(25), 9329–9339.

Skidmore-Roth, L. (2006a). Coenzyme Q10. In *Mosby's handbook of herbs & natural supplements* (pp. 315–319). St. Louis, MO: ElsevierMosby.

Skidmore-Roth, L. (2006b). Flax. In *Mosby's handbook of herbs & natural supplements* (pp. 450–454). St. Louis, MO: ElsevierMosby.

Skidmore-Roth, L. (2006c). Green tea. In *Mosby's handbook of herbs & natural supplements* (pp. 535–539). St. Louis, MO: ElsevierMosby.

Skidmore-Roth, L. (2006d). Turmeric. In *Mosby's handbook of herbs & natural supplements* (pp. 974–977). St. Louis, MO: ElsevierMosby.

Skidmore-Roth, L. (2006e). Licorice. In *Mosby's handbook of herbs & natural supplements* (pp. 659–665). St. Louis, MO: ElsevierMosby.

Snedeker, S. M. (2006). Chemical exposures in the workplace: Effect on breast cancer risk among women. *American Association of Occupational Health Nursing Journal, 54*(6), 270–279.

Stanton, A. L., Danoff-Burg, S., Sworowski, L. A., Collins, C. A., Branstetter, A. D., Rodri-
guez-Hanley, A., . . . Austenfeld, J. L. (2002). Randomized, controlled trial of written
emotional expression and benefit finding in breast cancer patients. *Journal of Clinical
Oncology, 20*(20), 4160–4168.

Stein, M. B., & Barrett-Connor, E. (2000). Sexual assault and physical health: Findings from
a population-based study of older adults. *Psychosomatic Medicine, 62*(6), 838–843.

Taylor, E. F., Burley, V. J., & Cade, J. E. (2007). Meat consumption and risk of breast cancer
in the UK Women's Cohort Study. *British Journal of Cancer, 96*(7), 1139–1146.

Technical University of Denmark. (2008). A little rosemary can go a long way to reducing acrylamide in food. *ScienceDaily*. Retrieved from http://www.sciencedaily.com
/releases/2008/02/080229142817.htm

Teitelbaum, S. L, Gammon, M. D., Britton, J. A., Neugut, A. I., Levin, B., & Stellman, S. D.
(2007). Reported residential pesticide use and breast cancer risk on Long Island, New
York. *American Journal of Epidemiology, 165*(6), 643–651.

University of Alberta. (2007, June 19). Simple steps make breast cancer survivors eager
to exercise, study shows. *ScienceDaily*. Retrieved from http://www.sciencedaily.com
/releases/2007/06/070613120937.htm

University of Pittsburgh School of the Health Sciences. (2007, November 9). Extracts of
catfish caught in polluted waters cause breast cancer cells to multiply. *ScienceDaily*.
Retrieved from http://www.sciencedaily.com/releases/2007/11/071107083910.htm

Wang, L., Chen, J., & Thompson, L. U. (2005). The inhibitory effect of flaxseed on the growth
and metastasis of estrogen receptor negative human breast cancer xenografts is attributed to both its lignan and oil components. *International Journal of Cancer, 116*(5),
793–798.

Warner, M. B., Eskenazi, B., Mocarelli, P., Gerthoux, P. M., Samuels, S., & Needham, L.
(2002). Serum dioxin concentrations and breast cancer risk in the Seveso Women's
Health Study. *Environmental Health Perspectives, 110*, 625–628.

World Health Organization. (2007). *Dioxins and their effects on human health*. Retrieved
from http://www.who.int/mediacentre/factsheets/fs225/en/print.html

World Health Organization. (2011). Electromagnetic fields and public health: Mobile phones.
Retrieved from http://www.who.int/mediacentre/factsheets/fs193/en/

Wu, A. H., Yu, M. C., Tseng, C. C., & Pike, M. C. (2008). Epidemiology of soy exposures and
breast cancer risk. *British Journal of Cancer, 98*(1), 9–14.

Xiao, J. X., Huang, G. Q., & Zhang, S. H. (2007). Soyasaponins inhibit the proliferation of
hela cells by inducing apoptosis. *Experimental Toxicology and Pathology, 59*(1), 35–42.

Yang, J. H. (2005). The effects of foot reflexology on nausea, vomiting and fatigue of breast
cancer patients undergoing chemotherapy. *Taehan Kanho Hakkoe, Chi 35*(1), 177–185.

Ye, L., Gho, W. M., Chan, F. L., Chen, S., & Leung, L. K. (2009). Dietary administration of
the licorice flavonoid isoliquiritigenin deters the growth of MCF-7 cells overexpressing
aromatase. *International Journal of Cancer, 124*(5), 1028–1036.

Zhang, S. M., Lee, I. M., Manson, J. E., Cook, N. R., Willett, W. C. & Buring, J. E. (2007).
Alcohol consumption and breast cancer risk in the Women's Health Study. *American
Journal of Epidemiology, 165*(6), 667–676.

Cervical Cancer

Environment

Environmental evidence-based practice for cervical cancer includes oral contraceptive use and smoking cessation.

1. *Oral contraception.* Use of oral contraceptives is linked to an increase in cervical cancer. The relative risk for cancer rises with increasing duration of oral contraceptive use; alternative methods may be prudent (Appleby et al., 2007).
2. *Smoking cessation.* Smoking is associated with an increased risk for cervical cancer (Tseng, Lin, Martin, Chen & Partridge, 2010).

Exercise

Evidence-based exercise/movement approaches for cervical cancer include yoga.

Yoga can reduce stress, improve activities of daily living, and enhance quality of life (Ulger & Yagli, 2010).

Herbs/Essential Oils

Herb evidence-based practice for cervical cancer includes using cactus pear and milk thistle.

1. *Cactus pear.* Arizona cactus fruit solution, the aqueous extract of cactus pear, inhibited cell growth in cervical epithelial cells, suppressed tumor growth in nude mice, and modulated expression of tumor-related genes. **Other considerations:** Effects of cactus pear were comparable with those caused by a synthetic retinoid currently used in chemoprevention trials (Zou et al., 2005).
2. *Milk thistle (silymarin, silibinin, or silybin).* Milk thistle at 200 to 400 mg a day inhibits cancer cell growth in human cervical cells. Preliminary evidence suggests that silybin may enhance the tumor-fighting effects of cisplatin and doxorubicin (Garcia-Maceira & Mateo, 2009; Post-White, Ladas, & Kelly, 2007).

Mind-Set

Mind-set evidence-based practice for cervical cancer includes cognitive behavioral group sessions.

Cognitive behavioral group sessions can reduce stress and may provide cancer preventive action (Antoni et al., 2008).

Nutrition

Nutrition evidence-based practice for cervical cancer includes the following:

1. *Cruciferous vegetables*. Consumption of these vegetables suppressed the proliferation of cervical tumor cells in initial clinical trials (Aggarwall & Ichikawa, 2005). Advise clients to eat half to 1 cup of one or more of the following vegetables: cabbage, radishes, cauliflower, broccoli, Brussels sprouts, and/or daikon. Except for daikon and radishes, which are eaten raw, cauliflower and broccoli florets and small heads of cabbage should be quartered and gently steamed for no more than 5 minutes to release the cancer-protective substances (Vallejo, Tomas-Barberan, & Garcia-Viguera, 2003).

2. *Folate*. Women with human papilloma viruses may reduce their risk of cervical cancer by increasing their intake of folate. Because national surveys revealed most people did not consume adequate folate, a grain fortification program is in place (Piyathilake, Macaluso, Brill, Heimburger & Partridge, 2007). Food sources of folate: Leafy green vegetables (like spinach and turnip greens), fruits (citrus fruits and juices), and dried beans and peas are all natural sources of folate that can help meet the suggested amount of 1,000 micrograms a day. Clients on diets who do not eat breads, cereals, or pasta; and who abuse alcohol; or take medications that interfere with folate absorption may not receive sufficient amounts of the nutrient and may need additional amounts. **Cautions:** Medications and medical conditions that increase the need for folate or result in an increased excretion of folate include anticonvulsant medications, metformin, sulfasalazine, triamterene, methotrexate, barbiturates, pregnancy and lactation, alcohol abuse, malabsorption, kidney dialysis, liver disease, and certain anemias. Because folate is a water-soluble B-vitamin, unneeded amounts will be eliminated in the urine. Instruct clients to avoid fortified foods as a source of folic acid; new research has shown the introduction of flour fortified with folic acid into common foods has been linked to colon cancer. **Other considerations:** Exceeding 1,000 micrograms per day of folate may trigger vitamin B_{12} deficiency (Blackwell Publishing, Ltd. 2007). To compensate, clients can take a multivitamin that contains B_{12} or eat at least one food daily that contains B_{12}, such as nutritional yeast (unless susceptible to *Candida*), clams, eggs, herring, kidney, liver, mackerel, seafood, milk, or dairy products.

3. *Selenium*. Selenium intake has been associated with a decreased risk of cancer (Ravn-Haren et al., 2008. Garlic and onions and members of the brassica family (broccoli, cauliflower, cabbage, Brussels sprouts, and kohlabri) are able to extract selenium from the soil, providing selenium-containing phytochemicals that show anticarcinogenic potentials.

Cautions: Most soils worldwide are deficient in this mineral. Counsel clients to eat as many of these foods as possible from selenium-rich soils, such as organic sources (Irion, 1999). Selenium can be toxic when taken as a supplement instead of in food. Avoid selenium marked "sodium selenite." Selenium labelled "l-selenomethionine" is less likely to cause side effects and will not react with vitamin C to block selenium absorption. Consult a physician before taking doses over 100 micrograms. Other food sources of selenium include shellfish, Brazil nuts, vegetables, eggs, brewer's yeast, broccoli, brown rice, chicken, dairy products, liver, molasses, salmon, tuna, vegetables, wheat germ, and whole grains. No harm has been reported from obtaining selenium via food.

4. *Soy.* Soyasaponins have been shown to inhibit the proliferation of cancer cells. **Cautions:** Nonfermented forms of soy foods may reduce assimilation of calcium, magnesium, copper, iron, and zinc due to their high levels of phytic acid (Xiao, Huang & Zhang, 2007). The best sources are organic fermented soy products are tempeh and miso.

5. *Other vegetables.* Results from previous studies have suggested that higher dietary consumption and circulating levels of certain micronutrients, such as vitamin A and carotenoids, may be protective against cervical cancer, as may watercress. Other vegetables that may be helpful include pumpkin, squash, cantaloupe, spinach, sweet potatoes, apricots, kale, broccoli, mangoes, cooked greens, sweet red peppers, turnip greens, and carrots (Hwang, Lee, Kim & Kim, 2010).

6. *Vitamin-rich foods* that contain vitamin A, B_{12}, D, and E have been shown to protect against cervical cancer. Vitamin A is available in animal livers, fish liver oils, apricot, asparagus, beet greens, broccoli, cantaloupe, carrots, collards, dandelion greens, garlic, kale, mustard greens, papayas, peaches, pumpkin, red peppers, spinach, sweet potatoes, Swiss chard, turnip greens, watercress, and yellow squash. Vitamin B_{12} is available in clams, eggs, herring, kidney, liver, mackerel, milk and dairy products, seafood, soybeans and soy products, and sea vegetables (dulse, kelp, kombu, and nori). Vitamin E is found in green, leafy vegetables, legumes (peanuts, dried beans, and peas), seeds (e.g., sunflower and pumpkin), whole grains, brown rice, cornmeal, eggs, soybeans, sweet potatoes, watercress, wheat, and wheat germ. Most vegetables, except spinach, should be cut and lightly steamed to obtain the most nutrients (Friedrich et al., 2002; Lwanbunjan, Saengkar, Cheeramakara, Tangjitgamol & Chitcharoenrung, 2006; Shannon et al., 2002; Siegel, 2007).

Stress Management

Stress management evidence-based practice for cervical cancer includes mindfulness-based stress reduction.

A weak immune system is one of the major factors that promotes cancer metastases after an operation, chemotherapy, or radiation therapy. Fear and stress weaken the immune system. Adequate stress management prior to and after medical treatment may help to prevent metastases (Tel Aviv University, 2008). Women with an abnormal pap smear participated in a stress reduction mindfulness-based stress reduction (MBSR) program for 2 hours a week over 6 consecutive weeks; it was evaluated very positively by participants, and there was a significant reduction in anxiety (Abercrombie, Zamora, & Korn, 2007). **Other considerations:** Websites that may be useful are http://www.mindfulnessmeditationcentre.org/breathingGathas.htm and http://www.meditationcenter.com

Supplements

Supplement evidence-based practice for cervical cancer includes cactus pear and mistletoe.

1. *Cactus pear.* Cactus pear inhibits growth of cervical cancer cells in cultured cells and in an animal model and modulates the expression of tumor-related genes; this is likely because it contains numerous antioxidants (Tesoriere, 2004). **Other considerations:** Cactus pear fruit can also be eaten; it is found in the produce section of grocery stores. Cactus pear effects are comparable with those caused by a synthetic retinoid currently used in chemoprevention trials (Zou, 2005).

2. *Mistletoe.* Mistletoe lengthens the survival time of women with cervical cancer and increases psychosomatic self-regulation more markedly than does conventional therapy alone (Grossarth-Maticek & Ziegler, 2006). **Cautions:** Because mistletoe is a uterine stimulant, it should not be used during pregnancy. Mistletoe should not be used by women who are hypersensitive to it, are lactating, or have progressive infections. Mistletoe is a toxic plant and should be kept out of reach of children. Possible adverse reactions include change in blood pressure and cardiac arrest, nausea, vomiting, anorexia, diarrhea, gastritis, and hepatitis. This supplement can also be used to reduce cancer-related fatigue (Sood, Barton, Bauer, & Loprinzi, 2007).

Touch

Touch evidence-based practice that may be helpful for cervical cancer includes foot reflexology and massage.

1. *Foot reflexology.* Foot reflexology has been shown to significantly reduce anxiety (Quattrin et al., 2006), nausea, vomiting, and fatigue of breast cancer patients undergoing chemotherapy (Jang, 2005).

2. *Massage.* Massage has been shown to help manage anxiety and depression in clients with cancer in a multicenter, randomized controlled trial (Wilkinson et al., 2007).

CERVICAL CANCER CASE STUDY

Ms. Miranda James, age 45, was just diagnosed with cervical cancer. She is terrified about what will happen to her; she is not sleeping and is depressed.

HEALTH PROMOTION CHALLENGE

Of all the interventions discussed for cervical cancer, which one do you think might be most helpful to Ms. James? What do you need to know or learn to use that intervention?

REFERENCES

Abercrombie, P. D., Zamora, A., & Korn, A. P. (2007). Lessons learned: Providing mindfulness-based stress reduction program for low-income multiethnic women with abnormal pap smears. *Holistic Nursing Practitioner, 21*(1), 26–34.

Aggarwall, B. B., & Ichikawa, H. (2005). Molecular targets and anticancer potential of indole-4-carbinol and its derivatives. *Cell Cycle, 4*(9), 1201–1215.

Antoni, M. H., Lechner, S. C., Kazi, A., Wimberly, S. R., Sifre. T., Urcuya. K. R. . . . Carver, C. S. (2006). How stress management improves quality of life after treatment for breast cancer. *Journal of Consulting and Clinical Psychology, 74*(6). 1143–1152.

Appleby, P., Beral, V., Berrington de Gonzalez, A., Colin, D., Franceschi, S., Goodhill, A., . . . Sweetland, S. (2007). Cervical cancer and hormonal contraceptives: Collaborative reanalysis of individual data for 16,573 women with cervical cancer and 35,509 women without cervical cancer from 24 epidemiological studies. *Lancet, 370*(9599), 1591–1592.

Blackwell Publishing Ltd. (2007, November 5). Folic acid linked to increased cancer rate, historical review suggests. *ScienceDaily*. Retrieved from http://www.sciencedaily.com/releases/2007/11/071102111956.htm

Friedrich, M., Villena-Heinsen, C., Axt-Fliedner, R., Meyberg, R., Tilgen, W., Schmidt, W. & Reichrath, J. (2002). Analysis of 25-hydroxyvitamin D3-1alpha-hydroxylase in cervical tissue. *Anticancer Research, 22*(1A), 183–186.

García-Maceira, P., & Mateo, J. (2009). Silibinin inhibits hypoxia-inducible factor-1alpha and mTOR/p70S6K/4E-BP1 signalling pathway in human cervical and hepatoma cancer cells: Implications for anticancer therapy. *Oncogene, 28*(3), 313–324.

Grossarth-Maticek, R., & Ziegler, R. (2006). Prospective controlled cohort studies on long-term therapy of cervical cancer patients with a mistletoe preparation. *Forschende Komplementärmedizin, 14*(3), 140–147.

Hwang, J. H., Lee, J. K., Kim, T. J., & Kim, M. K. (2010). The association between fruit and vegetable consumption and HPV viral load in high-risk HPV-positive women with cervical intraepithelial neoplasia. *Cancer Causes Control, 21*(1), 51–59.

Irion, C. W. (1999). Growing alliums and brassicas in selenium-enriched soils increases their anti-carcinogenic potentials. *Medical Hypotheses, 53*(3), 232–235.

Jang, J. H. (2005). The effects of foot reflexology on nausea, vomiting and fatigue of breast cancer patients undergoing chemotherapy. *Taehan Kanho Hakhoe Chi, 35*(1), 177–185.

Lwanbunjan, K., Saengkar, P., Cheeramakara, C., Tangjitgamol, S., & Chitcharoenrung, K. (2006). Vitamin B12 status of Thai women with neoplasia of the cervix uteri. *Southeast Asian Journal of Tropical Medicine and Public Health, 37*(Suppl 3), 178–183.

Piyathilake, C. J., Macaluso, M., Brill, I., Heimburger, D. C., & Partridge, E. E. (2007). Lower red blood cell folate enhances the HPV-16-associated risk of cervical intraepithelial neoplasia. *Nutrition, 23*(3), 203–210.

Post-White, J., Ladas, E. J., & Kelly, K. M. (2007). Advances in the use of milk thistle (*Silybum marianum*). *Integrative Cancer Therapy, 6*(2), 104–109.

Quattrin, R., Zanini, A., Buchini, S., Turello, D., Annunziata, M. A., Vidotti, C., . . . Brusaferro, S. (2006). Use of reflexology foot massage to reduce anxiety in hospitalized cancer patients in chemotherapy treatment: Methodology and outcomes. *Journal of Nursing Management, 14*(2), 96–105.

Ravn-Haren, G., Bugel, S., Krath, B. N., Hoac, T., Stagsted, J., Jorgensen, K., . . . Dragsted, L. O. (2008). A short-term intervention trial with selenate, selenium-enriched yeast and selenium-enriched milk: Effects on oxidative defense regulation. *British Journal of Nutrition, 99*(4), 883–892.

Shannon, J., Thomas, D. B., Ray, R. M., Kestin, M., Koetsawang, A., Koetsawang, S., . . . Kuypers, J. (2002). Dietary risk factors for invasive and in-situ cervical carcinomas in Bangkok, Thailand. *Cancer Causes and Control, 13*(8), 691–699.

Siegel, E. M., Craft, N. E., Duarte-Franco, E., Villa L. L., Franco, E. L. & Giuliano, A. R. (2007). Associations between serum carotenoids and tocopherols and type-specific HPV persistence: The Ludwig-McGill cohort study. *International Journal of Cancer, 120*(3), 672–680.

Sood, A., Barton, D. L., Bauer, B. A., & Loprinzi, C. I. (2007). A critical review of complementary therapies for cancer-related fatigue. *Integrative Cancer Therapies, 6*(1), 8–13.

Tel Aviv University. (2008, February 29). Stress and fear can affect cancer's recurrence. *Science-Daily*. Retrieved from http://www.sciencedaily.com/releases/2008/02/080227142656.htm

Tesoriere, L. (2004). Supplementation with cactus pear fruit decreases oxidative stress in healthy humans: A comparative study with vitamin C. *Journal of Clinical Nutrition, 80*(2), 391–395.

Tseng, T. S., Lin, H. Y., Martin, M. Y., Chen, T., & Partridge, E. E. (2010). Disparities in smoking and cessation status among cancer survivors and non-cancer individuals: A population-based study from National Health and Nutrition Examination Survey. *Journal of Cancer Survivorship, 4*(4):313–321

Vallejo, F., Tomas-Barberan, F. A., & Garcia-Viguera, C. (2003). Phenolic compounds content in edible parts of broccoli inflorescences after domestic cooking. *Journal of Science and Food Agriculture, 83*(14), 1151–1156.

Wilkinson, S. M., Love, S. B., Westcombe, A. M., Gambles, M. A. Burgess, C. C. Cargill, A., . . . Ramirez, A. J. (2007). Effectiveness of aromatherapy massage in the management of anxiety and depression in patients with cancer: A multicenter randomized controlled trial. *Journal of Clinical Oncology, 25*(5), 532–539.

Xiao, J. X., Huang, G. Q., & Zhang, S. H. (2007). Soyasaponins inhibit the proliferation of hela cells by inducing apoptosis. *Experimental Toxicology and Pathology, 59*(1), 35–42.

Zou, D. M., Brewer, M., Barcia, F., Feugang, J. M., Wang, J., Zang, R., . . . Zou, C. (2005). Cactus pear: A natural product in cancer chemoprevention. *Nutrition Journal, 8*(4), 25.

Colon and Rectal Cancer

Environment

Environmental evidence-based practice for colon and rectal cancer includes:

1. *Severe on-the-job aggravation.* In one study of a hospital and regional cancer registry of colorectal cancer (569 cases), severe on-the-job aggravation appeared to increase the risk of developing colon and rectal cancers by 5.5 times as compared to those who reported no such problems. Individuals who toil in high-pressure situations while processing little or no control over workplace decisions face the highest risks and may want to reduce their chance of colon or rectal cancer by finding a less stressful job (Courtney, Longnecker, Theorell, Gerhardsson, & deVerdier, 1993), and/or learning stress management methods.

2. *CT scans.* CT scans could be responsible for raising the risk of cancer. A typical CT scan delivers 50 to 100 times more radiation than a conventional X-ray. It is estimated that one-third of all CT scans might not be necessary. Safer options of ultrasound and magnetic resonance imaging should be considered because they do not expose clients to radiation (Brenner & Hall, 2007).

3. *Smoking.* Nicotine promotes colon tumor growth (Wong et al., 2007). Caution clients about the negative effects of smoking and discuss smoking cessation programs.

4. *Sunlight.* Studies show a strong correlation between high levels of circulating vitamin D and reduced risk of colorectal cancer (Jenab et al., 2010). For Caucasian clients, 10–15 minutes of direct midday sun at least twice a week on the face, arms, hands, or back is sufficient, according to the National Institutes of Health. Darker-skinned clients may require 3–6 times as much exposure. **Cautions:** More frequent exposure may result in skin cancer. Insufficient exposure to the sun can result in improper absorption of calcium and phosphorus, leading to imperfect skeletal formation as well as bone disorders. Help clients develop a plan for obtaining sufficient sunlight, depending on their lifestyle. Eating lunch outside when weather permits could be one solution. In

winter climes, women may need to ingest more cod liver oil, fatty fish and fish oils, and egg yolks. **Other considerations:** Vitamin D_2, found in fortified foods, especially breads and cereals, is poorly metabolized by the body. Certain drugs can interfere with vitamin D metabolism, including corticosteroids, phenytoin, heparin, cimetidine, isoniazid, rifampin, phenobarbital, and primidone. Counsel clients to find alternate medications whenever possible so they can metabolize vitamin D_3 (Demgrow, 2007; Jockers, 2007).

5. *Water.* Evidence exists of an inverse relationship between glasses of plain water per day and colon cancer risk (Shannon, White, Shattuck, & Potter, 1996; Simons et al., 2010). **Cautions:** Many tap water systems provide water that contains lead, coliform bacteria, carcinogenic byproducts of chlorination, arsenic, radioactive radon, pesticides, and byproducts of rocket fuel. In addition, many water systems are deteriorating due to old infrastructure and use out-of-date water treatment technologies (National Resources Defense Council, 2008). Counsel clients to drink 8, and preferably 10 glasses of distilled or reverse-osmosis water a day to reduce colon cancer risk.

Exercise

Exercise evidence-based practice for colon and rectal cancer includes leisure time physical activity.

Leisure time physical inactivity, high body mass (greater than 29 kg/m^2), and high waist-to-hip ratio have been linked to increased risk of colon cancer, while high physical activity is protective against colorectal cancer (Chan & Giovannucci, 2010). Counsel clients to complete a series of warm-up stretches prior to activity and cool-down stretches after physical activity to reduce risk of injury. For more information, go to: http://www.wellness.ma/adult-fitness/stretching-warmup.htm **Other considerations:** There is evidence for adverse effects of overweight and obesity on colon and rectal cancer (Johnson & Lund, 2007).

Herbs/Essential Oils

Herbs/essential oils evidence-based practice for colorectal cancer includes aromatherapy, curcumin, and licorice extract.

1. *Aromatherapy.* Laboratory and animal studies show that essential oils, such as Roman chamomile, geranium, lavender, and cedar wood, either inhaled or placed in a carrier oil and then on the skin, can improve the quality of life of women diagnosed with cancer by calming, energizing, and providing antibacterial qualities (Atsumi & Tonosaki, 2007).

2. *Curcumin.* This dietary spice, which can be used daily in stews, salad dressings, soups, and other foods, possess anti-inflammatory,

antioxidant, antiproliferative, and antiangiogenic activities. Effectiveness against colon cancer cells has been documented (Patel et al., 2010).

3. *Licorice extract.* Two hundred to five hundred milligrams of powdered licorice extract t.i.d. significantly inhibited tumor growth in mice inoculated with colon cancer cells (Lee, Park, Lim, Park, & Chung, 2007). **Cautions:** Women undergoing cisplatin therapy should avoid licorice extract. Lactating, pregnant, or hypertensive women should also avoid licorice. This herb should not be used by women with liver or kidney disease, heart arrhythmias, or congestive heart failure, or by those with sensitivity to licorice. Adverse reactions include possible hypertension, edema, headache, weakness, nausea, vomiting, and lack of appetite. Counsel clients to avoid using licorice concurrently with grapefruit juice, diuretics, cardiac glycosides, antihypertensives, antiarrhythmics, and corticosteroids. **Other considerations:** Women taking licorice extract for extended periods should take additional potassium (Skidmore-Roth, 2006e).

Mind-Set

Mind-set evidence-based practices for colorectal cancer include cognitive behavioral approaches.

A patient-controlled use of an MP3 player loaded with 12 cognitive-behavioral strategies (relaxation exercises, guided imagery, and nature sound recordings) helped reduce pain, fatigue, and sleep disturbances associated with colorectal cancer and its treatment (Kwekkeboom, Abbott-Anderson, & Wanta, 2010).

Nutrition

Nutrition evidence-based practice for colorectal cancer includes the following:

1. *Almonds.* Along with and other nuts (a handful a day in total), almonds may reduce cancer risk and do so via at least one lipid-associated component (Davis & Iwahashi, 2001). Counsel clients to choose unsalted and nonoiled brands. **Other considerations:** Clients who find almonds difficult to digest can eat them in cereal; crushed and put in smoothies, stews, soups, sauces; or placed on top of fish and baked.
2. *Berries.* Black raspberry and strawberry extracts showed the most significant ability to inhibit the growth of colon cancer cells (Seeram et al., 2006).
3. *Coffee.* Coffee intake is positively associated with rectal cancer in men (Simons et al., 2010). Counsel clients to eliminate coffee intake.
4. *Starchy-rich food patterns.* Eating many starchy foods is potentially an unfavorable indicator of risk for both colon and rectal cancer, whereas the vitamins and fiber pattern is associated with a reduced risk of rec-

tal cancer and the unsaturated fats patterns (animal and plant sources) with a reduced risk of colon cancer (Bravi et al., 2010). Counsel clients at risk for or already diagnosed with colon or rectal cancer to avoid eating starchy foods, including potatoes, corn, cereals, pasta, bagels, muffins, crackers, breads, waffles, pancakes, dried beans (especially pinto, kidney, and navy), tacos, cashews, cookies, cake, pies, fried foods, pizza, biscuits, burritos, nachos, chicken nuggets, fried chicken (and anything breaded), any kind of chips, corn puffs, granola bars, dumplings, egg rolls, lasagna, and macaroni and cheese.

5. *Fruits.* Plums/prunes, peaches, and cherries have been shown to kill and/or stop colon cancer cells from proliferating (Lea et al., 2008; Lee, Cha, et al., 2007; Mori et al., 2007).

6. *Garlic.* Researchers conducting one randomized controlled trial reported a statistically significant (29%) reduction in both size and number of colon adenomas in those taking aged garlic extract. Five of case control/cohort studies suggested a protective effect of high intake of raw/cooked garlic and 2 of 8 studies suggested a protective effect for distal colon. A published meta-analysis of 7 of these studies confirmed this inverse association, with a 30% reduction in relative risk. Eleven animal studies demonstrated a significant anticarcinogenic effect of garlic and/or its constituent. As number of portions of garlic rises, risk of colorectal cancer decreases (Galeone et al., 2006; Ngo, Williams, Cobiac & Head, 2007). **Cautions:** Advise clients to avoid use if they are sensitive to garlic. Garlic may interact with antiplatelet drugs. Encourage clients to use more garlic in cooking. Odorless garlic is also available. Organically grown garlic contains more cancer-fighting selenium (Irion, 1999). **Other considerations:** The methyl allyl trisulfide in garlic dilates blood vessel walls and inhibits blood clotting without the side effects of antiplatelet or anticoagulant therapy drugs. It improves circulation and food digestion, stimulates the immune system, is a natural antibiotic that does not kill "good digestive bacteria," and so it is not as disruptive to the body systems as antibiotics. Garlic treats fungal and viral infections. Garlic may be safe for clients on warfarin therapy (Macan et al., 2006).

7. *Flaxseed.* Flaxseed contains high levels of omega-3 fatty acids and lignans effective in preventing colon tumor development at 1–6 tablespoons a day by mouth as flaxseed meal or ground flaxseeds in cereal, salads, or smoothies or stirred into a glass of water (Bommareddy, Arasada, Mathees, & Dwivedi, 2006). **Cautions:** Flaxseed should not be used by women with bowel obstruction, dehydration, or sensitivity to flax. Adverse reactions include nausea, vomiting, anorexia, diarrhea, and flatulence. Flaxseeds can be ground at home using a small food processor or coffee grinder right before ingestion. **Other considerations:**

Flax may decrease absorption of medications if taken concurrently. Flax may increase (1) the risk of bleeding if taken with anticoagulants/antiplatelets, (2) the action of antidiabetes agents if taken concurrently, or (3) the action of laxatives, resulting in diarrhea.

8. *Green tea.* Numerous studies have shown the colon cancer preventive activity of green tea at 2–5 cups a day (Coppola & Malafa, 2007). **Cautions:** Green tea may decrease iron absorption. Dairy products may decrease the therapeutic effects of green tea. Women with kidney inflammation, gastrointestinal ulcers, insomnia, heart and blood vessel disease, or increased intraocular pressure should avoid caffeinated green tea (Skidmore-Roth, 2006). Decaffeinated green tea may decrease side effects such as the hypertension, anxiety, nervousness, or insomnia of the caffeinated versions. **Other considerations:** Green tea may interact with antacids, anticoagulants, beta-adrenergic blockers, benzodiazepines, bronchodilators, and MAOIs and should not be used concurrently with these agents. The digestive process affects anticancer activity of tea in gastrointestinal cells; advise clients to add citrus (such as lemon juice) or take ascorbic acid (vitamin C) to protect the catechins in green tea from digestive degradation (Espie et al., 2008).

9. *Low-carbohydrate diets.* Very-low-carbohydrate diets (such as the Atkins-type diets) may disrupt long-term gut health by reducing butyrate production; butyrates stop cancer cells from growing, thereby preventing colorectal cancer (Rowett, 2007). A normal maintenance diet should be composed of 13% protein, 52% carbohydrate and 35% fat. Encourage clients who eat low-carbohydrate diets to eat plenty of fiber-rich foods such as fruit and vegetables.

10. *Mediterranean diet.* The Mediterranean diet is linked with prevention of cancers (Mitrou et al., 2007). The diet consists of high daily intake of vegetables, legumes, antioxidants and antiproliferatives, whole grain foods (high fiber), fish, and unsaturated fatty acids such as olive oil; low intake of saturated fatty acids, dairy products, meat, and poultry; and low to moderate intake of alcohol. For more information, go to http://www.mayoclinic.com/health/mediteraneandiet/CL00011. **Cautions/adverse reactions:** Caution clients not to drink more than one 5-ounce glass of red wine a day; drinking more has been linked with health problems, including cancers. Excessive dietary intake of sugar, refined carbohydrates, and animal products (meat and dairy products with high content of saturated fat), also known as a traditional Western diet, is linked with cancer.

11. *Pomegranate.* Pomegranate may inhibit the incidence of colon adenocarcinomas (Sharma et al., 2010).

12. *Probiotics.* Lactic acid bacteria (LAB) are present in many foods such as yogurt with active organisms. Probiotics increase immune cell activity

and may suppress the growth of bacteria that convert procarcinogens into carcinogens (Matar & Perdigon, 2007).

13. *Soy.* Risk of colon cancer was reduced with an higher soy intake, e.g., a half cup of dried soybeans or 1 cup of tofu or 1–3 cups of miso soup a day (Oba et al., 2007). Counsel clients to replace portions of chicken or beef in stir-fry with small chunks of tofu, use soy burgers instead of beef burgers, and snack on 1/4 cup of soy nuts or 4 ounces of soy milk, preferably non-GMO versions that are not genetically engineered. Miso can also be used as a base for vegetable soups and stews.

14. *Sugars.* Sucrose and dextrin act as either a coinitiator or promoter of preneoplastic lesions in the colon (Poulsen, Molck, Thorup, Breinholt, & Meyer, 2001). Simple sugar foods and products include table sugar, candy, cookies, cake, pies, sugar-sweetened cereals, breads, sodas, toothpaste, vitamins, medications, and many canned and frozen items. Stevia, an herb, is an alternative sweetener that prevents DNA damage, can be used by women diagnosed with diabetes or hypoglycemia, and acts like a general tonic. Counsel clients to use this herb in either liquid or powder form (Ghanta, Banerjee, Poddar, & Chattopadyay, 2007).

15. *Selenium.* At no more than 400 micrograms per day, selenium is a chemopreventive agent that has shown efficacy in reducing colon cancer incidence (Decensi & Costa, 2000; Olejnik, Tomczyk, Kowalska, & Grajek, 2010). The highest level of selenium is found in Brazil nuts (275 micrograms/3–4 nuts), fish (20–68 micrograms/3 ounces), and whole wheat spaghetti (36 micrograms/cup).

16. *Vitamin C.* Intake of vitamin C in foods and supplements is associated with a 30–70% reduction in colon cancer risk (Satia-About et al., 2003; Hopkins, Fedirko, Jones, Terry, & Bostick, 2010). Counsel clients to increase their intake of vitamin C foods (asparagus, avocados, beet greens, black currants, broccoli, Brussels sprouts, cantaloupe, collards, dandelion greens, grapefruit, kale, lemons, mangoes, mustard greens, onions, oranges, papaya, green peas, sweet peppers, persimmons, pineapple, radishes, spinach, strawberries, Swiss chard, tomatoes, turnip greens, and watercress). **Other considerations:** Vitamin C aids in the production of interferon, an immune system chemical that kills bacteria and viruses.

17. *Vitamin E.* Both natural and synthetic analogues of vitamin E can be used effectively as anticancer therapy, either alone or in combination to enhance the therapeutic efficacy and reduce toxicity of other anticancer agents (Satia-About et al., 2003; Sylvester, 2007). Counsel clients to increase their daily intake of leafy green vegetables (collards, mustard greens, watercress, spinach), legumes, nuts, seeds, whole grains, brown rice, eggs, oatmeal, organ meats, sweet potatoes, and wheat germ if it is necessary to increase their vitamin E intake.

Stress Management

Stress management evidence-based practice for colorectal cancer includes mindfulness meditation.

A weak immune system is one of the major factors that promotes cancer metastases after an operation, chemotherapy, or radiation therapy. Fear and stress weaken the immune system. Adequate stress management prior to and after medical treatment may help to prevent metastases. Women who reported high stress had a 1.64-fold higher risk of colon cancer mortality (Kojima et al., 2005; Tel Aviv University, 2008). For information on using mindfulness meditation, go to http://www.stjohn.org/innerpage.aspx?PageID=1779 or http://www.mindfulnessmeditationcentre.org/breathingGathas.htm

Supplements

Supplement evidence-based practice that may help with colorectal cancer includes evidence pertaining to calcium and silymarin.

1. *Calcium.* Supplementation of 1,200 mg daily of calcium has been shown to decrease the risk of recurrence of colorectal adenomas in randomized trials and may extend for up to 5 years after cessation of 4 years of treatment (Grau et al., 2007). **Cautions/adverse reactions:** Advise clients to take calcium supplements with food to prevent the formation of kidney stones.
2. *Silymarin.* Milk thistle exhibits anticancer effects for colon cancer at 300 mg daily. It is also an anti-inflammatory that can reduce pain and counter the toxic effects of chemotherapy and radiation (Cheung, Gibbons, Johnson, & Nicol, 2010).

Touch

Touch evidence-based practices that may be helpful for colorectal cancer include:

1. *Acupressure.* This is a safe and effective tool for managing chemotherapy-induced nausea and vomiting. Stimulating the PC6 point (in the middle of the front of the forearm above the wrist crease) for at least 6 hours at the onset of chemotherapy reduced symptoms in 70% of women. (Gardani et al., 2006).
2. *Foot reflexology.* When performed by the partner of the client, foot reflexology resulted in an immediate reduction in pain and anxiety (Stephenson, Swanson, Dalton, Keefe, & Engelke, 2007).

COLORECTAL CANCER CASE STUDY ⬇ [www]

Sara Richards, 31, began to notice changes in her bowel habits, including gas, bloating, alternating diarrhea and constipation, extreme fatigue, vomiting, bright red blood in her stools, narrower stools, and abdominal cramps and fullness. She was diagnosed with colorectal cancer. The diagnosis was confirmed by a second physician at a different medical center. Sara received chemotherapy and radiation treatment for colorectal cancer. She is now on the mend, but extremely worried it may recur.

HEALTH PROMOTION CHALLENGE ☆ [www]

Reread the various health promotion approaches and the evidence provided for their use with clients like Sara. Develop a plan of care for Sara that includes at least four of the interventions you found. Provide a rationale for the ones you chose and develop a teaching plan that could be used with Sara and others like her who have a diagnosis of colorectal cancer.

REFERENCES

Atsumi, T., & Tonosaki, K. (2007). Smelling lavender and rosemary increases free radical scavenging activity and decreases cortisol level in saliva. *Psychiatry Research, 150*(1), 89–96.

Bommareddy, A., Arasada, B. L., Mathees, D. P., & Dwivedi, C. (2006). Chemopreventive effects of dietary flaxseed on colon tumor development. *Nutrition in Cancer, 54*(2), 216–222.

Bravi, F., Edefonti, V., Bosetti, C., Talamini, R., Montella, M., Giacosa, A et al. (2010). Nutrient dietary patterns and the risk of colorectal cancer: A case-control study from Italy. *Cancer Causes Control, 21*(11), 1911–1918.

Brenner, D., & Hall, E. J. (2007). Computed tomography, an increasing source of radiation exposure. *New England Journal of Medicine, 357*(22), 2277–2284.

Chan, A. T., & Giovannucci, E. L. (2010). Primary prevention of colorectal cancer. *Gastroenterology, 138*(6), 2029–2043.

Cheung, C. W., Gibbons, N., Johnson, D. W., Nicol, D. L. (2010). Silibinin—A promising new treatment for cancer. *Anticancer Agents in Medicinal Chemistry, 10*(3), 186–195.

Coppola, D., & Malafa, M. (2007). Green tea polyphenols in the prevention of colon cancer. *Frontiers in Bioscience, 12*, 2309–2315.

Courtney, J. G., Longnecker, M. P., Theorell, T., Gerhardsson, & deVerdier, M. (1993). Stressful life events and the risk of colorectal cancer. *Epidemiology, 4*(5), 407–414.

Davis, P. A., & Iwahashi, C. K. (2001). Whole almonds and almond fractions reduce aberrant crypt foci in a rat model of colon carcinogenesis. *Cancer Letters, 165*(1), 27–33.

Decensi, A., & Costa, A. (2000). Recent advances in cancer chemoprevention, with emphasis on breast and colorectal cancer. *European Journal of Cancer, 36*(6), 694–709.

Demgrow, M. (2007, June). High vitamin D: Treatment for cancer prevention? *The Clinical Advisor*, 54, 57.

Federation of American Societies for Experimental Biology (2008, April 10). Digestive process affects anti-cancer activity of tea in gastrointestinal cells. *ScienceDaily*. Retrieved from http://www.sciencedaily.com/releases/2008/04/080407172713.htm

Galeone, C., Pelucchi, C., Levi, F., Negri, E., Franceschi, S., Talamini, R., . . . LaVecchia, C. (2006). Onion and garlic use and human cancer. *American Journal of Clinical Nutrition*, 84(5), 1027–1032.

Gardani, G., Cerrone, R., Biella, C., Mancini, L., Proserpio, E., Casiraghi, M., . . . Lisoni, P. (2006). Effect of acupressure on nausea and vomiting induced by chemotherapy in cancer patients. *Minerva Medicine*, 97(5), 391–394.

Ghanta, S., Banerjee, A., Poddar, A., & Chattopadyay, S. (2007). Oxidative potential of *Stevia rebaudiana* (Bertoni) Bertoni, a natural sweetener. *Journal of Agricultural and Food Chemistry*, 55(26), 10962–10967.

Grau, M. V., Baron, J. A., Sandler, R. S., Wallace, K., Haile, R. W., Church, T. R., . . . Mandel, J. S. (2007). Prolonged effect of calcium supplementation on risk of colorectal adenomas in a randomized trial. *Journal of the National Cancer Institute*, 99(2), 129–136.

Hopkins, M. H., Fedirko, V., Jones, D. P., Terry, P. D., & Bostick, R. M. (2010). Antioxidant micronutrients and biomarkers of oxidative stress and inflammation in colorectal adenoma patients: Results from a randomized, controlled clinical trial. *Cancer Epidemiology, Biomarkers and Prevention*, 19(3), 850–858.

Irion, C. W. (1999). Growing alliums and brassicas in selenium-enriched soils increases their anticarcinogenic potentials. *Medical Hypotheses*, 53(3), 232–235.

Jenab, M., Bueno-de-Mesquita, H. B., Ferrari, P., van Duijnhoven, F. J., Norat, T., Pischon, T., . . . Riboli, E. (2010). Association between pre-diagnostic circulating vitamin D concentration and risk of colorectal cancer in European populations: A nested case-control study. *BMJ*. 340:b5500.

Jockers, B. S. (2007). Vitamin D sufficiency: An approach to disease prevention. *The American Journal for Nurse Practitioners*, 11(10), 43–50.

Johnson, I. T., & Lund, E. K. (2007). Review article: Nutrition, obesity and colorectal cancer. *Alimentary Pharmacology and Therapy*, 26(2), 161–181.

Kojima, M., Wakai, K., Tokudome, S., Tamakoshi, K., Toyoshima, H., Watanabe, Y., . . . Tamakoshi, A. (2005). Perceived psychologic stress and colorectal cancer mortality: Findings from the Japan Collaborative Cohort Study. *Psychosomatic Medicine*, 67, 72–77.

Kwekkeboom, K. L., Abbott-Anderson, K., & Wanta, B. (2010). Feasibility of a patient-controlled cognitive-behavioral intervention for pain, fatigue, and sleep disturbance in cancer. *Oncology Nursing Forum*, 37(3), E151–E159.

Lea, M. A., Ibeh, C., desBordes, C., Vizzotto, M., Cisneros-Zevallos, L., Byrne, D. H., . . . Moyer, M. P. (2008). Inhibition of growth and induction of differentiation of colon cancer cells by peach and plum phenolic compounds. *Anticancer Research*, 28(4B), 2067–2076.

Lee, B. B., Cha, M. R., Kim, S. Y., Park, E., Park, H. R., & Lee, S. C. (2007). Antioxidative and anticancer activity of extracts of cherry (*Prunus serrulata* var. spontanea) blossoms. *Plant Foods for Human Nutrition*, 62(2), 79–84.

Lee, C. K., Park, K. K., Lim, S. S., Park, J. H., & Chung, W. Y. (2007). Effects of the licorice extract against tumor growth and cisplatin-induced toxicity in a mouse xenograft model of colon cancer. *Biological Pharmacology Bulletin*, 30(11), 2191–2195.

Macan, H., Uykimpang, R., Clconcel, M., Takasu, J., Razon, R., Amagase, H., . . . Niihara, Y. (2006). Aged garlic extract may be safe for patients on warfarin therapy. *Journal of Nutrition*, 136(3 Suppl), 793S–795S.

Matar, C., & Perdigon, G. (2007). The application of probiotics in cancer. *British Journal of Nutrition* (Supplement 1), S105–S110.

Mitrou, P. N., Kipnis, V., Thiebaut, A. C., Reedy, J., Subar, A. F., Wirfalt, E., . . . Schatzkin, A. (2007). Mediterranean dietary pattern and prediction of all-cause mortality in a US population: Results from the NIH-AARP Diet and Health Study. *Archives of Internal Medicine, 167*(22), 2461–2468.

Mori, S., Sawada, T., Okada, T., Ohsawa, T., Adachi, M., & Keiichi, K. (2007). *World Journal of Gastroenterology, 13*(48), 6512–6517.

National Resources Defense Council. (2008). *What's on tap? Drinking water in U.S. cities.* Retrieved from http://www.nrdc.org/water/drinking/uscities/execsum.asp

Ngo, S. N., Williams, D. B., Cobiac, L., & Head, R. J. (2007). Does garlic reduce risk of colorectal cancer? A systematic review. *Journal of Nutrition, 137*(10), 2264–2269.

Oba, S., Nagata, C., Shimizu, N., Shimizu, H., Kametani, M., Takeyama, N., . . . Matsushita, S. (2007). Soy product consumption and the risk of colon cancer: A prospective study in Takayama, Japan. *Nutrition in Cancer, 57*(2), 151–157.

Olejnik, A., Tomczyk, J., Kowalska, K., & Grajek, W. (2010). The role of natural dietary compounds in colorectal cancer chemoprevention. *Postępy Higieny i Medycyny Doświadczalnej, 64*, 175–1787.

Patel, B. B., Gupta, D., Elliott, A. A., Sengupta, V., Yu, Y., & Majumdar, A. P. (2010). Curcumin targets FOLFOX-surviving colon cancer cells via inhibition of EGFRs and IGF-1R. *Anticancer Research, 30*(2), 319–325.

Poulsen, M., Molck, A. M., Thorup, I., Breinholt, V., & Meyer, O. (2001). The influence of simple sugars and starch given during pre- or post-initiation on aberrant crypt foci in rat colon. *Cancer Letters, 167*(2), 135–143.

Rowett Research Institute. (2007, June 20). Very low carbohydrate diets may disrupt long-term gut health. *ScienceDaily*. Retrieved from http://www.sciencedaily.com/releases/2007/06/070619173537.htm

Satia-About, J., Galanko, J. A., Martin, C. F., Potter, J., Ammerman, A., & Sandler, R. S. (2003). Associations of micronutrients with colon cancer risk in African Americans and whites: Results from the North Carolina Colon Cancer Study. *Cancer Epidemiological Biomarkers and Prevention, 12*(8), 747–754.

Seeram, N. P., Adams, L. S., Zhang, Y., Lee, R., Sand, D., Scheuller, H. S., & Heber, D. (2006). Blackberry, black raspberry, blueberry, cranberry, red raspberry, strawberry extract inhibit growth and stimulate apoptosis of human cancer cells in vitro. *Journal of Agriculture and Food Chemistry, 54*(25), 9329–9339.

Shannon, J., White, E., Shattuck, A. L., & Potter, J. D. (1996). Relationship of foods groups and water intake to colon cancer risk. *Cancer Epidemiology Biomarkers, 5*(7), 495–502.

Sharma, M., Li, L., Celver, J., Killian, C., Kovoor, A., & Seeram, N. P. (2010). Effects of fruit ellagitannin extracts, ellagic acid, and their colonic metabolite, urolithin A, on Wnt signaling. *Journal of Agricultural and Food Chemistry, 58*(7), 3965–3969.

Simons, C. C., Leurs, L. J., Weijenberg, M. P., Schouten, L. J., Goldbohm, R. A., & van den Brandt, P. A. (2010). Fluid intake and colorectal cancer risk in the Netherlands Cohort Study. *Nutrition and Cancer, 62*(3), 307–321.

Skidmore-Roth, L. (2006). Green tea. In *Herbs & natural supplements* (pp. 535–539). St. Louis, MO: ElsevierMosby.

Stephenson, N. L., Swanson, M., Dalton, J., Keefe, F. J., & Engelke, M. (2007). Partner-delivered reflexology: Effects on cancer pain and anxiety. *Oncology Nursing Forum, 34*(1), 127–132.

Sylvester, P. W. (2007). Vitamin E and apoptosis. *Vitamins and Hormones, 76*, 329–356.

Tel Aviv University. (2008, February 29). Stress and fear can affect cancer's recurrence. *Science-

Daily. Retrieved from http://www.sciencedaily.com/releases/2008/02/080227142656
.htm

Ulger, O., & Yagli, N. V. (2010). Effects of yoga on the quality of life in cancer patients. *Complementary Therapies in Clinical Practice, 16*(2), 60–63.

Wong, H. P., Yu, L., Lam, E. K., Tai, E. K., Wu, W. K., & Cho, C. H. (2007). Nicotine promotes colon tumor growth and angiogenesis through beta-adrenergic activation. *Toxicology Science, 97*(2), 279–287.

Depression

Environment

Environmental evidence-based practice for depression includes sunlight.

Vitamin D deficiency may play a role in depression. Studies show a strong correlation between high vitamin D intake (sunlight) and lower rates of depression (Bertone & Johnson, 2009). Routes/dosages/frequency: 10–15 minutes of direct midday sun at least twice a week on the face, arms, hands, or back is sufficient, according to the National Institutes of Health. Darker skinned clients may require 3–6 times as much exposure. Help clients develop a plan for obtaining sufficient sunlight, depending on their lifestyle. Eating lunch outside when weather permits could be one solution. In colder climes, clients can use short wavelength blue light or take a tablespoon of cod liver oil daily, and eat fatty fish, fish oils, and egg yolks. Supplements of vitamin D_3 (calciferol) may be necessary for certain clients. **Other considerations:** Vitamin D_2, found in fortified foods, especially breads and cereals, is poorly metabolized by the body. Certain drugs can interfere with vitamin D metabolism, including corticosteroids, phenytoin, heparin, cimetidine, isoniazid, rifampin, phenobarbital, and primidone. Counsel clients to find alternate medications whenever possible so they can metabolize vitamin D_3.

Exercise

Evidence-based practice for depression includes any form of exercise. Even a single workout is beneficial, although strength training and aerobic activity seem to have the most pronounced effects.

For information on warm-up and cool-down exercises, go to http://www.wellness.ma/adult-fitness/stretching-warmup.htm **Other considerations:** Depressed clients are more apt to report improvement from exercise than from either counseling or antidepressants (chiefly because of the adverse effects of the latter). Physical activity also boosts self-confidence, improves body image, and provides a sense of self-worth and strength. Study findings support the use of exercise in the acute treatment and in ongoing lifestyle management of individuals with mood disorders (Barbour, Edenfield, & Blumenthal, 2007). Halting exercise can also bring on depressive symptoms (Tucker, 2005). Computer-generated phone calls may be an effective, low-cost way to encourage sedentary clients to exercise (Stanford University Medical Center, 2007).

Herbs/Essential Oils

Herbs/essential oils evidence-based practice for depression includes sage and St. John's wort.

1. *Sage.* In a double-blind placebo-controlled crossover study, 600 mg once a week was shown to improve mood in healthy participants (Kennedy, 2006). **Cautions:** Sage is a uterine stimulant and should not be used during pregnancy; this herb should not be used during lactation or be given to children. Women with hypersensitivity to sage should not use it, and those diagnosed with diabetes and seizure disorders should be monitored closely. Adverse effects include nausea, vomiting, anorexia, stomatitis, cheilitis, dry mouth, oral irritation, and seizures.

2. *St. John's wort.* St. John's wort (300 mg with food three times a day) is a safe, inexpensive alternative to prescription medication for mild-to-moderate depression (Linde, Mulrow, Berner, & Egger, 2005; Mannel, Kuhn, Schmidt, Ploch, Murck, 2010). **Cautions:** St. John's wort causes milder unwanted effects (nausea, vomiting, diarrhea, dizziness, anxiety, dry mouth, confusion, and headache) than most prescription antidepressants. The herb can interfere with many of the antiretroviral agents used in HIV therapy, digoxin, warfarin, oral contraceptives, and some antidepressants. **Other considerations:** Women who are lactating or pregnant should avoid St. John's wort, as should men or women with severe depression, suicidal ideations or plans, and anyone with an allergy to plants and pollen (Sego, 2006).

Mind-Set

Mind-set evidence-based practices for depression include the following:

1. *Cognitive Behavioral Therapy (CBT).* CBT, in weekly sessions for 6 weeks, can be as helpful as antidepressants for clients with depression and is superior in preventing relapse. It may be helpful to ask clients to keep a diary of depression symptoms during the 6 weeks. Between-session assignments are often given to help clients apply concepts learned during sessions (DeRubeis, Hollon, Amsterdam, 2005). For more information, see the National Association of Cognitive-Behavioral Therapists, website, at www.nacbt.org/whatiscbt.htm

2. *Mindfulness meditation.* Mindfulness is the ability to live in the present moment. One way to practice this form of meditation is to label emo-

tions by saying them aloud, for example, "I'm feeling depressed right now," or "I'm feeling real low right now," or whatever the emotion is. During the labeling of emotions, the right ventrolateral prefrontal cortex of the brain is activated, which turns down activity in the amygdala and enhances mood (University of California, Los Angeles, 2007). Provide cue sheets or cards to remind clients to label their feelings.

3. *Prayer.* Intercessory prayer offered for the benefit of another person has been shown to have positive effects on depression (Hodge, 2007).

Nutrition

Nutrition evidence-based practice for depression includes the following:

1. *Folate.* Depressed clients often have low folate levels. Folic acid (the synthetic form of folate) is metabolized in the liver, while folate is metabolized in the gut, an easily saturated system. Fortification can lead to significant unmetabolized folic acid entering the bloodstream, with the potential to cause a number of health problems. Undigested folic acid accelerates cognitive decline in older adults with low vitamin B_{12} status. Vitamin B_{12} can be found in liver, fish, milk, eggs, tempeh, and vitamin B50 supplements. **Cautions:** Advise clients to avoid foods fortified with folic acid and eat foods high in folate instead. Good food sources of folate include leafy green vegetables (like spinach and turnip greens), fruits (like citrus fruits and juices), and dried beans and peas. **Other considerations:** Serotonin plays a role in the regulation of mood and depression. Decreased serotonin can be reversed by the administration of folate. The following medications can lead to B_{12} deficiencies and a need for more foods high in folate: H2 blockers (such as ranitidine), proton pump inhibitors (e.g., omeprazole), colchicines, zidovudine, nitrous oxide anesthesia, metformin, phenformin, and potassium supplements (Chambers, 2003; Wright, Dainty & Fingles, 2007).

2. *Omega-3 fatty acids.* Epidemiological and animal studies have suggested that dietary fish or fish oil rich in omega-3 fatty acids have positive effects on depressive symptoms (University of Pittsburgh Medical School, 2006). A study of older adults showed that eating fish once a week reduced levels of depression (Bountziouka et al., 2009). **Cautions:** Farmed fish contains more PCBs, and 11 other environmental toxins are present at higher levels than in wild fish. Farmed fish may also be less nutritious (Indiana University, 2004; Norwegian School of Veterinary Science, 2008). The following fish contain the most omega-3 fatty acids and are the least tainted: 6 ounces of wild Atlantic salmon (3.1 grams), 3 ounces of sardines in sardine oil (2.8 grams), 6 ounces of wild rainbow trout (1.7 grams), 3 ounces of mackerel (1.0 grams), and 6 ounces of specialty or gourmet canned Pacific Albacore tuna canned in water (1.35 grams).

3. *Sulfur foods* have clinical applications in the treatment of depression (Parcell, 2002). Foods to focus on include cabbage, peas, beans, cauliflower, Brussels sprouts, eggs, horseradish, shrimp, chestnuts, mustard greens, onions, and asparagus.

4. *Walnuts and molasses.* Walnuts (1 handful) and molasses (1 tablespoon/day) may have antidepressant effects (Neves, 2005).

5. *Vegetarian diets.* Vegetarian diets are associated with less depression (Beezhold, Johnston, & Daigle, 2010).

Stress Management

Stress management evidence-based practice for depression includes relaxation breathing exercises. Breathing retraining, with or without physical exercise, can decrease depression (Kim & Kim, 2005).

Supplements

Supplement evidence-based practice for depression includes the following:

1. *Vitamin B_6 and B_{12}.* A lack of these two vitamins is related to increases in depression. Higher total intakes, which included supplementation, of vitamins B_6 and B_{12} were associated with a decreased likelihood of incident depression for up to 12 years of follow-up, and each 10 additional milligrams of vitamin B_6 and 10 additional micrograms of vitamin B_{12} were associated with 2% lower odds of depressive symptoms per year. There was no association between depressive symptoms and food intakes of these vitamins (Skarupski, Tangney, Li, Ouyang, Evans, & Morris, 2010). Suggest depressed clients take one or more b-complex capsules daily after discussing the matter with their pharmacist.

2. *Chromium picolinate.* Chromium is an essential trace element required for proper metabolic functioning, especially the metabolism of glucose. It is available from dietary sources such as brown rice, brewer's yeast, molasses, brown sugar, tea, cheese, meat, chicken, corn, dairy products, eggs, mushrooms, and potatoes, as well as some wines and beers. Taking a chromium picolinate supplement can improve symptoms of appetite increase, increased eating, carbohydrate cravings, and diurnal variation in feelings, such as depression (Docherty, Sack, Roffman, Finch, & Komorwski, 2005).

Touch

Touch evidence-based practice for depression includes acupressure, massage, and reflexology.

1. *Acupressure with massage.* Acupressure can lead to greater improvements in depression than routine care (Cho & Tsay, 2004).

2. *Massage therapy.* Depressed pregnant women who received massage therapy reported lower levels of anxiety and depression and less pain than women participating in either progressive muscle relaxation or a control group that received standard prenatal care. Stroking, squeezing, and stretching techniques are used on the head, arms, legs, feet, and back. For techniques to use, go to http://altmedicine.about.com/od/massage/a/massage_types.htm and http://highered.mcgraw-hill.com/sites/dl/free/0073025828/461945/Chapter04.pdf. **Other considerations:** The offspring of pregnant women can benefit from massage therapy as demonstrated by reduced fetal activity and better neonatal outcome for the massage group (Field, Diego, Hernandez-Reif, Schanberg, & Kuhn, 2004).

3. *Reflexology.* Middle-aged clients who gave themselves a 40–60-minute self-foot reflexology massage reduced their depression and strengthened their immune system (Lee, 2006). **Cautions:** Pregnant women should avoid foot reflexology because certain manipulations can lead to premature labor. Those with foot problems, gout, arthritis, and vascular conditions such as varicose veins should be careful using this procedure. Focus on massaging the whole foot. For foot charts and a demonstration, go to http://www.littleepiphany.com/massage/foot-massage-chart.htm

ADOLESCENT DEPRESSION CASE STUDY

Timothy Stevens, age 16, has a history of self-mutilation (cutting). He recently was treated in the emergency room for a cut that was deeper than he intended. Several days later he was seen in the emergency room after reportedly taking about 30 aspirin and naproxen. He states he broke up with his girlfriend. He was diagnosed with major depressive disorder and is referred for outpatient evaluation for cognitive behavioral therapy and medication management.

This case study and health promotion challenge were developed by Pamela P DiNapoli, RN PhD, Associate Professor of Nursing, University of New Hampshire.

HEALTH PROMOTION CHALLENGE

Read the adolescent depression case study and then go to the Agency for Healthcare Research and Quality website at http://www.ahrq.gov/, and access the report number 09-05130-EF-1. What are the U.S. Preventive Services Task Force recommendations for the screening and treatment of adolescent depression in primary care of adolescent depression?

REFERENCES

Barbour, K. A., Edenfield, T. M., & Blumenthal, J. A. (2007). Exercise as a treatment for depression and other psychiatric disorders: A review. *Journal of Cardiopulmonary and Rehabilitation Prevention, 27*(6), 359–367.

Beezhold, B. L., Johnston, C. S., & Daigle, D. R. (2010). Vegetarian diets are associated with healthy mood states: A cross-sectional study in Seventh Day Adventist adults. *Nutrition Journal, 9,* 26.

Bertone-Johnson, E. R. (2009). Vitamin D and the occurrence of depression: Causal association or circumstantial evidence? *Nutrition Reviews, 67*(8), 481–492.

Bountziouka, V., Polychronopoulos, E., Zeimbekis, A., Papavenetiou, E., Ladoukaki, E., Papairakleous, N., . . . Panagiotakos, D. (2009). Long-term fish intake is associated with less severe depressive symptoms among elderly men and women: The MEDIS (MEDiterranean ISlands Elderly) epidemiological study. *Journal of Aging and Health, 21*(6), 864–880.

Chambers, K. H. (2003). *Health benefits of folic acid.* New York, NY: Medical Education Collaboration.

Cho, Y. C., & Tsay, S. L. (2004). The effect of acupressure with massage on fatigue and depression in patients with end-stage renal disease. *Journal of Nursing Research, 12*(1), 51–59.

DeRubeis, R. J., Hollon, S. D., & Amsterdam, J. D. (2005). Cognitive therapy vs. medications in the treatment of moderate to severe depression. *Archives of General Psychiatry, 62,* 409–416.

Docherty, J. P., Sack, D. A., Roffman, M., Finch, M., & Komorowski, J. R. (2005). A double-blind, placebo-controlled, exploratory trial of chromium picolinate in atypical depression: Effect on carbohydrate craving. *Journal of Psychiatric Practice, 11*(5), 302–314.

Field, T., Diego, M. A., Hernandez-Reif, M., Schanberg, S., & Kuhn, C. (2004). Massage therapy effects on depressed pregnant women. *Journal of Psychosomatic Obstetrical Gynecology, 25*(2), 115–122.

Hodge, D. R. (2007). A systematic review of the empirical literature on intercessory prayer. *Research on Social Work Practice, 17*(2), 174–187.

Indiana University. (2004, January 9). Farmed salmon more toxic than wild salmon, study finds. *ScienceDaily.* Retrieved from http://www.sciencedaily.com/releases/2004/01/040109072244.htm

Kennedy, D. O. (2006). Effects of cholinesterase inhibiting sage (*Salia officinalis*) on mood, anxiety and performance on a psychological stressor battery. *Neuropsychopharmacology, 31*(4), 845–852.

Kim, S., & Kim, H. A. (2005). Effects of relaxation breathing exercises on anxiety, depression and leukocytes in hemopoietic stem cell transplantation patients. *Cancer Nursing, 28*(1), 79–83.

Lee, Y. M. (2006). Effects of self-foot reflexology massage on depression, stress responses and immune functions of middle aged women. *Taehan Kanho Hakhoe Chi, 36*(1), 179–188.

Linde, K., Mulrow, C. D., Berner, M., & Egger, M. (2005). St. John's wort for depression. *Cochrane Database System of Reviews, 18*(2), CD000448.

Mannel, M., Kuhn, U., Schmidt, U., Ploch, M., & Murck, H. (2010). St. John's wort extract LI160 for the treatment of depression with atypical features—A double-blind, randomized, and placebo-controlled trial. *Journal of Psychiatric Research, 44*(12), 760–767.

Neves, L. (2005). *Food ingredients may be as effective as antidepressants: Researchers discover 'mood foods' relieve signs of depression.* Press release, February 10. Belmont, MA: McLean Hospital. Retrieved from http://www.mclean.harvard.edu/news/press/current.php?id=72

Norwegian School of Veterinary Science. (2008, February 28). Farmed fish fed cheap food may be less nutritious for humans. Retrieved from http://www.sciencedaily.com/releases/2008/02/080226164105.htm

Parcell, S. (2002). Sulfur in human nutrition and applications in medicine. *Alternative Medicine Review, 7*(1), 22–44.

Sego, S. (2006, July). St. John's wort. *The Clinical Advisor*, pp. 135–137.

Skarupski, K. A., Tangney, C., Li, H., Ouyang, B., Evans, D. A., & Morris, M. C. (2010). Longitudinal association of vitamin B-6, folate, and vitamin B-12 with depressive symptoms among older adults over time. *American Journal of Clinical Nutrition, 92*(2), 330–335.

Stanford University Medical Center (2007, December 5). Computer calls can talk couch potatoes into walking, study finds. *ScienceDaily*. Retrieved from http://www.sciencedaily.com/releases/2007/12/071204122000.htm

Tucker, M. E. (2005, September). Halt to exercise = depression. *Clinical Psychiatric News*, p. 33.

University of California, Los Angeles. (2007, June 22). Putting feelings into words produces therapeutic effects in the brain. *ScienceDaily*. Retrieved from http://www.sciencedaily.com/releases/2007/06/070622090727.htm

University of Pittsburgh Medical Center. (2006, March 4). Omega 3 fatty acids influence mood, impulsivity and personality, study indicates. *ScienceDaily*. Retrieved from http://www.sciencedaily.com/releases/2006/03//060303205050.htm

Wright, J., Dainty, J., & Fingles, P. (2007). Folic acid metabolism in human subjects: Potential implications for proposed mandatory folic acid fortification in the UK. *British Journal of Nutrition, 98*, 667–675.

Digestion (Constipation, Crohn's Disease, Diarrhea, Gastroesophageal Reflux Disease, Irritable Bowel Syndrome)

Environment

Environmental evidence-based practice for digestion includes hand washing.

Hand washing can reduce the incidence of diarrhea by up to 30%. Good hand washing technique includes washing with soap and water or an alcohol-based sanitizer. Antimicrobial cleaners are as good as soap and water, but not as effective as alcohol-based sanitizers. Antimicrobial cleaners also are harmful (Emerging Contaminants Work Group, 2006). **Other considerations:** Hand contact with ready-to-eat food consumed without further washing or cooking can transmit more germs than food that is prepared and cooked at home (Center for the Advancement of Health, 2008; Mayo Clinic, 2008).

Exercise/Movement

Exercise/movement evidence-based practice for digestion includes physical exercise.

Physical exercise, such as walking or swimming can be effective against constipation (Ostaszkiewicz, Hornby, Millar, & Ockerby, 2010). **Cautions:** Advise clients to avoid overexertion. Nonstrenuous exercise is best. For ideas on warm-up and cool-down exercises, go to http://www.wellness .ma/adult-fitness/stretching-warmup.htm. **Other considerations:** Use in combination with adequate hydration and dedicated bathroom time for best results.

Herbs

Herbal evidence-based practice for digestion includes the following:

1. *Chamomile.* An anti-inflammatory and antispasmodic used to treat digestive conditions such as irritable bowel syndrome, indigestion, colitis, and Crohn's disease, clients should drink 2–4 ounces of chamomile tea as needed (McKay & Blumberg, 2006a). **Cautions:** Chamomile should not be used during pregnancy or lactation or taken by clients sensitive to sunflowers, ragweed, echinacea, feverfew, or milk thistle. Advise clients to not take concurrently with sedatives or alcohol (Skidmore-Roth, 2006a).

2. *Fenugreek.* Fenugreek has a positive effect on constipation, dyspepsia, gastritis, and inflammatory bowel disease at 1 cup of tea one to three times a day (Langmead et al., 2002). **Cautions:** Fenugreek can cause premature labor. Because of the rapid rate at which this herb moves through the bowel and coats the gastrointestinal tract, fenugreek can reduce the absorption of all medications, foods, and supplements taken concurrently. There may be an increased risk for bleeding if taken with anticoagulants. Because fenugreek lowers blood glucose levels, hypoglycemia is a possibility when used concurrently with oral antidiabetes agents (Skidmore-Roth, 2006c).

3. *Milk thistle.* Also known as silymarin, milk thistle helps normalize liver functions when taken orally as capsules of between 420 and 800 mg per day in 3 doses (Shaker, Mahmoud, & Mnaa, 2010). **Cautions:** Though generally well tolerated, milk thistle can have a mild laxative effect and could worsen menstrual cramping. Pregnant women or women planning to become pregnant, lactating women, and children should not use milk thistle. Women sensitive to pollen-bearing plants should avoid silymarin. **Other considerations:** Milk thistle has been used to treat hepatotoxicity due to poisonous mushrooms, cirrhosis of the liver, chronic candidiasis, hepatitis C, exposure to toxic chemicals, and liver transplantation (Sego, 2007; Tamayo & Diamond, 2007).

4. *Peppermint tea.* Animal studies demonstrate a relaxation effect on gastrointestinal (GI) tissue. Suggested amount: 1–3 cups a day (McKay & Blumberg, 2006b).

Mind-Set

Mind-set evidence-based practice for digestion includes cognitive behavioral therapy and hypnosis.

1. *Cognitive behavioral therapy (CBT).* CBT works as well as standard care for irritable bowel syndrome (Ljótsson et al., 2010). For more information, go to http://www.mind.org.uk/Information/Booklets /Making+sense/MakingSenseCBT.htm. **Other considerations:** Routine clinical care may have adverse effects, while CBT does not.

2. *Hypnosis.* Hypnosis can provide a relaxed state for clients with irritable bowel syndrome (IBS), thereby modulating gastrointestinal physiology, perceived rectal distension, and improved mood. Some results lasted up to 6 years following treatment that included either listening to a hypnosis tape or visiting a practitioner who follows a specific protocol for IBS (Simren, 2006). Go to http://www.ibshypnosis.com/ for information about hypnosis.

Nutrition

Nutrition evidence-based practice for digestion includes the following:

1. *Cinnamon.* Used at 1–2 teaspoons added to food, cinnamon contains antibacterial and blood sugar controlling factors (Meades et al., 2010). **Cautions:** Until more research is conducted, avoid during pregnancy and lactation in large doses. Can be used safely as a spice, e.g., on oatmeal, rice, pears, stews, prunes, cereals, and soups.

2. *Cow's milk. Escherichia coli* is known to be present during Crohn's disease in greater numbers and may be due to ingesting milk and milk products. **Cautions:** This bacterium is a likely trigger for a circulating antibody protein (ASCA) that is found in about two-thirds of people with Crohn's disease, suggesting these clients may have been infected by *Mycobacterium* (University of Liverpool, 2007).

3. *Curcumin.* Turmeric is a natural dietary produce spice shown to significantly attenuate colitis and treat IBD. **Cautions:** Turmeric is considered safe for most adults. High doses or long-term use of turmeric may cause indigestion. Women with gallbladder disease should avoid using turmeric as a dietary supplement, as it may worsen the condition. The spice may be sprinkled on salads, baked potatoes, stews, soups, curries, rice, poultry, or fish and used in cooking (Deguchi et al., 2007).

4. *Fat, spices, and reflux.* Meals high in fat can provoke reflux, possibly through delayed gastric emptying. Additional spices, such as curry, do

not increase reflux (Schonfeld & Evans, 2007). Counsel clients to reduce or eliminate fatty animal products and to concentrate their meals on fruits, vegetables, grains, and fish.

5. *Overweight and gastroesophageal reflux disease (GERD).* In a meta-analysis of studies, six showed a statistically significant association between obesity and GERD. Overweight and obesity increase the risk of GERD and complications such as erosive esophagitis (Hamphel, Abraham, & El-Serag, 2005). Weight loss may help improve symptoms. **Cautions:** Postmenopausal hormone therapy in women strengthened the association between GERD symptoms and high body mass index, or BMI (overweight = 25 to 30; obese = greater than 30).

6. *Vitamins A, C, and E, and beta carotene.* In foods, these nutrients can decrease risk of cervical cancer (Kim et al., 2010). Good sources of these vitamins are fruits and vegetables, especially citrus, carrots, tomatoes, spinach, and cauliflower. Counsel clients to eat these foods daily.

7. *Water.* Drinking water replaces lost fluids while caffeinated beverages or alcohol increase fluid output, leeching out needed liquids, minerals and vitamins. Constipation can be a sign of inadequate fluid intake. At least 8 glasses a day of water is recommended. **Cautions:** Tap water and even bottled water can contain parasites, weed killers, nitrates (correlated with spontaneous miscarriage and blue-baby syndrome), *Salmonella*, *E. coli*, chlorine, fluoride, and other potentially dangerous substances. Counsel clients to drink (and cook with) only distilled water or reverse-osmosis filtered water. **Other considerations:** Fluid intake is probably adequate when thirst is rarely experienced and when urine is colorless or slightly yellow. As women age, they may experience less thirst. Counsel older adults to drink water before thirst sets in because by that time, dehydration may already have taken over (Mayo Clinic, 2007).

Stress Management

Stress management evidence-based practice for digestion includes cognitive behavioral therapy (CBT).

CBT-based self-management in the form of a structured manual and minimal therapist contact is an effective and acceptable form of treatment for primary-care IBS patients (Moss-Morris, McAlpine, Didsbury & Spence, 2010).

Supplements

Supplement evidence-based practice for digestion includes pycnogenol and probiotics.

1. *Pycnogenol.* Within 12 hours, pycnogenol significantly ameliorated inflammation in rats with inflammatory bowel disease (Mochizuki &

Hasegawa, 2004). The equivalent for humans is one capsule (50 mg) three times a day. **Cautions:** Theoretically, pycnogenol may interact with immunosuppressants and cause reduced blood platelet aggregation. No other adverse reactions are known. **Other considerations:** Advise clients to avoid using pycnogenol when lactating.

2. *Probiotics.* Usually two capsules a day with meals or a large glass of water, probiotics produce the "good bacteria" that render the digestive tract unfavorable for more aggressive bacteria and have been shown effective in reducing symptoms of inflammatory bowel disease. (Cary & Boullata, 2010). **Cautions:** Advise clients not to use concurrently with antibiotics; have them separate probiotics and antibiotics by 2 hours. Probiotics should not be used concurrently with immunosuppressants; they may decrease the action of warfarin. Probiotics may decrease the absorption of garlic; advise clients to separate probiotics and garlic use by 2 hours. **Other considerations:** This supplement also inhibits the growth of vaginal microorganisms. Multidophilus treats a variety of gastrointestinal conditions.

Touch

Touch evidence-based practice for digestion includes acupressure.

Except for clients with eye or nearby facial wounds, pressing on stomach meridians on the ridge of the cavity directly below the pupils (on for 5 seconds and off for 5) can positively affect gastric action by activating the signaling pathway, providing evidence for traditional Chinese medicine approaches such as acupressure (Yan et al., 2007). Pressing these points has also shown to be helpful for reflux symptoms (Wen, Hao, & Jin, 2010). **Other considerations:** For more information on using acupressure, go to http://www.eclecticenergies .com/acupressure/howto.php.

IRRITABLE BOWEL SYNDROME CASE STUDY

Mr. Schroeder, age 28, complained of loose stools with sticky mucus and undigested matter, bloating of the abdomen, and flatulence for the past 2 years ever since his wife died in a car accident and he was left to raise twins by himself. He reported getting very irritable over small things, but would never express it out loud, and getting depressed because he could not perform his work or family responsibilities to perfection. He was diagnosed with irritable bowel syndrome.

HEALTH PROMOTION CHALLENGE

Using the evidence available in this chapter, develop a plan of care and a teaching plan for Mr. Schroeder.

REFERENCES

Cary, V. A., & Boullata, J. (2010). What is the evidence for the use of probiotics in the treatment of inflammatory bowel disease? *Journal of Clinical Nursing, 19*(7–8), 904–916.

Center for the Advancement of Health. (2008, January 25). Handwashing can reduce diarrhea episodes by about one-third. *ScienceDaily*. Retrieved from http://www.sciencedaily.com/releases/2008/01/080122203221.htm

Deguchi, Y., Andoh, A., Inatomi, O., Yagi, Y., Bamba, S. Araki, Y., . . . Fujiyama, Y. (2007). Curcumin prevents the development of dextran sulfate sodium (DSS)-induced experimental colitis. *Digestive Diseases and Sciences, 52*(11), 2993–2998.

Emerging Contaminants Work Group. (2006). Retrieved from http://www.scbwmi.org/PDFs/WMI_Triclosan_FinalJan06.pdf

Hamphel, H., Abraham, N. S., & El-Serag, H. B. (2005). Meta-analysis of obesity and the risk of gastroesophageal reflux disease and its complications. *Annals of Internal Medicine, 143*, 199–211.

Kim, J., Kim, M. K., Lee, J. K., Kim, J. H., Son, S. K., Song, E. S. . . . Yun, Y. M. (2010). Intakes of vitamin A, C, and E, and beta-carotene are associated with risk of cervical cancer: a case-control study in Korea. *Nutrition in Cancer, 62*(2), 181–189.

Langmead, L., Dawson, C., Hawkins, C., Banna, N., Loo, S., & Rampton, D. S. (2002). Antioxidant effects of herbal therapies used by patients with inflammatory bowel disease. *Alimentary Pharmacology Therapy, 16*(2), 197–205.

Ljótsson, B., Falk, L., Vesterlund, A. W., Hedman, E., Lindfors, P., Rück, C., . . . Andersson, G. (2010). Internet-delivered exposure and mindfulness based therapy for irritable bowel syndrome—a randomized controlled trial. *Behaviour Research and Therapy, 48*(6), 531–9.

Mayo Clinic. (2007, August 13). How much water should you drink? It depends. Retrieved from http://www.mayoclinic.com/health/water/NU00283

Mayo Clinic. (2008). Hand washing: An easy way to prevent infection. Retrieved from http://www.mayoclinic.com/health/hand-washing/HQ00407

McKay, D. L., & Blumberg, J. B. (2006a). A review of the bioactivity and potential health benefits of chamomile tea. *Phytotherapy Research, 20*(7), 519–530.

McKay, D. L., & Blumberg, J. B. (2006b). A review of the bioactivity and potential health benefits of peppermint tea. *Phytotherapy Research, 20*(8), 619–633.

Meades, G. Jr., Henken, R. L., Waldrop, G. L., Rahman, M. M., Gilman, S. D., Kamatou, G. P., . . . Gibbons, S. (2010). Constituents of cinnamon inhibit bacterial Acetyl CoA Carboxylase. *Planta Medica, 6*(14), 1570–1575.

Mochizuki, M., & Hasegawa, N. (2004). Therapeutic efficacy of pycnogenol in experimental inflammatory bowel diseases. *Phytotherapy Research, 18*(12), 1027–1028.

Moss-Morris, R., McAlpine, L., Didsbury, L. P., & Spence, M. J. (2010). A randomized controlled trial of a cognitive behavioural therapy-based self-management intervention for irritable bowel syndrome in primary care. *Psychological Medicine, 40*(1), 85–94.

Ostaszkiewicz, J., Hornby, L., Millar, L., & Ockerby, C. (2010). The effects of conservative treatment for constipation on symptom severity and quality of life in community-dwelling adults. *Journal of Wound, Ostomy, and Continence Nursing, 37*(2), 193–198.

Schonfeld, J., & Evans, D. F. (2007). Fat, spices and gastro-eosophageal reflux. *Zeitschrift fur Gastroenterologie, 45*(2), 171–175.

Sego, S. (2007, June). Milk thistle. *The Clinical Advisor,* 136–137.

Shaker, E., Mahmoud, H., & Mnaa, S. (2010). Silymarin, the antioxidant component and *Silybum marianum* extracts prevent liver damage. *Food and Chemical Toxicology, 48*(3), 803–806.

Simren, M. (2006). Hypnosis for irritable bowel syndrome: The quest for the mechanism of action. *International Journal of Clinical Experimental Hypnosis, 5*(1), 65–84.

Skidmore-Roth, L. (2006a). Chamomile. In *Mosby's handbook of herbs & natural supplements* (pp. 264–268). St. Louis, MO: ElsevierMosby.

Skidmore-Roth, L. (2006b). Cinnamon. In *Mosby's handbook of herbs & natural supplements* (pp. 302–305). St. Louis, MO: ElsevierMosby.

Skidmore-Roth, L. (2006c). Fenugreek. In *Mosby's handbook of herbs & natural supplements* (pp. 435–439). St. Louis, MO: ElsevierMosby.

Tamayo, C., & Diamond, S. (2007). Review of clinical trials evaluating safety and efficacy of milk thistle. *Integrative Cancer Therapies, 6*(2), 146–157.

University of Liverpool. (2007, December 13). How bacteria in cows' milk may cause Crohn's disease. *ScienceDaily.* Retrieved from http://www.sciencedaily.com/releases/2007/12/071210104002.htm

Wen, N., Hao, J. D., & Jin, Z. G. (2010). Clinical observation on acupuncture for treatment of reflux esophagitis of heat stagnation of liver and stomach type. *Zhongguo Zhen Jiu, 30*(4), 285–288.

Yan, J., Yang, Z. B., Chang, X. R., Yi, S. X., Lin, Y. P., & Zhong, Y. (2007). Expressions of epidermal growth factor receptor signaling substances in gastric mucosal cells influenced by serum derived from rats treated with electroacupuncture at stomach meridian acupoints. *Zong Xi Yi Jie He Xue Bao, 5*(3), 338–342.

Endometrial Cancer

Environment

Environmental evidence-based practice for endometrial cancer includes the following:

1. *Alcohol.* Consuming two or more alcoholic beverages a day may double a woman's risk of endometrial cancer (University of Southern California, 2007b).

2. *Aromatherapy.* Laboratory and animal studies show that essential oils, such as Roman chamomile, geranium, lavender, and cedarwood can improve the quality of life of women diagnosed with cancer by calming, energizing, and providing antibacterial qualities (Atsumi & Tonosaki, 2007).

3. *CT scans.* A typical CT scan delivers 50 to 100 times more radiation than a conventional X-ray and could be responsible for raising cancer risk. **Cautions:** Brenner and Hall (2007) estimate that one-third of all CT scans might not be necessary. Suggest using the safer options of ultrasound and magnetic resonance imaging, which do not expose women to radiation. **Other considerations:** An estimated 62 million CT scans were performed in 2006, compared to only 3 million in 1980 (Brenner & Hall, 2007).

4. *Sunlight.* Researchers at the Moores Cancer Center at University of California, San Diego have shown a clear association between deficiency in exposure to sunlight—especially ultraviolet B (UVB)—and endometrial cancer (University of California, San Diego, 2007a). For Caucasian women, 10–15 minutes of direct midday sun at least twice a week on the face, arms, hands, or back is sufficient, according to the National Institutes of Health. Darker skinned women may require 3–6 times as much exposure. Help women develop a plan for obtaining sufficient sunlight, depending on their lifestyle. Eating lunch outside when weather permits could be one solution. In colder climes, women can take a tablespoon of cod liver oil daily, and eat fatty fish, fish oils, and egg yolks. Supplements of vitamin D_3 (calciferol) may be necessary for certain women. **Other considerations:** Vitamin D_2, found in fortified foods, especially breads and cereals, is poorly metabolized by the body. Certain drugs can interfere with vitamin D metabolism, including corticosteroids, phenytoin, heparin, cimetidine, isoniazid, rifampin, phenobarbital, and primidone. Counsel women to find alternate medications whenever possible so they can metabolize vitamin D_3 (Autoimmunity Research Foundation, 2008).

5. *Overweight/obesity.* Half of all cases of endometrial cancer are attributable to overweight or obesity (British Medical Journal, 2007).

6. *Talc.* Perineal talcum powder use increases the risk of endometrial cancer, particularly among postmenopausal women (Karageorgi, Gates, Hankinson, & Devivo, 2010).

Exercise/Movement

Epidemiologic and biologic evidence shows that vigorous activity, as well as light and moderate intensity activities such as housework, gardening, or walking for transportation, may reduce risk for endometrial cancer, with the strongest evidence for household activities. Inactive premenopausal women have the highest risk of endometrial cancer (Cust, Armstrong, Friedenreich, Slimani, & Bauman, 2007; Friedenreich et al., 2007). Encourage premenopausal women to increase their household activity if they are inactive. **Other considerations:**

Fourteen of eighteen studies of physical activity and endometrial cancer show a convincing or possible protective effect of physical activity on endometrial cancer risk.

Herbs/Essential Oils

Herbal evidence-based practice for endometrial cancer includes glycyrrhizin and milk thistle.

1. *Glycyrrhizin.* Licorice (but not the licorice candy), taken by mouth at 250–500 mg t.i.d. generated a significant decrease in the incidence of endometrial adenocarcinoma (Niwa et al., 2007). **Cautions:** Glycyrrhizin should not be used by pregnant or lactating women, given to children, or used by anyone diagnosed with liver or kidney disease, hypertension, arrhythmias, congestive heart failure, or anyone who is hypersensitive to the herb. **Other considerations:** Advise women to increase potassium intake if using licorice for extended periods.

2. *Milk thistle.* Silymarin, the active substance in milk thistle, stimulates detoxification pathways, inhibits the growth of certain cancer cell lines, exerts direct cytotoxic activity toward certain cancer cell lines, and may increase the efficacy of certain chemotherapy agents when taken at 200 to 400 mg per day (Cheung, Gibbons, Johnson, Nicol, 2010). **Cautions:** Adverse effects are rare, but may include stomach pain, nausea, vomiting, diarrhea, headache, rash, joint pain, and anaphylaxis in allergic women. Warn pregnant and lactating women or those who are hypersensitive (have a known sensitivity to ragweed, marigolds, chrysanthemums, or marigolds) not to use milk thistle. Milk thistle may protect against liver damage from chemotherapy and radiation (National Cancer Institute, 2010).

Nutrition

Nutrition evidence-based practice for endometrial cancer includes the following:

1. *Fiber.* Fiber intake is inversely related to endometrial cancer. Most Americans (95%) do not eat enough high fiber foods daily (15 grams vs. the recommended 25 grams for women and 38 grams for adult men) to meet the American Academy of Nutrition and Dietetics (2008) guidelines. To meet their guidelines means eating more legumes, 5–10 servings of vegetables and fruits every day, along with 4–6 servings of whole grain breads and cereals. Advise women who do not eat sufficient fiber to increase their intake of fiber to decrease risk of endometrial cancer (Bidoli et al., 2010).

2. *Folate.* Folate intake may decrease the risk of endometrial cancer and modify genotype (MTHFR) risk (Xu, Shrubsole, et al., 2007). Leafy, green vegetables (like spinach and turnip greens), fruits (citrus fruits and juices), and dried beans and peas are all natural sources of folate that can help meet the suggested amount of 1,000 micrograms a day (Office of Dietary Supplements, 2005). Clients on diets who do not eat breads, cereals, or pasta; who abuse alcohol; or who take medications that interfere with folate absorption may not receive sufficient amounts of the nutrient and may need additional amounts. **Cautions:** Medications and medical conditions that increase the need for folate or result in an increased excretion of folate include anticonvulsant medications, metformin, sulfasalazine, triamterene, methotrexate, barbiturates, pregnancy and lactation, alcohol abuse, malabsorption, kidney dialysis, liver disease, and certain anemias. Because folate is a water-soluble B-vitamin, unneeded amounts will be eliminated in the urine. Advise clients to avoid flour-fortified foods as a source of folic acid; research has shown the introduction of flour fortified with folic acid into common foods or taken as a supplement has been linked to colon cancer (Martinez et al., 2012). **Other considerations:** Exceeding 1,000 micrograms of folate per day may trigger vitamin B_{12} deficiency. To compensate, clients can take a multivitamin that contains B_{12} or eat at least one food daily that contains B_{12}, such as nutritional yeast (unless susceptible to *Candida*), clams, eggs, herring, kidney, liver, mackerel, seafood, milk, or dairy products.

3. *Garlic and brassica vegetables.* Garlic and brassica vegetables readily uptake inorganic and anticarcinogenic selenium from soil and incorporate it into bioactive organic chemicals (Gill et al., 2007; Irion, 1999). Garlic has been shown to have chemopreventive effects and to suppress the proliferation of tumor cells (Melino, Sabelli, & Paci, 2010), as have brassica vegetables (Vallejo, Tomas-Barberan, Garcia-Viguera, 2003). **Cautions:** Counsel clients to avoid microwaving vegetables; this method destroys most of their helpful antioxidants. Garlic can be baked in its skin or chopped and used in tomato sauce, stews, fish, tofu, and other diesh. Advise clients to cut the garlic into small pieces and lightly steam brassica vegetables for 5 minutes in a small amount of water to release all amino acids and antioxidants. If any liquids remain, clients can cool them and drink them later or use in cooking. **Other considerations:** Brassica vegetables include broccoli, cauliflower, Brussels sprouts, collards, kohlrabi, and kale, as well as more than 350 other plants, such as arugula, mustard, radish, daikon, watercress, horseradish, and wasabi.

4. *Soy and fiber.* Soy and fiber consumption from whole grains, vegetables, fruits, and seaweeds is associated with a reduced risk of endometrial

cancer (Dalvi, Canchola, & Horn-Ross, 2007; Goodman et al., 1997; Xu et al., 2004, 2007). Unless clients are allergic or sensitive, recommend they eat tofu, soybeans, tempeh, soy cheese, and/or drink soy milk along with 8–10 servings (half cup each) of vegetables and fruits daily. Advise them to use seaweeds as a source of minerals and taste for stews, salads, soups, and other dishes. **Other considerations:** Soy food intake is especially beneficial to women with a high body mass index and waist-to-hip ratio. Among nonusers of supplements, a diet comprised of sugar and sugary foods, refined carbohydrates, and animal products was associated with greater risk of endometrial cancer, regardless of fruit and vegetable consumption.

5. *Tea.* Drinking tea is inversely associated with endometrial cancer (American Association for Cancer Research, 2007). Counsel clients to choose decaffeinated teas. Digestive process affects anticancer activity of tea in gastrointestinal cells; advise clients to add citrus (such as lemon juice) or take ascorbic acid (vitamin C) to protect the catechins in green tea from digestive degradation (Federation of American Societies for Experimental Biology, 2008).

6. *Turmeric.* Curcumin, found in the spice turmeric, has been demonstrated to have an antitumor effect in endometrial cancer cells at 400–600 mg by mouth t.i.d., standardized to curcumin content (Yu & Shah, 2007). **Cautions:** Advise clients to avoid using turmeric if they are diagnosed with bile duct obstruction, peptic ulcer, hyperacidity, gallstones, bleeding disorders, or hypersensitivity to the herb. Advise clients to take turmeric on an empty stomach. **Other considerations:** Turmeric may interact with heparin, salicylates, warfarin, cyclosporine, and NSAIDS.

Stress Management

Evidence-based practice for endometrial cancer includes managing stress.

A weak immune system is one of the major factors that promotes cancer metastases after an operation, chemotherapy, or radiation therapy. Adequate stress management prior to and after medical treatment may help to prevent metastases. Fear and stress weaken the immune system (Tel Aviv University, 2008). For stress management teaching materials, go to: http:www.mindfulnessmeditationcentre.org/breathingGathas.htm, http://www.santosha.com/asanas/asana.html, and http://www.alternateheals.com/relaxationtherapy/home.relaxation.treatments.htm

Supplements

Supplement evidence-based practice for endometrial cancer includes vitamins A, C, and E.

Dietary intake of foods high in vitamins A, C, and E and/or vitamin supplementation may decrease the risk of endometrial cancer. When derived from plant sources, all three vitamins show an inverse relationship to this type of cancer. Dietary intake of animal origin nutrients was correlated with a high risk for endometrial cancer (Xu, Dai, Xianag, Xhao, et al., 2007).

Touch

Acupressure is a safe and effective tool for managing chemotherapy-induced nausea and vomiting. Stimulating PC6 point for at least 6 hours at the onset of chemotherapy reduced symptoms in 70% of women (Gardani et al., 2006). **Tips for use:** PC6 is situated in the middle of the front of the forearm above the wrist crease. Combining reflexology, aromatherapy, and foot soak significantly improved fatigue in women with advanced cancer (Kohara, 2004).

ENDOMETRIAL CANCER CASE STUDY

Ms. Shaw, a 33-year-old woman, married for 4 years, was evaluated in a local hospital for infertility and oligomenorrhea. Her cycles had been infrequent since menarche. Pelvic examination findings were normal. She had two episodes of profuse vaginal bleeding for which curettage was done by her physician, and she was referred for further treatment. Total hysterectomy with bilateral salpingo-oophorectomy and pelvic and paraaortic lymphadenectomy was done and Ms. Shaw received three courses of chemotherapy.

HEALTH PROMOTION CHALLENGE

Using the evidence presented for this condition, develop a health promotion plan of care and relevant teaching plan for Ms. Shaw.

REFERENCES

American Academy of Nutrition and Dietetics. (2008). Health implications of dietary fiber. *Journal of the American Academy of Nutrition and Dietetics, 108*(10), 1716–1731.

American Association for Cancer Research. (2007, August 12). Green tea boosts production of detox enzymes, rendering cancerous chemicals harmless. Retrieved from http://www.sciencedaily.com/releases/2007/08/070810194923.htm

Atsumi, T., & Tonosaki, K. (2007). Smelling lavender and rosemary increases free radical scavenging activity and decreases cortisol level in saliva. *Psychiatry Research, 150*(1), 89–96.

Autoimmunity Research Foundation. (2008, January 27). Vitamin D deficiency study raises new questions about disease and supplements. *ScienceDaily*. Retrieved from http://www.sciencedaily.com/releases/2008/01/080125223302.htm

Bidoli, E., Pelucchi, C., Zucchetto, A., Negri, E., Dal Maso, L., Polesel, J., . . . Talamini, R. (2010). Fiber intake and endometrial cancer risk. *Acta Oncologica, 49*(4), 441–446.

Brenner, D., & Hall, E. J. (2007). Computed tomography, an increasing source of radiation exposure. *New England Journal of Medicine, 357*(22), 2277–2284.

British Medical Journal. (2007, November 10). Overweight and obesity cause 6,000 cancers a year in UK. *ScienceDaily*. Retrieved from http://www.sciencedaily.com/releases/2007/11/071106174207.htm

Cheung, C. W., Gibbons, N., Johnson, D. W., & Nicol, D. L. (2010). Silibinin—A promising new treatment for cancer. *Anticancer Agents in Medicinal Chemistry, 10*(3), 186–195.

Cust, A. E., Armstrong, B. K., Friedenreich, C. M., Slimani, N., & Bauman, A. (2007). Physical activity and endometrial cancer risk: A review of the current evidence, biologic mechanisms and the quality of physical activity assessment methods. *Cancer Causes Control, 18*(3), 243–258.

Dalvi, T. B., Canchola, A. J., & Horn-Ross, P. L. (2007). Dietary patterns, Mediterranean diet, and endometrial cancer risk. *Cancer Causes Control, 18*(9), 957–966.

Federation of American Societies for Experimental Biology. (2008). Digestive process affects anti-cancer activity of tea in gastrointestinal cells. *ScienceDaily*. Retrieved from http://www.sciencedaily.com/releases/2008/04/080407172713.htm

Friedenreich, C., Cust, A., Lahmann, P. H., Steindorf, K., Boutron-Ruault, M. C., Clavel-Chapelon, F., . . . Riboli, E. (2007). Physical activity and risk of endometrial cancer: The European prospective investigation into cancer and nutrition. *International Journal of Cancer, 121*(2), 347–355.

Gardani, G., Cerrone, R., Biella, C., Mancini, L., Proserpio, E., Casiraghi, M., . . . Lissoni, P. (2006). Effect of acupressure on nausea and vomiting induced by chemotherapy in cancer patients. *Minerva Medicine, 97*(5), 391–394.

Gill, C. I., Haldar, S., Boyd, L. A., Bennett, R., Whiteford, J., Butler, M., . . . Rowland, I. R. (2007). Watercress supplementation in diet reduces lymphocyte DNA damage and alters blood antioxidant status in healthy adults. *American Journal of Clinical Nutrition, 85*(2), 504–510.

Goodman, M. T., Wilkens, L. R., Hankin, J. H., Lyu, L. C., Wu, A. H., & Kolonel, L. N. (1997). Association of soy and fiber consumption with the risk of endometrial cancer. *American Journal of Epidemiolpgy, 146*(4), 294–306.

Irion, C. W. (1999). Growing alliums and brassicas in selenium-enriched soils increases their anticarcinogenic potentials. *Medical Hypothesis, 53*(3), 232–235.

Karageorgi, S., Gates, M. A., Hankinson, S. E., & De Vivo, I. (2010). Perineal use of talcum powder and endometrial cancer risk. *Cancer Epidemiology, Biomarkers and Prevention, 19*(5), 1269–1275.

Kohara, H., Miyauchi, T., Suehiro, Y., Ueoka, H., Takeyama, H., & Morita, T. (2004). Combined modality treatment of aromatherapy, footsoak, and reflexology relieves fatigue in patients with cancer. *Journal of Palliative Medicine, 7*(6), 791–796.

Martinez, M. E., Jacobs, E. T., Baron, J. A., Marshall, J. R., & Byers, T. (2012). Dietary supplements and cancer prevention: Balancing potential benefits against proven harms. *Journal of the National Cancer Institute, 104*(10), 732.

Melino, S., Sabelli, R., & Paci, M. (2010). Allyl sulfur compounds and cellular detoxification system: Effects and perspectives in cancer therapy. *Amino Acids, 41*(1), 103–112.

National Cancer Institute. (2010). Milk thistle. Retrieved from http://www.cancer.gov/cancertopics/pdq/cam/milkthistle

Niwa, K., Lian, Z., Onogi, K., Yan, W., Tang, L., Mori, H., & Tamaya, T. (2007). Preventive effects of glycyrrhizin on estrogen-related endometrial carcinogenesis in mice. *Oncology and Reproduction, 17*(3), 617–622.

Office of Dietary Supplements. (2005). *Dietary supplement fact sheet: Folate.* Bethesda, MD: NIH Clinical Center, National Institutes of Health. Retrieved from http://ods.od.nih.gov

Tel Aviv University. (2008, February 29). Stress and fear can affect cancer's recurrence. *ScienceDaily.* Retrieved from http://www.sciencedaily.com/releases/2008/02/080227142656.htm

University of California–San Diego. (2007a, November 16). Deficiency to exposure to sunlight linked to endometrial cancer. *ScienceDaily.* Retrieved from http://www.sciencedaily.com/releases/2007/11/071114162728.htm

University of Southern California. (2007b, September 8). Frequent alcohol consumption increases cancer risk in older women. *ScienceDaily.* Retrieved from http://www.sciencedaily.com/releases/2007/09/070907150936.htm

Vallejo, F., Tomas-Barberan, F. A., & Garcia-Viguera, C. (2003). Phenolic compounds content in edible parts of broccoli inflorescences after domestic cooking. *Journal of Science and Food Agriculture, 83*(14), 1151–1156.

Xu, W. H., Dai, Q., Xiang, Y. B., Long, J. R., Ruan, Z. X., Cheng, J. R. . . . Shu, X. O. (2007). Interaction of soy food and tea consumption with CYP19A1 genetic polymorphisms in the development of endometrial cancer. *American Journal of Epidemiology, 166*(12), 1420–1430.

Xu, W. H., Dai, Q., Xiang, Y. B., Zhao, G. M., Ruan, Z. X., Cheng, J. R. . . . Shu, X. O. (2007). Nutritional factors in relation to endometrial cancer: A report from a population-based case-control study in Shanghai. *International Journal of Cancer, 120*(8), 1776–1881.

Xu, W. H., Shrubsole, M. J., Xiang, Y. B. Cai, Q., Zhao, G. M., Ruan, Z. X., . . . Shu, X. O. (2007). Dietary folate intake, MTHFR genetic polymorphisms, and the rise. Endometrial cancer among Chinese women. *Cancer Epidemiology Biomarkers Prevention, 16*(2), 281–287.

Xu, W. H., Zheng, W., Xiang, Y. B., Ruan, Z. X., Cheng, J. R., Dai, Q., . . . Shu, X. O. (2004). Soya food intake and risk of endometrial cancer among Chinese women in Shanghai population based case-control. *British Medical Journal, 328*(7451), 1285.

Yu, Z., & Shah, D. M. (2007). Curcumin down-regulates Ets-1 and Bcl-2 expression in human endometrial carcinoma HEC-1-A cells. *Gynecology Oncology, 106*(3), 541–548.

Falls

Environment

Environmental evidence-based practice for falls includes prevention.

Environmental actions clients can take to prevent falls include using nonpharmacological approaches instead of medications associated with dizziness (benzodiazepines and sleeping pills that increase risk of daytime sedation, falls, and cognitive and psychomotor impairment), using adequate daytime lighting, wearing nonslip footwear (light-weight tie shoe with a hard rubber sole is best), sitting on the edge of the bed and assessing strength prior to standing or walking (gently massaging the arms, chest, and head can bring needed oxygen to the brain), and obtaining assistance when getting out of bed or walking as needed (having a bell by the bedside to call for help). **Cautions:** Conventional and atypical antipsychotics should not be used as they are linked with increased risk of hospitalization for femur fracture (Conn & Madan, 2006; Cooper, Freeman, Cook, & Burfield, 2007; Gerber, 2007; Liperoti et al., 2007; Rubenstein, 2006). **Health tip:** Provide clients with a bell, flashlight, walker, nonslip footwear, and/or assistance when needed. **Other considerations:** Encourage clients to carry small loads and avoid laundry baskets and large boxes, concentrate on walking, arrange furniture to accomodate wide walking areas, keep clutter and tripping hazards off the floor, anchor all rugs and carpeting and remove throw rugs without nonskid backing, install mounted handrails on indoor and outdoor steps and teach clients to use them, and keep a phone next to the bed.

Exercise/Movement

Exercise evidence-based practice for falls includes supervised group exercise and yoga.

1. *Supervised group exercise.* Supervised group exercise (3 times a week for 8–16 weeks for 30–45 minutes each session) is more effective at reducing the risk factors related to falling among older residents living in a nursing home than is unsupervised home exercise. Although education and home safety assessment improved quality of life, only exercise training led to improvements in functional reach, balance, and fear of falling. Even a modest amount of gentle exercise can improve balance (Blackwell Publishing Ltd., 2007; Donat & Ozcan, 2007; Sullivan, 2005). Exercises include a set of stretching exercises to promote flexibility, simple leg raises, marching, lifting 2-pound weights or lighter, and using sensing exercises to promote balance such as dimming the room lights and asking participants to walk slowly on a treadmill or bend over and pick up a lit flashlight. For a sample active health kit, go to http://firststepto activehealth.com/samplekit/index.htm

2. *Yoga.* Yoga poses can prevent falls in women over age 65 (Temple University, 2008). Go to /http://www.yogajournal.com/health/1634?print=1

Nutrition

Nutrition evidence-based practice for falls includes the following:

1. *Blueberries.* Study participants who ate 1 cup a day of fresh or frozen berries came out on top in tests of balance and coordination (Joseph et al., 1999) and cognitive ability (Lau, Shukitt-Hall & Joseph, 2005). It may take up to 8 weeks to see a change in balance.

2. *Omega-3 fatty acids.* A high intake of omega-3s appears to preserve bone density, keeping bones stronger and protecting against falls and fractures (Ward & Fonseca, 2007). Counsel clients to consume up to 12 ounces of ocean-grown salmon, tuna, and Spanish mackerel each week in 3–4-ounce servings (about the size the palm of the hand when cooked). Have clients dip fish in soy flour or drink soy milk to make bone tissue even stronger and protect against falls. Use olive oil for salads and cooking. Eat beans and rice several times a week, along with a serving of winter squash (orange or yellow). Use ground flaxseeds in water, drinks, soups, salads, or as a coating food for tofu prior to baking, broiling, or sautéing. **Cautions:** Advise clients to steer clear of large fish such as shark, swordfish, and tilefish, which contain more mercury. Also, have them avoid farm-fed fish, as that may be less nutritious (Norwegian School of Veterinary Science, 2008). For clients who prefer not to eat fish, other sources of omega-3s are winter squash, walnuts, olive oil, beans (pinto, black, baked, etc.), and flaxseeds.

3. *Tea.* While drinking tea, especially green tea (1–6 cups a day), is associated with increased bone mineral density and protecting against falls and fractures, coffee is negatively associated with bone strength (Muraki et al., 2007). **Cautions:** Caffeinated tea can lead to jitteriness and insomnia in susceptible individuals. Counsel clients to use decaffeinated tea. **Other considerations:** The findings about tea strengthening bones are irrespective of smoking status, use of hormone replacement therapy, coffee drinking, and whether milk was added to tea (Shen, Yeh, Cao & Wang, 2009).

Supplements

Supplement evidence-based practice concerning falls includes vitamin D.

Nursing home residents who received high amounts of vitamin D (800 IU by mouth, daily) had a lower number of falls and a lower incidence rate of falls over 5 months than those taking lower amounts (Broe et al., 2007; JAMA and Archives Journals, 2008). Because of the potential for depressing the immune system when taking vitamin D supplements, it may be preferable to recommend exposure to sunshine (Autoimmunity Research Foundation, 2008). Caucasian clients must spend 5 minutes outside at noontime, exposing the face and hands to sunshine 3 times a week provide sufficient vitamin D. (Darker-skinned clients may need up to 40 minutes in the sun.)

CASE STUDY: A COMPARISON OF EXERCISE PROGRAMS TO PREVENT FALLS

Physically inactive adults often have losses of abilities to function in daily activities. This inactivity can result in decreased muscle mass, endurance, strength, balance, and/or flexibility. These losses often contribute to falls, feelings of anxiety, low mood, and decreased self confidence. Research suggests that low to moderate level physical exercise can promote well-being and improved health for seniors. Three annual exercise programs were conducted in a community church over a 3-year period. Participants ranged from 40 to 90 years old. The majority were female. Each 4–8-week group session had 6–18 attending participants. A trained exercise leader and parish nurse facilitated each 1.5 hour session. Handouts, workbooks, and exercise videos were made available. Topics of home safety, fall prevention, nutrition, and health were discussed. Group one focused on resistance training to strengthen muscles. Group two stressed movements for balance and strength. Group three emphasized fall prevention through discussion and chair exercises. Anecdotal outcome reports of participants included the following:

1. Increased motivation to exercise.
2. Choosing to participate in prescribed physical therapy.
3. Making home safety environmental changes.
4. Increased health awareness.

Future exercise group recommendations are to:

1. Conduct individual baseline and postparticipation balance/gait assessments.
2. Include all five exercise components of movement, strength, balance, endurance, and flexibility according to ability levels.

This case study and health promotion challenge were developed by Dr. Judith Gammonley, ARNP, B.C., Ed.D. Morton Plant Mease BayCare Health System.

HEALTH PROMOTION CHALLENGE

Read the previous case study, then go to PubMed (http://www.ncbi.nlm.nih.gov/pubmed/), type "falls" in the Search box, and click on the Search button. Find three abstracts that contain information you could use to help older adults prevent falls.

SOURCES:

Bird, M. L., Hill, K., Ball, M., & Williams, A. D. (2009). Effects of resistance and flexibility exercise interventions on balance and related measures in older adults [Abstract]. *Journal of Aging and Physical Activity, 4*, 444–454.

Costello, E., & Edelstein, J. E. (2008). Update on falls prevention for community-dwelling older adults: Review of single and multifactorial intervention programs [Abstract]. *Journal of Rehabilitation Research and Development, 45*(8), 1135–1152.

Jones, T. E., Stephenson, K. W., King, J. G., Knight, K. R., Marshall, T. L., & Scott, W. B. (2009). Sarcopenia mechanisms and treatments [Abstract]. *Journal of Geriatric Physical Therapy, 32*(2) 39–45.

REFERENCES

Autoimmunity Research Foundation. (2008, January 27). Vitamin D deficiency study raises new questions about disease and supplements. *ScienceDaily*. Retrieved from http://www.sciencedaily.com/releases/2008/01/080125223302.htm

Broe, K. E., Chen, T. C., Weinberg, J., Bischoff-Ferrari, H. A., Holick, M. F., & Kiel, D. P. (2007). A higher dose of vitamin D reduces the risk of falls in nursing home residents: A randomized, multiple-dose study. *Journal of the American Geriatrics Society, 55*(2), 234–239.

Conn, D. K., & Madan, R. (2006). Use of sleep-promoting medications in nursing home residents: Risks versus benefits. *Drugs and Aging, 23*, 271–287.

Cooper, J. W., Freeman, M. H., Cook, C. L., Burfield, A. H. (2007). Assessment of psychotropic and psychoactive drug loads and falls in nursing facility residents. *Consulting Pharmacist, 22*(6), 483–489.

Donat, H., & Ozcan, A. (2007). Comparison of the effectiveness of two programmes on older adults at risk of falling: Unsupervised home exercise and supervised group exercise. *Clinical Rehabilitation, 21*(3), 272–283.

Gerber, L. (2007, July 2). Keeping clients fall-free. *Nurse.com, 7*, 19.

JAMA and Archives Journals. (2008, January 15). Vitamin D2 supplements may help prevent falls among high-risk older women. *ScienceDaily*. Retrieved from http://www.sciencedaily.com/releases/2008/01/080114162516.htm

Joseph, J. A., Shukitt-Halle, B., Denisova, N. A., Bielinksi, D., Martin, A., McEwen, J. J., & Bickford, P. C. (1999). Reversals of age-related declines in neuronal signal transduction, cognitive, and motor behavioral deficits with blueberry, spinach or strawberry dietary supplementation. *Journal of Neuroscience, 19*(18), 8114–8121.

Lau, F. C., Shukitt-Hale, B., & Joseph, J. A. (2005). The beneficial effects of fruit polyphenols on brain aging. *Neurobiology of Aging, 26*(Suppl 1), 128–132.

Liperoti, R., Onder, G., Lapane, K. L., Mor, V., Friedman, J. H., Bernabei, R., & Gambassi, G. (2007). Conventional and atypical antipsychotics and the risk of femur fracture among elderly patients: Results of a case-control study. *Journal of Clinical Psychiatry, 68*(6), 929–934.

Muraki, S., Yamamoto, S., Ishibashi, H., Oka, H., Yoshimura, N., Kawaguchi, H., & Nakamura, K. (2007). Diet and lifestyle associated with increased bone mineral density: Cross-sectional study of Japanese elderly women at an osteoporosis outpatient clinic. *Journal Orthopedic Science, 12*(4), 317–320.

Norwegian School of Veterinary Science. (2008, February 28). Farmed fish fed cheap food may be less nutritious for humans. *ScienceDaily*. Retrieved from http://www.sciencedaily.com/releases/2008/02/080226164105.htm

Rubenstein, L. A. (2006). Falls in older people: Epidemiology, risk factors and strategies for prevention. *Age and Ageing, 35*(Supplement 2), ii37–ii41.

Shen, C. L., Yeh, J. K., Cao, J. J., & Wang, J. S. (2009). Green tea and bone metabolism. *Nutrition Research, 29*(7), 437–456.

Sullivan, M. G. (2005, September). Gentle exercises can lead to improved balance. *Clinical Psychiatry News*, p. 48.

Temple University. (2008, April 8). Yoga poses can prevent falls in women over 65, study suggests. *ScienceDaily*. Retrieved from http://www.sciencedaily.com/releases/2008/04/080404114445.htm

Ward, W. E., & Fonseca, D. (2007). Soy isoflavones and fatty acids: Effects on bone tissue postovariectomy in mice. *Molecular Nutrition and Food Research, 51*(7), 824–831.

Fatigue

Environment

Environmental evidence-based practice for fatigue includes blue light.

Six hours of blue light exposure may be a countermeasure for fatigue, particularly during the night. Women exposed to blue light were able to sustain a high level of alertness during the night. **Cautions:** Blue light, if misused, can cause damage to the eye, and exposures need to be carefully monitored. Blue light for shift workers could improve safety in potentially dangerous situations that may arise due to sleepiness on the job (Harvard Medical School, 2006). For more information on blue light therapy, go to http://sleep.med.harvard .edu/news/28/Blue+Light+May+Fight+Fatigue

Exercise/Movement

Exercise/movement evidence-based practice for fatigue includes yoga, progressive walking, strength training, and stretching.

Yoga, progressive walking, and simple strength training movements and stretching activities can relieve fatigue (Flegal, Kishiyama, Zajdel, Haas, & Oken, 2007; Ingram & Visovsky, 2007; Rooks et al., 2007). **Cautions:** Counsel clients to work their way into an exercise program, always using warm-ups prior to and after exercising See http://yoga.lifetips.com/cat/56770/yoga-cautions/ **Other considerations:** For more information on exercise, go to http://exercise .lifetips.com

Herbs/Essential Oils

Herbal evidence-based practice for fatigue includes garlic.

Garlic (one 1 clove by mouth daily) produces symptomatic improvement in women with fatigue, systematic fatigue due to cold, or lassitude of indefinite cause (Morihara et al., 2007). **Cautions:** Garlic can stimulate labor so it should be avoided by pregnant women. Garlic can also increase clotting time and irritate stomach inflammation. The herb should not be used by women hypersensitive to garlic. Drugs that may interact with garlic include anticoagulants, although aged garlic extract is relatively safe and poses no serious hemorrhagic risk when closely monitored during use of warfarin therapy (Macan et al., 2006), insulin, oral antidiabetes agents, and oral contraceptives. *Acidophilus* can decrease the absorption of garlic. Separate the 2 by 3 hours for best absorption (Skidmore-Roth, 2006).

Mind-Set

Mind-set evidence-based practice for fatigue includes cognitive behavioral therapy (CBT).

CBT for 8 weekly sessions is a clinically effective treatment for fatigue. Both CBT and relaxation training (RT) are clinically effective treatments, although the effects for CBT are greater than those for RT. Even after 6 months, both treatment groups reported levels of fatigue equivalent to those of the healthy comparison group (Van Kessel et al., 2008). For more information on RT, go to http://www.alternateheals.com/relaxation-therapy/home-relaxation-treatments.htm and http://www.mind.org.uk/Information/Booklets/Making+Sense/MakingSenseCBT.htm

Nutrition

Nutrition evidence-based practice for fatigue includes recommending clients eat fruits and vegetables.

Eating a healthy diet of 10 half-cup servings of fruits and vegetables and omega-3 and -6 fatty acids can provide needed vitamins and minerals and reduce fatigue (Huskisson, Maggini & Ruf, 2007; Yehuda, Rabinovitz, Mostofsky, 2005). For information on how to use telephone counseling, newsletters, and recipes to help clients change eating habits, go to http://www.healthyeating ucsd.org/pages/whelStudy.htm. For a discussion and listing of fatty acids, go to http://www.ific.org/publications/factsheets/omega3fs.cfm.

Touch

Women who received acupressure with massage (12 minutes per day, 3 days per week, for 4 weeks) showed significantly greater improvement in reducing fatigue than women who did not receive the treatment (Cho & Tsay, 2004).

FATIGUE CASE STUDY

Ms. Atchison, age 36, complains of fatigue even after a good night's sleep. She has chronic fatigue that has persisted for years. In addition to fatigue, she also complains of weakness, muscle aches and pains, excessive sleep, fever, sore throat, and impaired memory.

HEALTH PROMOTION CHALLENGE

Using the evidence in this section, develop a nursing care plan and teaching plan for Ms. Atchison.

REFERENCES

Cho, Y. C., & Tsay, S. L. (2004). The effect of acupressure with massage on fatigue and depression in patients with end-stage renal disease. *Journal of Nursing Research, 12*(1), 51–59.

Flegal, K. E., Kishiyama, S., Zajdel, D., Haas, M., & Oken, B. S. (2007). Adherence to yoga and exercise intervention in a 6-month clinical trial. *BMC Complementary and Alternative Medicine, 9*, 37.

Harvard Medical School. (2006). Blue light may fight fatigue. Retrieved from https://sleep.med .harvard.edu/news/28/Blue+Light+May+Fight+Fatigue

Huskisson, E., Maggini, S., & Ruf, M. (2007). The role of vitamins and minerals in energy metabolism and well-being. *Journal of International Medical Research, 35*(3), 277–289.

Ingram, C., & Visovsky, C. (2007). Exercise intervention to modify physiologic risk factors in cancer survivors. *Seminars in Oncology Nursing, 23*(4), 275–284.

Macan, H., Uykimpang, R., Alconcel, M. Takasu, J., Razon, R., Amagase, H., & Niihara, Y. (2006). Aged garlic extract may be safe for patients on warfarin therapy. *Journal of Nutrition, 136*(3 Suppl), 793S–795S.

Morihara, N., Nishihama, T., Ushijima, M., Ide, N., Takeda, H., & Hayama, M. (2007). Garlic as an anti-fatigue agent. *Molecular Nutrition and Food Research, 51*(11), 1329–1334.

Rooks, D. S., Gautam, S., Romeling, M., Cross, M. L., Stratigakis, D., Evans, B., . . . Katz, J. N. (2007). Group exercise, education, and combination self-management in women with fibromyalgia: A randomized trial. *Archives of Internal Medicine, 167*(20), 2192–3000.

Skidmore-Roth, L. (2006). Garlic. In *Mosby's handbook of herbs & natural supplements* (pp. 471–477). St. Louis, MO: ElsevierMosby.

Van Kessel, K., Moss-Morris R., Wiloughby, E., Chalder, T., Johnson, M. H., & Robinson, E. (2008). A randomized controlled trial of cognitive behavior therapy for multiple sclerosis fatigue. *Psychosomatic Medicine, 70*(2), 205–213.

Yehuda, S., Rabinovitz, S., & Mostofsky, D. I. (2005). Mixture of essential fatty acids lowers test anxiety. *Nutrition and Neuroscience, 8*(4), 265–267.

Fibroids

Environment

Environmental evidence-based practice for fibroids includes avoiding perineal talc.

Researchers conclude that nonhormonal factors influence risk of uterine fibroids, including use of talc powder on the perineum. Risk of uterine leiomyoma (fibroids) is associated in a graded fashion with the frequency of perineal talc use. No use is best (Faerstein, Szklo & Rosenshein, 2001). **Cautions:** Counsel women not to use talc powder on their perineum and that each time they do, they increase their risk for fibroids. Corn starch is a good alternative to using talc.

Exercise

Evidence-based practice for fibroids includes exercise.

Exercise may help prevent fibroids. Regular exercise, daily if possible, is best (Baird, Dunson, Hill, Cousins, & Schectman, 2007).

Nutrition

Nutrition evidence-based practice for fibroids includes soy.

Soy (preferably 1–2 servings per day) may block leiomyoma (fibroid) cell growth (Shushan, Ben-Bassat, Mishani, Laufer, & Klein, 2007).

Touch

Touch evidence-based practice for fibroids includes Chinese approaches.

Of 37 women with symptomatic fibroids treated with acupuncture, Chinese herbs, nutritional therapy, pelvic body work, meditation, and guided imagery, 22 saw their fibroids disappear, shrink, or stay stable compared with only 32 in 37 who received the conventional hormonal manipulation and nonsteroidal anti-inflammatory medication (Mehl-Madrona, 2002).

FIBROIDS CASE STUDY

Mrs. Wilcox, age 40, 185 pounds, is experiencing very heavy and frequent menstrual periods. In a concerned voice, she told the nurse that the bleeding lasted as long as 7 days and was occurring every 2 weeks. She was using 8 or more pads a day and had noticed that she was passing clots. She also felt quite tired. Her condition was distressing enough to interfere with her ability to function at home and at her job as a data analyst for a computer company.

The nurse told her about having a hysterectomy—surgical removal of the entire uterus—as one of her options. The nurse also told her abdominal surgery is much riskier in patients who are as heavy as Mrs. Wilcox. There is a greater chance of damage to other pelvic tissues and organs during the procedure. Afterwards, there is a risk of serious bleeding, phlebitis, or improper healing of the wounds. Mrs. Wilcox asked what other options she had.

HEALTH PROMOTION CHALLENGE

What would you tell Mrs. Wilcox? Based on information in this section as well as what you can find by going to PubMed (http://www.ncbi.nlm.nih.gov /pubmed/) and searching for fibroids, compose a response and a teaching plan, if necessary.

REFERENCES

Baird, D. D., Dunson, D. B., Hill, M. C., Cousins, D., & Schectman, J. M. (2007). Association of physical activity with development of uterine leiomyoma. *American Journal of Epidemiology, 165*(2), 157–163.

Faerstein, E., Szklo, M., & Rosenshein, N. B. (2001). Risk factors for uterine leiomyoma: A practice-based case-control study. II. *American Journal of Epidemiology, 153*(1), 11–19.

Mehl-Madrona, L. (2002). Complementary medicine treatment of uterine fibroids: A pilot study. *Alternative Therapies in Health and Medicine, 8*(2), 38–40, 44–46.

Shushan, A., Ben-Bassat, H., Mishani, E., Laufer, N., & Klein, B. Y. (2007). Inhibition of leiomyoma cell proliferation in vitro by genistein and the protein tyrosine kinase inhibitor TKS050. *Fertility and Sterilization, 87*(1), 127–135.

Gastric Cancer

Environment

Environmental evidence-based practice for gastric cancer includes:

1. *Agricultural exposures.* Gastric cancer in Hispanic farm workers in California is associated with work in the citrus fruit industry and among those who work in fields treated with 2, 4-D; chlordane; propargite; and trifluin. **Other considerations:** These findings may have larger public health implications, especially in those areas of the country where these pesticides are heavily used and where they may be found in the ambient atmosphere (Mills & Yang, 2007).

2. *Aromatherapy.* Inhalation or skin application of chamomile, geranium, and lavender essential oils has been shown to reduce anxiety and depression related to cancer and can enhance quality of life (Wilkinson et al., 2007). **Other considerations:** Suggest clients either inhale a specific essential oil(s) or add a few drops to bath oil or pillow.

3. *CT scans.* CT scans could be responsible for raising the risk of cancer. A typical CT scan delivers 50 to 100 times more radiation than a conventional X-ray (Brenner & Hall, 2007). **Cautions:** Brenner and Hall estimate that one-third of all CT scans might not be necessary. Suggest the safer options of ultrasound and magnetic resonance imaging, which do not expose clients to radiation.

4. *Hexavalent chromium in drinking water.* Hexavalent chromium (Cr+6) in drinking water is linked with all cancers (Beaumont et al., 2008; Sedman et al., 2006). **Cautions:** Counsel clients to have their drinking water checked by a reliable source. As a preventive measure, advise clients to drink and use either distilled water or water that has passed through a reverse-osmosis water filter. **Other considerations:**

Cr+6 has been found in 38% of municipal sources of drinking water in California and is widely used in electroplating, stainless steel production, leather tanning, textile manufacturing, and wood preservation in the United States, which is the greatest producer of chromium compounds. For more information, go to http://ntp.niehs.nih.gov/files /NTPHexaVChrmFactR5.pdf

Herbs/Essential Oils

Herbal evidence-based practice for gastric cancer includes aloe vera and basil leaf.

1. *Aloe vera (cape aloe).* Aloe vera is an anti-inflammatory, antibacterial, antifungal protective for the liver and inhibits growth of tumors when 1–3 ounces are consumed three times a day after meals (Kametani et al., 2008). Advise clients to only buy aloe vera gel from a health food store, to buy the herb in a glass container if possible, and to never drink the juice or gel from home aloe plants because that can lead to diarrhea. Other considerations: Aloe contains vitamins A, B-complex, E, carboxypeptidase (anti-inflammatory enzyme), magnesium, potassium, calcium, magnesium, manganese, copper, zinc, chromium, iron, glucomannans (immunomodulator), saponins (antiseptic), anthraquinone (aids absorption in the gastrointestinal tract), salicylic acid (anti-inflammatory), and amino acids (protein building blocks) (Skidmore-Roth, 2006a).

2. *Basil leaf.* Basil leaf extract has tumor inhibition and immune-stimulant characteristics. It is taken by mouth, either fresh or powdered as a spice in food (Dasgupta, Rao, & Yadava, 2004). **Cautions:** Warn pregnant women not to take basil in large amounts; dietary uses are safe. Basil can have mutagenic effects on fetuses. Clients diagnosed with diabetes should use basil cautiously, as it can increase the hypoglycemic effects of insulin and oral antidiabetes agents; advise clients not to use concurrently (Skidmore-Roth, 2006b). **Other considerations:** Because of its mutagen ability, advise clients to avoid using basil for long periods of time.

Nutrition

Nutritional evidence-based practice for gastric cancer includes the following:

1. *Folate.* Dietary folates are protective against cancer, but folic acid fortification is associated with cancer. Because national surveys revealed most Americans did not consume adequate folate, a grain fortification program is in place (Blackwell Publishing, 2007). Leafy green vegetables (like spinach and turnip greens), broccoli, fruits (citrus fruits

and juices), and dried beans and peas are all natural sources of folate that can help meet the suggested amount of 1,000 micrograms a day. Clients who do not eat breads, cereals, or pasta; who abuse alcohol; or who take medications that interfere with folate absorption may not receive sufficient amounts of the nutrient and may need additional amounts (Office of Dietary Supplements, 2005). **Cautions:** Medications and medical conditions that increase the need for folate or result in an increased excretion of folate include anticonvulsant medications, metformin, sulfasalazine, triamterene, methotrexate, barbiturates, pregnancy and lactation, alcohol abuse, malabsorption, kidney dialysis, liver disease, certain anemias. Because folate is a water-soluble B-vitamin, unneeded amounts will be eliminated in the urine. Advise clients to avoid flour-fortified foods as a source of folic acid; new research has shown the introduction of flour fortified with folic acid into common foods has been linked to cancer (Blackwell Publishing, 2007). **Other considerations:** Exceeding 1,000 micrograms per day of folate may trigger vitamin B_{12} deficiency. To compensate, clients can take a multivitamin that contains B_{12} or eat at least one food daily that contains B_{12}, such as nutritional yeast (unless susceptible to *Candida*), clams, eggs, herring, kidney, liver, mackerel, seafood, and milk or dairy products.

2. *Fruit, vegetables, and whole grains.* Fruit, vegetable and whole grain consumption (5–10 servings a day) is linked to a decreased risk for cancers. Consuming one serving of raw tomatoes per week reduced the risk of all cancers by 50% for older women (Friedman et al., 2007). Watercress is linked to a reduced risk of cancer via decreased damage to DNA (Gill et al., 2007). For more information, go to http://www.cooks.com/rec /ch/vegetables.html **Other considerations:** Fruits and vegetables contain a plethora of anticarcinogenic substances including carotenoids, vitamins C and E, selenium, dietary fiber, flavonoids, polyphenols, and many other health-producing compounds. Grains to avoid: cornflakes, enriched macaroni or spaghetti, couscous, grits, pretzels, white bread, rye bread, and white rice (Hord, 2005).

3. *Green tea.* Two to five cups of decaffeinated tea daily is protective against cancer before disease occurs and after onset, possibly by creating a detoxifying effect (American Association for Cancer Research, 2007). **Cautions:** Green tea may decrease iron absorption, so separate iron-rich foods or iron pills by at least 2 hours from green tea ingestion. Caffeinated green tea can interact with MAOIs and lead to a hypertensive crisis. Counsel clients not to take green tea with anticoagulants/ antiplatelets (may increase risk of bleeding), beta-adrenergic blockers (can lead to increased inotropic effects), or benzodiazepines (may increase sedation). (Skidmore-Roth, 2006c). **Other considerations:** Dairy products may decrease the therapeutic effects of green tea so

advise clients to separate their intake by several hours. Digestive process affects anticancer activity of tea in gastrointestinal cells; have clients add citrus (such as lemon juice) or have them take ascorbic acid (vitamin C) to protect the catechins in green tea from digestive degradation (Federation of American Societies for Experimental Biology, 2008).

4. *Maitake mushrooms.* Animal and human studies have supported the use of maitake MD-fraction for cancer (Masuda et al., 2009). This mushroom is an immune modulator that helps to normalize the immune system (Kodama, Komuta, & Nanba, 2002). **Cautions:** Advise clients to avoid maitake mushrooms if they are sensitive to this food. They may interact with immunosuppressants and antidiabetes agents. Advise clients to store maitake in a clean, dry place, away from moisture and heat. For recipes and ways to use maitake, go to http://theforagerpress .com/fieldguide/maitake/maitake-recipes.htm **Other considerations:** Maitake and other mushrooms have been used for thousands of years in Asia for many purposes. Maitake is also available in capsules or as an extract.

5. *Red and processed meat; onions and garlic.* Advise clients to avoid red and processed meat and increase intake of onions and garlic raw and cooked, as tolerated. Baked or broiled, they go well with vegetable burgers and vegetables; raw and diced, they make a salad tasty. Consumption of red and processed meat is positively associated with noncardia stomach cancer, while onions and garlic reduce the risk of stomach cancer (Gonzalez & Riboli, 2006). **Other considerations:** Garlic and onions are toxic for many animals. Counsel clients to keep garlic and onions away from their pets.

Stress Management

Stress management evidence-based practice for gastric cancer strengthens the immune system.

A weak immune system is one of the major factors that promotes cancer metastases after an operation, chemotherapy, or radiation therapy. Fear and stress weaken the immune system. Adequate stress management prior to and after medical treatment may help to prevent metastases (Tel Aviv University, 2008). For teaching materials, go to http://www.mindfulnessmeditationcentre. org/breathingGathas.htm

Supplements

Supplement evidence-based practice for gastric cancer includes beta-carotene, vitamin E, and selenium.

Daily supplementation of beta-carotene, vitamin E, and selenium reduced gastric cancer incidence, mortality, and overall cancer mortality in poorly nourished women (Huang, 2006). **Other considerations:** It is usually safer to obtain vitamins and minerals from food. Sources of beta-carotene include: sweet potatoes, carrots, kale, spinach, turnip greens, winter squash, collard greens, cilantro, and fresh thyme. Food sources of vitamin E include sunflower seeds, almonds, filberts, turnip greens, tomato paste, pine nuts, peanut butter, wheat germ, avocados, carrot juice, olive oil, spinach, dandelion greens, sardines, blue crab, Brazil nuts, and pickled herring. Food sources of selenium include Brazil nuts (dried, unblanched), light tuna (canned in oil, drained), cooked beef, spaghetti with meat sauce, cod (cooked), turkey (light meat, roasted), beef chuck roast (lean only, roasted), chicken breast (meat only, roasted), egg (whole), and oatmeal.

GASTRIC CANCER CASE STUDY

Ms. Jameson, age 21, talks to you about her family and tells you her father, uncle, aunt, and cousin died of stomach cancer. Although she has no symptoms, she is afraid she might develop gastric cancer too, and asks you if she should have her stomach surgically removed so she will not get cancer. She also asks if there are alternatives.

HEALTH PROMOTION CHALLENGE

Based on the information in this section on gastric cancer and studies you find by searching PubMed (http://www.ncbi.nlm.nih.gov/pubmed/), come up with an answer for Ms. Jameson and any related teaching/learning materials.

REFERENCES

American Association for Cancer Research. (2007, August 12). Green tea boosts production of detox enzymes, rendering cancerous chemicals harmless. Retrieved from http://www.sciencedaily.com/releases/2007/08/070810194923.htm

Beaumont, J. J., Sedman, R. M., Reynolds, S. D., Sherman, C. D., Li, L. H., Howd, R. A., . . . Alexeeff, G. V. (2008). Cancer mortality in a Chinese population exposed to hexavalent chromium in drinking water. *Epidemiology, 19*(1), 12–23.

Blackwell Publishing Ltd. (2007, November 5). Folic acid linked to increased cancer rate, historical review suggests. *ScienceDaily*. Retrieved from http://www.sciencedaily.com/releases/2007/11/07/071102111956.htm

Brenner, D., & Hall, E. J. (2007). Computed tomography, an increasing source of radiation exposure. *New England Journal of Medicine, 357*(22), 2277–2284.

Dasgupta, T., Rao, A. R., & Yadava, P. K. (2004). Chemomodulatory efficacy of basil leaf on drug metabolizing and antioxidant enzymes, and on carcinogen-induced skin and forestomach papillomagenesis. *Phytomedicine, 11*(2–3), 139–151.

Federation of American Societies for Experimental Biology. (2008, April 10). Digestive process affects anti-cancer activity of tea in gastrointestinal cells. *ScienceDaily.* Retrieved from http://www.sciencedaily.com/releases/2008/04/080407172713.htm

Friedman, M., Levin, C. E., Lee, S. U., Kim, H. J., Lee, I. S., Byun, J. O., & Kozukue, N. (2009). Tomatine-containing green tomato extracts inhibit growth of human breast, colon, liver, and stomach cancer cells. *Journal of Agricultural and Food Chemistry, 57*(13), 5727.

Gill, C. I., Haldar, S., Boyd, L. A., Bennett, R., Whiteford, J., Butler, M., . . . Rowland, I. R. (2007). Watercress supplementation in diet reduces lymphocyte DNA damage and alters blood antioxidant status in healthy adults. *American Journal of Clinical Nutrition, 85*(2), 504–510.

Gonzalez, C. A., & Riboli, E. (2006). Diet and cancer prevention: Where we are, where we are going. *Nutrition in Cancer, 56*(2), 225–231.

Hord, N. G. (2005). The role of dietary factors in cancer prevention: Beyond fruits and vegetables. *Nutrition in Clinical Practice, 20*(4), 451–459.

Huang, H. Y., Caballero, B., Chang, S., Alberg, A., Semba, R., Schneyer, C., . . . Bass, E. B. (2006). Multivitamin/mineral supplements and prevention of chronic disease. *Evidence Reports and Technology Assessments 139,* 1–117.

Kodama, N., Komuta, K., & Nanba, H. (2002). Can maitake MD-fraction aid cancer patients? *Alternative Medical Review, 7*(3), 236–239.

Masuda, Y., Matsumoto, A, Toida T., Oikawa. T., Ito, K., & Nanba, H. (2009). Characterization and antitumor effect of a novel polysaccharide from *Grifola frondosa. Journal of Agricultural and Food Chemistry, 57*(21), 10143–10149.

Mills, P. K., & Yang, R. C. (2007). Agricultural exposures and gastric cancer risk in Hispanic farm workers in California. *Environmental Research, 104*(2), 282–289.

Office of Dietary Supplements. (2005). *Dietary supplement fact sheet: Folate.* Bethesda, MD: NIH Clinical Center. National Institutes of Health. Available at http://ods.od.nih.gov

Sedman, R. M., Beaumont, J., McDonald, T. A., Reynolds, S., Krowech, G., & Howd, R. (2006). Review of the evidence regarding the carcinogenicity hexavalent chromium in drinking water. *Journal of Environmental Science and Health Part C, 24*(1), 155–182.

Skidmore-Roth, L. (2006a). Aloe. In *Mosby's handbook of herbs & natural supplements* (pp. 30–35). St. Louis, MO: ElsevierMosby.

Skidmore-Roth, L. (2006b). Basil. In *Mosby's handbook of herbs & natural supplements* (pp. 84–88). St. Louis, MO: ElsevierMosby.

Skidmore-Roth, L. (2006c). Green tea. In *Mosby's handbook of herbs & natural supplements* (pp. 535–539). St. Louis, MO: ElsevierMosby.

Tel Aviv University. (2008, February 29). Stress and fear can affect cancer's recurrence. *ScienceDaily.* Retrieved from http://www.sciencedaily.com/releases/2008/02/080227142656.htm

Wilkinson, S. M., Love, S. B., Westcombe, A. M., Gambles, M. A., Burgess, C. C., & Cargill, A. (2007). Effectiveness of aromatherapy massage in the management of anxiety and depression in patients with cancer: A multicenter randomized controlled trial. *Journal of Clinical Oncology, 25*(5), 532–539.

Heart/Blood Vessels

Environment

Environmental evidence-based practice for heart/blood vessels includes social support and sunshine.

1. *Social support.* Casting a wide net when it comes to friends and family appears to be associated with a dramatically lower risk of suffering a heart attack, landing in a hospital, or dying from heart disease (Ross, 2005). Counsel clients to join a group or class focused on a valued activity. Church or recreational or work groups may also provide friendship opportunities.

2. *Sunshine.* Vitamin D from sun exposure may protect against cardiovascular disease. (American Heart Association, 2008; Jockers, 2007; Martins et al., 2007). Taking vitamin D supplements may not be the answer (Autoimmunity Research Foundation, 2008).

Exercise/Movement

Exercise/movement evidence-based practice for heart/blood vessels includes the following:

1. *Aerobic exercise.* Training consisting of a 10-minute warm-up, exercise on a stationary bicycle, followed by 35 minutes of fast walking and jogging can decrease cardiovascular risk (Blumenthal et al., 2005). **Cautions:** Only clients with stable ischemic heart disease should participate in such intense exercise. Computer-generated phone calls may be an effective, low-cost way to encourage sedentary adults to exercise as well as stand instead of sitting while performing household chores, shopping, typing, and more (University of Missouri-Columbia, 2007; Stanford University Medical Center, 2007). For information on warm-ups and cool-downs prior to and after exercising, go to http://www.wellness.ma/adult-fitness/stretching-warmup.htm **Other considerations:** Even moderate exercise can reduce the incidence of and length of rehabilitation from cardiovascular diseases by 49% (Kruk, 2007) and lower LDL cholesterol (Kodama et al., 2007).

2. *Sports participation.* Participating in sports at least once a week reduces the risk of developing a blood clot in a lung artery by 46% and a blood clot in a leg vein by 24% (Blackwell Publishing Ltd., 2007). **Cautions:** Go to http://www.lasting-weight-loss.com/dangers.html **Other considerations:** Obese clients (with a body mass index of 30 or greater) who did not participate in sports were more than four times as likely to develop a blood clot than lean clients (with a body mass index of less than 25) (Blackwell Publishing Ltd., 2007).

3. *Resistance training.* Clients with chronic congestive heart failure (CHF) must maintain and/or increase muscle mass and strength. Dynamic resistance exercise is well tolerated in chronic stable CHF when (1) initial contraction intensity is low, (2) small muscle groups are involved, (3) work phases are kept short, (4) a small number of repetitions per set is performed, and (5) the work/rest ratio is ≥ 1:2. With resistance training programs lasting 12 weeks, maximal strength could be improved by 15–50%. No differences were found between combined resistance/aerobic training and resistance training alone. Thus, resistance exercise can be assumed to be as safe as aerobic exercise in clinically stable CHF (Meyer, 2006). For information on strength training, go to http://www2 .gsu.edu/~wwwfit/strength.html **Other considerations:** By following a 12-week resistance program, maximum exercise time and peak Vo2 were between 10% and 18% (Meyer, 2006).

4. *Tai chi.* Tai chi class participation twice weekly for 1 hour improved quality of life in clients with heart failure, increased results on a 6-minute walk test, and improved B-type natriuretic peptide levels in women with heart failure more than a control group in a study by Kirn (2004). For directions on tai chi, go to http://www.everyday-taichi.com/ tai-chi-instruction.html

5. *Yoga.* The practice of Hatha yoga in a 30–60-minute-per-week class or by using a yoga tape (search the Internet) can improve strength and flexibility and may help control such physiological variables as blood pressure, respiration and heart rate, and metabolic rate to improve overall exercise capacity for clients with cardiopulmonary disease (Pullen et al., 2008; Raub, 2002). **Cautions:** Go to http://yoga.lifetips.com /cat/56770/yoga-cautions/ For more information about yoga, go to http://www.yogajournal.com/video/173

Herbs/Essential Oils

Herbal evidence-based practice for heart and blood vessels includes the following:

1. *Chamomile tea.* Drinking 1–2 cups of chamomile tea a day shows significant antiplatelet activity in vitro. Animal model studies indicate potent anti-inflammatory action and cholesterol-lowering activities, as well as antispasmodic and anxiolytic effects (McKay & Blumberg, 2006). **Cautions:** Advise clients to avoid chamomile tea if they are sensitive to flowers. Advise clients to avoid concurrent use of chamomile with anticoagulants and central nervous system depressants. Clients must avoid chamomile tea during pregnancy; it is a known abortifacient.

2. *Fenugreek.* A cup of fenugreek tea daily for up to 6 weeks can lower blood lipid levels, reduce LDL cholesterol, and improve blood vessels

and circulation (Xue et al., 2007). **Cautions:** This herb rapidly coats the intestinal system and may reduce absorption of medications used concurrently. Counsel pregnant women not to use fenugreek; it may cause premature labor.

3. *Garlic.* One half to one clove of garlic per day has been associated with anticlotting, cholesterol lowering, and reducing the atherogenic properties of cholesterol (Tapsell, et al., 2006; Zahid, Hussain & Fahim, 2005). **Cautions:** Large amounts of garlic can stimulate labor and cause colic in infants. Dietary amounts are safe. Avoid using prior to surgery as garlic can increase clotting time. **Other considerations:** Garlic can replace less desirable ingredients such as salt, sugar, and added saturated fat in marinades and dressings, stir-fry dishes, casseroles, soups, curries, and Mediterranean-style dishes.

4. *Flax.* In one study, 22 hyperlipidemic (elevated cholesterol) men and 7 postmenopausal hyperlipidemic women participated in a randomized, crossover trial. Participants were given flaxseed (experimental group) or wheat bran (control group) muffins. The flaxseed muffins effectively lowered LDL cholesterol while the wheat bran muffins did not. Other studies have confirmed that the addition of flax to the diet reduces risk for coronary artery disease (Bassett et al., 2011), thrombotic disorders (Sano et al., 2003), and cerbrovascular accident (Prasad, 2005).

5. *Green tea.* Consumption of 2–3 cups of green tea a day (preferably noncaffeinated) is associated with improved myocardial function and reduced mortality due to cardiovascular disease (Hirai et al., 2007; Kuri-yama et al., 2006).

6. *Hawthorn.* At 100 to 250 mg t.i.d., hawthorn produces a significant benefit in symptom control and physiologic outcomes as a treatment for chronic heart failure (Pittler, Guo, & Ernst, 2008). **Cautions:** Advise clients to avoid hawthorn if they are sensitive to it or if they are pregnant or lactating. Adverse effects to watch for include low blood pressure, arrhythmias, fatigue, nausea, vomiting, and loss of appetite. Hawthorn may increase the effects of antihypertensives, cardiac glycosides, and central nervous system depressants; advise clients to avoid using these concurrently with hawthorn. This herb may increase the absorption of iron salts; clients should separate iron salts and hawthorn by 2 hours (Skidmore-Roth, 2006c). **Other considerations:** Hawthorn increases blood supply to the heart, increases the force of contractions, and indirectly inhibits angiotensin-converting enzyme (ACE). The herb also stabilizes collagen, reduces atherosclerosis, and decreases cholesterol (Pittler, Guo & Ernst, 2008).

Mind-Set

Mind-set evidence-based practice for heart and blood vessels includes cognitive behavioral therapy (CBT).

An 8-week program of individual CBT improves post-coronary artery bypass graft surgery depression in women (DeRubeis, Hollon, & Amsterdam, 2005). For more information on CBT, go to the National Association of Cognitive-Behavioral Therapists, website, at www.nacbt.org/whatiscbt.htm

Nutrition

Nutritional evidence-based practice for heart and blood vessels includes the following:

1. *Animal protein; antioxidant foods.* Antioxidants prevent cardiovascular disease naturally, and cholesterol changes can be made through dietary changes alone (Gardner et al., 2005; University of Michigan Health System, 2008). Heme iron from red meat, fish, and poultry is associated with heart disease (Qi, van Dam, Rexrode, & Hu, 2007) as are ham, salami, and butter, but not eggs (Djousse & Gaziano, 2008).

   Foods containing high amounts of heart-protective antioxidants include beans (small red, kidney, pinto, and black); fruits (apples with peels, berries, avocados, cherries, green and red pears, fresh or dried plums, pineapple, oranges, and kiwi); vegetables (artichokes, spinach, red cabbage, red and white potatoes with peels, sweet potatoes, and broccoli); green tea; nuts (especially walnuts, pistachios, pecans, hazelnuts, and almonds); oats; ground cloves, cinnamon, or ginger; dried oregano leaf; and turmeric powder (Jenkins et al., 2003). Encourage clients to eat 5–10 servings of fruits and vegetables/day. **Other considerations:** A low-fat diet rich in vegetables, fruits, whole grains, and beans has twice the cholesterol-lowering power as a conventional low-fat diet. Apples, berries, and onions are especially associated with reduced risk of coronary heart disease because they contain quercetin. The American Heart Association adds soy protein and nuts to round out an eating regimen found to be as effective as taking statin medication, and with none of the side effects. The more soy isoflavones clients eat, the lower their risk for cerebral and myocardial infarctions (Kokubo et al., 2007). Eating soy as tempeh allows for higher protein digestibility (Lee, Park, Choi, Ha, & Ryu, 2007).

2. *Calcium foods.* Foods high in calcium increase the "good" (HDL) cholesterol (Drouillet et al., 2007). Suggest clients eat at least a half a cup daily of the following foods to enhance calcium intake: soy drinks, tofu, soybeans, sardines, collards, spinach, turnip greens, ocean perch, and oatmeal. Advise clients to take several tablespoons of blackstrap molasses

a day. It can be placed in drinks, used instead of sugar in cooking or baking, or eaten off the spoon; it is also high in iron.

3. *Cinnamon.* Two and a half teaspoons of cinnamon (used as a spice in a bowl of oatmeal, other cereal, or rice) lowers total cholesterol and triacylgycerol levels (Bjorgell & Almer, 2007; Skidmore-Roth, 2006a).

4. *Coffee, tea and soft drinks.* Green tea is associated with a lowered heart disease risk (even for smokers), lowers the "bad" cholesterol, increases the heart-protective HDL cholesterol, and can reduce the risk of cardiovascular disease in diabetes, with a significant improvement in lipid metabolism (Anandh Babu, Sabitha, & Shyamaladevi, 2006; Chacko, Thambi, Kuttan, & Nishigaki, 2010; Kapoor, 2008). Coffee (black or decaffeinated) elevates cholesterol. Habitual coffee consumption is associated with heightened acute inflammatory response to mental stress in the blood vessels (Hamer, Eilliams, Vuononvirta, Gibson, & Steptoe, 2006), and elevated cholesterol (Baylor College of Medicine, 2007). Use of soft drinks is linked to increase in risk factors for heart disease, including obesity (American Heart Association, 2007). **Cautions:** Caffeinated green tea should not be used by clients with hypersensitivity to green tea or by those with kidney inflammation, gastrointestinal ulcers, insomnia, cardiovascular disease, or increased intraocular pressure. High doses of caffeinated green tea can result in palpitations and irregular heartbeat, anxiety, nervousness, insomnia, nausea, and heartburn, and it increases stomach acid. The decaffeinated form may be a better choice for these reasons (Skidmore-Roth, 2006b). **Other considerations:** Antacids may decrease the therapeutic effects of green tea, and green tea may interact with anticoagulants/antiplatelets, increasing risk of bleeding. Advise clients to avoid drinking green tea while taking MAOIs or bronchodilators (Skidmore-Roth, 2006b).

5. *Magnesium-rich foods.* Magnesium has been shown to significantly decrease plasma lipids such as cholesterol, triglycerides, and phospholipids (Obarzanek et al., 2010; Takeda & Nakamura, 2008). Counsel clients to eat magnesium-rich foods including 1 ounce of roasted pumpkin and squash seeds, almonds, Brazil nuts, pine nuts, or bran cereal; 3 ounces of halibut or tuna; half cup cooked spinach, soybeans, black or white beans, artichoke hearts, lima beans, and beet greens.

6. *Pomegranate juice.* An ounce of pomegranate juice a day may improve stress-induced myocardial ischemia in clients who have coronary heart disease (Sumner et al., 2005). **Cautions:** Pomegranate is an abortifacient; caution women not to use during the first trimester of pregnancy. Pomegranate should also not be used by clients who are hypersensitive to it.

7. *Sucrose.* Table sugar, also called sucrose, is found in many desserts, sodas, and other sweet products. Sucrose and sucrose-laden sweets are

significantly correlated with blood lipid levels known to increase cardiovascular disease risk (Welsh et al., 2010).

8. *Trans fat, low fat, low carbohydrate diets.* High trans fat consumption is a significant risk factor for coronary heart disease. Low-fat diets are more effective in preserving and promoting a healthy cardiovascular system than low-carbohydrate, Atkins-like diets, which are high in saturated fats and dietary cholesterol. The more trans fat consumed, the more detrimental the diet is to heart health, putting the dieter at risk of atherosclerosis (hardening of the arteries) because low-carbohydrate diets do not contain enough folic acid to lower homocysteine (Medical College of Wisconsin, 2008; Sun et al., 2008). Counsel clients to read labels carefully and avoid partially hydrogenated vegetable oils, which are produced by the food industry to create solid fats from liquid oils to increase the shelf life of products; examples include margarines; high-fat baked goods, especially doughnuts, cookies, and cakes; and any product that has a label that says, "partially hydrogenated vegetables oils." Assess intake of an Atkins-like diet. **Other considerations:** French fries and potato chips may also contain partially hydrogenated vegetable oils.

9. *Turmeric (curcumin).* Turmeric, eaten as a spice, can prevent heart failure, relax blood vessels, and reduce the atherogenic properties of cholesterol (Anand, Kunnumakkara, Newman & Aggarwal, 2007; Morimoto et al., 2008).

10. *Walnuts, pecans, and olive oil.* Walnuts and olive oil lessen the sudden inflammation and oxidation in the arteries after a meal of animal fat, including a salami and cheese sandwich and full-fat yogurt (Cortez et al., 2006). Pecans may inhibit unwanted oxidation of blood lipids, helping reduce the risk of heart disease (Halton et al., 2006). **Other considerations:** Walnuts preserve the elasticity and flexibility of the arteries, regardless of cholesterol level. Pecans are especially rich in one form of vitamin E (gamma tocopherol), which protects fats from oxidation and lowers levels of LDL cholesterol by 16.5 (Loma Linda University, 2006).

Stress Management

Stress management includes laughter, stress management training, and yoga.

1. *Laughter.* Along with an active sense of humor, laughter can help protect against a heart attack, whereas mental stress is associated with impairment of the endothelium, the protective barrier lining the blood vessels. Stress sets up a series of inflammatory reactions that lead to fat and cholesterol buildup in the coronary arteries and ultimately to a heart attack (Miller, 2005). Counsel clients to watch comedies, find humor in life situations, and make it a point to laugh at least five times a day. Discuss their favorite comedies and what makes the show/movie funny

for them. **Other considerations:** For more humor ideas, go to http://www.healthliteracy.com/article.asp?PageID=3797; www.aath.org, and www.worldlaughtertour.com

2. *Stress management training.* In one study, participating in 1.5 hours of stress management training a week for 16 weeks, along with an education component with skill training, group interaction, and social support, resulted in improvements on several cardiovascular risk markers. The education component included information about ischemic heart disease and myocardial ischemia, structure and function of the heart, traditional risk factors, and emotional stress. The skill training included ways to reduce the affective, behavioral, cognitive, and physiological components of stress. The risk markers included improvements in flow-mediated dilation and baroreflex sensitivity, smaller reduction in left ventricular ejection fraction during mental stress and exercise testing, and reduced wall motion abnormalities (Blumenthal et al., 2005). **Cautions:** Only clients with stable ischemic heart disease and exercise-induced myocardial ischemia should participate. For more information on developing stress management programs, go to http://www.mindtools.com/smpage.html

3. *Yoga.* A yoga lifestyle program reduces risk factors for cardiovascular disease (serum total cholesterol, low-density lipoprotein [LDL] cholesterol, the ratio of total cholesterol to high density lipoprotein [HDL] cholesterol, and total triglycerides), and raises the "good" HDL cholesterol (Bijlani et al., 2005). **Cautions:** Go to http://yoga.lifetips.com/cat/56770/yoga-cautions/. For more information, go to http://www.yogajournal.com/video/173

Supplements

Supplements for heart and blood vessels include the following:

1. *Coenzyme Q10 (CoQ10).* CoQ10 helps cells regenerate and improves the survival of heart cells during and after a infarct (heart attack). It has also been shown to reduce heart size in congestive heart failure in doses of 50–120 mg daily in an oil-filled capsule (Kalenikova, Gorodetskaya, Kolokolchikova, Shashurin & Medvedev, 2007; Molyneux, 2009). Have clients start at a low dosage and gradually build if needed to obtain effect. **Other considerations:** CoQ10 may reduce the toxic effects on the heart caused by the chemotherapy medications daunorubicin and doxorubicin, enhance the effect of blood pressure medications, and reduce the heart-related side effects of timolol drops, a beta-blocker used to treat glaucoma (Sego, 2007).

2. *Pycnogenol.* Pycnogenol was effective in decreasing the number of deep venous thrombosis and superficial vein thrombosis cases during long-haul flights (Belcaro et al., 2004). By mouth, 150–200 mg daily for 8

weeks, the supplement has also been shown superior to Daflon multivitamin for treating chronic venous insufficiency and venous microangiopathy (Cesarone et al., 2006).

3. *Psyllium.* Psyllium lowers serum LDL cholesterol concentrations without affecting HDL cholesterol and is inversely associated with cardiovascular disease (Theuwissen & Mensink, 2008). Stir 1 teaspoon of psyllium husks into a glass of water and drink before it gels. Separate use from vitamins, minerals, herbs, and drugs to ensure adequate absorption. **Cautions:** Drink sufficient water, preferably 8–10 glasses a day, when increasing fiber.

4. *Vitamins and minerals.* The intake of vitamins B (up to 100 mg b.i.d.), E (up to 1,000 IU daily), and selenium (200–400 micrograms daily) is associated with reducing the inflammatory process underlying atherosclerosis (Scheurig, Thorand, Fischer, Heier & Hoenig, 2008).

Touch

Touch evidence-based practice for heart and blood vessels includes acupressure.

In a 2003 study, clients who used continuous wristband acupressure points experienced significantly lower incidence of nausea and/or vomiting postacute myocardial infarction compared with placebo. The severity of symptoms and the need for antiemetic drugs were also reduced in the acupressure group (Dent, Dewhurst, Mills, & Willoughby, 2003). Acupressure to the lower limb blood flow for the treatment of peripheral arterial occlusive diseases caused a significant increase in lower limb blood flow (Li et al., 2007). For more information on using acupressure, go to http://www.agelessherbs.com/acupressure points.html

CARDIOVASCULAR CASE STUDY

Mr. Adams, age 35, tells you his family has a history of heart and blood vessel conditions. His father died of a heart attack and so did two of his uncles. His uncle recently had a quadruple bypass, and his grandmother died of a stroke. He tells you he would like to do whatever possible so that he can to prevent getting any heart condition.

HEALTH PROMOTION CHALLENGE

Using the information in this section and other ideas you can find by searching on PubMed (http://www.ncbi.nlm.nih.gov/pubmed/), develop a teaching/ learning program for Mr. Adams.

REFERENCES

American Heart Association. (2007, July 25). Diet and regular soft drinks linked to increase in risk factors for heart disease. *ScienceDaily*. Retrieved from http://www.sciencedaily.com/releases/2007/07/070723163526.htm

American Heart Association. (2008, January 8). Lack of vitamin D may increase heart disease risk. *ScienceDaily*. Retrieved from http://www.sciencedaily.com/releases/2008/01/080107181600.htm

Anand, P., Kunnumakkara, A. B., Newman, R. A., & Aggarwal, B. B. (2007). Bioavailability of curcumin: Problems and promises. *Molecular Pharmacology, 4*(6), 807–818.

Anandh Babu, P. V., Sabitha, K. E., & Shyamaladevi, C. S. (2006). Green tea extract impedes dyslipidaemia and development of cardiac dysfunction in streptozotocin-diabetic rats. *Clinical Experimental Pharmacology and Physiology, 33*(12), 1184–1189.

Autoimmunity Research Foundation. (2008, Jamuary 27). Vitamin D deficiency study raises new questions about disease and supplements. *ScienceDaily*. Retrieved from http://www.sciencedaily.com/releases/2008/01/080125223302.htm

Bassett, C. M., McCullough, R. S., Edel, A. L., Patenaude, A., LaVallee, R. K., & Pierce, G. N. (2011). The a-linolenic acid content of flaxseed can prevent the atherogenic effects o f dietary transfat. *American Journal of Physiology of the Heart and Circulation Physiology, 301*(6), H2220-6.

Baylor College of Medicine. (2007, June 15). How coffee raises cholesterol. *ScienceDaily*. Retrieved from http://www.sciencedaily.com/releases/2007/06/070614162223.htm

Belcaro, G., Cesarone, M. R., Rohdewald, P., Ricci, A., Ippolito, E., Dugall, M., . . . Cerritelli, F. (2004). Prevention of venous thrombosis and thrombophlebitis in long-haul flights with pycnogenol. *Clinical Application of Thrombosis and Hemostasis, 10*(4), 373–377.

Bijlani, R. L., Vempati, R. P., Yadav, R. K., Ray, R. B., Gupta, V., Sharma, R., . . . Mahapatra, S. C. (2005). A brief but comprehensive lifestyle education program based on yoga reduces risk factors for cardiovascular disease and diabetes mellitus. *Journal of Alternative and Complementary Medicine, 11*(2), 267–274.

Bjorgell, O., & Almer, L. O. (2007). Effect of cinnamon on postprandial blood glucose, gastric emptying, and satiety in healthy subjects. *American Journal of Clinical Nutrition, 85*(6), 1552–1556.

Blackwell Publishing Ltd. (2007, November 21). Regular exercise reduces risk of blood clots, study suggests. *ScienceDaily*. Retrieved from http://www.sciencedaily.com/releases/2007/11/071120124245.htm

Blumenthal, J. A., Sherwood, A., Babyak, M. A., Watkins, L. L., Waugh, R., Georgiades, A., . . . Hinderliter, A. (2005). Effects of exercise and stress management training on markers of cardiovascular risk in patients with ischemic heart disease. *Journal of Journal of the American Medical Association, 293*(1), 1126–1634.

Cesarone, M. R., Belcaro, G., Rohdewald, P., Pellegrini, L., Ledda, A., Vinciguerra, G., . . . Corsi, M. (2006). Comparison of pycnogenol and Daflon in treating chronic venous insufficiency: prospective, controlled study. *Clinical Application of Thrombosis and Hemostasis, 12*(2), 205–212.

Chacko, S. M., Thambi, P. T., Kuttan, R., & Nishigaki, I. (2010). Beneficial effects of green tea: a literature review. *Chinese Medicine, 6*(5), 13.

Cortes, B., Nunez, I., Cofan, M., Gilabert, R., Perez-Heras, A. Casals, E., . . . Ros, E. (2006). Acute effects of high-fat meals enriched with walnuts or live oil on postprandial endothelial function. *Journal American College of Cardiology, 48*(8), 1666–1671.

Dent, H. E., Dewhurst, N. G., Mills, S. Y., & Willoughby, M. (2003). Continuous PC6 wristband acupressure for relief of nausea and vomiting associated with acute myocardial infarction: A partially randomized, placebo-controlled trial. *Complementary Therapy in Medicine, 11*(2), 72–77.

DeRubeis, R. J., Hollon, S. D., & Amsterdam, J. D. (2005). Cognitive therapy vs. medications in the treatment of moderate to severe depression. *Archives of General Psychiatry, 62,* 409–416.

Djousse, L., & Gaziano, J. M. (2008). Egg consumption in relation to cardiovascular disease and mortality: The Physicians' Health Study. *American Journal of Clinical Nutrition, 87*(4), 964–969.

Drouillet, P., Balkau, B., Charles, M. A. Vol, S., Bedouet, M., & Ducimetiere, P. (2007). Calcium consumption and insulin resistance syndrome parameter. *Nutrition and Metabolism in Cardiovascular Disease, 17*(7), 486–492.

Gardner, C. D., Coulston, A., Chatterjee, L., Rigby, A., Spiller, G., & Farquhar, J. W. (2005). The effect of a plant-based diet on plasma lipids in hypercholesterolemic adults: A randomized trial. *Annals of Internal Medicine, 142*(9), 725–733.

Halton, T. L., Willett, W. C., Liu, S., Manson, J. E., Albert, C. M., Rexrode, K. & Hu, H. B. (2006). Low-carbohydrate-diet score and the risk of coronary heart disease in women. *New England Journal of Medicine, 355*(19), 1991–2002.

Hamer, M., Eilliams, E. D., Vuononvirta, R., Gibson, E. L., & Steptoe, A. (2006). Association between coffee consumption and markers of inflammation and cardiovascular function during mental stress. *Journal of Hypertension, 24*(11), 2191–2197.

Hirai, M., Hotta, Y., Ishikawa, N., Wakida, Y., Fukuzawa, Y., Isobe, F., . . . Kawamura, N. (2007). Protective effects of EGCg or GCg, a green tea catechin epimer, against postischemic myocardial dysfunction in guinea-pig hearts. *Life Science, 80*(11), 1020–1032.

Jenkins, D. J., Kendall, C. W., Vidgen, E., Agarwal, S., Rao, A. V., Rosenberg, R. S. . . . Cunnane, S. C. (1999). Health aspects of partially defatted flaxseed, including effects on serum lipids, oxidative measures, and ex vivo androgen and progestin activity: a controlled crossover trial. *American Journal of Clinical Nutrition, 69*(3), 395–402.

Jenkins, D. J., Kendall, C. W., Marchie, A., Faulkner, D. A., Wong, J. M., de Souze, R., . . . Connelly, P. W. (2003). Effects of a dietary portfolio of cholesterol lowering foods vs. lovastatin on serum lipids and C-reactive protein. *Journal of American Medical Association, 290*(4), 502–510.

Jockers, B. (2007). Vitamin D sufficiency: An approach to disease. *Prevention. The American Journal for Nurse Practitioners, 11*(10), 43–50.

Kalenikova, E. I., Gorodetskaya, E. A., Kolokolchikova, E. G., Shashurin, D. A., Medvedev, O. S. (2007). Chronic administration of coenzyme Q10 limits postinfarct myocardial remodeling in rats. *Biochemistry, 72*(3), 332–338.

Kapoor, S. (2008). Green tea: Beneficial effects on cholesterol and lipid metabolism besides endothelial function. *European Journal of Cardiovascular Prevention and Rehabilitation, 15*(4), 497.

Kirn, T. (2004, February). Tai chi improves quality of life in heart failure. *Clinical Psychiatry,* p. 90.

Kodama, S., Tanaka, S., Saito, K., Shu, M., Sone, Y., Onitake, F., . . . Sone, H. (2007). Effect of aerobic exercise training on serum levels of high-density lipoprotein cholesterol: A meta-analysis. *Archives of Internal Medicine, 167*(10), 999–1008.

Kokubo, Y., Iso, H., Ishihara, J., Okada, K., Inoue M., & Tsugane, S. (2007). Association of dietary intake of soy, beans and isoflavones with risk of cerebral and myocardial infarctions in Japanese populations: The Japan Public Health Center-based (JPHC) study cohort. *Circulation, 116*(22), 2553–2562.

Kruk, J. (2007). Physical activity in the prevention of the most frequent chronic diseases:

An analysis of the recent evidence. *Asian Pacific Journal of Cancer Prevention, 8*(3), 325–338.

Kuriyama, S., Shimazu, T., Ohmori, K., Kikuchi, N., Nakaya, N., Nichino, Y., . . . Tsuji, I. (2006). Green tea consumption and mortality due to cardiovascular disease, cancer and all causes in Japan. *Journal of the American Medical Association, 296*(10), 1255–1265.

Lee, J. O., Park, M. H., Choi, Y. H., Ha, Y. L., & Ryu, C. H. (2007). New fermentation technique for complete digestion of soybean protein. *Journal of Microbiology and Biotechnology, 17*(11), 1904–1907.

Li, S., Hirokawa, M., Inoue, Y., Sugano, N., Qian, S., & Iwai, T. (2007). Effects of acupressure on lower limb blood flow for the treatment of peripheral arterial occlusive diseases. *Surgery Today, 37*(2), 103–108.

Loma Linda University. (2006, October 3). Antioxidant-rich pecans can protect against unhealthy oxidation. *ScienceDaily.* Retrieved from http://www.sciencedaily.com /releases/2006/09/060929093646.htm

Martins, D., Wolf, M., Pan, D., Zadshir, A., Tareen, N., Thadhani, R., . . . Norris, K. (2007). Prevalence of cardiovascular risk factors and the serum levels of 250 hydroxyvitamin D in the United States: Data from the Third National Health and Nutrition Examination Survey. *Archives of Internal Medicine, 167*(11), 1159–1165.

McKay, D. L., & Blumberg, J. B. (2006). A review of the bioactivity and potential health benefits of chamomile tea (*Matricaria recutita L.*) *Phytotherapy research, 20*(7), 519–530.

Medical College of Wisconsin. (2008, March 3). Low-fat diets more likely to reduce risk of heart disease than low-carb diets. *ScienceDaily.* Retrieved from http://www.science daily.com/releases/2008/02/080229141756.htm

Meyer, K. (2006). Resistance exercise in chronic heart failure—landmark studies and implications for practice. *Clinical Investigations in Medicine, 29*(3), 166–169.

Miller, M. (2005, March). Laughter helps blood vessels function better. Presented at the American Heart Association's 78th Scientific Sessions, Orlando, FL. Details available at www.umm.edu/news/releases/laughter2.htm

Molyneux, S. L., Florkowski, C. M., Richards, A. M., Lever, M., Young, J. M., & George, P. M. (2009). Coenzyme Q10; an adjunctive therapy for congestive heart failure? *The New Zealand Medical Journal, 122*(1305), 74–79.

Morimoto, T., Sunagawa, Y., Kawamura, T., Takaya, T., Wada, H., Nagasawa, A., Hasegawa, K. (2008). The dietary compound curcumin inhibits p300 histone acetyltransferase activity and prevents heart failure in rats. *Journal of Clinical Investigation, 118*(3), 868–878.

Obarzanek, E., Wu, C. O., Cutler, J. A., Kavey, R. E., Pearson, G. D., & Daniels, S. R. (2010). Prevalence and incidence of hypertension in adolescent girls. *Journal of Pediatrics, 57*(3), 461–467

Pittler, M., Guo, R., & Ernst, E. (2008). Hawthorn extract for treating chronic heart failure. *Cochrane Database System of Reviews*, 1:CD005312.

Prasad, K. (2005). Hypocholesterolemic and antiatherosclerotic effect of flax lignan complex isolated from flaxseed. *Atherosclerosis, 179*(2), 269–275.

Pullen, P. R., Nagamia, S. H., Mehta, P. K., Thompson, W. R., Benardot, D., Hammoud, R., . . . Khan, B. V. (2008). Effects of yoga on inflammation and exercise capacity in patients with chronic heart failure. *Journal of Cardiac Failure, 14*(5), 407–413.

Qi, L., van Dam, R. M., Rexrode, K., & Hu, F. B. (2007). Heme iron from diet as a risk factor for coronary heart disease in women with type 2 diabetes. *Diabetes Care, 30*(1), 101–106.

Raub, J. A. (2002). Psychophysiologic effects of Hatha yoga on musculoskeletal and cardiopulmonary function: A literature review. *Journal of Alternative and Complementary Medicine, 8*(6), 797–812.

Ross, M. F. (2005). *Size, strength of social networks influence heart disease risk.* [Press release.] Gainesville: University of Florida Office of News & Communication.

Sano, T., Oda, E., Yamashita, T., Shiramasa, H., Lijiri, Y., Yamashita, T., & Yamamoto, J. (2003). Antithrombic and anti-atherogenic effects of partially defatted flaxseed meal using a laser-induced using a laser-induced thrombosis test in apolipoprotein E and low-density lipoprotein receptor deficient mice. *Blood Coagulation and Fibrinolysis, 14*(8), 707–712.

Scheurig, A. C., Thorand, B., Fischer, B., Heier, M., & Hoenig, W. (2008). Association between the intake of vitamins and trace elements from supplements and C-reactive protein: Results of the MONICA/KORA Augsburg study. *European Journal of Clinical Nutrition, 62*(1), 127–137.

Sego, S. (2007, October). Coenzyme Q10. *The Clinical Advisor,* 126–128.

Skidmore-Roth, L. (2006a). Cinnamon. In *Mosby's handbook of herbs & natural supplements* (pp. 302–305). St. Louis, MO: ElsevierMosby.

Skidmore-Roth, L. (2006b). Green tea. In *Mosby's handbook of herbs & natural supplements* (pp. 535–539). St. Louis, MO: ElsevierMosby.

Skidmore-Roth, L. (2006c). Hawthorn. In *Mosby's handbook of herbs & natural supplements* (pp. 555–559). St. Louis, MO: ElsevierMosby.

Stanford University Medical Center. (2007, December 5). Computer calls can talk couch potatoes into walking, study finds. *ScienceDaily.* Retrieved from http://www.science daily.com/releases/2007/12/071204122000.htm

Sumner, M. D., Elliott-Eller, M., Weidner, G., Daubenmier, J. J., Chew, M. H., Marlin, R., . . . Ornish, D. (2005). Effects of pomegranate juice consumption on myocardial perfusion in patients with coronary heart disease. *American Journal of Cardiology, 96*(6), 810–814.

Sun, Q., Jing, M., Campos, H., Hankinson, S. E., Manson, J. E., Stampfer, M. J., . . . Hu, F. B. (2008). A prospective study of trans fatty acids in erythrocytes and risk of coronary heart disease. *Circulation, 115,* 1858–1865.

Takeda, R., & Nakamura, T. (2008). Effects of high magnesium intake on bone mineral status and lipid metabolism in rats. *Journal of Nutritional Science and Vitaminology, 54*(1), 66–75.

Tapsell, L. C., Hemphill, I., Cobiac, L., Patch, C. S., Sullivan, D. R., Fenech, M., . . . Inge, K. E. (2006). Health benefits of herbs and spices: The past, the present, the future. *Medical Journal of Australia, 185*(Suppl), S4–S24.

Theuwissen, E., & Mensink, R. P. (2008). Water-soluble dietary fibers and cardiovascular disease. *Physiology and Behavior, 94*(2), 285–92.

University of Michigan Health System. (2008, March 6). Many patients can reach LDL cholesterol goal through dietary changes alone, study shows. *ScienceDaily.* Retrieved from http://www.sciencedaily.com/releases/2008/03/080304105817.htm

University of Missouri-Columbia. (2007, November 20). Sitting may increase risk of disease. *ScienceDaily.* http://www.sciencedaily.com/releases/2007/11/071119130734.htm

Welsh, J. A., Sharma, A., Abramson, J. L., Vaccarino, V., Gillespie, C., & Vos, M. B. (2010). Caloric sweetener consumption and dyslipidemia among US adults. *JAMA, 303*(15), 1490–1497.

Xue, W. L., Li, S. X., Zhang, J., Liu, Y. H., Wang, Z. L., & Zhang, R. J. (2007). Effect of *Trigonella foenum-graecum* (fenugreek) extract on blood glucose, blood lipid and hemorheaological properties in streptozotocin-induced diabetic rats. *Asia Pacific Journal of Clinical Nutrition, 16*(Suppl 1), 422–426.

Zahid, A. M., Hussain, M. E., & Fahim, M. (2005). Antiatherosclerotic effects of dietary supplementations of garlic and turmeric: Restoration of endothelial function in rats. *Life Science, 77*(8), 837–857.

Incontinence

Environment

Environmental evidence-based practice for incontinence includes going outdoors.

Going outdoors after age 70 is associated with fewer complaints of urinary incontinence. Not going out daily at age 70 is predictive of subsequent urinary incontinence (Jacobs et al., 2008).

Exercise/Movement

Exercise/movement evidence-based practice for incontinence includes physical activity and Kegel exercises and bladder training.

1. *Physical activity.* In a community-based study of men and women, habitual physical activity levels (walking, moderate and vigorous activities) were assessed along with the prevalence of urinary incontinence (UI). The researchers found an inverse association between UI and walking, which has important implications for the prevention and treatment of this distressing condition (Lee & Hirayama, 2012). Suggest clients choose more than one activity and vary them to reduce boredom.

2. *Kegel exercises and bladder training.* Kegel exercises, or pelvic floor muscle training, and bladder training resolve urinary incontinence. Teach clients to empty their bladder and then hold the muscle that voluntarily stops the stream of urine for a count of 10 then relax for another count of 10 to a daily total of 35. The bladder can be trained by resisting a premature signal to void and holding urine 5 minutes longer, adding 5 minutes each week until 4 hours elapse between urinations. Vaginal weights can also be purchased to help identify and use the correct muscles (Shamliyan, Kane, Wyman, & Wilt (2008).

Nutrition

1. *Irritating foods and fluids.* Too little or too much fluid consumption (more than 1,500 ml a day), caffeinated and carbonated drinks, artificial sweeteners, honey, tomato products, nicotine, spicy foods, alcohol, and acidic juices can irritate the bladder and are correlated with urination urge (Bradley, Kennedy, & Nygaard, 2005).

2. *Vitamin D, protein, potassium.* Nutrients that may decrease overactive bladder include vitamin D, protein, and potassium. Niacin and vitamin B_6 are also associated with decreased risk, but not significantly. Individuals living at latitudes north of 35°, who may not receive exposure to the sun, or who are older than 49 years may need to take a tablespoon of cod liver oil daily. Foods rich in potassium include baked and sweet

potatoes, white beans, and bananas. Dietary surveys indicate 15–25% of older adults do not consume enough niacin. Foods rich in niacin (vitamin B_3) include peanuts, white chicken meat, tuna, corn grits, and peanut butter. Foods rich in pyridoxine (vitamin B_6) include baked potatoes with skins, bananas, garbanzo beans, oatmeal, rainbow trout, and sunflower seeds (Dallosso, McGrother, Matthews, Donaldson, & Leicestershire, M.R.C., 2004).

Stress Management

Stress management evidence-based practice for incontinence includes cognitive-behavioral therapy.

Audio-taped cognitive strategies and a voiding diary, designed to augment the effects of an education program on urinary frequency and incontinence, provided improved control over urination and enhanced comfort in two studies (Dowd & Dowd, 2006; Garley & Unwin, 2006).

Touch

Touch evidence-based practice for incontinence includes reflexology.

Foot reflexology (twice a week for 40 minutes) resulted in a more significant change in the daytime frequency of urination when compared to a foot massage group in a study by Bradley, Kennedy, and Nygaard (2005). **Cautions:** Pregnant women should avoid foot reflexology because certain manipulations can lead to premature labor. Those with foot problems, gout, arthritis, and vascular conditions such as varicose veins should be careful using this procedure. For foot charts, see http://www.reflexologyinstitute .com/reflex_chart.php

INCONTINENCE CASE STUDY

Ms. Linden, 52, has a 2-year history of urge-related urinary incontinence. For the past 2 years, she has been wearing urinary pads to prevent wetting her clothes if she cannot reach a toilet in time. Previous urinalysis revealed no evidence of bladder infection. She is not being treated for any diagnosed illnesses and does not take medication on a regular basis.

She is a consultant for the state education department, and her job involves extensive driving. To stay awake, she drinks large quantities of coffee and caffeinated sodas.

A vaginal exam revealed atrophic external genitalia and vaginal tissues. She had good anatomic support of her bladder and was able to perform a weak voluntary contraction of pelvic floor muscles.

She says she wants to learn new ways to control her bladder urgency.

HEALTH PROMOTION CHALLENGE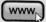

Use the information in this section as well as from searching PubMed (http://www.ncbi.nlm.nih.gov/pubmed/) for urinary incontinence and prepare a teaching/learning program for Ms. Linden.

REFERENCES

Bradley, C. S., Kennedy, C. M., & Nygaard, I. E. (2005). Pelvis floor symptoms and life style factors in older women. *Journal of Women's Health, 14*(2), 128–135.

Dowd, T., & Dowd, E. T. (2006). A cognitive therapy approach to promote continence. *Journal of Wound, Ostomy, and Continence Nursing, 33*(1), 63–68.

Garley, A., & Unwin, J. (2006). A case series to pilot cognitive behaviour therapy for women with urinary incontinence. *British Journal of Health Psychology, 11*(Pt 3), 373–386.

Jacobs, J. M., Cohen, A., Hammerman-Rozenberg, R., Azoulay, D., Maaravi, Y., & Stessman, J. (2008). Going outdoors daily predicts long-term functional and health benefits among ambulatory older people. *Journal of Aging and Health, 20*(3), 259–272.

Lee, A. H., & Hirayama, F. (2012). Physical activity and urinary incontinence in older adults: a community-based study. *Current Aging Science, 5*(1), 35–40.

Shamliyan, T. A., Kane, R. L., Wyman, J., & Wilt, T. J. (2008). Systematic review: Randomized, controlled trials of nonsurgical treatments for urinary incontinence in women. *Annals of Internal Medicine, 148*(6), 459–473.

Insomnia

Environment

Environmental evidence-based practice for insomnia includes the following:

1. *Aromatherapy.* Women receiving either lavender or sweet almond essential oil via an aroma-stream device, which diffused it through the air, showed an improvement and less insomnia. (Lewith, Godfrey, & Prescott, 2005).

2. *Environmental behavioral training.* A master's level adult psychiatric and primary care nurse practitioner provided four individually tailored instructions to women suffering from insomnia: (1) reduce the time spent in bed to closely match the number of hours of sleep, (2) get up at the same time every day of the week, (3) not to go to bed unless they were sleepy, and (4) not to stay in bed unless they were asleep. Participating in this program significantly improved scores on the Pittsburgh Sleep Quality Index (PSQ), decreased the time it took to fall asleep,

and decreased the amount of wake time after sleep onset (Finn, 2007; Germain, 2006).

3. *Music therapy and progressive relaxation.* Music therapy paired with progressive relaxation (as compared to a control group) produced a more significant effect on sleep quality in a 2005 study. Listening to participant-selected music for at least five consecutive nights resulted in improved sleep (Hernandez-Reuiz, 2005).

Exercise/Movement

Exercise (50–60 minutes a day or as tolerated) is an inexpensive, safe means of improving sleep (Youngstedt, 2005).

Herbs/Essential Oils

Herb evidence-based practice for insomnia includes black cohosh and chamomile.

1. *Black cohosh.* Black cohosh (40–80 mg/day) may be a useful treatment for insomnia, especially for menopausal women (Mahady, 2005). **Cautions:** Transient adverse events such as nausea, vomiting, headaches, dizziness, mastalgia, and weight gain have been observed in clinical trials. **Other considerations:** The most recent data suggest black cohosh is not estrogenic.
2. *Chamomile.* Chamomile is classified as a mild sleep aid or sedative by the German Commission on Herbal Medicines (Blumenthal, Hall, Rister, & Steinhoff, 1996). A cup of chamomile tea prior to bedtime is recommended. **Cautions:** No known adverse reactions unless sensitive to dried chamomile.

Mind-Set

Mind-set evidence-based practice for insomnia includes CBT.

An 8-week program of CBT self-help treatment decreased total wake time by 52 minutes to help taper off the chronic use of sleep hypnotics. Using hypnosis alone increased total wake time by 17 minutes (Belleville, Guay, Guay, & Morin, 2007). For more information, go to http://www.mind.org.uk/Information/Booklets/Making+sense/MakingSenseCBT.htm

Touch

Touch evidence-based practice for insomnia includes acupressure and back massage.

1. *Acupressure massage.* Acupressure massage improves the quality of sleep and does so in a noninvasive way (Sun, Sung, Huang, Cheng &

Lin, 2010). In one study, sleep log data revealed the acupressure group significantly decreased wake time and improved quality of sleep (Tsay, Rong, & Lin, 2003. For more information on acupressure, go to http://www.agelessherbs.com/acupressurepoints.html

2. *Back massage.* A review of 16 studies indicated that back massage nightly for 5–15 minutes promotes relaxation and sleep (Schiff, 2006).

INSOMNIA CASE STUDY

Mr. Quartero, age 47, complains of inability to sleep. Most nights he lies in bed for hours, unable to sleep. When he does fall asleep, he wakes in about 2 hours. Even though he spends many hours in bed, he always wakes up fatigued.

He has tried many medications and found they helped for a while, but he is looking for something with no side effects.

HEALTH PROMOTION CHALLENGE

Based on what you learned in this section, what could you tell Mr. Quartero?

REFERENCES

Belleville, G., Guay, C., Guay, B., & Morin, C. M. (2007). Hypnotic tapes with or without self-help treatment of insomnia: A randomized clinical trial. *Journal of Consulting and Clinical Psychology, 75*(2), 325–335.

Blumenthal, M., Hall, T., Rister, R., and Steinhoff, B. (Eds.). (1996). *The complete German Commission E monographs: Therapeutic guide to herbal medicines* (pp. 573–575). Austin, TX: American Botanical Council.

Finn, R. (2007, March). Brief behavioral training improves insomnia. *Clinical Psychiatry News,* 21.

Germain, A., Moul, D. E., Franzen, P. L., Miewald, J. M., Reynolds, C. F. 3rd, Monk, T. H., . . . Buysse, D. J. (2006). Effects of a brief behavioral treatment for late-life insomnia: Preliminary findings. *Journal of Clinical Sleep Medicine, 2*(4), 403–406.

Hernandez-Reuiz, E. (2005). Effect of music therapy on the anxiety levels and sleep patterns of abused women in shelters. *Journal of Music Therapy, 42*(2), 140–158.

Lewith, G. T., Godfrey, A. D., & Prescott, P. (2005). A single-blinded, randomized pilot study evaluating the aroma of *Lavandula augustifolia* as a treatment for mild insomnia. *Journal of Alternative and Complementary Medicine, 11*(4), 631–637.

Mahady, G. B. (2005). Black cohosh (*Actaea/Cimicifuga racemosa*): Review of the clinical data for safety and efficacy in menopausal symptoms. *Treatment in Endocrinology, 4*(3), 177–184.

Schiff, A. (2006). Literature review of back massage and similar techniques to promote sleep in elderly people. *Pflege, 19*(3), 163–173.

Sun, J. L., Sung, M. S., Huang, M. Y., Cheng, G. C., & Lin, C. C. (2010). Effectiveness of acupressure for residents of long-term care facilities with insomnia: a randomized controlled trial. *International Journal of Nursing Studies, 47*(7), 798–805.

Tsay, S. L., Rong, J. R., & Lin, P. F. (2003). Acupoints massage in improving the quality of sleep and quality of life in patients with end-stage renal disease. *Journal of Advanced Nursing, 42*(2), 134–142.

Youngstedt, S. D. (2005). Effects of exercise on sleep. *Clinical Sports Medicine, 24*(2), 355–365.

Kidneys

Environment

Environmental evidence-based practice for kidneys includes aromatherapy, sunlight, and vitamin D.

1. *Aromatherapy.* Laboratory studies and animal studies have shown that certain essential oils have antibacterial, calming, or energizing effects. Aromatherapy may work by sending chemical messages to the part of the brain that affects moods and emotions. Lavender and rosemary protect the body from oxidative stress by decreasing the stress hormone, cortisol, and provide a calming effect when the oil is sniffed for 5 minutes. Clients with kidney cancer may use aromatherapy mainly to improve their quality of life (Atsumi & Tonosaki, 2007).

2. *Sunlight.* Researchers at the Moores Cancer Center at University of California, San Diego (UCSD) showed a clear association between deficiency in exposure to sunlight, specifically ultraviolet B (UVB), and kidney cancer (University of California–San Diego, 2006). For Caucasian clients, 10–15 minutes of direct midday sun at least twice a week on the face, arms, hands, or back is sufficient, according to the National Institutes of Health. Darker skinned clients may require 3–6 times as much exposure. Help clients develop a plan for obtaining sufficient sunlight, depending on their lifestyle. Eating lunch outside when weather permits could be one solution. In colder climes, women can take a tablespoon of cod liver oil daily and eat fatty fish and fish oils and egg yolks. Supplements of vitamin D_3 (calciferol) may be necessary for certain women. **Other considerations:** Vitamin D_2, found in fortified foods, especially breads and cereals, is poorly metabolized by the body. Certain drugs can interfere with vitamin D metabolism, including corticosteroids, phenytoin, heparin, cimetidine, isoniazid, rifampin, phenobarbital, and primidone. Counsel clients to find alternate medications whenever possible so they can metabolize vitamin D.

3. *Vitamin D.* Taking vitamin D supplements can actually block VDR activation, the opposite effect to that of sunshine. Quite nominal amounts
of ingested vitamin D can suppress the proper operation of the immune
system (Autoimmunity Research Foundation, 2008; Demgrow, 2007;
Jockers, 2007).

Exercise/Movement

Exercise/movement evidence-based practice for kidneys includes aerobic exercise, resistance training, and regular exercise.

1. *Aerobic exercise and resistance training.* Working out 3 days a week,
working up to 30–60 minutes per session, during kidney dialysis
improves muscle strength, work output, cardiac fitness, and possibly
dialysis adequacy (Moinuddin & Leehey, 2008).

2. *Regular exercise.* Regular exercise leads to better blood pressure control,
lower levels of blood fats (cholesterol and triglycerides), better, deeper
sleep, and better weight control. High blood pressure, high blood fats,
kidney disease and being overweight increase risk of developing heart
disease, while exercise may lessen this risk. Exercise may also help to
prevent a weakening of bones—a problem that women who undergo
kidney dialysis and transplant often have. **Cautions:** Go to http://
ktda.org/Exercise.pdf **Other considerations:** For pre- and post-exer-
cise stretching exercises, go to http://www.wellness.ma/adult-fitness
/stretching-warmup.htm

Herbs

Herb evidence-based practice for kidneys includes basil leaf extract and milk
thistle.

1. *Basil leaf extract.* Basil leaf extract (1–2 milliliters taken 3–5 times a day)
was highly effective in inhibiting carcinogen-induced tumors in the kidney in one study (Dasgupta, Rao, & Yadava, 2004). The dried leaf can
also be used in cooking. **Cautions:** Except when used in cooking, basil
leaf extract in large amounts may increase the hypoglycemic effects of
insulin and oral antidiabetes agents; advise clients to avoid using concurrently. Basil leaf extract is not recommended for therapeutic use during
pregnancy and lactation (Skidmore-Roth, 2006). **Other considerations:**
Basil has been used to increase immunity and metabolic function.

2. *Milk thistle.* Milk thistle (*Silybum marianum*), or silymarin, at 200–400
mg a day protects the kidney cells from cancer and the toxic effects of
chemotherapy (Post-White, Ladas, & Kelly, 2007). **Cautions:** Adverse
effects are rare, but may include stomach pain, nausea, vomiting, diarrhea, headache, rash, joint pain, and anaphylaxis in allergic clients.

Warn pregnant and lactating women or those who are hypersensitive (have a known sensitivity to ragweed, marigolds, chrysanthemums, or marigolds) not to use milk thistle.

Nutrition

Nutrition evidence-based practice for kidneys includes the following:

1. *Garlic.* Garlic protects the kidneys against oxidative damage. The high-protein Atkins diet is associated with reduced kidney function. Over time, individuals who consume very large amounts of protein, particularly animal protein, risk significant kidney damage (Kabasakal, 2005).

2. *Animal protein.* High intake of animal protein is linked to kidney stones. The American Academy of Family Physicians notes that high animal protein intake is largely responsible for the high prevalence of kidney stones in the United States and other developed countries and recommends protein restriction for the prevention of recurrent kidney stones (Allon & Friedman, 2004).

3. *Carbonated beverages.* Cola, along with other carbonated beverages, may increase the risk of chronic kidney disease (Saldana, Basso, Darden, & Sandler, 2007).

4. *Green tea.* Drinking green tea may help strengthen metabolic defense against toxins capable of causing cancer. Homocysteine, a normal by-product of protein metabolism, derived primarily from meat and dairy products, is linked to kidney disease (American Association for Cancer Research, 2007).

5. *The Mediterranean diet.* A diet high in vegetables, legumes, fruits, nuts, whole grains and fish, also known as the Mediterranean diet, is associated with reduced deaths due to kidney cancer (Divisi, Di Tommaso, Salvemini, Garramone, & Crisci, 2006; Mitrou et al., 2007).

Stress Management

Daily practice of stress management procedures prior to and after medical treatment may help to prevent metastases. A weak immune system is one of the major factors that promote cancer metastases after an operation, chemotherapy, or radiation therapy. Fear and stress weaken the immune system (Tel Aviv University, 2008). Go to http://www.webmd.com/balance/stress-management /features/blissing-out-10-relaxation-techniques-reduce-stress-spot.

Supplements

Supplement evidence-based practice for kidneys includes quercetin.

Quercetin (400 mg b.i.d.) shows antihypertensive, protective, and antioxidant effects in renovascular hypertension (Garcia-Saura et al., 2005) and toxicity (Zal, Mostafavi-Pour, & Vessal, 2007). In combination with 400 IU of vitamin E, it may even ameliorate the chronic toxic effects of the immuno-suppressive drug cyclosporine A for renal transplants (Behling et al., 2006). **Cautions:** Advise clients to avoid taking quercetin in the first trimester of pregnancy. For clients who are taking blood thinners, discuss the use of vitamin E with their primary care practitioners.

Touch

Touch evidence-based practice for kidneys includes acupressure and reflexology.

1. *Acupressure.* Women with end-stage renal disease who received acupoint massage for 12 minutes per day, 3 days per week, for 4 weeks showed significantly greater improvement in fatigue and depression than women in a control group (Cho & Tsay, 2004). A meta-analysis of randomized clinical trials examining the treatment of clinical symptoms in kidney disease concluded that acupressure was superior to regular care, sleep medication, and unspecified control interventions (Kim, Lee, Kang, & Choi, 2010). For more information on acupressure, go to http://www.agelessherbs.com/acupressurepoints.html

2. *Foot reflexology.* Life satisfaction was significantly improved in the experimental group after foot reflexology in a study by Kohara and colleagues (2004). Combined with aromatherapy and foot soak (warm water and lavender oil for 3 minutes), reflexology also relieves fatigue in women with cancer. Twice a week for 4 weeks, foot reflexology (with jojoba oil containing lavender) or self-foot reflexology also significantly enhances and strengthens the immune system so it can catch and eliminate cancer cells and prevent tumors from developing (Kohara et al., 2004). For a reflexology charts, go to http://www.reflexology-research.com/charts.htm

   Other considerations: Quality of life is the most important predictor of survival for advanced cancer patients (Fox Chase Cancer Center, 2007).

KIDNEYS CASE STUDY

Mrs. Rodriguez, a 42-year-old Hispanic woman, has a 15-year history of type 2 diabetes. Her blood pressure is 130/80 and she is a nonsmoker. She is 5'4" and weighs 189 lb. Worried about her weight, she put herself on the latest high-protein diet (i.e., the Atkins diet). She lost 20 pounds, her blood pressure decreased to 110/76, and she developed stage 1 chronic kidney disease.

HEALTH PROMOTION CHALLENGE

If Mrs. Rodriguez were your patient, what could you tell Mrs. Rodriguez that might help her reduce her kidney disease risk?

REFERENCES

Allon, N., & Friedman, M. D. (2004). High-protein diets: Potential effects on the kidney in renal health and disease. *American Journal of Kidney Diseases, 44*(6), 950–962.

American Association for Cancer Research. (2007, August 12). Green tea boosts production of detox enzymes, rending cancerous chemicals harmless. Retrieved from http://www.sciencedaily.com/releases/2007/08/070810194923.htm

Atsumi, T., & Tonosaki, K. (2007). Smelling lavender and rosemary increases free radical scavenging activity and decreases cortisol level in saliva. *Psychiatry Research, 150*(1), 89–96.

Autoimmunity Research Foundation. (2008, January 27). Vitamin D deficiency study raises new questions about disease and supplements. *ScienceDaily*. Retrieved from http://www.sciencedaily.com/releases/2008/01/080125223302.htm

Behling, E. B., Sendao, M. C., Fancescato, H. D., Antunes, L. M., Costa, R. S., & Bianchi, M. L. (2006). Comparative study of multiple dosage of quercetain against cisplatin-induced nephrotoxicity and oxidative stress in rat kidneys. *Pharmacology Reports, 58*(4), 526–532.

Cho, Y. C., & Tsay, S. L. (2004). The effect of acupressure with massage on fatigue and depression in patients with end-stage renal disease. *Journal of Nursing Research, 12*(1), 51–59.

Dasgupta, T., Rao, A. R., & Yadava, P. K. (2004). Chemodulatory efficacy of basil leaf (*Ocimum basilicum*) on drug metabolizing and antioxidant enzymes, and on carcinogen-induced skin and forestomach papillomagenesis. *Phytomedicine, 11*(2), 139–151.

Demgrow, M. (2007, June). High vitamin D: Treatment for cancer prevention? *The Clinical Advisor, 54*, 57.

Divisi, D., Di Tommaso, S., Salvemini, S., Garramone, M., & Crisci, R. (2006). Diet and cancer. *Acta Biomedica, 77*(2), 118–123.

Fox Chase Cancer Center. (2007, November 1). Quality of life is the most important predictor of survival for advanced cancer patients. *ScienceDaily*. Retrieved from http://www.sciencedaily.com/releases/2007/10/071030170208.htm

Garcia-Saura, M. F., Galisteo, M., Villar, I. C., Bermejo, A., Zarzuelo, A., Vargas, F., & Duarte, J. (2005). Effects of chronic quercetin treatment in experimental renovascular hypertension. *Molecular Cell Biochemistry, 270*(1–2), 147–155.

Jockers, B. S. (2007). Vitamin D sufficiency: An approach to disease prevention. *The American Journal for Nurse Practitioners, 11*(10), 43–50.

Kabasakal, L., Sehirli, O., Cetinel, S., Cikler, E., Gedik, N., & Sener, G. (2005). Protective effect of aqueous garlic extract against renal ischemia/reperfusion injury in rats. *Journal of Medicinal Food, 8*(3), 319–326.

Kim, K. H, Lee, M. S., Kang, K. W., & Choi, S. M. (2010). Role of acupressure in symptom management in patients with end-stage renal disease: A systematic review. *Journal of Palliative Medicine, 13*(7), 885–922.

Kohara, H., Miyauchi, T., Suehiro, Y., Ueoka, H., Takeyama, H., Morita, T. (2004). Combined modality treatment of aromatherapy, footsoak, and reflexology relieves fatigue in patients with cancer. *Journal of Palliative Medicine, 7*(6), 791–6.

Mitrou, P. N., Kipnis, V., Thiebaut, A. C., Reedy, J., Subar, A. F., Wirfalt, E., & Schatzkin, A. (2007). Mediterranean dietary pattern and prediction of all-cause mortality in a US population: Results from the NIH-AARP diet and health study. *Archives of Internal Medicine, 167*(22), 2461–2468.

Moinuddin, I., & Leehey, D. J. (2008). A comparison of aerobic exercise and resistance training in patients with and without chronic kidney disease. *Advance Chronic Kidney Disease, 15*(1), 83–96.

Post-White, J., Ladas, E. J., & Kelly, K. M. (2007). Advances in the use of milk thistle (*Silybum marianum*). *Integrative Cancer therapy, 2*, 104–109.

Saldana, T. M., Basso, O., Darden, R., & Sandler, D. P. (2007). Carbonated beverages and chronic kidney disease. *Epidemiology, 18*(4), 501–506.

Skidmore-Roth, L. (2006). Basil. In *Mosby's handbook of herbs & natural supplements* (pp. 84–88). St. Louis, MO: ElsevierMosby.

Tel Aviv University. (2008, February 29). Stress and fear can affect cancer's recurrence. *ScienceDaily*. Retrieved from http://www.sciencedaily.com/releases/2008/02/080227142656.htm

University of California–San Diego. (2006, September 19). Global view shows strong link between kidney cancer, sunlight exposure. *ScienceDaily*. Retrieved from www.sciencedaily.com/releases/2006/09/060918164649.htm

Zal, F., Mostafavi-Pour, Z., & Vessal, M. (2007). Comparison of the effectsof vitamin E and/or quercetin in attenuating chronic cyclosporine A-induced nephrotoxicity in male rats. *Clinical Experimental Pharmacology Physiology, 34*(8), 720–724.

Liver

Environment

Environmental evidence-based practice for the liver includes aromatherapy and sunlight.

1. *Aromatherapy.* Laboratory and animal studies have shown that certain essential oils have antibacterial, calming, or energizing effects. Aromatherapy may work by sending chemical messages to the part of the brain that affects moods and emotions. Lavender and rosemary protect the body from oxidative stress by decreasing the stress hormone, cortisol. Clients with liver cancer may use aromatherapy (sniffing essential lavender and rosemary oils for 5 minutes) mainly to improve their quality of life and enhance relaxation (Atsumi & Tonosake, 2007).

2. *Sunlight.* Studies show a strong correlation between adequate exposure to sunlight (10–40 minutes, depending on darkness of skin color, twice a week to the face, arms, hands, or back) and a lower risk of cancer

(Autoimmunity Research Foundation, 2007; Demgrow, 2007; Jockers, 2007).

Exercise/Movement

Exercise can enhance the health of clients with liver disease. A good beginning regimen might include 10–20 minutes of aerobic exercise, followed by a few weight-bearing exercises, three times a week. Even standing instead of sitting while using the computer, watching TV, reading, or talking on the phone can improve health. Physical inactivity throughout the day stimulates disease-promoting processes, while moving and standing stimulates enzymes that optimize metabolism (University of Missouri-Columbia, 2007, 2008). **Cautions:** When a client is in an acute phase of hepatitis or experiencing a severe exacerbation or relapse of disease, any form of intense exertion should be avoided. The liver has only so much energy to distribute to the rest of the body, so it is never wise to overdo it. Counsel clients prior to commencing any exercise program to discuss the prospect with their healthcare practitioner. Clients diagnosed with liver disease should drink at least six 8-ounce glasses of water per day. It is especially important for clients with chronic hepatitis B or C who are on interferon therapy to stay well hydrated. These clients should probably increase their water intake to at least twelve 8-ounce glasses of water per day. Clients with liver disease often find that drinking abundant amounts of water helps give them an improved sense of well-being, and patients on interferon often find that liberal water consumption helps them with some of side effects of the medication. On the other hand, individuals with ascites (the accumulation of fluid in the peritoneal cavity) are prone to excessive water retention. These individuals are advised to restrict their water intake to approximately three to four 8-ounce glasses of water per day, depending upon the degree of fluid accumulation present. When drinking bottled mineral water, it is important to take note of the water's sodium content. In some instances, the sodium content may present a problem for individuals on sodium-restricted diets. Counsel clients to warm up prior to exercise and cool down afterward. For more information, go to: http://www.wellness.ma/adult-fitness/stretching-warmup.htm and http://www.liverdisease.com/exercise_hepatitis.html

Herbs/Essential Oils

Herbal evidence-based practice for liver disease includes milk thistle and spearmint.

1. *Milk thistle.* Silymarin, the active substance in milk thistle, stimulates detoxification pathways, inhibits the growth of certain cancer cell lines, exerts direct cytotoxic activity toward certain cancer cell lines, and may increase the efficacy of certain chemotherapy agents. Milk thistle also

protects the liver from drug- or alcohol-related injury. Silibinin, a compound of milk thistle, may even prevent the development of liver cancer at 200 to 400 mg per day (Abenavoli, Capasso, Milic, & Capasso, 2010).

2. *Spearmint.* When brewed in hot water for 5 minutes, spearmint possesses antimutagenic qualities that inhibit carcinogen activation (Yu, Xu, & Dashwood, 2004).

Nutrition

1. *Curcumin.* Found in turmeric, curcumin exerts antiproliferative effects on various tumor cell lines but leaves normal human tissue alone. Because of its qualities, curcumin may prevent the spread of liver cancer (Novak, Grbesa, Ivkic, Katdare, & Gall-Troselj, 2008). Advise clients to sprinkle this spice in soups and stews, add to fish or chicken marinades, use in egg salads to add a rich yellow color, or make a tasty yellow rice pilaf.

2. *Folate.* Dietary folates protect against cancer, but folic acid fortification is associated with cancer (Ebbing et al., 2009). Leafy green vegetables (like spinach and turnip greens), broccoli, fruits (citrus fruits and juices), and dried beans and peas are all natural sources of folate that can help meet the suggested amount of 1,000 micrograms a day. Clients who do not eat breads, cereals, or pasta; who abuse alcohol; or take medications that interfere with folate absorption may not receive sufficient amounts of the nutrient and may need additional amounts (Office of Dietary Supplements, 2005). **Cautions:** Medications and medical conditions that increase the need for folate or result in an increased excretion of folate include anticonvulsant medications, metformin, sulfasalazine, triamterene, methotrexate, barbiturates, pregnancy and lactation, alcohol abuse, malabsorption, kidney dialysis, liver disease, and certain anemias. Because folate is a water-soluble B-vitamin, unneeded amounts will be eliminated in the urine. Advise clients to avoid flour-fortified foods as a source of folic acid; new research has shown the introduction of flour fortified with folic acid into common foods has been linked to cancer.

3. *Fruits, vegetables, and whole grains.* Fruits and vegetables (5–10 servings a day) and whole grains (5 servings a day) are linked to a decreased risk for cancer. Tomatoes are especially helpful, as they show a consistent pattern of protection when eaten raw and often. Consuming one serving of raw tomatoes per week reduced the risk of all cancers by 50% for older women. Watercress is linked to a reduced risk of cancer via decreased damage to DNA and possible modulation of antioxidant status by increasing carotenoid concentration (Gill et al., 2007; Hord, 2005).

4. *Green tea.* Green tea is protective against cancer before disease occurs and after onset, possibly by creating a detoxifying effect at 2–5 cups of decaffeinated tea daily (American Association of Cancer Research, 2007). **Cautions:** May decrease iron absorption, so separate iron-rich foods or iron pills by at least 2 hours from green tea ingestion. Caffeinated green tea can interact with MAOIs and lead to a hypertensive crisis. Counsel clients not to take green tea with anticoagulants/antiplatelets (may increase risk of bleeding), beta-adrenergic blockers (can lead to increased inotropic effects), or benzodiazepines (may increase sedation). Dairy products may decrease the therapeutic effects of green tea, so separate their intake by several hours (Skidmore-Roth, 2006). The digestive process affects anticancer activity of tea in gastrointestinal cells; instruct clients to add citrus (such as lemon juice) or take ascorbic acid (vitamin C) to protect the catechins in green tea from digestive degradation (Federation of American Societies for Experimental Biology, 2008).

5. *Pomegranate juice.* Pomegranate juice can reduce liver stress (Faria, Monteiro, Mateus, Azevedo & Calhau, 2007).

Supplements

Supplement evidence-based practice for liver disease includes aged garlic extract.

Aged garlic extract at 4 milliliters daily attenuated histological liver damage and oxidative stress (Kodai et al., 2007). **Cautions:** Should not be used medicinally during pregnancy because this extract can stimulate labor. Dietary amounts of garlic are acceptable. **Other considerations:** Instruct clients to discontinue use of garlic prior to undergoing any invasive procedure, and during pregnancy, monitor CBC and coagulation (when using extract at a high level) and seek supervision by a qualified herbalist if the client is taking garlic extract long term.

Touch

Touch evidence-based practice for liver disease includes acupressure and foot reflexology.

1. *Acupressure.* Acupressure can reduce nausea and vomiting induced by chemotherapy (Gardani et al., 2006).

2. *Foot reflexology.* Life satisfaction, depression, and fatigue was significantly improved in after foot reflexology twice a week for 4 weeks (Kohara et al., 2004). Combined with aromatherapy and foot soak, reflexology also relieves fatigue in patients with cancer. Foot reflexology

or self-foot reflexology also significantly enhances and strengthens the immune system so it can catch and eliminate cancer cells and prevent tumors from developing (Fox Chase Cancer Center, 2007; Lee, 2006). For foot charts, see http://www.reflexology-research.com/charts.htm

LIVER CASE STUDY   www.

Mr. Gerard has been experiencing jaundice, weakness, anorexia, nausea, weight and muscle loss, itching, bruising, black stools, and a swollen abdomen. His physician told him he had liver disease that was caused by drinking too much alcohol over time. He is on the list for a transplant, but Mr. Gerard wants to try other approaches while he waits.

HEALTH PROMOTION CHALLENGE   www.

Based on what you learned in this section, what could you suggest to Mr. Gerard if he were your client? Develop a teaching/learning plan you could use that allows for client input.

REFERENCES

Abenavoli, L., Capasso, R., Milic, N., & Capasso, F. (2010). Milk thistle in liver diseases: Past, present, future. *Phytotherapy Research, 24*(10), 1423–1432.

American Association for Cancer Research. (2007, August 12). Green tea boosts production of detox enzymes, rendering cancerous chemicals harmless. Retrieved from http://www.sciencedaily.com/releases/2007/08/070810194923.htm

Atsumi, T., & Tonosaki, K. (2007). Smelling lavender and rosemary increases free radical scavenging activity and decreases cortisol level in saliva. *Psychiatry Research, 150*(1), 89–96.

Autoimmunity Research Foundation. (2008, January 27). Vitamin D deficiency study raises new questions about disease and supplements. *ScienceDaily*. Retrieved from http://www.sciencedaily.com/releases/2008/01/080125223302.htm

Demgrow, M. (2007, June). High vitamin D: Treatment for cancer prevention? *The Clinical Advisor, 54*, 57.

Ebbing, M., Bonaa, K. H., Nygard, O., Arnesen, E., Ueland, P. M., Nordrehaug, J. E., . . . Vollset, S. E. (2009). Cancer incidence and mortality after treatment with folic acid and vitamin B12. *Journal of the American Medical Association, 302*(19), 2119–2126.

Faria, A., Monteiro, R., Mateus, N., Azevedo, I., & Calhau, C. (2007). Effect of pomegranate (*Punica granatum*) juice intake on hepatic oxidative stress. *European Journal of Nutrition, 46*(5), 271–278.

Federation of American Societies for Experimental Biology. (2008, April 10). Digestive process affects anti-cancer activity of tea in gastrointestinal cells. *ScienceDaily*. Retrieved from http://www.sciencedaily.com/releases/2008/04/080407172713.htm

Fox Chase Cancer Center. (2007, November 1). Quality of life is the most important predictor of survival for advanced cancer patients. *ScienceDaily*. Retrieved from http://www.sciencedaily.com/releases/2007/10/071030170208.htm

Gardani, G., Cerrone, R., Biella, C., Mancini, L., Proserpio, E., Casiraghi, M., . . . Lissoni, P. (2006). Effect of acupressure on nausea and vomiting induced by chemotherapy in cancer patients. *Minerva Medicine, 97*(5), 391–394.

Gill, C. I., Haldar, S., Boyd, L. A., Bennett, R., Whiteford, J., Butler, M., . . . Rowland, I. R. (2007). Watercress supplementation in diet reduces lymphocyte DNA damage and alters blood antioxidant status in healthy adults. *American Journal of Clinical Nutrition, 85*(2), 504–510.

Hord, N. G. (2005). The role of dietary factors in cancer prevention: Beyond fruit and vegetables. *Nutrition in Clinical Practice, 20*(4), 451–459.

Jockers, B. S. (2007). Vitamin D sufficiency: An approach to disease prevention. *The American Journal for Nurse Practitioners, 11*(10), 43–50.

Kohara, H., Miyauchi, T., Suehiro, Y., Ueoka, H., Takeyama, H., & Morita, T. (2004). Combined modality treatment of aromatherapy, footsoak, and reflexology relieves fatigue in patients with cancer. *Journal of Palliative Medicine, 7*(6), 791–796.

Lee, Y. M. (2006). Effect of self-foot reflexology massage on depression, stress responses and immune functions of middle aged women. *Taehan Kanho Hakhoe Chi, 36*(1), 179–188.

Novak, K. R., Grbesa, I., Ivkic, M., Katdare, M., & Gall-Troselj, K. (2008). Curcumin downregulates H19 gene transcription in tumor cells. *Journal of Cell Biochemistry, 104*(5), 1781–1792.

Office of Dietary Supplements. (2005). *Dietary supplement fact sheet: Folate.* Bethesda, MD: NIH Clinical Center, National Institutes of Health.

Skidmore-Roth, L. (2006). Green tea. In *Mosby's handbook of herbs & natural supplements* (pp. 535–539). St. Louis, MO: ElsevierMosby.

University of Missouri-Columbia. (2007, November 20). Sitting may increase risk of disease. *ScienceDaily*. Retrieved from http://www.sciencedaily.com/releases/2007/11/071119130734.htm

University of Missouri-Columbia. (2008, March 23). Killer stairs? Taking the elevator could be worse for your body. *ScienceDaily*. Retrieved from http://www.sciencedaily.com/releases/2008/03/080318182741.htm

Yu, T. W., Xu, M., & Dashwood, R. H. (2004). Antimutagenic activity of spearmint. *Environmental Molecular Mutagens, 44*(5), 387–393.

Lung Conditions

Environment

Environmental advice for lungs pertains to aromatherapy and sunlight.

1. *Aromatherapy.* Lavender and rosemary essential oils protect the body from stress and may improve quality of life for clients diagnosed with lung cancer (Atsumi & Tonosaki, 2007).

2. *Sunlight.* Researchers at the Moors Cancer Center at the University of California, San Diego showed a clear association between deficiency in exposure to sunlight, specifically ultraviolet B (UVB) and cancer. According to the National Institutes of Health, 10–15 minutes of direct midday sun at least twice a week on the face, arms, hands, or back is sufficient for Caucasians; darker skinned clients may require 3–6 times as much exposure. Eating lunch outside when weather permits could be one solution. In colder climes, clients can take a tablespoon of cod liver oil daily, eat fatty fish and fish oils, and egg yolks. Supplements of vitamin D_3 (calciferol) may be necessary for certain clients (Demgrow, 2007; Jockers, 2007).

Herbs/Essential Oils

Herbal evidence-based practice for lungs includes milk thistle.

Silymarin, the active substance in milk thistle, stimulates detoxification pathways, inhibits the growth of certain cancer cell lines, exerts direct cyto-toxic activity toward certain cancer cell lines, and may increase the efficacy of certain chemotherapy agents. Milk thistle also protects the liver from drug- or alcohol-related injury. Silibinin, a compound of milk thistle, may even prevent the development of liver cancer when 200 to 400 mg of silymarin is taken daily (Cheung, Gibbons, Johnson, & Nicol, 2010).

Nutrition

Nutrition evidence-based practice for lungs includes the following:

1. *Dietary fats.* Preservation of lung health with aging is an important health issue in the general population, as loss of lung function with aging can lead to the development of obstructive lung disease and is a predictor of all-cause and cardiovascular mortality. Inflammation is increasingly linked to loss of lung function, and evidence suggests that consumption of dietary fat exacerbates inflammation (Wood, Attia, McElduff, McEvoy, & Gibson, 2010).

2. *Curcumin.* Curcumin, found in turmeric, exerts an antiproliferative effect on various tumor cell lines, but leaves normal human tissue alone. Because of its qualities, curcumin may prevent the spread of liver cancer (Novak, Grbesa, Ivkic, Katdarek & Gall-Troselj, 2008).

3. *Fruits, vegetables, and whole grains.* The consumption of fruits and vegetables and whole grains is linked to a decreased risk for cancers, including lung cancer. Raw tomatoes are especially helpful (Hord, 2005).

4. *Green tea.* Green tea (2–5 cups daily, decaffeinated) is protective against cancer before disease occurs and after onset, possibly by creating a detoxifying effect (American Association for Cancer Research, 2007).

Cautions: Green tea may decrease iron absorption, so separate iron-rich foods or iron pills by at least 2 hours from green tea ingestion.

5. *Red and processed meat, onions and apples.* Consumption of red and processed meat is positively associated with lung cancer (Cross et al., 2007), while onions, garlic, and apples may reduce risk (Galeon, 2006; Gonzalez & Riboli, 2006; Hung, 2007).

Stress Management

A weak immune system is one of the major factors that promotes cancer metastases after an operation, chemotherapy, or radiation therapy. Fear and stress weaken the immune system. Adequate stress management prior to and after medical treatment may help to prevent metastases (Tel Aviv University, 2008). For stress management techniques, go to: http://www.mindtools.com/pages /main/newMN_TCS.htm

Supplements

Supplement evidence-based practice for lungs includes use of silymarin.

Silymarin (silibinin) is an anticancer and anti-inflammatory agent that can also counter the negative effects of chemotherapy and radiation, as it cleanses and strengthens the liver and kidneys (Cheung, Gibbons, Johnson, & Nicol, 2010).

Touch

1. *Acupressure.* Acupressure can reduce nausea and vomiting induced by chemotherapy (Gardani et al., 2006). The PC6 point in the middle of the front of the forearm above the wrist crease is stimulated. Wristbands are available to stimulate this point. The point can be stimulated every 2–3 hours or as needed. For more information on using acupressure, go to http://www.eclecticenergies.com/acupressure/howto.php and http:// www.agelessherbs.com/acupressurepoints.html

2. *Foot reflexology.* When delivered by a partner, foot reflexology can relieve anxiety and pain of lung cancer patients (Stephenson, Swanson, Dalton, Keefe, Engelke, 2007). For foot reflexology information, go to http://www.how-to-do-reflexology.com/footreflexology.html

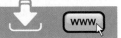

LUNG CASE STUDY

Mrs. Amory, a 68-year-old woman, diagnosed with pulmonary hypertension secondary to congenital heart disease, came to the emergency department with chest pain. She was on therapy with calcium channel blockers and an ACE inhibitor. She was started on inhaled iloprost.

HEALTH PROMOTION CHALLENGE ☆ ⟨www⟩

What health promotion procedures that complement her medical treatment could you recommend to Mrs. Amory based on what you read in this section?

REFERENCES

American Association for Cancer Research. (2007, August 12). Green tea boosts production of detox enzymes, rendering cancerous chemicals harmless. Retrieved from http://www.sciencedaily.com/releases/2007/08/070810194923.htm

Atsumi, T., & Tonosaki, K. (2007). Smelling lavender and rosemary increases free radical scavenging activity and decreases cortisol level in saliva. *Psychiatry Research, 150*(1), 89–96.

Cheung, C. W., Gibbons, N., Johnson, D. W., & Nicol, D. L. (2010). Silibinin—a promising new treatment for cancer. *Anticancer Agents in Medicinal Chemistry, 10*(3), 186–195.

Cross, A. J., Leitzann, M. E., Gail, M. H., Hollenbeck, A. R., Schatzkin, A., & Sinha, R. (2007). A prospective study of red and processed meat intake in relation to cancer risk. *PLoS Medicine, 4*(12), e325.

Demgrow, M. (2007, June). High vitamin D: Treatment for cancer prevention? *The Clinical Advisor, 54*, 57.

Galeon, C. (2006). Onion and garlic use and human cancer. *American Journal of Clinical Nutrition, 84*, 1027–1032.

Gardani, G., Cerrone, R., Biella, C., Mancini, L., Proserpio, E., Casiraghi, M., . . . Lissoni, P. (2006). Effect of acupressure on nausea and vomiting induced by chemotherapy in cancer patients. *Minerva Medicine, 97*(5), 391–394.

Gonzalez, C. A., & Riboli, E. (2006). Diet and cancer prevention: Where we are, where we are going. *Nutrition in Cancer, 56*(2), 225–231.

Hord, N. G. (2005). The role of dietary factors in cancer prevention: Beyond fruits and vegetables. *Nutrition in Clinical Practice, 20*(4), 451–459.

Hung, H. (2007). Dietary quercetin inhibits proliferation of lung carcinoma cells. *Forum of Nutrition, 60*, 146–57.

Jockers, B. S. (2007). Vitamin D sufficiency: An approach to disease prevention. *The American Journal for Nurse Practitioners, 11*(10), 43–50.

Novak, K. R., Grbesa, I., Ivkic, M., Katdare, M., & Gall-Troselj, K. (2008). Curcumin downregulates H19 gene transcription in tumor cells. *Journal of Cell Biochemistry, 104*(5), 1781–1792.

Stephenson, N. L., Swanson, M., Dalton, J., Keefe, F. J., Engelke, M. (2007). Partner-delivered reflexology: Effects on cancer pain and anxiety. *Oncology Nursing Forum, 34*(1), 127–132.

Tel Aviv University. (2008, February 29). Stress and fear can affect cancer's recurrence. *Science-Daily*. Retrieved from http://www.sciencedaily.com/releases/2008/02/080227142656.htm

Wood, L. G., Attia, J., McElduff, P., McEvoy, M., Gibson, P. G. (2010). Assessment of dietary fat intake and innate immune activation as risk factors for impaired lung function. *European Journal of Clinical Nutrition, 64*(8), 818–825.

Menopause

Environment

Environmental evidence-based practice for menopause includes conjugated estrogens/medroxyprogesterone.

Postmenopausal women who take conjugated estrogens/medroxyprogesterone (Prempro, Premarin, or Premique) for breakthrough bleeding have a significant increase in cardiovascular events including CFD, venous thromboembolism, unstable angina requiring hospitalization, heart attack, or sudden coronary death. Discontinuing hormones can also lead to an increased risk of breast cancer and heart disease (Nelson, Walker, Zakher & Mitchell, 2012), so it might be best never to start taking them (Alper, 2008).

Exercise/Movement

Exercise/movement evidence-based practice for menopause includes brisk walking and preventing bone loss.

1. *Brisk walking.* Women in pre- and postmenopause who walked regularly every week reduced oxidative stress, thereby improving their sleep status and their perceived mood, including anxiety and depression. The most beneficial reactions occurred in women who walked for an hour and a half at least five times a week. Women who walked five times a week for 40 minutes also benefited, but not as much (Wilbur, Miller, McDevitt, Wang, & Miller, 2005). **Cautions:** Go to http://exercise .lifetips.com/cat/7281/injuryprevention/index.html **Other considerations:** Counsel women that they need not go to the gym. They can walk outside on city blocks or in shopping malls (Temple University, 2008a, 2008b).

2. *Resistance training and hormones for preventing bone loss.* Weight lifting (resistance training, using the squat and deadlift 2 days a week) alone was as effective as hormones for early postmenopausal women in preventing spinal bone loss, with no side effects (Maddalozzo et al., 2006). **Cautions:** Continue to breathe while lifting weights to prevent increased blood pressure. For more information, go to http://www.bodybuilding .com/fun/south30.htm

Herbs/Essential Oils

Herb evidence-based practice for menopause includes black cohosh and spearmint.

1. *Black cohosh.* Black cohosh can reduce menopause symptoms as well as conjugated estrogens at a daily oral dose of 40 mg, black cohosh vs.

0.6 mg/day of conjugated estrogens (Geller & Studee, 2006), but with none of the dangerous side effects of hormones (stroke, thromboembolic events, gallbladder disease, and urinary incontinence; estrogen plus progestin increased breast cancer and probable dementia (Nelson, Walker, Zakher, & Mitchell, 2012).) Counsel women to take only standardized products. **Other considerations:** Structurally, black cohosh more closely resembles estriol, which researchers believe offers protection against cancer of the endometrium, ovaries, and breast (Lupu et al., 2003).

2. *Spearmint.* Tea made from spearmint tea can be an alternative to antiandrogenic treatment for excessive growth of hair. **Cautions:** Women with hiatal hernia or a gallstone attack should avoid spearmint (Akdogan et al., 2007).

Nutrition

Nutrition evidence-based practice for menopause includes soy, red meat, and vitamin K.

1. *Soy.* High soy isoflavone intake (half cup of soy nuts divided into 3–4 portions spaced throughout the day; 1–2 glasses of soy milk, 1 cup cooked soybeans, 1 soy burger, or soy cheese to a total of 100 mg isoflavones/day) reduces the risk of cerebral and myocardial infarctions, osteoporosis, hot flashes, and bone fracture, and improves memory and sexuality in postmenopausal women (Kokubo et al., 2007; Welty, Lee, Lew, Nasca & Zhou, 2007; Zhang et al., 2005). **Cautions:** Many nonorganic soy beans have been genetically modified (never researched for their long-term effects) and may be treated with dangerous chemicals, so they should be avoided. The best sources of soy are organic fermented products like tempeh or miso because they are more easily digested.

2. *Red meat.* Consumption of heme iron from red meat may increase cardiovascular health risk among postmenopausal women compared to premenopausal women, especially for women with diabetes. The higher the consumption, the higher the risk (Qi, van Dam, Rexrode, & Hu, 2007).

3. *Vitamin K foods.* An analysis of 13 clinical trials showed that vitamin K reduces postmenopausal fracture rates (Alper, 2007). Counsel postmenopausal women to eat daily servings of asparagus, blackstrap molasses, broccoli, Brussels sprouts, cabbage, cauliflower, dark green leafy vegetables, egg yolks, liver, oatmeal, soybeans, and wheat.

Stress Management

Stress management evidence-based practice for menopause includes cognitive behavioral group intervention.

In one study, a cognitive behavioral group intervention resulted in women showing significant improvements in anxiety, depression, partnership relations, sexuality, hot flashes, and cardiac complaints from pre- to postintervention. The women, all suffering from climacteric symptoms, participated in psychoeducation, group discussion, and coping skills training (Alder et al., 2006). **Cautions:** This pilot study points at possible effectiveness. Future studies are needed to use random assignment and a control group. For more information see http://www.mind.org.uk/Information/Booklets/Making+sense/MakingSenseCBT.html

Supplements

Supplement evidence-based practice for menopause includes flaxseed, magnolia extract, magnesium, and pycnogenol.

1. *Flaxseed.* A daily dose of 4 tablespoons of flaxseed, crushed and placed in food or water, decreased hot flashes by 50% over 6 weeks in postmenopausal women (Pruthi et al., 2007). Suggest clients with hot flashes start with 1/2 a teaspoon of flax seeds to make sure they don't have an allergic reaction. If that amount is well-tolerated, slowly work up to 4 tablespoons daily. **Cautions:** Should not be used by women with a bowel obstruction. Flax can interact with all oral medications; absorption of medications may be decreased if taken concurrently with flax, so take them at different time of the day. Flax may increase risk of bleeding if clients are taking anticoagulants. Flax may increase the action of antibetic agents (Skidmore-Roth, 2006a).

2. *Magnolia extract and magnesium.* In a study by Mucci and colleagues (2006), magnolia extract (60 mg) and magnesium (50 mg) showed a significant effect on flushing, nocturnal sweating, palpitations, insomnia, asthenia, anxiety, mood depression, irritability, vaginal dryness, pain during intercourse, and loss of libido as opposed to taking soy isoflavones, lactobacilli, calcium, and vitamin D_3.

3. *Pycnogenol.* Pycnogenol (200 mg daily) improves all menopause symptoms (Yang, Liao, Zhu, Liao, & Rohdewald, 2007).

MENOPAUSE CASE STUDY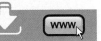

Ms. Orengo, age 50, is searching for information on how to relieve her hot flashes, irritability, emotionality, insomnia, skin changes, thinning hair, and sexual discomfort. She has been taken off hormones by her nurse practitioner because of the cancer and heart-related issues involved. Ms. Orengo asks to talk to someone about health promotion interventions with no side effects.

HEALTH PROMOTION CHALLENGE

Using the information in this section as well as what you find at PubMed (http://www.ncbi.nlm.nih.gov/pubmed/), develop a teaching/learning plan for Ms. Orengo.

REFERENCES

Akdogan, M., Tamer, M. N., Cure, E., Cure, M. C., Koroglu, B. K., & Delibas, N. (2007). Effect of spearmint (*Mentha spicata Labiatae*) teas on androgen levels in women with hirsutism. *Phytotherapy Research, 21*(5), 444–447.

Alder, J., Eymann, B. K., Armbruster, U., Decio, R., Gairing, A., Kang, A., & Bitzer, J. (2006). Cognitive-behavioural group intervention for climacteric syndrome. *Psychotherapy and Psychosomatics, 75*(5), 298–303.

Alper, B. S. (2007, January). Vitamin K appears to reduce post-menopausal fracture rates. Evidence-based medicine. *The Clinical Advisor*, p. 127.

Alper, B. S. (2008, January). Evidence-based medicine. HRT increases risk of cardiovascular disease in older women. *The Clinical Advisor*, p. 97.

Geller, S. E., & Studee, I. (2006). Contemporary alternatives to plant estrogens for menopause. *Maturitas, 55*(Suppl1), S3–S13.

Kokubo, Y., Iso, H., Ishihara, J., Okada, K., Inoue, M., & Tsugane, S. (2007). Association of dietary intake of soy, beans, and isoflavones with risk of cerebral and myocardial infarctions in Japanese populations: The Japan Public Health Center-based (JPHC) study cohort. *Circulation, 116*(22), 2553–2562.

Lupu, R., Mehmi, I., Atlas, E., Tsai, M. S., Pisha, E., . . . Kronenberg, F. (2003, November). Black cohosh, a menopausal remedy, does not have estrogenic activity and does not promote breast cancer cell growth. *International Journal of Oncology, 5*(23), 1407–1412.

Maddalozzo, G. F., Widrick, J. J., Cardinal, B. J., Winters-Stone, K. M., Hoffman, M. A., & Snow, C. M. (2006). The effects of hormone replacement therapy and resistance training on spine bone mineral density in early postmenopausal women. *Bone, 40*(5), 1244–1251.

Mucci, M., Carraro, C., Mancino, P., Monti, M., Papadia, L. S., Volpini, G., & Benvenuti, C. (2006). Soy isoflavones, lactobacilli, magnolia bark extract, vitamin D3 and calcium. Controlled clinical study in menopause. *Minerva Ginecology, 58*(4), 323–334.

Nelson, H. D., Walker, M., Zakher, B., & Mitchell, J. (2012). Menopausal hormone therapy for the primary prevention of chronic conditions: Systematic Review to Update the 2002 and 2005 U.S. Preventive Services Task Force Recommendations. Rockville (MD): Agency for Healthcare Research and Quality (US); 2012 May. Report No.: 12-05168-EF-1. U.S. Preventive Services Task Force Evidence Syntheses, formerly Systematic Evidence Reviews.

Pruthi, S., Thompson, S. L., Novotny, P. J., Barton, D. L., Kottschade, L. A. Tan, A. D., . . . Loprinzi, C. L. (2007). Pilot evaluation of flaxseed for the management of hot flashes. *Journal of the Society for Integrative Oncology, 5*(3), 106–112.

Qi, L., van Dam, R. M., Rexrode, K., & Hu, F. B. (2007). Heme iron from diet as a risk factor for coronary heart disease in women with type 2 diabetes. *Diabetes Care, 30*(1), 101–106.

Skidmore-Roth. (2006a). Flax. In *Mosby's handbooks of herbs & natural supplements* (pp. 450–454). St. Louis, MO: Elsevier Mosby.

Temple University. (2008a, March 20). Reducing heart disease risk naturally post-menopause. *ScienceDaily*. Retrieved from http://www.sciencedaily.com/releases/2008/03/080318084333.htm

Temple University. (2008b, January 4). Walk away menopausal anxiety, stress and depression. *ScienceDaily*. Retrieved from http://www.sciencedaily.com/releases/2008/01/080103090651.htm

Welty, F. K., Lee, K. S., Lew, N. S., Nasca, M., & Zhou, J-R. (2007). The association between soy nut consumption and decreased menopausal symptoms. *Journal of Women's Health, 16*(3), 361–369.

Wilbur, J., Miller, A. M., McDevitt, J., Wang, E., & Miller, J. (2005). Menopausal status, moderate-intensity walking, and symptoms in midlife women. *Research and Theory in Nursing Practice, 19*(2), 163–180.

Yang, H. M., Liao, M. F., Zhu, S. Y., Liao, M. N., & Rohdewald, P. (2007). A randomized, double-blind, placebo-controlled trial on the effect of pycnogenol on the climacteric syndrome in peri-menopausal women. *Acta obstetricia et Gynecologica Scandinavica, 86*(8), 978 985.

Zhang, X., Shu, X.-O., Honglan, L., Yang, G., Qi, L., Yu-Tang, G., et al. (2005). Prospective cohort study of soy food consumption and risk of bone fracture among post-menopausal women. *Archives of Internal Medicine, 165*, 1890–1895.

Migraines

Exercise/Movement

Exercise/movement evidence-based practice for migraines includes yoga.

A significant reduction in migraine headache frequency and associated clinical features occurred in women who participated in 60-minute yoga sessions over 3 months (John, Sharma, Sharma, & Kankane, 2007). **Cautions:** Go to http://yoga.lifetips.com/cat/56770/yoga-cautions/

Herbs/Essential Oils

Herbal evidence-based practice for migraines includes butterbur.

Butterbur significantly decreased migraine attack frequency per month by 48% more than placebo when taken orally as an extract of 75 mg (Lipton, Gobel, Einhaupl, Wilks, & Mauskop, 2004). **Cautions:** The most frequently reported adverse reactions were mild gastrointestinal events, predominantly burping.

Stress Management

Stress management evidence-based practice for migraines includes cognitive behavioral therapy, relaxation training, and autogenic training.

1. *Cognitive behavioral therapy and relaxation training.* In one study, three or more sessions of behavioral treatments enabled women with recurrent headaches to handle related stress, modify reactions to their condition, and reduce migraine occurrence significantly (approximately 32–49% as opposed to 5% reduction in a control group). The effects appear to be sustained over time with or without further contacts or booster sessions (Symvoulakis, Clark, Dowson, Jones, & Leone, 2007). **Other considerations:** The U.S. Headache Consortium recommended that relaxation training and cognitive behavioral therapy be considered as treatment options for the prevention of migraine (grade A evidence).

2. *Autogenic training.* In a study, long-term autogenic training (every evening, preferably prior to going to sleep) proved to be a significantly effective preventive intervention in migraine sufferers (Juhasz et al., 2007). **Cautions:** Go to http://www.autoaura.com/autogenic.html

Supplements

Supplement evidence-based practice for migraines includes coenzyme Q10.

Compared to placebo, CoQ10 (100 mg t.i.d. for 3 months) was superior for attack frequency, headache days, and days with nausea in a 2005 study (Sandor et al., 2005). **Cautions:** Well tolerated, but mild gastrointestinal reactions have been reported, including nausea, anorexia, diarrhea, and epigastric pain. CoQ10 may decrease the action of anticoagulants; advise clients to avoid using CoQ10 and anticoagulants concurrently. Drugs that can decrease the action of coenzyme Q10 include beta-blockers, HMG-CoA reductase inhibitors, chlorpromazine, and tricyclic antidepressants.

Touch

Touch evidence-based practice for migraines includes acupuncture and massage therapy.

1. *Acupuncture.* In a multicentral, randomized, and controlled trial, acupuncture was significantly more effective than treatment with flunarizine tablets. The total effective rates for stopping pain after treatment and 3 months and 6 months after treatment in the acupuncture group were 93.0%, 93.0%, and 87.7%, respectively, which were better than 85.6%, 86.5%, and 69.2% in the Western medication group (all $P < 0.01$). One year later, the stability of the therapeutic effect in the acupuncture group was better than that in the Western medicine group ($P < 0.05$); the adverse reaction and the compliance in the acupuncture group were significantly superior to those in the Western medicine group (Zhong et al., 2009). A review of more than 12 additional studies suggests that acupuncture is at least as effective as, or possibly more effective than,

prophylactic drug treatment, and it has fewer adverse effects. Acupuncture should be considered a treatment option for patients willing to undergo this treatment (Linde et al., 2009).

2. *Massage therapy.* Compared to control participants, massage participants in weekly massage sessions exhibited greater improvements in migraine frequency and sleep quality (Lawler & Cameron, 2006). Massaging over the greater occipital nerve can reduce the intensity for migraine attacks (Piovesan et al., 2007). **Cautions:** The aged, extremely ill, or dying individual may require a gentle massage. The head is also a sensitive area and only gentle sweeping motions are used, and energy is not concentrated in that area or in an area where cancer resides. Go to http://www.wikihow.com/Do-a-Hard-Core-Advanced-Therapeutic-Massage

MIGRAINE CASE STUDY

Mr. Humphries, age 47, has migraines once a month and had had 3 attacks in the past 60 days. Symptoms associated with his migraines include ice cold extremities, dizziness, vomiting, diarrhea, and off-balance walking. He has a prominent aura that precedes his headaches. He has tried various pain medications, but they only make the migraines come back even worse. He wants to know if there are more health-promoting approaches to his migraines.

HEALTH PROMOTION CHALLENGE

Based on this section and doing a search on PubMed (http://www.ncbi.nlm.nih.gov/pubmed/) for migraines, develop a teaching/learning program for Mr. Humphries.

REFERENCES

John, P. J., Sharma, N., Sharma, C. M., & Kankane, A. (2007). Effectiveness of yoga therapy in the treatment of migraine without aura: A randomized controlled trial. *Headache, 47*(5), 654–661.

Juhasz, G., Zsombok, T., Gonda, X., Nagyne, N., Modosne, E., & Bagdy, G. (2007). Effects of autogenic training on nitroglycerin-induced headaches. *Headaches, 47*(3), 371–383.

Lawler, S. P., & Cameron, L. D. (2006). A randomized, controlled trial for massage therapy as a treatment for migraine. *Annals of Behavioral Medicine, 32*(1), 50–59.

Linde, K., Allais, G., Brinkhaus, B., Manheimer, E., Vickers, A., & White, A. R. (2009). Acupuncture for migraine prophylaxis. *Cochrane Database System of Reviews, 21*(1), CD001218.

Lipton, R. B., Gobel, H., Einhaupl, K. M., Wilks, K., & Mauskop, A. (2004). Petasites ybridus root (butterbur) is an effective preventive treatment for migraine. *Neurology, 63*(12), 2240–2244.

Piovesan, E. J., Di Stani, F., Kowacs, P. A., Mulinari, R. A., Radunz, V. H., Utiumi, M., & Werneck, L. C. (2007). Massaging over the greater occipital nerve reduces the intensity of migraine attacks: Evidence for inhibitory trigemino-cervical convergence mechanisms. *Arquivos de neuro-psiquiatria, 65*(3A), 599–604.

Sandor, E. S., Di Clemente, L., Coppola, G., Saenger, U., Fumal, A., Magis, D., . . . Schoenen, J. (2005). Efficacy of coenzyme Q10 in migraine prophylaxis: a randomized controlled trial. *Neurology, 64*(4), 713–715.

Symvoulakis, E. K., Clark, L. V., Dowson, A. J., Jones, R., & Leone, R. (2007). Headache: A suitable case for behavioural treatment in primary care? *British Journal of General Practice, 57*(536), 231–237.

Zhong, G. W. Li, W., Luo, Y. H., Wang, S. E., Wu, Q. M., Zhou, B., . . . Liu, B. L. (2009, April). Acupuncture at points of the liver and gallbladder meridians for treatment of migraine: A multi-center randomized and controlled study. *Zhongguo Zhen Jiu, 29*(4), 259–263.

Osteoporosis/Osteopenia

Environment

Environmental evidence-based practice for osteoporosis/osteopenia includes the following:

1. *Antidepressants.* Antidepressant use is associated with increased risk of fractures at the spine and sites other than the hip or wrist, and clients taking fluoxetine (Prozac), paroxetine (Paxil), and sertraline (Zoloft) are more prone to bone loss (Oregon Health and Science University, 2007; Spangler et al., 2008).

2. *Dieting.* Clients whose diet does not supply enough energy to fuel their exercise level may harm their body's ability to form bone. Thousands of women severely restrict their diet and practice rigorous exercise programs (2 hours a day) for weight control (Ohio University, 2007).

3. *Low vitamin D.* Clients with low levels of vitamin D have a 77% increased risk of hip fracture (University of Pittsburgh Schools of the Health Sciences, 2007). Vitamin D is available in fish liver oil or is produced in Caucasians by 4–10 minutes of exposure of face, arms, or back to the noonday sun, and by 60–80 minutes of exposure for darker skinned individuals. Clients living at latitudes north of 35°, who do not receive exposure to the sun, or who are older than 49 years may need to take a tablespoon of cod liver oil daily (Jockers, 2007). Vitamin D_2 that is added to fortified foods and many multivitamins and is usually written in prescriptions is inefficiently metabolized in humans; only 20–40% is metabolized into biologically active vitamin D_3.

4. *Smoking.* Smoking is linked with osteoporosis. The more women smoke, the more the risk for osteoporosis (Aran-Arri, Gutierrez-Ibarluzea, Ecenarro, & Asua Batarrita, 2007). For smoking cessation ideas, go to http://www.helpguide.org/mental/quit_smoking_cessation.htm or www.cdc.gov/tobacco/how2quit.htm

Exercise/Movement

Exercise/movement evidence-based practice for osteoporosis includes physical activity and weighted exercises.

1. *Physical activity.* There is an inverse relationship between physical activity and hip fracture. Intense, high-impact programs are the most effective (Schmitt, Schmitt, & Doren, 2009).

2. *Weighted exercises.* Using weights (8–12 repetitions of 2–3 sets performed over 1 year) can help maintain bone mineral density (BMD) in postmenopausal women and increase BMD of the spine and hip in women with osteopenia and osteoporosis (Zehnacker & Bemis-Doughtery, 2007). Clients in long-term care institutions are especially at risk for osteoporotic fractures owing to their lack of mobility, poor nutrition, and limited sun exposure. A comprehensive exercise program combined with vitamin D and calcium, been recommended by the Quebec symposium for the treatment of osteoporosis in long-term care institutions (Duque et al., 2007). For information on weight training, go to http://www.exrx.net/Exercise.html, http://www.exrx.net/WeightTraining/Instructions.html, and http://treadmarkz.wordpress.com/2008/02/16/wheelchair-weightlifting-tips-and-cautions/

Nutrition

Nutrition evidence-based practice for osteoporosis includes the following:

1. *Acidic dietary patterns.* Metabolic acidosis can have a negative effect on bone density. In a 2007 study, those with the greatest potential renal acid load (PRAL) had higher intakes of meat, fish, eggs, and cereal and lower intakes of fruit and vegetables. PRAL was inversely associated with bone ultrasound measures in women. Fruits and vegetables provide magnesium, a mineral associated with an alkaline environment that reduces calcium excretion, thereby improving bone density (Kitchin & Morgan, 2007). Encourage clientso eat a half cup of 5–10 fruits and/or vegetables daily to increase bone density (Welch, Bingham, Reeve, & Khaw, 2007).

2. *Calcium.* Calcium has been found beneficial for bone health (Tucker, 2009). Good sources of calcium include salmon with bones, sardines, seafoods, cooked green leafy vegetables, broccoli, cabbage, figs, oatmeal, prunes, and low-fat yogurt. Oxalic acid (found in almonds, beet

greens, cashews, chard, cocoa, kale, rhubarb, soybeans, and spinach) can interfere with calcium absorption when used in large amounts. Phytic acid, found in the bran of whole grains, nuts, and the skins of legumes, can bind to calcium to block its intake. A diet high in protein, fat, and/or sugar affects calcium uptake. The average American diet of meats, refined grains, and soft drinks (high in phosphorus) leads to increased excretion of calcium. Consuming alcoholic beverages, coffee, junk foods, excess salt, and/or white flour products also leads to loss of calcium from the body (Frasetto, Morris, Sellmety, & Sebastian, 2008).

3. *Coffee.* In two studies, drinking four or more cups of coffee a day significantly increased the risk of fracture for older women, but tea did not, probably because of its high level of flavonoids (Hallstrom, Wolk, Glynne & Michaelsson, 2006; Muraki et al., 2007). Assist clients to reduce or eliminate their coffee intake by drinking half caffeinated and half decaffeinated coffee. Counsel them to switch to drinking black or green tea, but not the instant form (Washington University School of Medicine, 2008).

4. *Chocolate.* Chocolate's oxalate content blocks calcium absorption and its sugar content boosts calcium excretion, making a negative impact on women's bone density and strength for total hip, femoral neck, tibia, and heel bones. The greatest risk to bone density and strength is when chocolate is eaten daily. The more frequently chocolate is eaten, the greater the risk (Hodgson, Devine, Burke, Dick, & Prince, 2008). Counsel clients to switch to carob; it has a natural sweetness and three times more calcium than milk.

5. *Colas.* Intake of colas, but not other carbonated soft drinks, is associated with low bone mineral density at each hip site, but not the spine, in women. In a 2006 study, the mean bone mineral density of those with daily cola intake was 3.7% lower at the femoral neck and 5.4% lower at Ward's area than of those who consumed less than one serving of cola a month. Similar results were seen for diet cola, although weaker, and for decaffeinated cola (Tucker et al., 2006). Counsel clients to drink water, fruit juices, or teas that do not compromise bone mineral density.

6. *Curcumin.* Curcumin elicits unique signaling pathways to orchestrate bioeffects in bone (Anand, Kunnumakkara, Newman & Aggarwall, 2007; Jurutka et al., 2007). Found the curry spice turmeric, curcumin possesses potent antioxidant and anti-inflammatory properties and can be used daily to season salad dressings, baked potatoes, stews, soups, vegetables, meats, fish, and sauces.

7. *Homocysteine and vitamin B_{12}.* Older adults with high homocysteine (an amino acid produced by the body as a byproduct of consuming meat or drinking five or more cups of coffee) and low vitamin B_{12} levels

have a 70% greater risk of hip fracture (Dhonukshe-Rutten et al., 2005; McClean et al., 2008).

8. *Magnesium.* Foods rich in magnesium significantly improve bone density. Good sources of magnesium include dry-roasted pumpkin and squash seed kernels, Brazil nuts, halibut, spinach, dry-roasted cashews, cooked soybeans, and pine nuts (Takeda & Nakamura, 2008). Caution clients to use the non-oil-added brands of nuts and seeds if weight maintenance or loss is an issue.

9. *Soy, omega-3 fatty acids, and fruit.* Omega-3 long chain fatty acids, such as those in fish oil, may be integral to preventing bone loss. When added to fish oil (in salmon, sardines, tuna, mackerel or other cold water fish), soy made vertebrae more resistant to fracture (Ho et al., 2003; Ward & Fonseca, 2007). High fruit intake is associated with higher bone mineral density (Zalloua, 2007). A daily diet containing soy, omega-3 fatty acids, and fruit may be ideal to prevent bone loss. Other sources of omega-3 include winter squash, walnuts, olive oil, beans, and flaxseeds. Sources of soy include soy milk, soy cheese or soy meat, soy nuts, tempeh, and miso soup.

10. *Tea.* Instant teas can contain dangerous levels of fluoride (Whyte, Essmyer, Gannon, & Reinus, 2005). Suggest clients make their own tea, not use instant versions.

11. *Vitamin K.* Vitamin K reduced bone loss in 12 of 13 trials and was associated with reduced postmenopausal fracture rates in all 7 trials that evaluated this outcome (Borrelli & Ernst, 2010; "Vitamin K," 2007). Daily ingestion of vitamin K-rich foods can strengthen bones. Foods to focus on include asparagus, blackstrap molasses (a tablespoon a day or use in cooking), broccoli, Brussels sprouts, cabbage, cauliflower, green leafy vegetables, egg yolks, liver, and oatmeal. **Cautions:** Coumarin-based anticoagulants adversely affect vertebral bone mineral density and increase fracture risk (Pearson, 2007).

Supplements

Supplement evidence-based practice for osteoporosis includes calcium.

Adults over 50 who take calcium supplements (1,500 mg/day) suffer fewer fractures and enjoy a better quality of life. Older adults in long-term care institutions, where osteoporosis is underdiagnosed and undertreated, are especially at risk for osteoporotic fractures due to their immobility, poor nutrition, and limited sun exposure. These clients should receive vitamin D (via sunshine or tablet), calcium, and a comprehensive exercise program (see "Exercise" previously in this section). **Other considerations:** The positive effects of daily calcium and vitamin D supplements have the potential to reduce the risk of fracture in older adults by almost one-fourth (Duque et al., 2007; Tang, et al., 2007).

OSTEOPOROSIS CASE STUDY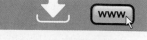

Mrs. Vickers, a 60-year-old postmenopausal grandmother, started taking an estrogen-progestin for to prevent osteoporosis. She recently found out about the dangers of taking hormones and worries she is at risk cancer or heart disease. As a result, she has decided to stop taking hormone replacement therapy and to find more health-promoting approaches to prevent osteoporosis.

HEALTH PROMOTION CHALLENGE

What would you tell Mrs. Vickers? Develop a teaching/learning plan for her.

REFERENCES

Anand, P., Kunnumakkara, A. B., Newman, R. A., & Aggarwal, B. B. (2007). Bioavailability of curcumin: Problems and promises. *Molecular Pharmacology, 4*(6), 807–818.

Aran-Arri, E., Gutierrez-Ibarluzea, I., Ecenarro, M. A., & Asua Batarrita, J. (2007). Prevalence of certain osteoporosis-determining habits among post menopausal women in the Basque country, Spain, in 2003. *Revista Espanola de Salud Publica, 81*(6), 647–656.

Borrelli, F., & Ernst, E. (2010). Alternative and complementary therapies for the menopause. *Maturitas, 66*(4), 333–343.

Dhonukshe-Rutten, R. A., Pluijm S. M., de Groot, L. C., Lips, P., Smit, J. H., & van Staveren, W. A. (2005). Homocysteine and vitamin B12 status relate to bone turnover markers, broadband ultrasound attenuation, and fractures in healthy elderly people. *Journal of Bone Mineral Research, 20*(6), 921–929.

Duque, G., Mallet, L., Roberts, A., Gingrass, S., Kremer, R., Sainte-Marie, L. G., & Kiel, D. P. (2007). To treat or not to treat, that is the question: Proceedings of the Quebec symposium for the treatment of osteoporosis in long-term care institutions. *Journal of Medical Directors Association, 8*(3 Suppl 2), e67–e73.

Frasetto, L. A., Morris, R. C., Jr., Sellmety, D. E., & Sebastian, A. (2008). Adverse effects of sodium chloride on bone in the aging human population resulting from habitual consumption of typical American diets. *Journal of Nutrition, 138*(2), 419S–422S.

Hallstrom, H., Wolk, A., Glynne, A., & Michaelsson, K. (2006). Coffee, tea and caffeine consumption in relation to osteoporotic fracture risk in a cohort of Swedish women. *Osteoporosis International, 17*(7), 1055–1064.

Ho, S. C., Woo, J., Lam, S., Chen, Y., Sham, A., & Lau, J. (2003). Soy protein consumption and bone mass in early postmenopausal Chinese women. *Osteoporosis International, 14*(10), 835–842.

Hodgson, J. M., Devine, A., Burke, V., Dick, I. M., & Prince, R. L. (2008). Chocolate consumption and bone density in older women. *American Journal of Clinical Nutrition, 8*(1), 175–180.

Jockers, B. S. (2007). Vitamin D sufficiency: An approach to disease prevention. *The American Journal for Nurse Practitioners, 11*(10), 43–50.

Jurutka, P. W., Bartik, L., Whitfield, G. K., Mathern, D. R., Barthel, T. K., Gurevich, M., . . . Haussler, M. R. (2007). Vitamin D receptor: key roles in bone mineral pathophysiology, molecular mechanism of action, and novel nutritional ligands. *Journal of Bone and Mineral Research, 22*(Suppl 2), V2–V10.

Kitchin, B., & Morgan, S. L. (2007). Not just calcium and vitamin D: Other nutritional considerations in osteoporosis. *Current Rheumatology Reports, 9*(1), 85–92.

McClean, R. R., Jacques, P. F., Selhub, J., Fredman, L., Tucker, K. L., Samuelson, E. J., . . . Hannan, M. T. (2008). Plasma B vitamins; homocysteine and their relation with bloss and hip fracture in elderly men and women. *Journal of Clinical Endocrinology and Metabolism, 93*(6), 2206–2212.

Muraki, S., Yamamoto, S., Ishibashi, H., Okra, H. Yoshimura, N., Kawaguchi, H., & Nakamura, K. (2007). Diet and lifestyle associated with increased bone mineral density cross-sectional study of Japanese elderly women at an osteoporosis outpatient clinic. *Journal of Orthopedic Science, 12*(4), 317–320.

Ohio University. (2007, June 5). Women up to age 30 at risk for bone loss, study finds. *ScienceDaily.* Retrieved from http://www.sciencedaily.com/releases/2007/06/070604123853.htm

Oregon Health & Science University. (2007, June 27). Antidepressants linked to bone loss, study suggests. *ScienceDaily.* Retrieved from http://www.sciencedaily.com/releases/2007/06/070626115436.htm

Pearson, D. A. (2007). Bone health and osteoporosis: The role of vitamin K and potential antagonism by anticoagulants. *Nutrition in Clinical Practice, 22*(5), 517–544.

Schmitt, N. M., Schmitt, J., & Dören, M. (2009). The role of physical activity in the prevention of osteoporosis in postmenopausal women—An update. *Maturitas, 63*(1), 34–38.

Spangler, L., Scholes, D., Brunner, R. L., Robbins, J., Reed, S. D., Newton, K. M., . . . Lacroix, A. Z. (2008, February 20). Depressive symptoms, bone loss, and fractures in postmenopausal women. *Journal of General Internal Medicine.* doi:10.1007.s11606-008-0525-0

Takeda, R., & Nakamura, T. (2008). Effects of high magnesium intake on bone mineral status and lipid metabolism in rats. *Journal of Nutritional Science and Vitaminology, 54*(1), 66 75.

Tang, B. M., Eslick, G. D., Nowson, C., Smith, C., & Bensoussan, A. (2007). Use of calcium or calcium in combination with vitamin D supplementation to prevent fractures and bone loss in people age 50 years and older: a meta-analysis. *Lancet, 370*(9588), 657–666.

Tucker, K. L. (2009). Osteoporosis prevention and nutrition. *Current Osteoporosis Reports, 7*(4), 111–117.

Tucker, K. L., Morita, K I., Qiao, N., Hannan, M. T., Cupples, L. A., & Kiel, D. P. (2006). Colas, but not other carbonated beverages, are associated with low bone mineral density in older women: The Framingham Osteoporosis Study. *The American Journal of Clinical Nutrition, 84*(4), 936–942.

University of Pittsburgh Schools of the Health Sciences. (2007, September 21). Low vitamin D linked to higher risk of hip fracture. *ScienceDaily.* Retrieved from http://www.sciencedaily.com/releases/2007/09/070920111402.htm

Vitamin K appears to reduce post-menopausal fracture rates. (2007, January). *The Clinical Advisor,* p. 127.

Ward, W. E., & Fonseca, D. (2007). Soy isoflavones and fatty acids: Effects on bone tissue postovariectomy in mice. *Molecular Nutrition and Food Research, 51*(7), 824–831.

Welch, A. A., Bingham, S. A., Reeve, J., & Khaw, K. T. (2007). More acidic dietary acid-base load is associated with reduced calcaneal broadband ultrasound attenuation in women but not in men: Results from the EPIC-Norfolk cohort study. *American Journal of Clinical Nutrition, 85*(4), 1134–1141.

Whyte, M. P., Essmyer, K. E., Gannon, F. H., Reinus, W. R. (2005). Skeletal fluorosis and instant tea. *American Journal of Medicine, 118*(1), 78–82.

Zalloua, P. A., Hsu, Y. H., Terwedow, H., Zang, T., Wu, D., Tang, G., . . . Xu, X. (2007). Impact of seafood and fruit consumption on bone mineral density. *Maturitas, 56*(11), 1–11.

Zehnacker, C. H., & Bemis-Doughtery, A. (2007). Effect of weighted exercises on bone mineral density in post menopausal women: A systematic review. *Journal of Geriatric Physical Therapy, 30*(2), 79–88.

Ovarian Cancer

Environment

Environmental evidence-based practice for ovarian cancer concerns CT scans and sunlight.

1. *CT scans.* CT scans could be responsible for raising the risk of cancer. A typical CT scan delivers 50 to 100 times more radiation than a conventional X-ray. **Cautions:** Brenner and Hall (2007) estimate that one-third of all CT scans might not be necessary. Suggest using the safer options of ultrasound and magnetic resonance imaging, which do not expose women to radiation.

2. *Sunlight.* A deficiency of vitamin D is linked to increased incidence of ovarian cancer (University of California, San Diego, 2006). For Caucasian clients, 10–15 minutes of direct midday sun at least twice a week on the face, arms, hands, or back is sufficient, according to the National Institutes of Health (2011). Darker skinned clients may require 3–6 times as much exposure.

Exercise/Movement

Exercise/movement evidence-based practice for ovarian cancer includes recreational exercise.

High levels of moderate, recreational exercise are associated with a reduced risk of ovarian cancer. In addition, women with jobs that require moderate or strenuous activity experienced a lower ovarian cancer risk compared with those who worked in sedentary occupations (Pan, Ugnat, & Mao, 2005).

Herbs/Essential Oils

Herbal evidence-based practice for ovarian cancer includes milk thistle.

Milk thistle (silymarin), at 200 to 300 mg/day, stimulates detoxification pathways, inhibits the growth of certain cancer cell lines, exerts direct cytotoxic activity toward certain cancer cell lines, and may increase the efficacy of certain chemotherapy agents. Milk thistle also protects the liver from drug- or alcohol-related injury (Lah, Cui, & Hu, 2007; Post-White, Ladas, & Kelly, 2007).

Nutrition

Nutrition evidence-based practice for ovarian cancer includes watercress.

Watercress (one bowl/day) protects against DNA damage in blood cells, which is considered to be an important trigger in cancer development (Gill et al., 2007).

Touch

Touch evidence-based practice for ovarian cancer includes foot reflexology.

Self-foot reflexology (four 40-minute treatments) can enhance natural killer cells and IgG, strengthening the immune system against cancer and possibly preventing tumor development (Lee, 2006). For information on reflexology, go to: http://www.how-to-do-reflexology.com/reflexologyfootmap .html. **Other considerations:** Foot reflexology has been shown to significantly improve life satisfaction, the most important predictor of survival for women with advanced cancer (Fox Chase Cancer Center, 2007).

OVARIAN CANCER CASE STUDY

Ms. Moland, age 24, has been having abdominal pain. An ultrasound indicated a mass on her right ovary. Her physician recommended both ovaries be removed, followed by chemotherapy and radiation. Ms. Moland is terrified of having surgery. Her mother died on the operating table while being operated on for a damaged heart valve. Ms. Moland asks you if there is something else she can try other than surgery.

HEALTH PROMOTION CHALLENGE

Based on what you have read in this section and on any other new studies you find by going to PubMed (http://www.ncbi.nlm.nih.gov/pubmed/) and searching for ovarian cancer, prepare a teaching/learning program for Ms. Moland.

REFERENCES

Brenner, D., & Hall, E. J. (2007). Computed tomography, an increasing source of radiation exposure. *New England Journal of Medicine, 357*(22), 2277–2284.

Fox Chase Cancer Center. (2007, November 1). Quality of life is the most important predictor of survival for advanced cancer patients. *ScienceDaily.* Retrieved from http://www.sciencedaily.com/releases/2007/10/071030170208.htm

Gill, C. I., Haldar, S., Boyd, L. A., Bennett, R., Whiteford, J., Butler, M., . . . Rowland, I. R. (2007). Watercress supplementation in diet reduces lymphocyte DNA damage and alters blood antioxidant status in healthy adults. *American Journal of Clinical Nutrition, 85*(2), 504–510.

Lah, J. J., Cui, W., & Hu, K. Q. (2007). Effects and mechanisms of silibinin on human hepatoma cell lines. *World Journal of Gastroenterology, 13*(40), 5299–5305.

Lee, Y. M. (2006). Effect of self-foot reflexology massage on depression, stress responses and immune functions of middle aged women. *Taehan Kanho Hakhoe Chi, 36*(1), 179–188.

National Institutes of Health. (2011). Vitamin D. Accessed from http://ods.od.nih.gov/factsheets/VitaminD-HealthProfessional/

Pan, S. Y., Ugnat, A.-M., & Mao, Y. (2005). Physical activity and the risk of ovarian cancer: a case-control study in Canada. *International Journal of Cancer, 117*(2), 300–307.

Post-White, J., Ladas, E. J., & Kelly, K. M. (2007). Advances in the use of milk thistle (*Silybum marianum*). *Integrative Cancer Therapy, 6*(2), 104–109.

University of California, San Diego. (2006, November 2). Deficiency in exposure to sunlight linked to ovarian cancer. *ScienceDaily.* Retrieved from http://www.sciencedaily.com/releases/2006/11/061102092052.htm

Overweight/Obesity

Environment

Environmental evidence-based practice for overweight/obesity includes a social network.

A client's social network can affect weight gain. When a friend becomes obese, the chances of the client also becoming obese goes up to 57%. Among mutual friends, the effect is even stronger, with chances increasing 171%. Among siblings, if one becomes obese, the likelihood for the other to become obese increases 40%; among spouses, the likelihood is 37%.

Distance does not affect weight; a friend who is 500 miles away has just as much impact on a woman's obesity as one who lives next door. People come to think that it is okay to be bigger since those around them are bigger. The social network effects extend to a client's friends' friends' friends. Any intervention should consider the network of a client's friends. **Other considerations:** When a practitioner helps one woman lose weight, the whole social network could benefit. Not only may obesity be contagious, thinness may be also. Encouraging obese clients to find thin friends may be beneficial (Christakis & Fowler, 2007).

Exercise/Movement

Exercise/movement evidence-based practice for overweight/obesity includes the following:

1. *Aerobic exercise.* One session of 45 minutes on a treadmill followed by 45 minutes on a cycle increases storage of fat in muscle, which improves insulin sensitivity by 25% over base level of inactivity. By increasing their physical activity, clients can prevent the weight gain associated with aging by at least two times when compared to clients who are inactive (Kruk, 2007; Schenck & Horowitz, 2007).

2. *Walking.* In one study, daily walking and consuming 1,200 calories/ day resulted in 100-pound weight loss. One in four persons who participated in an intensive weight loss program went on to lose over 100 pounds (University of Kentucky, 2007). **Cautions:** Although this program is demanding, it has much lower risks than surgery, which can lead to memory loss and confusion (due to vitamin deficiency), inability to coordinate movement, vomiting, seizures, deafness, psychosis, muscle weakness, and pain or numbness in the feet or hands (American Academy of Neurology, 2007). **Other considerations:** The positive results of the behavioral program went beyond losing 100 pounds. Weight loss was accompanied by improvements in blood pressure, cholesterol levels, diabetes, sleep apnea, and other conditions. Sixty-six percent of participants were able to discontinue medications for high blood lipids, high blood pressure, diabetes, or degenerative joint disease, saving an average of $100 a month (University of Kentucky, 2007).

3. *Dieting without exercise.* Dieting without concurrent exercise causes bone loss. In a 1-year program of calorie restriction, without exercise, the diet group lost significant mass in the hip and spine, two common sites of fracture ("Dieting Without Exercise," 2007; John Wiley, 2007).

4. *Focus on health benefits, not appearance.* Young women reported they enjoyed a step aerobics class (45 minutes 3–4 times/week) more when the instructor focused on the health-related aspects of the workout, telling them how exercise will make them more fit overall, as opposed to being told how exercise would tone their legs or other body parts. Body mass index (BMI) is not a significant factor in mortality risk, but physical fitness is (Ohio State University, 2007). Reinforce client preference for exercise feedback.

5. *Splitting up exercise bouts.* Repeated bouts of exercise burn more fat than one long exercise session. The American College of Sports Medicine recommends moderate exercise for the duration of 45 to 60 minutes to ensure a sufficient amount of energy is depleted in obese clients. **Cautions:** Go to http://exercise.lifetips.com Encourage clients to break up their workout with a 20-minute break after 30 minutes of exercise, followed by another 30 minutes of exercise. **Other considerations:** To reduce the intimidation of starting an exercise program, suggest clients walk 15–30 minutes away from home to a friend's house or park, rest for 20 minutes, and then return home. Walking just 30 minutes three times a week can result in a significant reduction in waist and hip girth, overall fitness, and even lowered systolic blood pressure. Other ideas to consider when teaching clients are to counsel them to walk instead of drive; use stairs rather than elevators; and mix aerobic, flexibility, and strength-training exercises to reduce the chance of being bored (American Physiological Society, 2007).

Mind-Set

Mind-set evidence-based practice for overweight/obesity includes the following:

1. *Counseling and engagement in weight-loss strategies.* In a 2008 study, a personal-contact intervention (monthly person-to-person telephone calls of 5–15 minutes and a face-to-face meeting of 45–60 minutes every 4th month, without any Internet contact) was more effective than Internet contact at preventing or reducing weight regain, but an interactive Web-based intervention was more effective before 30 months (Barclay & Lie, 2008).

2. *Denial about children's weight problems.* While 87% of the children surveyed in a Vanderbilt Medical Center (2008) study were obese by the most recent Centers for Disease Control and Prevention (CDC) standards, only 41% of parents and 35% of the children reported themselves "very overweight." Among parents who reported their child's weight as "about right," 40% had children who actually were at or over the 95th percentile for weight and were considered obese by government standards. Girls were more likely than boys to underestimate their weight. Because it may be a challenge to treat obesity if many of the parents of overweight or obese children do not even recognize the problem, work on shared communication, using more clear language, goal setting with families about key behavior changes, identifying barriers to change, and setting goals. Provide parents with information about the definition of overweight and obesity and ask them to evaluate themselves and their

family members based on these definitions, and set reasonable goals for weight loss (Vanderbilt Medical Center, 2008).

Nutrition

Nutrition evidence-based practice for overweight/obesity includes the following:

1. *Cinnamon.* Two and a half teaspoons of cinnamon in a bowl of oatmeal or rice can lower blood glucose levels by 50% and steady blood sugar, reducing the tendency to overeat (Hlebowicz, Darwiche, Bjorgell, & Almer, 2007).

2. *Fat and fiber intake.* Decreased fat intake and increased fruit/vegetable/fiber consumption is associated with reductions in BMI. Daily ingestion of 5–10 fruits or vegetables and a bowl or more of high-fiber cereal are suggested (Linde et al., 2006). **Caution:** High fiber intake can reduce absorption of valuable minerals (Prynne, McCarron, Wadsworth, & Stephen, 2010). A multimineral tablet may need to be taken between high-fiber meals to ensure sufficient amounts of zinc, copper, and magnesium are ingested. To increase fiber and satiety, add blueberries or strawberries to cereal, mango or peach slices to a slice of bread smothered with peanut butter, or eat a bowl of broth-based vegetable soup or a leafy green salad.

3. *Fructose.* Foods prepared with high fructose corn syrup and table sugar causes uric acid levels to spike, blocking the ability of insulin to regulate how body cells use and store sugar and other nutrients for energy, leading to obesity. One of the biggest sources of fructose is soft drinks. The fructose in an apple is as problematic as the high fructose corn syrup in soda, but the fruit also provides necessary fiber and cancer-fighting antioxidants. Fructose has no healthy nutritional properties. While one apple may be healthful, eating multiple apples in one sitting could send the body over the fructose edge (University of Florida, 2007). Counsel clients to check labels of processed foods including sodas (which has 10.5 teaspoons of sugar per serving), low-fat yogurts with fruit (10 teaspoons of sugar per serving), Mott's applesauce (5 teaspoons of sugar per serving), and ketchup (1 teaspoon of sugar per tablespoon of ketchup).

4. *Magnesium.* Eating high amounts of magnesium-rich foods may impose a significant body weight decline (Takeda & Nakamura, 2008). Counsel clients to increase intake of halibut, spinach, cooked soybeans, raw pumpkin seeds, Brazil nuts, cashews, and pine nuts.

5. *Seaweed alginate and pectin.* In a 2007 study, alginate-pectin (2.8 g), ingested twice a day (once before breakfast and once midafternoon),

reduced food intake at dinner by signaling satiety in overweight and obese women with low rigid restraint scores; these women consumed 12% less energy during the day and 22% less for the evening snack compared with the control condition (Pelkman, Navia, Miller, & Pohle, 2007). **Cautions:** To eliminate the dangers of mineral loss from high-fiber diets, a daily multimineral may be necessary and should be taken with the noon meal.

6. *Sesame oil.* In a 2005 study, sesame oil used daily as the only oil for foods and cooking (up to 2 tablespoons/day) for 45 days led to a significant reduction in body weight and BMI (Ramesh, Saravanan, & Pugalendi, 2005). **Health tip:** Two types of sesame oil are available: one for cooking and the other for salads and noncooking purposes.

7. *Targeted dietary advice.* In a 2007 study, dietary advice targeted to obese women to increase the intake of vegetables and fruit contributed to weight reduction (Svendsen, Blomhoff, Holme, & Tonstad, 2007).

8. *Vegetarian diets.* In a 2006 study, vegetarian diets were effective for weight control in women who adhered to a lacto-ovo (milk and eggs, but no meat or fish) vegetarian diet for 6 months (Burke et al., 2006). **Cautions:** Vegetarians must eat eggs, sea vegetables (dulse, kelp, kombu and nori), and soybeans and soy products (especially tempeh and miso, which are more easily digestible), or take a B-complex capsule daily to ensure adequate intake of vitamin B_{12}. For information on vegetarian eating principles, go to http://www.tryveg.com/cfi/toc/ or http://www.medicinenet.com/script/main/art.asp?articlekey=61183

Stress Management

Stress management evidence for overweight/obesity concerns binge eating.

Binge eating is often related to stress and low self-esteem. In a study comparing self-help/bibliotherapy, interpersonal therapy, and behavior weight loss, interpersonal therapy (twenty 60-minute sessions over a 24-week period) was superior to the two other treatment options. In a study by Lovinger (2007), women with high negative affect (as measured by the Beck Depression Inventory), were more likely to do poorly when the behavioral weight loss approach was used. **Cautions:** Dieting can also lead to bingeing and weight gain, while restricting foods can lead to bouts of overeating; these repeated cycles lead to weight gain (Finn, 2003). For information on interpersonal therapy, go to http://psychservices.psychiatryonline.org/cgi/content/full/51/6/825-a For information on behavioral weight loss therapy, go to http://www.nhlbi.nih.gov/guidelines/obesity/e_txtbk/txgd/4323.htm For information on bibliotherapy, go to http://www.minddisorders.com/A-Br/Bibliotherapy.html

Other considerations: For information on the Beck Depression Inventory, go to http://www.ibogaine.desk.nl/graphics/3639b1c_23.pdf

Supplements

Supplements evidence-based practice for overweight/obesity concerns the following:

1. *Pomegranate leaf extract.* Pomegranate leaf extract (standardized to 250 mg and 1 capsule taken daily) can inhibit the development of obesity (Lei et al., 2007). Counsel women to avoid pomegranate leaf extract during first trimester of pregnancy and teach men and women to avoid the extract when sensitive to pomegranate.

2. *Vinegar.* Fermented and pickled products reduce postprandial responses and increase the subjective rating of satiety due to vinegar and its high acetic acid level (Ostman, Granfeldt, Perrson, & Bjorck, 2005). Clients who feel full are less likely to overeat.

3. *Water.* Drinking two glasses of water prior to a meal increases metabolic rate by 30% and can aid in weight loss regimes. Drinking 8 cups of water daily is recommended to augment energy expenditure and aid in weight loss. Distilled water or water that has passed through a reverse osmosis filter can protect against unwanted substances.

OVERWEIGHT/OBESITY CASE STUDY

Ms. Sommers, age 34, is 50 pounds overweight. She has been dieting since age 11 and has gained and lost those 50 pounds 20 times. She has tried countless diets and countless diet pills and still can not keep the weight off. She asks you if you have any ideas to help her.

HEALTH PROMOTION CHALLENGE

Using the information in this chapter and by searching PubMed (http://www.ncbi.nlm.nih.gov/pubmed/) for overweight and nutrition and overweight and supplements, develop a teaching/learning program for Ms. Sommers.

REFERENCES

American Academy of Neurology. (2007, March 13). Obesity surgery can lead to memory loss, other problems. *ScienceDaily*. Retrieved from http://www.sciencedaily.com/releases/2007/03/070312161244.htm

American Physiological Society. (2007). Exercise, exercise, rest, repeat—how a break can help your workout. Retrieved from http://www.sciencedaily.com/releases/2007/07/070718001504.htm

Barclay, L., & Lie, D. (2008). Behavioral intervention may help overweight, obese patients lose and maintain weight. Retrieved from www.medscape.com/viewarticle/571544

Burke, L. E., Styn, M. A., Steenkiste, A. R., Music, E., Warziski, M., & Choo, J. (2006). A randomized clinical trial testing treatment preference and two dietary options in behavioral weight management: Preliminary results of the impact of diet at 6 months—PREFER study. *Obesity, 14*(11), 2007–2011.

Christakis, N. A., & Fowler, J. H. (2007). The spread of obesity in a large social network over 32 years. *New England Journal of Medicine, 357*(4), 370–379.

Dieting without exercise causes bone loss. (2007, February). *The Clinical Advisor*, 12.

Finn, R. (2003, December). Dieting results in bingeing, weight gain. *Clinical Psychiatry News*, 22.

Hlebowicz, J., Darwiche, G., Bjorgell, O., & Almer, L. O. (2007). Effect of cinnamon on postprandial blood glucose, gastric emptying, and satiety in healthy subjects. *American Journal of Clinical Nutrition, 85*(6), 1552–1556.

John Wiley & Sons, Inc. (2007, July 18). Losing weight after pregnancy: Diet and exercise better than diet alone. *ScienceDaily*. Retrieved from http://www.sciencedaily.com /releases/2007/07/070718002456.htm

Kruk, J. (2007). Physical activity in the prevention of the most frequent chronic diseases: An analysis of the recent evidence. *Asian Pacific Journal of Cancer Prevention, 8*(3), 325–333.

Lei, F., Zhang, X. N., Wang, W., Xing, D. M., Xie, W. D., Su, H., & Du, L. J. (2007). Evidence of anti-obesity effects of the pomegranate leaf extract in high-fat diet induced obese mice. *International Journal of Obesity, 31*(6), 1023–1029.

Linde, J. A., Utter, J., Jeffery, R. W., Sherwood, N. E., Pronk, N. P., & Boyle, R. G. (2006). Specific food intake, fat and fiber intake, and behavioral correlates of BMI among overweight and obese members of a managed care organization. *International Journal of Behavior Nutrition and Physical Activity, 3*, 42.

Lovinger, S. P. (2007, March). Large study of binge-eating disorder is a first. *Clinical Psychiatry News*, 41.

Ohio State University. (2007, August 13). Some women benefit more from exercise when emphasis is on health, not appearance. *ScienceDaily*. Retrieved from http://www .sciencedaily.com/releases/2007/08/070809125804.htm

Ostman, E., Granfeldt, Y., Persson, L., & Bjorck, I. (2005). Vinegar supplementation lowers glucose and insulin responses and increases satiety after a bread meal in healthy subjects. *European Journal of Clinical Nutrition, 59*(9), 983–988.

Pelkman, C. L., Navia, J. L., Miller, A. E., & Pohle, R. J. (2007). Novel calcium-gelled, alginate-pectin beverage reduced energy intake in nondieting overweight and obese women: Interactions with dietary restraint status. *American Journal of Clinical Nutrition, 86*(6), 1595–1602.

Prynne, C. J., McCarron, A., Wadsworth, M. E., & Stephen, A. M. (2010). Dietary fibre and phytate—a balancing act: Results from three time points in a British birth cohort. *British Journal of Nutrition, 103*(2), 274–280.

Ramesh, B., Saravanan, R., & Pugalendi, K. V. (2005). Influence of sesame oil on blood glucose, lipid peroxidation, and antioxidant status in streptozotocin diabetic rats. *Journal of Medicinal Food, 8*(3), 377–381.

Schenck, S., & Horowitz, J. F. (2007). Dramatic health benefits after just one exercise session. *Journal of Clinical Investigation, 117*(5), 1690–1698. Available at http://content .jci.org/articles/view/30566

Svendsen, M., Blomhoff, R., Holme, I., & Tonstad, S. (2007). The effect of an increased intake of vegetables and fruit on weight loss, blood pressure and antioxidant defense in subjects with sleep related breathing disorders. *European Journal of Clinical Nutrition, 61*(11), 1301–1311.

Takeda, R., & Nakamura, T. (2008). Effects of high magnesium intake on bone mineral status and lipid metabolism in rats. *Journal of Nutritional Science and Vitaminology, 54*(1), 66–75.

University of Florida. (2007, December 14). Too much fructose could leave dieters sugar shocked. *ScienceDaily*. Retrieved from http://www.sciencedaily.com/releases/2007/12/071212201311.htm

University of Kentucky. (2007, August 27). 100-pound weight loss possible with behavioral changes. *ScienceDaily*. Retrieved from http://www.sciencedaily.com/releases/2007/08/070824180608.htm

Vanderbilt Medical Center. (2008, March 5). Parents in denial about their children's weight problems, study finds. *ScienceDaily*. Retrieved from http://www.sciencedaily.com/releases/2008/03/080304173130.htm

Pain

Environment

Environmental evidence-based practice for pain includes the following:

1. *Floating.* Relaxing in large, sound- and light-proof tanks with high-salt water is an effective way to alleviate long-term stress related to pain of fibromyalgia and whiplash. Twelve treatments over 7 weeks activates the body's own system for recuperation and healing.

   To help clients overcome their fears of water or darkness, go to http://www.guidetopsychology.com/sysden.htm **Other considerations:** If no tanks are available, consider filling a large bathtub with warm salty water in a quiet environment and ask the client to wear an eye mask during treatment (Swedish Research Council, 2007).

2. *Ginger compresses.* Ginger compresses can produce (1) meditative-like stillness and relaxation of thoughts; (2) constant penetrating warmth throughout the body; (3) positive change in outlook; (4) increased energy and interest in the world; (5) a deeply relaxed state that progresses to a gradual shift in pain and increased interest in others; (6) increased suppleness within the body; and (7) comfortable, flexible joint mobility. The essential experience of ginger compresses exposes the unique qualities of heat, stimulation, anti-inflammation, and analgesia (Therkleson, 2010).

3. *Mirror treatment.* Compared to mental visualization or viewing a covered mirror, phantom limb pain in women who had a foot or leg amputed was reduced significantly when they viewed themselves in a mirror daily for a month in a 2007 study (Uniformed Services

University of the Health Sciences, 2007). One hundred percent of the mirror group reported less phantom pain; only 17% reported a pain decrease and 50% reported worsening pain in the covered mirror group, and 67% reported worsening pain in the mental visualization group.

4. *Music.* Listening to classical music during colonoscopy helps reduce the dose of sedative medications, as well as anxiety, pain, and dissatisfaction during the procedure (Ovayoulu et al., 2006). Listening to music during a C-clamp procedure after percutaneous coronary interventions reduced heart rate, respiratory rate, and oxygen saturation, and produced a lower pain score than the control group in a study by Chan and Kiang (2007).

5. *Sitz baths.* Women who received sitz baths (in lukewarm water for 10 minutes once after defecation in the morning, and again at bedtime, for 4 weeks) and psyllium husk (as opposed to no sitz bath and psyllium husk) reported a lower pain score (Gupta, 2006).

6. *Vitamin D deficiency.* Deficient levels of vitamin D are linked with pain, especially chronic back pain (Denison, 2005; De Torrente de la Jara, Picoud & Favrat, 2004; Plotnikoff & Quigley, 2003). Vitamin D_3 is produced in Caucasians by 4–10 minutes of exposure of face, arms, or back to the noonday sun and by 60–80 minutes of exposure for darker skinned individuals. Individuals living at latitudes north of 35°, those who may not receive exposure to the sun, or those who are older than 49 years may need to take a tablespoon of cod liver oil daily. **Cautions:** Taking amounts over 100,000 IU of vitamin D/day as a supplement may be toxic; signs of toxicity include anorexia, nausea/vomiting, polyuria, polydipsia, weakness, nervousness, and pruritus. Vitamin D supplements can suppress the proper operation of the immune system (Autoimmunity Research Foundation, 2008). Vitamin D_2 that is added to fortified foods and many multivitamins and is usually written in prescriptions is inefficiently metabolized in humans; only 20–40% is metabolized into biologically active vitamin D_3. **Other considerations:** Clients using corticosteroids may require additional vitamin D.

Exercise/Movement

Exercise/movement evidence-based practice for pain includes the following:

1. *Hydrotherapy and land-based exercise.* Although land-based exercise improved knee function and reduced pain, hydrotherapy was superior in relieving pain due to osteoarthritis of the knee before and after walking 50 feet daily for 18 weeks (Silva et al., 2008). For more information on water- and land-based exercise, go to http://exercise.lifetips.com; for information on measuring pain, visit: http://ergonomics.about.com/od/ergonomicbasics/ss/painscale_6.htm

2. *Supervised exercise vs. standard treatment.* Clients with low back pain will do better with supervised exercise (1-hour sessions twice a week for an average of 7 weeks) than with standard treatment (Staal et al., 2004). **Other considerations:** In Staal's study, clients who exercised used half the analgesics that the traditional-care group did. Eighty five percent of the time it is impossible to determine the cause of back pain. Most of the time the pain goes away without treatment (Staal et al., 2004).

3. *Tai chi.* The sun-style 24 forms of tai chi exercise (for 60 minutes, twice a week for at least 12 weeks) is effective in decreasing pain (Lee & Lee, 2008). For directions, go to http://www.everyday-taichi.com/tai-chi-instruction.html **Other considerations:** Tai chi is also effective for decreasing stiffness and fear of falling and improves balance, rising time, and knee joint motion.

4. *Yoga.* Pregnant women who participated in a yoga program had a shorter duration of the first stage of labor, shorter total time of labor, and higher levels of maternal comfort outcomes after participating in six 1–hour sessions. Yoga (12-week session, experimental group) was superior to the book and exercise control groups at 12 weeks. No significant differences in symptom bothersomeness were found between any two groups at 12 weeks or at 26 weeks. For nonpregnant women, a yoga group was superior to a book group for symptom bothersomeness, possibly due to instructor motivation (Chuntharapat, Petpichetchian & Hatthakit, 2008).

   In a study by Williams and colleagues (2009), after 24 weeks, the yoga group had reductions in functional disability, pain intensity, and depression that were more statistically significant than those who received standard medical care (control group) that lasted for 6 months postintervention. The yoga group also reduced their pain medication usage compared to the control group. For more about yoga, go to http://www.yogajournal.com

Herbs/Essential Oils

Herbal evidence-based practice for pain includes peppermint oil.

Two or three drops of essential peppermint oil massaged into herpes zoster-(shingles) affected skin areas 3–4 times may work better than any offerings from a pain clinic to relieve pain (Davis, Harding, & Baranowski, 2002). **Cautions:** Peppermint oil should not be used on the face, especially near the eyes; mucous membranes; or abrasions. Counsel clients to dilute peppermint oil in almond oil (1:5 ratio) if any redness occurs at treatment sites. Dilution of essential oil may reduce pain relief. An occasional supplement of full-strength oil is recommended.

Mind-Set

Mind-set evidence-based practice for pain includes psychological treatments.

A meta-analysis of psychological studies for pain suggests that the effects of psychological treatments for fibromyalgia are relatively small but robust and comparable to those reported for other pain and drug treatments used for this disorder. Cognitive-behavioral therapy was associated with the greatest effect (Glombiewski et al., 2010). For more information about cognitive-behavioral therapy, go to: http://www.mind.org.uk/help/medical_and_alternative_care/making_sense_of_cognitive_behaviour_therapy

Nutrition

Nutrition evidence-based practice for pain includes cherry juice.

In a study conducted by Connolly and colleagues (2006), pain and strength loss were significantly less in the cherry juice trial (versus placebo) for muscle damage. Twelve fluid ounces of cherry juice blend was ingested twice a day for 8 consecutive days. **Other considerations:** Numerous antioxidant and anti-inflammatory agents have been identified in tart cherries (Connolly, McHugh, Padilla-Zakour, Carlson, & Sayres, 2006).

Stress Management

Stress management evidence-based practice for pain includes the following:

1. *Breathing therapy.* Clients suffering from chronic low back pain improved significantly (over physical therapy) with 6–8 weeks (12 sessions) of breathing therapy (Mehling, Hamel, Acree, Byl, & Hecht, 2005). For information on breathing therapy, go to http://www.breathaware.com/breathing.html

2. *Guided imagery with relaxation.* Guided imagery can significantly reduce osteoarthritis pain and increase quality of life (Baird & Sands, 2006). For more information on using guided imagery, go to http://holisticonline.com/guided-imagery.htm

3. *Hypnotherapy.* A hypnotherapy group that used direct and indirect hypnotic suggestions showed significantly lower pain ratings than the control group and reported a significant reduction in pain from baseline for burn participants in a study by Jensen and Patterson (2006). In another study, a significant reduction in trauma reexperience scores occurred in the hypnotherapy group but not the control group (Shakibaei, Harandi, Gholamrezaei, Samoei, & Salehi, 2008). For more information on hypnosis, go to http://www.ehow.com/how_7949_self-hypnosis.html

4. *Mindfulness-based stress reduction.* Mindfulness-based stress reduction is more effective in reducing pain than cognitive-behavioral stress reduction (Smith et al., 2008). An 8-week course using meditation,

gentle yoga, and body scanning exercises led to increased mindful-ness. For information on mindfulness, go to http://www.ehow.com/how_2101306_practice-mindfulness.html

Supplements

Supplement evidence-based practice for pain includes peppermint oil and silymarin.

1. *Peppermint oil.* In one study, taking two enteric-coated peppermint oil capsules twice a day for 4 weeks for irritable bowel syndrome pain resulted in a 50% reduction of symptoms (Cappello, Spezzaferro, Grossi, Manzoli, & Marzio, 2007). **Cautions:** Peppermint should not be used by clients with hypersensitivity to it or by those with gallblad-der inflammation, severe hepatic disease, gastroesophageal reflux dis-ease, or obstruction of bile ducts. Avoid during pregnancy or lactation. **Other considerations:** In another study, peppermint oil internally also reduced diarrhea, constipation, feeling of incomplete evacuation, and urgency at defecation (Skidmore-Roth, 2006).

2. *Silymarin.* Silymarin, at 300 mg daily, has anti-inflammatory effects that reduce knee pain associated with osteoarthritis as well as piroxicam or meloxicam (Hussain, Jassim, Numan, Al-Khalifa, & Abdullah, 2009).

Touch

Touch evidence-based practice for pain includes the following:

1. *Acupressure.* In a 2009 study, acupressure at Sanyinjiao point (SP6) for 30 minutes reduced the duration and severity of pain of the active phase of labor, cesarean section rates, and necessity and amount of oxytocin (Kashanian & Shahali, 2009). Pain during transportation is a common phenomenon in emergency medicine. Acupressure was performed either at true points or at sham points during the study. Lang and col-leagues (2007) found that acupressure in the prehospital setting effectively reduced pain and anxiety in patients with distal radial trauma. Taylor, Miakowski, and Kohn (2002) found that 90% of women wearing an acu-pressure garment obtained at least a 25% reduction in menstrual pain severity compared to only 8% of the control group, and pain medication dropped to two pills per day for the Relief Brief group but remained at six pills for the control group. For more information on the Relief Brief, con-tact Diana.Taylor@nursing.ucsf.edu Acupressure can be an effective, cost-free, self-care intervention for relieving pain. For more information on acupressure, go to http://www.agelessherbs.com/acupressurepoints.html

2. *Aromathery and abdominal massage.* Topically applied lavender (two drops), clary sage (one drop), and rose (one drop), all stirred into 5 cc almond oil and massaged into the abdomen, is effective in decreasing

menstrual pain (Han, Hur, Buckle, Choi, & Lee, 2006). **Other considerations:** Lavender, when inhaled, produces a sedative effect.

3. *Massage.* Twenty minutes of back massage every evening for up to 5 postoperative days improves pain management and postoperative anxiety among women who experience unrelieved postoperative pain (Barclay & Murata, 2007). For more on back massage, go to http://www.easyvigour.net.nz/backpain/h_BackMassage.htm

4. *Therapeutic touch.* Compared with those who received usual care in a 2010 study, participants who received therapeutic touch had significantly lower level of pain, lower cortisol level, and higher natural kill cells (NKC) level, a measure of immune system competence (Coakley & Duffy, 2010).

PAIN MANAGEMENT CASE STUDY

Jason Smith, age 28, was admitted to the emergency department with a deep laceration of his left thigh. A holistic nurse was assigned to his care. On exam, his height was 73 inches, body weight 210 pounds, blood pressure 142/90 mmHg, heart rate 84 beats per minute, and respirations 20 per minute. Jason was noticeably fidgety, inattentive, and speaking at a very fast pace. An intravenous solution of 0.9% sodium chloride was started and infused at 125 cc/hour. Jason complained of severe pain, and after the physician checked for drug allergies, the physician ordered 2 mg morphine sulfate to ease the pain. As the physician was suturing Jason's laceration, Jason told the holistic nurse that he is generally an anxious person and is very frightened of hospitals. The holistic nurse used the tools of authentic presence and soothing touch to help Jason calm his fears. After a few minutes, Jason commented on how the touch really helped and wanted to know if the nurse could teach him other things to help him manage his anxiety.

This case study and health promotion challenge were developed by Susanne M. Tracy, PhD, RN, Assistant Professor of Nursing University of New Hampshire, Department of Nursing.

HEALTH PROMOTION CHALLENGE

Go to PubMed (http://www.ncbi.nlm.nih.gov/pubmed/), type "soothing touch" in the search box at the top of the page, and click on the Search button. Select each of the four holistic pain management tools below and explain how each of these tools would have helped Jason reduce his anxiety and promote healing.

1. Soothing touch
2. Music
3. Self-guided imagery
4. Authentic presence

REFERENCES

Autoimmunity Research Foundation. (2008, January 27). Vitamin D deficiency study raises new questions about disease and supplements. *ScienceDaily*. Retrieved from http://www.sciencedaily.com/releases/2008/01/080125223302.htm

Baird, C. L., & Sands, L. P. (2006). Effect of guided imagery with relaxation on health-related quality of life in older women with osteoarthritis. *Research in Nursing and Health, 29*(5), 442–451.

Barclay, L., & Murata, P. (2007). Massage may help relieve acute postoperative pain. *Archives of Surgery, 142*, 1158–1167.

Cappello, G., Spezzaferro, M., Grossi, L., Manzoli, L., & Marzio, L. (2007). Peppermint oil (mint oil) in the treatment of irritable bowel syndrome: A prospective double blind placebo-controlled randomized trial. *Digestion and Liver Disease, 39*(6), 530–536.

Chan, M. F., & Kiang, W. (2007). Effects of music on patients undergoing a C-clamp procedure after percutaneous coronary interventions: A randomized controlled trial. *Heart and Lung, 36*(6), 431–439.

Chuntharapat, S., Petpichetchian, W., & Hatthakit, U. (2008). Yoga during pregnancy: Effects on maternal comfort, labor pain and birth outcomes. *Complementary Therapies in Clinical Practice, 14*(2), 105–115.

Coakley, A. B., & Duffy, M. E. (2010). The effect of therapeutic touch on postoperative patients. *Journal of Holistic Nursing, 28*(3), 193–200.

Connolly, D. A., McHugh, M. P., Padilla-Zakour, O. I., Carlson, L., & Sayres, S. P. (2006). Efficacy of a tart cherry juice blend in preventing the symptoms of muscle damage. *British Journal of Sports Medicine, 40*(8), 679–683.

Davis, S., Harding, L., & Baranowski, A. P. (2002). A novel treatment of post herpetic neuralgia using peppermint oil. *Clinical Journal of Pain, 18*(3), 200–202.

De Torrente de la Jara, G. P., Picoud, A., & Favrat, B. (2004). Musculoskeletal pain in female asylum seekers and hypovitaminosis D3. *British Medical Journal, 329*, 156–157.

Denison, N. (2005, summer). Easing pain with vitamin D. *On Wisconsin*, 39.

Glombiewski, J. A., Sawyer, A. T., Gutermann, J., Koenig, K., Rief, W., & Hofmann, S. G. (2010, August 18). Psychological treatments for fibromyalgia: A meta-analysis. *Pain, 151*(2), 280–295.

Gupta, P. (2006). Randomized, controlled study comparing sitz-bath and no-sitz-bath treatments in patients with acute anal fissures. *ANZ Journal of Surgery, 76*(8), 718–721.

Hussain, S. A., Jassim, N. A., Numan, I. T., Al-Khalifa, I. I., & Abdullah, T. A. (2009). Anti-inflammatory activity of silymarin in patients with knee osteoarthritis. A comparative study with piroxicam and meloxicam. *Saudi Medical Journal, 30*(1), 98–103.

Jensen, M., & Patterson, D. R. (2006). Hypnotic treatment of chronic pain. *Journal of Behavioral Medicine, 29*(1), 95–124.

Kashanian, M., & Shahali, S. (2009). Effects of acupressure at the Sanyinjiao point (SP6) on the process of active phase of labor in nulliparous women. *Journal of Maternal-Fetal Neonatal Medicine, 15*, 1–4.

Lee, H. Y., & Lee, K. J. (2008). Effects of tai chi exercise in elderly with knee osteoarthritis. *Taehan Kanho Hakhoe Chi, 38*(1), 11–18.

Lang, T., Hager, H., Funovits, V., Barker, R., Steinlechner, B., Hoerauf, K., & Kober, A. (2007). Prehospital analgesia with acupressure at the Baihui and Hegu points in patients with radial fractures: A prospective, randomized, double-blind trial. *The American Journal of Emergency Medicine, 25*(8), 887–893.

Mehling, W. E., Hamel, K. A., Acree, M., Byl, N., & Hecht, F. M. (2005). Randomized controlled trial for breath therapy for patients with chronic low-back pain. *Alternative Therapies in Health and Medicine, 11*(4), 44–52.

Ovayolu, N., Ucan, O., Pehlivan, S., Pehlivan, Y., Buyukhatipoglu, H., Savas, M. C., & Gulsen, M. T. (2006). Listening to Turkish classical music decreases patients' anxiety, pain, dissatisfaction and the dose of sedative and analgesic drugs during colonoscopy: A prospective randomized controlled trial. *World Journal of Gastroenterology, 12*(46), 7532–7536.

Plotnikoff, G. A., & Quigley, J. M. (2003). Prevalence of severe hypovitaminosis D in patients with persistent, nonspecific musculoskeletal pain. *Mayo Clinic Proceedings, 78*, 1463–1470.

Shakibaei, F., Harandi, A. A., Gholamrezaei, A., Samoei, R., & Salehi, P. (2008). Hypnotherapy in management of pain and reexperiencing of trauma in burns. *International Journal of Clinical Experimental Hypnosis, 56*(2), 185–197.

Silva, L. E., Valim, V., Pessanha, A. P., Oliveira, L. M., Myamoto, S., Jones, A., & Natour, J. (2008). Hydrotherapy versus conventional land-based exercise for the management of pain. *Physical Therapy, 88*(1), 12–21.

Skidmore-Roth, L. (2006). Peppermint. In *Mosby's handbook of herbs & natural supplements* (pp. 821–825). St. Louis, MO: ElsevierMosby.

Smith, B. W., Shelley, B. M., Dalen, J., Wiggins, K., Tooley, E., & Bernard, J. (2008). A pilot study comparing the effects of mindfulness-based and cognitive-behavioral stress reduction. *The Journal of Alternative and Complementary Medicine, 14*(3), 251–258.

Staal, J. B., Hlobil, H., Twisk, J. W. R., Smid, T., Koke, J. A., & van Mechelen, W. (2004). Graded activity for low back pain in occupational health care a randomized, controlled trial. *Annals of Internal Medicine, 140*(2), 77–84.

Swedish Research Council. (2007, November 6). Floating effective for stress and pain, research suggests. *ScienceDaily*. Retrieved from http://www.sciencedaily.com/releases/2007/11/071105120604.htm

Taylor, D., Miaskowski, C., & Kohn, J. (2002). A randomized clinical trial of the effectiveness of an acupressure device (relief brief) for managing symptoms of dysmenorrhea. *Journal of Alternative and Complementary Medicine, 8*(3), 357–370.

Therkleson, T. (2010). Ginger compress therapy for adults with osteoarthritis. *Journal of Advanced Nursing, 66*(10), 2225–2233.

Uniformed Services University of the Health Sciences. (2007, November 24). Phantom limb pain may be reduced by simple mirror treatment. *ScienceDaily*. Retrieved from http://www.sciencedaily.com/releases/2007/11/071123195218.htm

Williams, K., Abildso, C., Steinberg, L., Doyle, E., Epstein, B., Smith, D., . . . Cooper, L. (2009). Evaluation of the effectiveness and efficacy of Iyengar yoga therapy on chronic low back pain. *Spine (Phila Pa 1976), 34*(19), 2066–2076.

Pancreatic Cancer

Environment

Environmental evidence-based practice for pancreatic cancer includes the following:

1. *CT scans.* CT scans could be responsible for raising the risk of pancreatic cancer. A typical CT scan delivers 50 to100 times more radiation

than a conventional X-ray. Brenner and Hall (2007) estimate that one-third of all CT scans might not be necessary and suggest using the safer options of ultrasound and magnetic resonance imaging, which do not expose clients to radiation.

2. *Organochlorines.* In a study by Hardell and colleagues (2007), survival of clients with high concentrations of persistent organic pollutants in their adipose tissue who are diagnosed with pancreatic cancer was significantly less than those with low concentrations. Organic pollutants include motor vehicle emissions, exposure to petroleum and chemical industries, emissions from waste incinerators and service stations, domestic solid fuel and gas combustion, spray painting, dry cleaning and other solvent usage, pesticide use, and cigarette smoke. Help clients assess their exposure to organic pollutants, eliminate as many as possible, and lose weight if they are overweight. See "Overweight/Obesity," previously in this appendix, for ideas.

3. *Sunlight/vitamin D.* Geographic regions with more sunlight exposure have lower incidences and mortality for cancer. Skinner and colleagues (2006) found that participants who met the U.S. Recommended Daily Allowance of vitamin D (400 IU) had a 43% lower risk of pancreatic cancer. Vitamin D_3 is produced in Caucasians by 4–10 minutes of exposure of face, arms, or back to the noonday sun, and by 60–80 minutes of exposure for darker skinned individuals. Individuals living at latitudes north of 35°, who may not receive exposure to the sun, or who are older than 49 years may need to take a tablespoon of cod liver oil daily (Jockers, 2007). **Cautions:** Vitamin D supplements can suppress the proper operation of the immune system, especially in those who are already ill (Autoimmunity Research Foundation, 2008). Vitamin D_2 that is added to fortified foods and many multivitamins and is usually written in prescriptions is inefficiently metabolized in humans; only 20–40% is metabolized into biologically active vitamin D_3. **Other considerations:** Clients using corticosteroids may require additional vitamin D.

Exercise/Movement

Exercise/movement evidence-based approaches for pancreatic cancer concern obesity and physical activity.

By virtue of their influence on insulin resistance, obesity and physical inactivity may increase risk of pancreatic cancer. In one study (Arslan et al., 2010), obesity significantly increased the risk of pancreatic cancer. Physical activity appears to decrease the risk of pancreatic cancer among those who are overweight. Centralized weight deposit, especially in women, increases risk for pancreatic cancer (Arslan et al.). Counsel clients who are overweight to increase their activity level and lose weight to reduce their risk for pancreatic cancer. If nothing else, suggest they walk a few flights instead of taking the elevator (University of Missouri-Columbia, 2008). For exercise tips, go to http://exercise.lifetips.com For obesity/overweight suggestions, see "Overweight/Obesity," previously in this appendix.

Herbs/Essential Oils

Herbal evidence-based practice for pancreatic cancer includes milk thistle and curcumin.

1. *Milk thistle.* Milk thistle (silymarin 200 to 400 mg/day) stimulates detoxification pathways, inhibits the growth of certain cancer cell lines, exerts direct cytotoxic activity toward certain cancer cell lines, may increase the efficacy of certain chemotherapy agents, and also protects the liver from drug or alcohol-related injury (Lah, Cui & Hu, 2007; Post-White, Ladas, & Kelly, 2007).

2. *Curcumin (turmeric).* Curcumin (turmeric) has antiproliferative and antiangiogenic activities that make it therapeutically efficacious for pancreatic cancer when given by mouth daily for 2 months at a dose of 8 grams. It has been shown to stabilize, reduce tumor size, and provide partial remission in survivors (Anand, Kunnumakkara, Newman, & Aggarwal, 2007; Dhillon et al., 2006; Kujundzic, Grbesa, Ivkic, Katdare, & Gall-Troselj, 2006; Shehzad, Wahid, & Lee, 2010). No toxicities were found in the Anand et al. study, but clients should be monitored for hypersensitivity reactions, including dermatitis, and coagulant studies for long-term use of the herb.

Nutrition

Nutrition evidence-based practice for pancreatic cancer includes the following:

1. *Dietary fats of animal origin and other saturated fats.* Men and women who consumed high amounts of total animal fats had 53% and 23% higher relative rates of pancreatic cancer, respectively, compared with men and women who had the lowest animal fat consumption. Participants who consumed high amounts of saturated fats had 36% higher relative rates of pancreatic cancer compared with those who consumed low amounts (Thiébaut et al., 2009).

2. *Flavonols.* A diet rich in flavonols from foods such as onions, apples, and berries may cut the risk of developing pancreatic cancer by about 25%, a multiethnic study reports. Daily ingestion of kaempferols (spinach and cabbage) are associated with the largest risk reduction (22% among all participants), while quercetin (found in onions and applies), and myricetin (found in red onions and berries) also reduce pancreatic cancer risk (Nothings, Murphy, Wilkens, Henderson, & Kolonel,

2007). Advise clients to strive for organic, local produce. **Other considerations:** The advantages for smokers may be even more profound—a risk reduction of 59%.

3. *Folate.* Results of a large study found that increased intake of folate from food sources was statistically significantly inversely associated with risk of pancreatic cancer. Daily consumption of folate-rich foods, especially leafy green vegetables (like spinach and turnip greens), fruits (citrus fruits and juices), and dried beans and peas that can help meet the suggested amount of 1,000 micrograms a day, may reduce risk for pancreatic cancer. Clients who do not eat breads, cereals, or pasta; who abuse alcohol; or who take medications that interfere with folate absorption may not receive sufficient amounts of the nutrient. **Other considerations:** Folate from supplements was not associated with pancreatic cancer protection (Bravi et al., 2010; Larsson, Hakansson, Giovannucci & Wolk, 2006).

4. *Green tea.* Decaffeinated green tea (2–5 cups daily) is protective against pancreatic cancer before disease occurs and after onset, possibly by creating a detoxifying effect (Shankar, Ganapathy, Hingorani, & Srivastava, 2008). **Cautions:** May decrease iron absorption, so separate iron-rich foods or iron pills by at least 2 hours from green tea ingestion. Caffeinated green tea can interact with MAOIs and lead to a hypertensive crisis. Counsel women not to take green tea with anticoagulants/antiplatelets (may increase risk of bleeding), beta-adrenergic blockers (can lead to increased inotropic effects), or benzodiazepines (may increase sedation). Dairy products may decrease the therapeutic effects of green tea, so separate their intake by several hours (Skidmore-Roth, 2006). The digestive process affects anticancer activity of tea in gastrointestinal cells; advise clients to add citrus (such as lemon juice) or take ascorbic acid (vitamin C) to protect the catechins in green tea from digestive degradation (Purdue University, 2007).

5. *Omega-3 fatty acids.* Omega-3 fatty acids in fish, dried beans, winter squash, walnuts, and flax may inhibit proliferation of pancreatic cancer cells (Hering et al., 2007). **Cautions:** Farmed fish contains more PCBs, and 11 other environmental toxins are present at higher levels than in wild fish. Farmed fish may also be less nutritious (Indiana University, 2004). The following fish contain the most omega-3 fatty acids and are the least tainted: wild Atlantic salmon, sardines in sardine oil, wild rainbow trout, mackerel, and specialty or gourmet Pacific albacore tuna canned in water. **Other considerations:** Smaller, family-owned tuna fisheries fresh freeze their fish and only cook it once, preserving their natural juices and fats. The larger commercial canneries cook their fish twice, during which time natural juices and fats are lost (Norwegian School of Veterinary Science (2008).

6. *Starchy diet.* A diet high in starchy foods (high glycemic index) may increase the risk of pancreatic cancer in clients who are overweight and sedentary. Eating foods such as potatoes, rice, white bread, and fructose daily is associated with pancreatic cancer (Dana-Farber Cancer Institute, 2002). **Cautions:** Clients who are obese and inactive tend to be insulin resistant, causing them to produce large amounts of insulin to compensate and putting themselves at greater risk for pancreatic cancer. Counsel clients to substitute less starchy vegetables such as broccoli for potatoes and rice, and to snack on fruit to reduce pancreatic cancer risk.

7. *Sugar and sugar-sweetened foods.* Emerging evidence indicates that hyperglycemia and hyperinsulinemia due to eating sugar and sugar-sweetened foods may be implicated in the development of pancreatic cancer (Jiao et al., 2009; Larsson, Bergkvist & Wolk, 2006). **Health tip:** Counsel clients to use safer sweeteners. Stevia, a herb sweetener that prevents DNA damage, can be used by clients diagnosed with diabetes or hypoglycemia, and acts like a general tonic. It can be used in either liquid or powder form (Ghanta, Banerjee, Poddar, & Chattopadyay (2007).

8. *Watercress.* Watercress has been linked to a reduced risk of cancer via decreased damage to DNA and possible modulation of antioxidant status by increasing carotenoid concentrations. Eating a bowlful of watercress every day for 8 weeks resulted in blood triglyceride levels being reduced by 10% and blood levels of the antioxidants lutein and beta-carotene to increase by 100% and 33%, respectively. **Other considerations:** Cruciferous vegetable consumption is associated with a reduced risk of several cancers in epidemiologic studies (Gill et al., 2007).

9. *Western diet.* Epidemiological evidence on the relationship between nutrition and pancreatic cancer found consistently positive associations between the intakes of meat, carbohydrates, and dietary cholesterol and pancreatic cancer. Nutrition and food patterns explain 35% of all cases in the etiology of pancreatic cancer (Wang & Li, 2006). Good carbs include whole grain breads, cereals, brown rice, bulgur, wheat berries, millet, hulled barley, whole wheat pasta, dried beans (e.g., black, pinto, kidney), and lots of fruits and vegetables. Recommend that clients eat potatoes only occasionally, and steer clear of processed cereals, breads, and white rice. Good fats include olive oil and peanut oil; cashews, almonds, peanuts, and most other nuts; avocados; and up to one egg a day. Sources of bad fats include whole milk, butter, cheese, ice cream, red meat, chocolate, coconuts, coconut milk and oil, poultry skin, palm oil and palm kernel oil, most margarines, vegetable shortening, partially hydrogenated vegetable oil, deep fried chips, many fast foods, and most commercial baked goods (Harvard School of Public Health, 2007).

Stress Management

Stress management evidence-based practice for pancreatic cancer concerns a weak immune system.

A weak immune system is one of the major factors that promotes cancer metastases after an operation, chemotherapy, or radiation therapy. Fear and stress weaken the immune system (Tel Aviv University, 2008). Regular stress-management practice prior to and after medical treatment may help to prevent metastases. For stress management tools, go to http://www.mindtools.com /pages/main/newMN_TCS.htm

Supplements

Supplement evidence-based practice for pancreatic cancer includes the use of aloe, vitamins A, C, and E, and fatty acids.

1. *Aloe.* Animal studies have shown that 3 ounces by mouth of aloe prevents pancreatic neoplasia (Furukawa, 2002). Aloe has also been shown to increase chemotherapy efficacy in terms of both tumor regression rate and survival time (Lissoni et al., 2009). **Cautions:** None unless the client is hypersensitive to aloe. Caution clients not to use their own aloe plants; diarrhea can result if aloe is taken from the wrong leaf area.

2. *Vitamins A, C, and E and fatty acids.* A high intake of saturated and certain monounsaturated fatty acids may increase the risk of pancreatic cancer, whereas greater intake of omega-3 fatty acids and vitamins C and E may reduce the risk (Gong, Holly, Wang, Chan & Bracci, 2010).

Touch

Touch evidence-based practice for pancreatic cancer includes acupressure and foot reflexology.

1. *Acupressure.* Acupressure can relieve nausea, vomiting, and retching associated with chemotherapy (Dribble et al., 2007; Gardani, et al., 2006). Finger acupressure treatment is given bilaterally at the acupressure points P6 and ST36, located on the forearm and by the knee, every 2–3 hours. Gentle acupressure means holding the spot with three middle fingers until a strong pulsation is felt (signaling a blockage has opened) and then moving to the next spot. For more information on using acupressure, go to http://www.eclecticenergies.com/acupressure/howto.php.

2. *Foot reflexology.* Four 40-minute foot reflexology self-treatments enhance natural killer cells and IgG, strengthening the immune system against cancer and possibly preventing tumor development. For more information on reflexology, go to http://www.how-to-do-reflexology

.com/ **Other considerations:** Foot reflexology has been shown to significantly improve life satisfaction, the most important predictor of survival for clients with advanced cancer (Fox Chase Cancer Center, 2007).

PANCREATIC CANCER CASE STUDY

Ted Baxter, age 56, has been diagnosed with pancreatic cancer. He is frightened and unsure about his treatment. He asks for information about health-promoting procedures that could complement his physician's plan.

HEALTH PROMOTION CHALLENGE

Using the information in this section as well as from doing an updated search at PubMed (http://www.ncbi.nlm.nih.gov/pubmed/), develop a teaching/learning program for Mr. Baxter.

REFERENCES

Anand, P., Kunnumakkara, A. B., Newman, R. A., & Aggarwal, B. B. (2007). Bioavailability of curcumin: Problems and promises. *Molecular Pharmacology, 4*(6), 807–818.

Arslan, A. A., Helzlsouer, K. J., Kooperberg, C., Shu, X. O., Steplowski, E., Bueno-de-Mesquita, H. B., . . . Patel, A. V. (2010). Anthropometric measures, body mass index, and pancreatic cancer: A pooled analysis from the Pancreatic Cancer Cohort Consortium (PanScan). *Archives of Internal Medicine, 170*(9), 791–802.

Autoimmunity Research Foundation. (2008, January 27). Vitamin D deficiency study raises new questions about disease and supplements. *ScienceDaily*. Retrieved from http://www.sciencedaily.com/releases/2008/01/080125223302.htm

Bravi, F., Polesel, J., Bosetti, C., Talamini, R., Negri, E., Dal Maso, L., . . . La Vecchia, C. (2010). Dietary intake of selected micronutrients and the risk of pancreatic cancer: An Italian case-control study. *Annals of Oncology, 22*, 202–206.

Brenner, D., & Hall, E. J. (2007). Computed tomography, an increasing source of radiation exposure. *New England Journal of Medicine, 357*(22), 2277–2284.

Dana-Farber Cancer Institute. (2002, September 4). Study suggests a possible link between high-starch diet and pancreatic cancer. *ScienceDaily*. Retrieved from http://www.sciencedaily.com/releases/2002/09/020904073950.htm

Dhillon, N., Aggarwal, B. B., Newman, R. A., Wolff, R. A., Kunnumakkara, A. B., Abbruzzese, J. L., . . . Kurzrock, R. (2008). Phase II clinical trial of curcumin in patients with advanced pancreatic cancer. *Journal of Clinical Oncology, 24*(18S June 20 Supplement), 14151.

Dribble, S. L., Luce, J., Cooper, B. A., Israel, J., Cohen, M., Nussey, B., & Rugo, H. (2007). Acupressure for chemotherapy-induced nausea and vomiting: A randomized clinical trial. *Oncology Nursing Forum, 34*(4), 813–820.

Fox Chase Cancer Center (2007, November 1). Quality of life is the most important predictor of survival for advanced cancer patients. *ScienceDaily*. Retrieved from www.science daily.com/releases/2007/10/071030170208.htm

Furukawa, F., Nishikawa, A., Chihara, T., Shimpo, K., Beppu, H., Kuzuya, H., . . . Hirose, M. (2002). Chemopreventive effects of *Aloe arborescens* on N-nitrosobis (2-oxopropyl) amine-induced pancreatic carcinogenesis in hamsters. *Cancer Letter, 178*(2), 117–122.

Gardani, G., Cerrone, R., Biella, C., Mancini, L., Proserpio, E., Casiraghi, M., . . . Lissoni, P. (2006). Effect of acupressure on nausea and vomiting induced b chemotherapy in cancer patients. *Minerva Medicine, 97*(5), 391–394.

Ghanta, S., Banerjee, A., Poddar, A., & Chattopadyay, S. (2007). Oxidative potential of *Stevia rebaudiana (Bertoni) Bertoni*, a natural sweetener. *Journal of Agricultural and Food Chemistry, 55*(26), 10962–10967.

Gill, C. I., Haldar, S., Boyd, L. A., Bennett, R., Whiteford, J., Butler, M., . . . Rowland, I. R. (2007). Watercress supplementation in diet reduces lymphocyte DNA damage and alters blood antioxidant status in healthy adults. *American Journal of Clinical Nutrition, 85*(2), 504–510.

Gong, Z., Holly, E. A., Wang, F., Chan, J. M., & Bracci, P. M. (2010). Intake of fatty acids and antioxidants and pancreatic cancer in a large population-based case-control study in the San Francisco Bay area. *International Journal of Cancer, 127*(8), 1893–1904.

Hardell, L., Carlberg, M., Hardell, K., Bjornfoth, H., Wickbom, G., Ionescu, M., . . . Lindstrom, G. (2007). Decreased survival in pancreatic cancer patients with high concentrations of organochlorines in adipose tissue. *Biomedical Pharmacotherapy, 61*(10), 659–664.

Harvard School of Public Health. (2007). *Good carbs guide the way*. Retrieved from http://www.hsph.harvard.edu/nutritionsource/what-should-you-eat/carbohydrates-full-story/

Hering, J., Garrean, S., Dekoj, T. R., Razzak, A., Saied, A., Trevino, J., . . . Espat, N. J. (2007). Inhibition of proliferation by omega-3 fatty acids in chemoresistant pancreatic cancer cells. *Annals of Surgical Oncology, 14*, 3620–3628.

Indiana University (2004, January 9). Farmed salmon more toxic than wild salmon, study finds. *ScienceDaily*. Retrieved from http://www.sciencedaily.com/releases/2004/01/040109072244.htm

Jiao, L., Flood, A., Subar, A. F., Hollenbeck, A. R., Schatzkin, A., & Stolzenberg-Solomon, R. (2009). Glycemic index, carbohydrates, glycemic load, and the risk of pancreatic cancer in a prospective cohort study. *Cancer Epidemiology, Biomarkers and Prevention, 18*(4), 1144–1151.

Jockers, B. S. (2007). Vitamin D sufficiency: An approach to disease prevention. *The American Journal for Nurse Practitioners, 11*(10), 43–50.

Kujundzic, N., Grbesa, R., Ivkic, I., Katdare, M., & Gall-Troselj, K. (2006). Curcumin downregulates H19 gene transcription in tumor cells. *Journal of Cellular Biochemistry, 104*(5), 1781–1792.

Lah, J. J., Cui, W., & Hu, K. Q. (2007). Effects and mechanisms of silibinin on human hepatoma cell lines. *World Journal of Gastroenterology, 13*(40), 5299–5305.

Larsson, S. C., Bergkvist, L., & Wolk, A. (2006). Consumption of sugar and sugar-sweetened foods and the risk of pancreatic cancer in a prospective study. *American Journal of Clinical Nutrition, 84*(5), 1171–1176.

Larsson, S. C., Hakansson, N., Giovannucci, E., & Wolk, A. (2006). Folate intake and pancreatic cancer incidence: A prospective study of Swedish women and men. *Journal of National Cancer Institute, 98*(6), 407–413.

Lissoni, P., Rovelli, F., Brivio, F., Zago, R., Colciago, M., Messina, G., . . . Porro, G. (2009). A randomized study of chemotherapy versus biochemotherapy with chemotherapy plus Aloe arborescens in patients with metastatic cancer. *In Vivo, 23*(1), 171–175.

Norwegian School of Veterinary Science (2008, February 28). Farmed fish fed cheap food may be less nutritious for humans. *ScienceDaily.* Retrieved from http://www.science daily.com/releases/2008/02/080226164105.htm

Nothings, U., Murphy, S. P., Wilkens, L. R., Henderson, B. E., & Kolonel, L. N. (2007). Flavonols and pancreatic cancer risk—the Multiethnic Cohort Study. *American Journal of Epidemiology, 166*(8), 924–931.

Post-White, J., Ladas, E. J., & Kelly, K. M. (2007). Advances in the use of milk thistle (*Silybum marianum*). *Integrative Cancer Therapy, 6*(2), 104–109.

Purdue University. (2007). Citrus juice, vitamin C give staying power to green tea antioxidants. Retrieved from http://news.uns.purdue.edu/x/2007b/071113FerruzziTea.html

Shankar, S., Ganapathy S, Hingorani, S. R., Srivastava, R. K. (2008). EGCG inhibits growth, invasion, angiogenesis and metastasis of pancreatic cancer. *Front Bioscience, 13*, 440–452.

Shehzad, A., Wahid, F., & Lee, Y. S. (2010, August 19). Curcumin in cancer chemoprevention: Molecular targets, pharmacokinetics, bioavailability, and clinical trials. *Archiv der Pharmazie (Weinheim).* [Advance online publication]. Retrieved from http://www .unboundmedicine.com/medline/ebm/record/20726007/abstract/Curcumin_in _Cancer_Chemoprevention:_Molecular_Targets_Pharmacokinetics_Bioavailability _and_Clinical_Trials_August 29, 2010.

Skinner, H. G., Michaud, D. S., Giovannucci, E., Willett, W. C., Colditz, G. A., & Fuch, C. S. (2006). Vitamin D intake and the risk for pancreatic cancer in two cohort studies. *Cancer Epidemiology Biomarkers and Prevention, 15*, 1688–1695.

Skidmore-Roth, L. (2006). Green tea. *Mosby's handbook of herbs & natural supplements*, pp. 525–539. St. Louis: ElsevierMosby.

Tel Aviv University. (2008, February 29). Stress and fear can affect cancer's recurrence. *ScienceDaily.* Retrieved from http://www.sciencedaily.com/releases/2008/02/080227142656 .htm

Thiébaut, A. C. M., Li Jiao, D. T., Silverman, A. J., Cross, F. E., Thompson, J., Subar, A. F., . . . Stolzenberg-Solomon, R. Z. (2009). Dietary fatty acids and pancreatic cancer in the NIH-AARP Diet and Health Study. *Journal of the National Cancer Institute, 101*(14), 1001–1011.

University of Missouri-Columbia. (2008, March 21). Killer stairs? Taking the elevator could be worse for our body. *ScienceDaily.* Retrieved from http://www.sciencedaily.com /releases/2008/03/080318182741.htm

Wang, L., & Li, H. (2006). Advances in research on genetic epidemiology of pancreatic cancer. *Acta Academiae Medicinae Sinicae, 28*(2), 289–293.

Premenstrual Syndrome

Environment

Exercise/movement evidence-based practice for premenstrual syndrome (PMS) includes qi gong.

The slow, gentle movements of qi gong can reduce negative feeling, pain, water retention, and total PMS symptoms more effectively than placebo controls (Jang & Lee, 2004). **Health tip:** For a gentle movement exercise that can help with PMS, go to http://www.everyday-taichi.com/qigong-instructions.html

Herbs/Essential Oils

Chaste tree (*Vitex agnes-castus*) was more effective than placebo in the treatment of 17 moderate-to-severe PMS symptoms (Ma et al., 2010).

Nutrition

Nutrition evidence-based practice for PMS includes the following:

1. *Calcium and vitamin D.* Blood calcium and vitamin D levels are lower in women with PMS, and the intake of calcium and vitamin D from food is inversely related to PMS (Bertone-Johnson, et al., 2005). Women need between 1,000 and 1,500 mg of calcium and 400 IU or more IU of vitamin D daily. Vitamin D supplements can suppress the proper operation of the immune system and vitamin D_2-fortified foods are inefficiently metabolized (Autoimmunity Research Foundation, 2008). Foods high in calcium that may be more easily metabolized include sardines in oil including bones, canned pink salmon including bones, boiled soybeans, cooked collards, cooked turnip greens, tofu, and dried figs. Besides spending time in the sun (15 minutes for fair-skinned and 45 minutes for darker-skinned women), clients can be counseled to eat egg yolks, saltwater fish, and/or take a tablespoon of cod liver oil every day. **Other considerations:** Women using corticosteroids may require additional vitamin D.

2. *Fat, carbohydrate, simple sugars, protein and alcohol.* In one study, overweight women with PMS showed a more significant increase in intake of fat, simple sugars (including cereals, cakes, desserts, and high-sugar foods), and alcohol, and a greater decrease in protein consumption, premenstrually (as compared to women without PMS). The study found a significant increase in episodes of eating premenstrually. Women who increase their nutrient intake during the premenstrual phase may benefit from more frequent reminders to eat more protein and fewer sugary foods (Bryant, Truesdale, & Dye, 2006).

3. *Obesity.* Obesity is a risk factor for PMS. One study found that obese women had a threefold greater risk for PMS as compared to nonobese women (Masho, Adera, & South-Paul, 2005). Go to "Overweight/Obesity," previously in this appendix, for more information.

4. *Soy isoflavones.* Soy isoflavones (25 grams daily) have a beneficial effect on certain menstrual symptoms (Kim, Kwon, Kim, & Reame, 2006). Counsel women to eat up to 25 grams daily, including several of the following:
   - 4 oz. firm tofu = 13 g soy protein
   - 4 oz. soft or silken tofu = 9 g soy protein
   - 1 soy-based burger = 10 to 12 g soy protein
   - 8 oz. plain soy milk = 10 g soy protein
   - 1 soy protein bar = 14 g soy protein
   - Half cup cooked soybeans = 16 g soy protein

   Fermented soy products (miso, tempeh) are more digestible than other forms.

Supplements

Supplement evidence-based practice for PMS includes the following:

1. *Calcium carbonate.* A double-blind clinical trial was designed to evaluate the effect of calcium supplement therapy on PMS symptoms. The study groups were selected from young female college students, based on PMS criteria. The subjects were divided in two groups; one group received placebo and the other received 500 mg of calcium carbonate twice daily for 3 months. The severity and intensity of symptoms, including early fatigability, changes in appetite, and depression, were evaluated using a standard questionnaire. Symptoms were compared before and after treatment. The mean age was 21.4 +/– 3.6 years. Early tiredness, appetite changes, and depressive symptoms were significantly improved in the group receiving calcium treatment compared with the placebo group (Ghanbari, Haghollahi, Shariat, Foroshani, & Ashrafi, 2009).

2. *Pyridoxine (vitamin B$_6$).* In a control group, 20 women were kept on ferrous sulphate tablets (100 mg for 3 months), as placebo. There was no significant change in the premenstrual symptoms score at the end of the study period in the control group. In two more groups of 20 women each, bromocriptine 2.5 mg twice a day and pyridoxine 100 mg/day showed a significant reduction in the mean premenstrual symptom score after 3 months of treatment. It is concluded that both of the drugs are effective for treatment of premenstrual syndrome, but pyridoxine showed significantly higher response rate and lesser incidence of side effects than bromocriptine (Sharma, Kulshreshtha, Singh, & Ghagoliwal, 2007).

3. *Vitamin E.* Compared to placebo, vitamin E (200 IU b.i.d. taken 2 days before the expected start of menstruation) resulted in greater relief of symptoms in a study by Rasgon & Yargin (2005).

Touch

Touch evidence-based practice for PMS includes reflexology.

In women who were taught self-foot massage, there is a statistically significant difference indepression and perceived stress. This suggests that a self-foot reflexology massage could be utilized as an effective nursing intervention to reduce depression and stress responses and to strengthen immune systems (Lee, 2006). For more information on foot reflexology, go to http://www .how-to-do-reflexology.com/

PMS CASE STUDY

Ms. Winstead, age 28, has been suffering from PMS since she began menstruating at age 13. She has tried medications but found them unsatisfactory. She asks you for ideas of things she can do to have less distressing periods.

HEALTH PROMOTION CHALLENGE

Use the information in this section and complete an updated search at PubMed (http://www.ncbi.nlm.nih.gov/pubmed/) using PMS in the search box. Develop a teaching/learning program for Ms. Winstead.

REFERENCES

Autoimmunity Research Foundation. (2008, January 27). Vitamin D deficiency study raises new questions about disease and supplements. *ScienceDaily*. Retrieved from http://www.sciencedaily.com/releases/2008/01/080125223302.htm

Bertone-Johnson, E. R., Hankinson, S. E., Bendich, A., Johnson, S. R., Willett, W. C., & Manson, J. E. (2005). Calcium and vitamin D intake and risk of incident premenstrual syndrome. *Archives of Internal Medicine, 165*(11), 1246–1252.

Bryant, M., Trucsdale, K. P., & Dye, L. (2006). Modest changes in dietary intake across the menstrual cycle: Implications for food intake research. *British Journal of Nutrition, 96*(5), 888–894.

Ghanbari, Z., Haghollahi, F., Shariat, M., Foroshani, A. R., & Ashrafi, M. (2009). Effects of calcium supplement therapy in women with premenstrual syndrome. *Taiwan Journal of Obstetrics and Gynecology, 48*(2), 124–129.

Jang, H. S., & Lee, M. S. (2004). Effects of qi therapy (external qigong) on premenstrual syndrome: A randomized placebo-controlled study. *Journal of Alternative and Complementary Medicine, 10*(3), 456–462.

Kim, H. W., Kwon, M. K., Kim, N. S., & Reame, N. E. (2006). Intake of dietary soy isoflavones in relation to perimenstrual symptoms of Korean women living in the USA. *Nursing Health Science, 8*(2), 108–113.

Lee, Y. M. (2006). Effect of self-foot reflexology massage on depression, stress response and immune functions of middle aged women. *Taehan Kanho Hakkoe Chi, 36*(1), 179–188.

Ma, L., Lin, S., Chen, R., Zhang, Y., Chen, F., & Wang, X. (2010). Evaluating therapeutic effect in symptoms of moderate-to-severe premenstrual syndrome with *Vitex agnus* castus (BNO 1095) in Chinese women. *Australian and New Zealand Journal of Obstetrics and Gynaecology, 50*(2), 189–193.

Masho, S. W., Adera, T., & South-Paul, J. (2005). Obesity as a risk factor for premenstrual syndrome. *Journal of Psychsomatics and Obstetric Gynaecology, 26*(1), 33–39.

Rasgon, N. L., & Yargin, K. N. (2005). Vitamin E for the treatment of dysmenorrhea. *BJOG, 112*(8), 1164.

Sharma, P., Kulshreshtha, S., Singh, G. M., & Bhagoliwal, A. (2007). Role of bromocriptine and pyridoxine in premenstrual tension syndrome. *Indian Journal of Physiology and Pharmacology, 51*(4), 368–74.

Polycystic Ovary Syndrome

Exercise/Movement

Exercise/movement evidence-based practice for polycystic ovary syndrome (PCOS) includes daily exercise and nutritional counseling.

Daily exercise and nutritional counseling for at least 12 weeks may benefit the metabolic and reproductive abnormalities associated with PCOS (Bruner, Chad, & Chizen, 2006). **Health tip:** For more information on exercise, go to http://exercise.lifetips.com

Herbs/Essential Oils

Herbal evidence-based practice for PCOS includes Chinese herbs.

Chinese herbs for nourishing yin to reduce fire can significantly reduce the serum levels of testosterone and insulin in women with PCOS. Chinese herbs for invigorating spleen and replenishing qi can significantly reduce the serum level of insulin in women with PCOS (Jia & Wang, 2006). **Cautions:** Consult a Chinese medicine practitioner before using any herbs.

Mind-Set

Mind-set evidence-based practice for PCOS includes a manual-based cognitive behavioral therapy approach.

In a 2009 study, a manual-based cognitive behavioral therapy approach to treat depression in adolescents with PCOS and obesity helped decrease depression and increase weight loss (Rofey et al., 2009).

Nutrition

Nutrition evidence-based practice for PCOS includes dietary counseling.

Women diagnosed with PCOS may consume significantly more white bread and fried potatoes than a control group. Several different scenarios of diets appear to work well with PCOS. A diet of 1,200–1,400 calories/day (25% protein, 25% fat, 50% carbohydrates plus 25–30 grams of fiber per week) ameliorated hyperinsulinemia and hyperandrogenemia in a study. In another study, a moderate reduction in dietary carbohydrate (43%) reduced the fasting and postchallenge insulin concentrations. Over time, these concentrations may improve reproductive/endocrine outcomes. An eating pattern similar to the type 2 diabetes diet, including an a decrease in refined carbohydrates, as well as a decrease in trans and saturated fats and an increase in anti-inflammatory compounds (omega-3 fatty acids, vitamin E, fiber, and red wine) can improve the androgen profile of women with PCOS (Douglas et al., 2006; Liepa, Sengupta, & Karsie, 2008; Qublan, Yannakoula, Al-Qudah, & El-Uri, 2007).

Supplements

Inositol at 100 mg b.i.d. improves ovarian function in women with oligomenorrhea and polycystic ovaries. As opposed to a control group, significant weight loss (and leptin reduction) was recorded in the inositol group. **Other considerations:** This substance is found in many foods, including whole grain cereals, nuts, beans, and fruit, especially cantaloupe melons and oranges. Inositol is not considered a vitamin because it can be synthesized by the body (Gerli, Mignosa, & Di Renzo, 2003).

PCOS CASE STUDY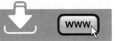

Ms. Torneadu, age 35, has been diagnosed with PCOS. She has gained 40 pounds in the past year and wants some ideas about how to lose weight and feel more comfortable.

HEALTH PROMOTION CHALLENGE

Using the information in this section, as well as by doing a search for PCOS at PubMed (http://www.ncbi.nlm.nih.gov/pubmed/), develop a teaching/learning program for Ms. Torneadu.

REFERENCES

Bruner, B., Chad, K., & Chizen, D. (2006). Effects of exercise and nutiriton counseling in women with polycystic ovary syndrome. *Applied Physiological Nutrition and Metabolism, 31*(4), 384–391.

Douglas, C. C., Gower, B. A., Darnell, B. E., OValle, F., Oster, R. A., & Azziz, R. (2006). Role of diet in the treatment of polycystic ovary syndrome. *Fertility and Sterility, 85*(3), 679–688.

Gerli, S., Mignosa, M., & Di Renzo, G. C. (2003). Effects of inositol on ovarian function and metabolic factors in women with PCOS: A randomized double blind placebo-controlled trial. *European Review of Medical Pharmacology and Science, 7*(6), 151–159.

Jia, L. N., & Wang, X. J. (2006). Clinical observation on treatment of 43 women with polycystic ovary syndrome based on syndrome differentiation. *Zhong Xi Yhi Jie He Xue Bao, 4*(6), 585–588.

Liepa, G. U., Sengupta, A., & Karsie, D. (2008). Polycystic ovary syndrome (PCOS) and other androgen excess-related conditions: Can changes in dietary intake make a difference? *Nutrition in Clinical Practice, 23*(1), 63–71.

Qublan, H. S., Yannakoula, E. K., Al-Qudah, M. A., & El-Uri, F. I. (2007). Dietary intervention versus metformin to improve the reproductive outcome in women with polycystic ovary syndrome. A prospective comparative study. *Saudi Medical Journal, 28*(11), 1694–1699.

Rofey, D. L., Szigethy, E. M., Noll, R. B., Dahl, R. E., Lobst, E., & Arslanian, S. A. (2009). Cognitive-behavioral therapy for physical and emotional disturbances in adolescents with polycystic ovary syndrome: A pilot study. *Journal of Pediatric Psychology, 34*(2), 156–163.

Pregnancy/Labor/Delivery

Environment

Environmental evidence-based practice for pregnancy/labor/delivery concerns the following:

1. *Air pollution.* Air pollution is linked to premature birth in pregnant women. Being exposed to vehicle traffic can increase the likelihood of having a preterm baby by 10–25% over women who lived in less polluted areas. This is especially true for women who breathed polluted air during the first trimester or during the last months and weeks of pregnancy (University of California, Los Angeles, 2007).

2. *Aromatherapy.* A drop of essential oil placed on a pillow or T-shirt, in a footbath, in a massage oil, or in a compress can optimize a woman's coping skills during labor, helping to release endorphins and reducing the use of oxytocin to help with contractions. Women who used aromatherapy were significantly less likely to have epidural anesthesia, irrespective of parity and labor onset. Aromatherapy also altered the

culture of the maternity unit, making people more kind to each other. Drops of essential oils are used as needed. Lavender, frankincense, rose, jasmine, and chamomile essential oils can be used for anxiety; peppermint for nausea and vomiting; and clary sage to assist contractions and enhance labor (Liptak, 2002; Tillett & Ames, 2010).

3. *Breastfeeding-friendly practices in hospitals.* Breastmilk and breastfeeding are recognized as the ideal choices of nutrition and feeding for infants. Breastfeeding-friendly practices in hospitals following birth can significantly improve long-term breastfeeding success. Nearly two-thirds of mothers who followed available supportive practices were still breastfeeding 4 months after going home. Supportive practices included (1) initiating breastfeeding within 1 hour of delivery, (2) keeping infants in the mother's hospital room (rooming in), (3) feeding infants only breastmilk in the hospital, (4) prohibiting pacifier use in the hospital, and (5) providing a telephone number to call for breastfeeding help after hospital discharge. **Other considerations:** In addition to receiving essential nutrients, breastfed infants have lower rates of ear infections, gastroenteritis, asthma, obesity, and diabetes. Benefits for mothers include decreased incidence of breast and ovarian cancer. National goals in the United States are a breastfeeding initiation rate of 75% (with an exclusive breastfeeding rate for the first 3 months of 60%), and continuation of 50% at 6 months of age, with 25% exclusively breastfeeding (Blackwell Publishing Ltd., 2007).

4. *Centering pregnancy for pregnant adolescents.* This 20-hour program over 28 weeks provides a holistic approach toward prenatal care and is well suited to adolescents because it also considers their developmental need for socializing and peer support. This program is associated with a greater improvement in birth outcomes when compared with traditional or adult-focused care (Grady & Bloome, 2004). This approach is most useful to teens because it allows them to focus on adjustment to pregnancy; share their fears and concerns with peers; and learn about fetal development, nutrition, exercise, the dangers of substance abuse and appropriate referral, preparation for childbirth (including relaxation and breathing methods), infant breastfeeding, baby care and coping techniques, parenting techniques and self-esteem building, contraception and postpartum depression, physical and sexual abuse, sexuality, and communication (Moeller, Vezeau & Carr, 2007).

5. *Cesarean sections.* Turning fetuses that are in a breech presentation can prevent unnecessary Cesarean sections, which increase the risk for potentially fatal complications. A physician or midwife uses his or her hands to manipulate the mother's abdomen and help the baby turn in a somersault-like motion (external cephalic version or ECV) at 34 to 36 weeks' gestation. **Cautions:** Turning a breech baby at 37 to 38 weeks

(the current procedure) is less successful (McMaster University, 2007). Except in breech births, women having a nonemergency cesarean birth have double the risk of illness or even death compared to a vaginal birth. Overweight pregnant women have greater risk for infection (including death due to wound infection), delayed wound healing, and blood clots. All pregnant women who undergo cesarean section have a greater risk of infection, hemorrhage, reaction to anesthesiology, and other surgical risks (British Medical Journal, 2007; Chettle, 2008; Huiras, 2008). The fetus is in breech position about once in every 25–30 full-term births. Counsel women with fetuses in breech position to ask for ECV at 34 to 36 weeks. For illustrations and a video on the procedure, go to: http://www.medicalnewstoday.com/articles/74317.php.

6. *Dental X-rays.* Both high and low-dose radiation exposure in women during pregnancy are associated with term low-birth-weight infants. **Cautions:** In one study, exposure to radiation higher than 0.4 Gy was associated with an increased risk (about double) of low-birth-weight infants (Hujoel, Bollen, Noonan, & del Aguila, 2004). Counsel clients to avoid dental X-rays during pregnancy.

7. *Dioxin.* Intrauterine dioxin exposure can disrupt the develop of mammary glands and predispose offspring to mammary cancer. Women are exposed to dioxin primarily through consumption of animal products, including meat, poultry, dairy products, and human breastmilk. **Cautions:** Dioxin is formed by the incineration of products containing PVC (polyvinyl chloride), PCBs, and other chlorinated compounds. Dioxin also comes from industrial processes that use chlorine and the combustion of diesel and gasoline, which contain chlorinated additives (World Health Organization, 2007). Counsel pregnant women and lactating women to avoid eating animal products, pumping gasoline into their vehicles, or being near vehicle exhaust whenever possible. **Other considerations:** Dioxins are known human carcinogens and hormone mimickers. Very low levels are found in the air and plants. Encourage pregnant women and lactating women to eat vegetables, fruits, dried beans, and whole grains and fewer or no animal products.

8. *Home visitors.* Receiving care from a health visitor trained in identification and psychological intervention methods prevents depression 6–18 months postnatally in women who are not depressed 6 weeks postnatally (Brugha, Morrell, Slade, & Walters, 2010).

9. *Kneeling for labor.* Kneeling on a cushion facing the head of the delivery bed vs. sitting position with the head of bed raised at least 60° in the second stage of labor until the child's head crowns is associated with shorter duration of the second stage of labor and several other benefits. These benefits include fewer in assisted deliveries; fewer episiotomies; less reporting of severe pain during second-stage labor; fewer abnormal

fetal heart rate patterns; and significantly reduced feelings of discomfort, vulnerability, exposure, difficulty, and postpartum perineal pain. **Cautions:** Kneeling position may increase risk of blood loss and perineal tears (Ragnar, Altman, Tyden, & Olsson, 2006). Encourage women to give birth in the position they find most comfortable.

10. *Methylmercury and polychlorinate biphenyls (PCBs).* Methylmercury and PCBs may interact when they cross the placenta and enter the developing brain of the fetus. **Cautions:** Human health studies indicate that: (1) reproductive function may be disrupted by exposure to PCBs; (2) neurobehavioral and developmental deficits occur in newborns and continue through school-aged children who had in-utero exposure to PCBs; (3) other systemic effects (e.g., self-reported liver disease and diabetes, and effects on the thyroid and immune systems) are associated with elevated serum levels of PCBs; and (4) increased cancer risks, e.g., non-Hodgkin's lymphoma, are associated with PCB exposures (U.S. Public Health Service and the Environmental Protective Agency, 2008). Counsel women to eat saltwater fish only. (See "Nutrition" later in this section.)

11. *Nonstick chemicals.* In one study, fetuses exposed to chemicals used in nonstick cookware were born at significantly lower body weight (Vanderbilt University, 2007). Advise clients to avoid nonstick cookware.

12. *Household exposure to pesticides.* Maternal exposure to household pesticides during pregnancy was significantly associated with childhood hematopoietic malignancies, the most common childhood cancers (leukemia, Hodgkin's lymphoma, and non-Hodgkin's lymphoma). The use of professional pest control services at any time from 1 year before birth to 3 years after was associated with a significantly increased risk of childhood leukemia. Pesticides used at home, on pets, or for garden crops were also significantly associated with childhood cancer in two studies (Rudant et al., 2007; Turner, Wigle, & Krewski, 2010). **Cautions:** Caution women not to use professional pest control services or use pesticides themselves in the home, on pets, or in the garden if pregnant or contemplating becoming pregnant. For information on safe alternatives to pesticides, go to http://www.wtv-zone.com/infchoice/no_tox.html

13. *Smoking.* Pregnant women who smoke are five times more likely to develop eclampsia. If women give up smoking before or even during pregnancy, they can significantly reduce this risk (University of Nottingham, 2008). Support women in quitting at every stage of pregnancy. For smoking cessation information, go to http://www.helpguide.org/mental/quit_smoking_cessation.htm

14. *SSRIs.* Maternal use of selective serotonin reuptake inhibitors during pregnancy may be associated with an increased risk of major birth defects, such as tetralogy of Fallot. According to one study, the risk was highest with paroxetine (Paxil) (Alwan, 2005). Teach women safer

approaches to insomnia, anxiety, depression, and stress. See "Nutrition," "Exercise," and "Stress Management" in this section for ideas.

15. *Vitamin D deficiency.* Low levels of vitamin D early in pregnancy is associated with a fivefold increased risk of preeclampsia, also known as toxemia, which is the leading cause of premature delivery and maternal and fetal illness and death worldwide. Even a small decline in vitamin D concentration more than doubled the risk of preeclampsia. Because a newborn's vitamin D stores are completely reliant on vitamin D from the mother, low vitamin levels also were observed in the umbilical cord blood of newborns from mothers with preeclampsia. **Cautions:** Vitamin D deficiency early in life is associated with rickets, as well as increased risk for type 1 diabetes, asthma, and schizophrenia (Jocker, 2007; University of Pittsburgh Schools of Health Science, 2007). Daily sensible sun exposure (4–10 minutes with face and arms exposed for light-skinned women and 40–80 minutes for darker-skinned women) can most often provide the needed amount of vitamin D. Sun exposure should be at solar noon when UVB rays are most directly penetrating. **Other considerations:** Women residing at latitudes north of 35° may have a difficult time obtaining sufficient sunshine in the wintertime. They may need to take a tablespoon of cod liver oil daily, eat fatty fish several times a week, eat eggs several times a week (the yolks are the portion that contain vitamin D), and/or take fish oil supplements. A vitamin D supplement may not be advised (Autoimmunity Research Foundation, 2008.).

Exercise/Movement

Exercise/movement evidence for pregnancy/labor/delivery:

1. *Aerobic exercise.* Significantly lower heart rates occur among fetuses exposed to maternal exercise. Moderate-to-heavy intensity aerobic activity for 30 minutes per session three times per week can keep the mom's and the baby's heart healthy (American Physiological Society, 2008). Go to http://exercise.lifetips.com for information on how to coach pregnant women.

2. *Kegel exercises.* Kegel exercises strengthen the pelvic floor and can calm an overactive bladder or stress incontinence (Shamliyan, Kane, Wyman, & Wilt, 2008).

3. *Yoga.* Compared to a control group in a 2008 study, pregnant women who participated in yoga (six 1-hour sessions at prescribed weeks during pregnancy) experienced higher levels of maternal comfort during labor and 2 hours postlabor, less subject-evaluated labor pain, a shorter first stage of labor, and a shorter total time of labor (Chuntharapat, Petpichetchian & Hatthakit, 2008). **Cautions:** Go to http://yoga

.lifetips.com/cat/56770/yoga-cautions/ For more information on yoga, go to www.yogajournal.com

Herbs/Essential Oils

Herbal evidence-based practice for pregnancy/labor/delivery pertains to ginger.

Ginger effectively treats stomach upset, nausea, and vomiting at least as effectively as medical treatment (central nervous system anticholinergics) and without any side effects (Smith, 2010). Fresh ginger, available in supermarkets, is recommended by the American College of Obstetricians and Gynecologists. Fresh ginger can be scraped into tea water, stews, soups, salads, oatmeal, and other cereals, or even sandwiches. **Other considerations:** The new antiemetics for nausea and vomiting are very costly; ginger is a very inexpensive, safe, healthy, and tasty alternative.

Nutrition

Nutrition evidence-based practice for pregnancy/labor/delivery includes the following:

1. *Caffeine.* Caffeinated coffee, tea, soda, and hot chocolate are associated with an increased risk of miscarriage. Women who consumed 2 or more cups of regular coffee or five 12-ounce cans of caffeinated soda had twice the miscarriage risk as women who consumed no caffeine (Kaiser Permanente Division of Research, 2008).

2. *Calcium.* In 12 studies comparing at least 1 gram of calcium daily during pregnancy with placebo, calcium reduced the rate of preeclampsia and reduced the rare occurrence of the outcome of maternal death or serious morbidity. Adequate dietary calcium before and in early pregnancy may be needed to prevent underlying pathology responsible for preeclampsia (Hofmeyr, Duley, & Atallah, 2007). **Cautions:** Without adequate daily calcium, high blood pressure, maternal death, and serious morbidity can result. Counsel women to eat high-calcium foods daily. For a list of foods high in calcium, go to www.health.gov /dietaryguidelines/dga2005/document/html/appendixB.htm and scroll to Non-Dairy Food Sources of Calcium. **Other considerations:** Some of the highest sources of nondairy calcium include soy beverages, sardine, tofu, and pink salmon with bones.

3. *Copper.* Copper within certain enzymes in the brain helps form key neurotransmitters that allow brain cells to "talk" to one another. Adequate amounts of copper are critical to the fetus during pregnancy, but 8–12% of childbearing-age women have inadequate copper intakes. Eating a balanced diet containing a variety of nutritious foods is the best approach to getting adequate copper, including beef liver, mushrooms,

trail mix, barley, and canned tomato puree (U.S. Department of Agriculture, 2007). **Cautions:** Without adequate copper, the fetus's brain may not develop. **Other considerations:** The areas of the brain most affected by low-copper diets are the gyrus and hippocampal areas of the brain, most important to higher brain functions, such as learning.

4. *Fiber.* Fiber intake during the second trimester of pregnancy is important to fetal and maternal health (Bang & Lee, 2009). Good sources of fiber include fruits, vegetables, whole grains, nuts, and seeds.

5. *Fish.* More than 90% of women consume less than the FDA recommended amount of fish. This leads to an inadequate intake of omega-3 fatty acids, resulting in risks to their health and the health of their unborn children. Some data show a connection with reduced preterm labor and postpartum depression in mothers who ate ocean fish when pregnant. A fish-rich diet in pregnancy can help to protect children from asthma and allergies (British Medical Journal, 2008). Counsel pregnant women to eat a minimum of 12 ounces per week of fish, including salmon, tuna, sardines, and Spanish mackerel, which are the least contaminated with mercury. Teach women that although fish may contain some mercury, they also contain selenium, an essential mineral that appears to protect against the toxicity from trace amounts of mercury (National Healthy Mothers, Healthy Babies Coalition, 2007).

6. *Folate.* Folic acid foods eaten during pregnancy reduce the risk of recurrent early pregnancy loss, birth defects in newborns, and preeclampsia in pregnant women, and they may protect offspring from colorectal cancer (American Association for Cancer Research, 2008). Low-carb diets (e.g., the Atkins diet) take a toll on women's folate levels ("Low Carb, Low Folate?" 2007). Leafy green vegetables (like spinach and turnip greens), fruits (citrus fruits and juices), and dried beans and peas are all natural sources of folate that can help meet the suggested amount per day of 400 micrograms. **Cautions:** In addition to pregnancy, medications and conditions that increase the need for folate or result in an increased excretion of folate include anticonvulsant medications, metformin, sulfasalazine, triamterene, methotrexate, barbiturates, lactation, alcohol abuse, malabsorption, kidney dialysis, liver disease, and certain anemias. Because folate is a water-soluble B-vitamin, unneeded amounts will be eliminated in the urine. Counsel clients to avoid flour-fortified foods as a source of folic acid; new research has shown the introduction of flour fortified with folic acid into common foods has been linked to colon cancer. Folate can be lost from foods during cooking so counsel women to serve fruits and vegetables raw whenever possible and to store vegetables in the refrigerator. Have clients eat whole grain cereals, breads, and pasta to avoid fortified flours (Willianne et al., 2007). For a fact sheet on folate, go to http://ohioline.osu.edu/hyg-fact/5000/5553

.html **Other considerations:** Exceeding 1,000 micrograms per day of folate may trigger vitamin B_{12} deficiency. To compensate, women can take a multivitamin that contains B_{12} or eat at least one food daily that contains B_{12}. Such foods include nutritional yeast (unless the client is susceptible to *Candida*), clams, eggs, herring, kidney, liver, Spanish mackerel, seafood, milk, and dairy products.

7. *Iron, phosphorus, and vitamin B_6.* When ingested in adequate amounts by pregnant women, iron, phosphorus, and vitamin B_6 improve maternal and fetal health (Bang & Lee, 2009). Iron is not easily assimilated in the body. Good sources of iron are food cooked in iron pots and pans and blackstrap molasses. Phosphorus is widely available in daily products and meat. For ideas, go to http://lpi.oregonstate.edu/infocenter/minerals/phosphorus/ Vitamin B_6 is available in bananas, turkey or chicken, baked potatoes, cooked spinach, and dry-roasted hazelnuts. For more information, go to http://lpi.oregonstate.edu/infocenter/vitamins/vitaminB6/

8. *Trans fat, sugar, and fertility.* Women who ate less trans fats and sugar from carbohydrates, consumed more protein from vegetables (not animals), ate more fiber and iron, took more multivitamins, weighed less, exercised for longer periods of time each day, and consumed more high-fat dairy products (not low-fat) were 89% more fertile. In a Harvard study, researchers found a sixfold difference in ovulatory infertility risk occurred between groups of women following five or more low-risk dietary and lifestyle habits and those following none. The more fertility factors followed, the more infertility risk drops (Harvard School of Public Health, 2007). To lower trans fat, advise clients to avoid fried foods; anything that has partially hydrogenated fat in it; and most donuts, chips, crackers, cookies, margarine, candy bars, and many other frozen and convenience foods. Instruct clients to read labels carefully and remind them that even if it says zero, there may be up to 0.5 gram of trans fat per serving, which can quickly add up.

9. *Eating and weight patterns prior to pregnancy.* Eating junk food while pregnant and breastfeeding may lead to obese offspring. Maternal obesity prior to pregnancy is associated with birth defects, greater risk of having hyperactive children, and difficulty breastfeeding. Gaining weight between pregnancies can result in preeclampsia, diabetes, pregnancy-induced high blood pressure, high birth weight, and stillbirths (JAMA and Archives Journals, 2007; Jevitt, Hernandez & Groer, 2007; Upsala University, 2007; Wellcome Trust, 2007). Losing weight prior to becoming pregnant and changing to healthier eating patterns can have significant effects on women and their offspring. **Cautions:** Losing weight between pregnancies can lead to giving birth prematurely. Assist women to attain a healthy weight prior to their first pregnancy.

Encourage women to avoid junk food while pregnant. For more information, go to http://www.weightlossresources.co.uk/diet/diet_tips.htm

Stress Management

Stress management evidence-based practice for pregnancy/labor/delivery concerns the following:

1. *Anxious or depressed mothers-to-be.* In one study, mothers classified as clinically anxious or depressed 18 weeks into pregnancy, compared to their nondepressed or nonanxious counterparts, were about 40% more likely to have an 18-month-old who refused to go to bed, woke up early, and kept crawling out of bed. The child's behavior often persisted until age 30 months (University of Rochester Medical Center, 2007). Chronic mild stress in pregnant mothers may increase the risk that their offspring will develop cerebral palsy (Society for Neuroscience, 2007). Go to www.mindtools.com for ways to help pregnant women reduce their stress.

2. *Hypnotherapy for labor.* Hypnosis has been shown to reduce labor length and pain levels, increase enjoyment of labor, and stop preterm labor (Brown & Hammond, 2007). **Cautions:** Go to http://www.ncpamd.com/medical_hypnosis.htm#Contraindications_for_Hypnosis For more information about hypnosis, go to http://psychceu.com/peterson/hypnosis.html

Supplements

Supplement evidence-based practice for pregnancy/labor/delivery includes the following:

1. *Multivitamins.* In one study, women taking a multivitamin tablet or capsule with low iron every day before conception through week 12 of pregnancy experienced significantly reduced nausea and vomiting (Ahn et al., 2006). Counsel women to take other steps to reduce nausea and vomiting, including the following:

   - Eat frequently and in small amounts
   - Eat complex carbohydrates (fruits, vegetables, dried beans, dried peas, whole grains)
   - Eat low-fat foods, except for 1–2 tablespoons of extra virgin olive oil on salads or to use in low-heat cooking
   - Eat high-protein foods, especially nonanimal foods (soy burgers, soy chips, soy milk, soy cheese, tempeh, beans, and rice)
   - Avoid spicy foods and any offensive smells
   - Drink clear liquids such as lemonade and ginger ale
   - Lie down and rest as needed

- Change position slowly, especially when rising
- Get outside and breathe in fresh air
- Brush teeth an hour after eating to avoid nausea and vomiting due to excess salivation or smell of toothpaste (Hunter, Sullivan, Young, & Weber, 2007)

2. *Probiotics. Listeria monocytogenes* is particularly dangerous during pregnancy. A probiotic taken during pregnancy could provide protection in a form that would be acceptable to expectant mothers (Corr et al., 2007). *Lactobacillus salivarius* is available as a supplement at health foods stores. Pregnant women should take 1 to 10 billion organisms by mouth. **Cautions:** A nondairy form should be used by women hypersensitive to milk. Advise clients to keep probiotics in the refrigerator and to follow directions on the bottle.

3. *Pycnogenol.* Thrombotic events (blood clots in the legs) are the leading cause of death in pregnant women (James, Jamison, Brancazio, & Myers, 2006). Pycnogenol (two or three 100 mg capsules per day with a glass of water) has been shown to prevent venous thrombosis and thrombophlebitis in moderate- to high-risk women (Belcaro et al., 2004). **Cautions:** Pycnogenol can cause reduced blood platelet aggregation (clotting). Otherwise this supplement is safe except for women who are hypersensitive to pine, as pycnogenol is a mixture of bioflavonoids found in pine bark.

4. *Vitamin B$_6$.* Vitamin B$_6$ (10 to 25 mg t.i.d.) can create a significant reduction in vomiting and severe nausea (Hunter, Sullivan, Young, & Weber, 2007; Smith, 2010). **Cautions:** Advise clients not to exceed 75 mg a day.

Touch

Touch evidence-based practice for pregnancy/labor/delivery includes acupressure and massage.

1. *Acupressure to point SP6.* In a study, acupressure at Sanyinjiao point SP6, above the ankle, reduced the duration and severity of pain of the active phase of labor, cesarean section rates, and necessity and amount of oxytocin (Kashanian & Shahali, 2009).

2. *Acupressure to point P6.* In a 2008 study, applying acupressure bands to P6 acupoint reduced the symptoms of nausea and vomiting during pregnancy more than acupressure to a sham point on the top of the wrist (Gurkan & Arslan, 2008). Two types of acupressure bands are available online.

3. *Massage therapy.* Pregnancy massage reduces prematurity, low birth weight, and postpartum depression. Pregnant women diagnosed with major depression were given 12 weeks of twice-per-week massage therapy by their significant other or only standard treatment as a control group in

a 2009 study. The massage therapy group women not only had reduced depression by the end of the therapy period, but they also had reduced depression and cortisol levels during the postpartum period. Their newborns were also less likely to be born prematurely and have low birth weight, and they had lower cortisol levels and performed better on the Brazelton Neonatal Behavioral Assessment habituation, orientation, and motor scales (Field, Diego, Hernandez-Reif, Deeds, & Figueiredo, 2009).

PREGNANCY CASE STUDY

Ms. Stanislow is contemplating becoming pregnant. She told her nurse that her dream is to have a healthy baby even though she is overweight, hypertensive, and has a history of infertility.

HEALTH PROMOTION CHALLENGE

Using the information in this section as well as by doing a search for updated studies at PubMed (http://www.ncbi.nlm.nih.gov/pubmed/), develop a teaching/learning program that would help for Ms. Stanislow to help her achieve her dream if she were your client.

REFERENCES

Ahn, E., Pairaudeau, N., Pairaudeau, N., Jr., Cerat, Y., Couturier, B., Fortier, A., . . . Koren, G. (2006). A randomized cross over trial of tolerability and compliance of a micronutrient supplement with low iron separated from calcium vs high iron combined with calcium in pregnant women. *BiomedCentral, 4*(6), 10.

Alwan, S. (2005, September). Use of SSRIs linked with birth defects. Annual meeting of the Teratology Society, St. Petersburg Beach, FL.

American Association for Cancer Research. (2008, April 16). Folic acid supplementation provided in utero, but not after birth, may protect offspring from colorectal cancer. *ScienceDaily*. Retrieved from http://www.sciencedaily.com/releases/2008/04/080413183000.htm

American Physiological Society. (2008, April 10). Exercise during pregnancy leads to a healthier heart in moms and babies-to-be. *ScienceDaily*. Retrieved from http://www.sciencedaily.com/releases/2008/04/080407114630.htm

Autoimmunity Research Foundation. (2008, January 27). Vitamin D deficiency study raises new questions about disease and supplements. *ScienceDaily*. Retrieved from http://www.sciencedaily.com/releases/2008/01/080125223302.htm

Bang, S. W., & Lee, S. S. (2009). The factors affecting pregnancy outcomes in the second trimester pregnant women. *Nutrition Research and Practice, 3*(2), 134–140.

Belcaro, G., Cesarone, M. R., Rohdewald, P., Ricci, A., Ippolito, E., Dugall, M., . . . Cerritelli, F. (2004). Prevention of venous thrombosis and thrombophlebitis in long-haul flights with pycnogenol. *Clinical and Applied Thrombosis/Hemostasis, 10*(4), 373–377.

Blackwell Publishing, Ltd. (2007, August 30). Hospital practices affect long-term breast-feeding success. *ScienceDaily*. Retrieved from http://www.sciencedaily.com /releases/2007/08/070828154929.htm

British Medical Journal. (2007b, July 30). Weight gain or weight loss can affect unborn baby. *ScienceDaily*. Retrieved from http://www.sciencedaily.com /releases/2007/07/070726193820.htm

British Medical Journal. (2008, January 16). Mediterranean diet in pregnancy helps ward off childhood asthma and allergy. *ScienceDaily*. Retrieved from http://www.sciencedaily .com/releases/2008/01/080115170113.htm

Brown, D. C., & Hammond, D. C. (2007). Evidence-based clinical hypnosis for obstetrics, labor and delivery, and preterm labor. *International Journal of Clinical Hypnosis, 55*(3), 355–371.

Brugha, Morrell, C. J., Slade, P., & Walters, S. J. (2010). Universal prevention of depression in women postnatally: Cluster randomized trial evidence in primary care. *Psychological Medicine, 41*(4), 739–748.

Chettle, C. C. (2008, April). Shocking high rates: Surgical site infections remain a constant threat. *Nursing Spectrum*, (FL), 24–28.

Chuntharapat, S., Petpichetchian, W., & Hatthakit, U. (2008). Yoga during pregnancy: Effects on maternal comfort, labor pain and birth outcomes. *Complementary Therapies in Clinical Practice, 14*(2), 105–115.

Corr, S. C., Li, Y., Riedel, C. U., O'Toole, P. W., Hill, C., & Gahan, C. G. M. (2007). Bacteriocin production as a mechanism for the antiinfective activity of *Lactobacillus salivarius* UCC118. *Proceedings of the National Academy of Sciences, 104*(18), 7617–7621.

Field, T., Diego, M., Hernandez-Reif, M., Deeds, O., & Figueiredo, B. (2009). Pregnancy massage reduces prematurity, low birthweight and postpartum depression. *Infant Behavior and Development, 32*(4), 454–460.

Grady, M. A., & Bloom, K. C. (2004). Pregnancy outcomes of adolescents enrolled in a Centering Pregnancy program. *Journal of Midwifery and Women's Health, 49*, 412–420.

Gurkan, O., & Arslan, H. (2008). Effect of acupressure on nausea and vomiting during pregnancy. *Complementary Therapies in Clinical Practice, 14*(1), 46–52.

Harvard School of Public Health. (2007, November 4). Diet and lifestyle changes may help prevent infertility from ovulatory disorders. *ScienceDaily*. Retrieved from http://www .sciencedaily.com/releases/2007/10/071031114319.htm

Hofmeyr, G. J., Duley, L., & Atallah, A. (2007). Dietary calcium supplementation for prevention of pre-eclampsia and related problems: A systematic review and commentary. *British Journal of Gynecology, 114*(8), 933–934.

Huiras, R. (2008, April 21). Maternal death rate increases. *Nursing Spectrum*, (Florida,) 20–21.

Hujoel, P. P., Bollen, A. M., Noonan, C. J., & del Aguila, M. A. (2004). Antepart dental radiography and infant low birth weight. *Journal of the American Medical Association, 28*(16), 1987–1993.

Hunter, L. P., Sullivan, C. A., Young, R. E., & Weber, C. E. (2007). Nausea and vomiting of pregnancy: Clinical management. *The American Journal for Nurse Practitioners, 11*(8), 57–67.

JAMA and Archives Journals. (2007, August 9). Maternal obesity prior to pregnancy associated with birth defects. *ScienceDaily*. Retrieved from http://www.sciencedaily .com/releases/2007/08/070806164539.htm

James, A., Jamison, M., Brancazio, L., & Myers, E. (2006). Venous thromboembolism during pregnancy and the postpartum period: Incidence, risk factors, and mortality. *American Journal of Obstetrics and Gynecology, 194*(5), 1311–1315.

Jevitt, C., Hernandez, I., & Groer, M. (2007). Lactation complicated by overweight and obesity: Supporting the mother and newborn. *Journal of Midwifery and Women's Health, 52*(6), 606–613.

Jocker, B. S. (2007). Vitamin D sufficiency: An approach to disease prevention. *The American Journal for Nurse Practitioners, 11*(10), 43–60.

Kaiser Permanente Division of Research. (2008, January 22). Caffeine is linked to miscarriage risk, new study shows. *ScienceDaily*. Retrieved from http://www.sciencedaily.com/releases/2008/01/080121080402.htm

Kashanian, M., & Shahali, S. (2009). Effects of acupressure at the Sanyinjiao point (SP6) on the process of active phase of labor in nulliparous women. *Journal of Maternal-Fetal and Neonatal Medicine, 15*, 1–4.

Liptak, E. (2002, September/October). Aromatherapy in childbirth: Lightening the labor. *Integrative Nursing*, 10.

McMaster University. (2007, June 20). When to turn breech babies. *ScienceDaily*. Retrieved from http://www.sciencedaily.com/releases/2007/06/070614151740.htm

Moeller, A. H., Vezeau, T. M., & Carr, K. C. (2007). Centering Pregnancy: A new program for adolescent prenatal care. *The American Journal for Nurse Practitioners, 11*(5), 48–56.

Low carb, low folate? (2007). *Clinican Reviews, 17*(2), 14.

National Healthy Mothers, Healthy Babies Coalition. (2007, October 5). Pregnant women should eat fish after all, experts urge. *ScienceDaily*. Retrieved from http://www.sciencedaily.com/releases/2007/10/071004133313.htm

Ragnar, I., Altman, D., Tyden, T., & Olsson, S. E. (2006). Comparison of the maternal experience and duration of labour in two upright delivery positions—a randomized controlled trial. *British Journal of Gynecology, 113*(2), 165–170.

Rudant, J., Menegaux, F., Leverger, G., Baruchel, A., Nelken, B., Bertrand, Y., Patte, C., . . . Clavel, J. (2007). Household exposure to pesticides and risk of childhood hematopoietic malignancies: The ESCALE Study (SFCE). *Environmental Health Perspectives, 115*(12), 1787–1793. Retrieved from http://www.ehponline.org/docs/2007/10596/abstract.html

Shamliyan, T. A., Kane, R. L., Wyman, J., & Wilt, T. J. (2008). Systematic review: Randomized, controlled trials of nonsurgical treatments for urinary incontinence in women. *Annals of Internal Medicine, 148*(6), 459–473.

Smith, C. (2010). Ginger reduces severity of nausea in early pregnancy compared with vitamin B6, and the two treatments are similarly effective for reducing number of vomiting episodes. *Evidence-Based Nursing, 13*(2), 40.

Society for Neuroscience. (2007, July 12). Mild stress in the womb may worsen risk of cerebral palsy. *ScienceDaily*. Retrieved from http://www.sciencedaily.com/releases/2007/07/070711105828.htm

Tillett, J., & Ames, D. (2010). The uses of aromatherapy in women's health. *Journal of Perinatal & Neonatal Nursing, 24*(3), 238–245.

Turner, M. C., Wigle, D. T., & Krewski, D. (2010). Residential pesticides and childhood leukemia: A systematic review and meta-analysis. *Environmental Health Perspectives, 118*(1), 33–41.

University of California, Los Angeles. (2007, August 27). Air pollution linked to premature birth in pregnant women. *ScienceDaily*. Retrieved www.sciencedaily.com/releases/2007/08/070823150343.htm

University of Nottingham. (2008, February 23). Smoking during pregnancy can put mothers and babies at risk. *ScienceDaily*. Available at http://www.sciencedaily.com /releases/2008/02/080111095354.htm

University of Pittsburgh Schools of the Health Sciences. (2007, September 11). Low vitamin D during pregnancy linked to pre-eclampsia. *ScienceDaily*. Retrieved from http://www .sciencedaily.com/releases/2007/09/070907102114.htm

University of Rochester Medical Center. (2007, July 30). Prenatal stress keeps infants, toddlers up at night, study says. *ScienceDaily*. Retrieved from http://www.sciencedaily .com/releases/2007/07/070727122926.htm

Upsala University. (2007, November 1). Overweight mothers run greater risk of having hyperactive children. *ScienceDaily*. Retrieved from http://www.sciencedaily.com /releases/2007/11/071101092754.htm

U.S. Department of Agriculture. (2007, October 9). Copper: An important nutrient for fetal brain development. *ScienceDaily*. Retrieved from http://www.sciencedaily.com /releases/2007/10/071006084704.htm

U.S. Public Health Service and the Environmental Protective Agency. (2008). Public Health implications of exposure to polychlorinate biphenyls (PCBs). Retrieved from http:// www.epa.gov/waterscience/fish/pcb99.html

Vanderbilt University. (2007, August 24). Non-stick chemicals linked to low birth weight. *ScienceDaily*. Retrieved from http://www.sciencedaily.com/releases/2007/08/ 070823171709.htm

Wellcome Trust. (2007, August 15). Eating junk food while pregnant and breastfeeding may lead to obese offspring. *ScienceDaily*. Retrieved from http://www.sciencedaily.com /releases/2007/08/070814212154.htm

Willianne, L., Nelen, D. M., Blom, H. J., Steegers, E. A. P., Heijer, M. D., Wright, J., . . . Fingles, P. (2007). Folic acid metabolism in human subjects: Potential implications for proposed mandatory folic acid fortification in the UK. *British Journal of Nutrition, 98*, 667–675.

World Health Organization. (2007). Dioxins and their effect on human health. Retrieved from http://www.who.int/mediacentre/factsheets/fs225/en/print.html

Prostate Cancer

Exercise/Movement

Exercise evidence-based practice for prostate cancer includes vigorous physical activity.

As little as 15 minutes of exercise a day can reduce overall mortality rates in patients with prostate cancer, according to findings presented at the American Association for Cancer Research Frontiers in Cancer Prevention Research Conference, December 6–9, 2009.

Mind-Set

Mind-set evidence-based practice for prostate cancer includes cognitive behavioral therapy. Espie and colleagues (2008) conducted a randomized, controlled two-center 2008 trial of cognitive behavioral therapy (CBT) versus treatment as usual (TAU). 150 participants (103 females, mean age 61 years) who had completed active therapy for cancer, reported cognitive behavioral therapy reduced their wakefulness 55 minutes per night and significantly reduced daytime fatigue compared to usual treatment, and these outcomes were sustained for 6 months after treatment.

Nutrition

Nutrition evidence-based practice for prostate cancer includes the following:

1. *Broccoli.* Eating one or more portions of broccoli every week can reduce both the risk of prostate cancer and the risk of localized cancer becoming more aggressive. Besides eating broccoli every week, the researchers suggest eating plenty of other cruciferous vegetables, including Brussels sprouts, cauliflower, cabbage, rocket, watercress, garden cress, kale, bok choy, radish, horseradish, and wasabi (Traka et al., 2010).

2. *High-fat diet.* A high-fat diet causes proliferation, inflammation, and oxidative stress that can lead to benign prostatic hyperplasia, prostatitis, and cancer of the prostate, some of the most common disorders affecting adult men (Case Western Reserve University, 2010).

3. *Polyunsaturated fats and n-6 fatty acids.* High intake of polyunsaturated fats (sunflower and safflower oil, margarine) and n-6 fatty acids (baked goods, soybean oil, canola oil) increase prostate cancer risk (Kristal et al., 2010).

Supplements

Supplement evidence-based practice for prostate cancer includes quercetin and silymarin.

1. *Quercetin.* A dietary flavonoid available in health food stores, quercetin inhibited cell proliferation and modulated the expression of genes involved in DNA repair, matrix degradation and tumor invasion, angiogenesis, apoptosis, cell cycle, metabolism, and glycolysis (Noori-Daloii et al., 2010). No cytotoxicity of quercetin on PC-3 cells was observed. Taken together, as shown by the issues of the study, the manifold inhibitory effects of quercetin on PC-3 cells may introduce quercetin as an efficacious anticancer agent in order to be used in the future nutritional transcriptomic investigations and multitarget therapy to overcome the therapeutic impediments against prostate cancer.

2. *Silymarin.* Silymarin (silibinin), at 300 mg daily, can exert anticancer effects. It also is an anti-inflammatory and can protect the liver and kidney from the negative effects of chemotherapy and radiation (Cheung, Gibbons, Johnson, & Nicol, 2010).

PROSTATE CANCER CASE STUDY

Mr. Jacobsen, age 68, has been diagnosed with prostate cancer. He has many questions about what he can do to complement his medical treatment.

HEALTH PROMOTION CHALLENGE

Based on information in this section and by doing a search at PubMed (http://www.ncbi.nlm.nih.gov/pubmed/), develop a teaching/learning program for Mr. Jacobsen.

REFERENCES

American Association for Cancer Research. (2009, December 8). Exercise reduces death rate in prostate cancer patients. *ScienceDaily*. Retrieved from http://www.sciencedaily.com/releases/2009/12/091207200911.htm

Case Western Reserve University. (2010, July 16). Mechanism for link between high fat diet and risk of prostate cancer and disorders unveiled. *ScienceDaily*. Retrieved from http://www.sciencedaily.com/releases/2010/07/100714151751.htm

Cheung, C. W., Gibbons, N., Johnson, D. W., & Nicol, D. L. (2010). Silibinin—a promising new treatment for cancer. *Anticancer Agents in Medicinal Chemistry, 10*(3), 186–195.

Espie, C. A., Fleming, L., Cassidy, J., Samuel, L., Taylor, L. M., White, C. A., et al. (2008). Randomized controlled clinical effectiveness trial of cognitive behavior therapy compared with treatment as usual for persistent insomnia in patients with cancer. *Journal of Clinical Oncology, 26*(28), 4651–4658.

Kristal, A. R., Arnold, K. B., Neuhouser, M. L., Goodman, P., Platz, E. A., Albanes, D., & Thompson, I. M. (2010). Diet, supplement use, and prostate cancer risk: Results from the prostate cancer prevention trial. *American Journal of Epidemiology, 172*(5), 566–577.

Noori-Daloii, M. R., Momeny, M., Yousefi, M., Shirazi, F. G., Yaseri, M., Motamed, N., Kazemialiakbar, N., & Hashemi, S. (2010, July 2). Multifaceted preventive effects of single agent quercetin on a human prostate adenocarcinoma cell line (PC-3): Implications for nutritional transcriptomics and multi-target therapy. *Medical Oncology, 28*(4), 1395–404.

Traka, M., Gasper, A. V., Antonietta, M., Bacon, J. R., Needs, P. W., Frost, V., et al. (2008). Broccoli consumption interacts with GSTM1 to perturb oncogenic signalling pathways in the prostate. *Plos One, 3*(7), e2568.

Stroke

Environment

Environmental evidence for stroke pertains to water, music, and a social network.

1. *Water.* Drinking water replaces lost fluids while caffeinated beverages or alcohol increase fluid output, leeching out needed liquids, minerals, and vitamins. Dehydration has been linked to stroke. Drinking at least 8 glasses a day of water is recommended (Manz, 2007). **Cautions:** Tap water and even bottled water can contain parasites, weed killers, nitrates (correlated with spontaneous miscarriage and blue-baby syndrome), *Salmonella*, *Escherichia coli*, chlorine, fluoride, and other potentially dangerous substances (Doull et al., 2006). Counsel clients to drink and cook with only distilled water or reverse-osmosis filtered water. **Other considerations:** Fluid intake is probably adequate when thirst is rarely experienced and when urine is colorless or slightly yellow. As adults age, they may experience less thirst. Counsel older adults to drink water before thirst sets in because by that time, dehydration may already have taken over.

2. *Music.* In recovery from a stroke, members of a daily music listening group improved verbal memory by 60% (as compared to 18% in audio book listeners and 29% in nonlisteners), improved their ability to control and perform mental operations and resolve conflicts among responses improved by 17% (as compared to zero for the other two groups), and experienced fewer depressed and confused moods than the control group who received care as usual. Members of the music listening group chose their own music. Suggest clients choose music with lyrics. Research suggests it is the combination of music and voice that plays a crucial role in improved recovery (University of Helsinki, 2008). **Other considerations:** Other ways listening to music can help with stroke recovery include enhanced arousal (alertness), attention, and mood, mediated by a dopaminergic mesocorticolimbic system that gives feelings of reward, pleasure, and arousal; directly stimulating damaged areas of the brain; and stimulating general areas of brain plasticity and helping the brain to repair itself (University of Helsinki).

3. *Social network.* Having many friends and family appears to be associated with a dramatically lower risk of suffering a stroke.
   a. **Routes/dosages/frequency:** This can be an intense relationship with one or two other close friends or significant others and can be developed in church groups, work groups, or recreational groups.
   b. **Cautions:** Encourage clients to think of disease as more than a physical condition.
   c. **Assessments:** Assess psychological and environmental characteristics that make clients more prone to be socially isolated.

Encourage clients to spend time developing friends and a social network as a way of preventing or recovering from a stroke. **Other considerations:** Some theories include the idea that socioeconomic factors, such as being socially isolated, feed into worse health outcomes. Clients who cannot afford a bus pass and are relatively tied to their home cannot go out to lunch with friends for financial reasons and can become more socially isolated. This can lead to not having friends check on them or be available to bring them for care when their health fails (Lui, Ross, & Thompson, 2005).

Exercise/Movement

Exercise evidence-based practice for stroke concerns physical activity and occupational therapy.

1. *Physical activity.* A high level of daily leisure time physical activity (20–30 minutes) reduces the risk of all subtypes of stroke (Goldstein, 2010). Daily active commuting also reduces the risk of ischemic stroke (Hu et al., 2006). For more information on counseling clients on exercise, go to http://exercise.lifetips.com

2. *Occupational therapy.* In nine randomized trials, occupational therapy reduced poststroke deterioration in eating, dressing, bathing, toileting, and moving about in social activities more than usual care did (Alper, 2008). Assess need for occupational therapy poststroke and refer as needed. For more information about occupational therapy, go to http://stroke.about.com/b/2006/10/26/occupational-therapy-in-stroke-rehabilitation.htm

Herbs/Essential Oils

Herbal evidence-based practice for stroke includes garlic.

Aged garlic extract (three-quarters of a teaspoon daily) or 1–3 cloves of garlic exerts inhibition on platelet aggregation and adhesion that may be important in the development of stroke (Atif, Yousuf, & Agrawal, 2009). **Cautions:** Advise clients to avoid concurrent use with anticoagulants. Garlic extract should not be used during pregnancy or lactation, but dietary amounts are acceptable. Aged garlic extract should not be used by clients with stomach inflammation or hypersensitivity to this herb.

Nutrition

Nutrition evidence-based practice for stroke concerns the following:

1. *DASH diet.* Greater daily intake of fruits, vegetables, whole grains, nuts, and legumes is associated with a lower risk for stroke, while a greater

intake of red and processed meats, sweetened beverages, and sodium is associated with increased risk for stroke (JAMA and Archives Journals, 2008). Counsel clients to reduce or eliminate intake of red and processed meats, sweetened beverages, and sodium to reduce risk for stroke. For diet-changing ideas to share with clients, go to http://nutrition.about .com/od/changeyourdiet/Diet.htm

2. *Flavonoids and quercetin.* Eating foods high in flavonoids daily, especially fruits and vegetables, and quercetin-rich foods (especially apples, berries, and onions) is associated with decreased risk of stroke (Edwards et al., 2007; Mursu, Voutilainen, Tuomainen, Kurl, & Salonen, 2008). For a list of foods high in flavonoids, go to http://www.nal.usda.gov /fnic/foodcomp/Data/Flav/flav.pdf

3. *Overweight/obesity.* Overweight/obesity is linked to stroke increase among middle-aged women. The women in the NHANES nutritional survey were significantly more obese than women a decade prior, with an average BMI of 28.67 kg/m^2 versus 27.11 kg/m^2 the decade prior. (A BMI of 25 to 30 is considered overweight; 30.1 or more is considered obese) (American Heart Association, 2008). **Cautions:** The more overweight a client, the greater the risk for stroke. For information on helping clients lose weight, go to http://weightloss.about.com /library/100tips/bltip6.htm

4. *Green or black tea.* The more tea consumed, the better the odds of staving off a stroke. In one study, by drinking 3 cups of tea a day, the risk of a stroke was reduced by 21%. It did not matter if it was green or black tea (University of California, Los Angeles, 2009). **Considerations:** There are very few known ways to reduce the risk of stroke. Developing medications for stroke victims is particularly challenging, given that the drug has to get to the stroke-damaged site quickly because damage occurs so fast. Arab said that by the time a stroke victim gets medical care, it is nearly too late to impede the damage. **Cautions:** Caffeinated tea should be avoided by clients with hypersensitivity to tea or by those with kidney inflammation, gastrointestinal ulcers, insomnia, cardiovascular disease, or increased intraocular pressure. High doses of caffeinated tea can result in palpitations and irregular heartbeat, anxiety, nervousness, insomnia, nausea, heartburn, and increased stomach acid. The decaffeinated form may be a better choice for these reasons. Antacids may decrease the therapeutic effects of green tea, and green tea may interact with anticoagulants/antiplatelets, increasing risk of bleeding. Counsel clients to avoid drinking green tea while taking MAOIs or bronchodilators (Kuriyama et al., 2006).

5. *Salt.* Reduction of salt intake (by not ingesting salty foods or adding salt to meals) in women over 65 years of age can help prevent stroke

(Cook et al., 2007). For more information about salt intake, Go to http://dietbites.com/Sodium-In-Foods/index.html

6. *Soybean lecithin.* Soybean lecithin (10 g capsules t.i.d.) is more effective in treatment of acute cerebral infarction compared to usual treatment (Shi, Zhou, & Meng, 2001).

7. *Vitamin C.* The level of vitamin C may serve as a biological marker of lifestyle or other factors associated with reduced stroke risk. Eating plenty of fruits and vegetables high in vitamin C is associated with lower prevalence of stroke (Myint et al., 2008). **Caution:** Insufficient intake of vitamin C may lead to stroke. Foods rich in vitamin C include guava, red bell pepper, papaya, orange juice, oranges, broccoli, green bell pepper, kohlrabi, strawberries, and grapefruit. For more foods and ways to preserve vitamin C in meal production, go to http://ohioline.osu.edu/hyg-fact/5000/5552.html

Stress Management

Stress management evidence-based practice for stroke concerns faith.

Emotional distress is common in the aftermath of stroke and can impact negatively on the outcome. The strength of religious beliefs influences the ability to cope after a stroke event, with stronger religious beliefs acting as a possible protective factor against emotional distress (Giaquinto, Spiridigliozzi, & Caracciolo, 2007). Provide needed support.

Touch

Touch evidence-based practice for stroke includes aromatherapy acupressure.

Aromatherapy acupressure for 20 minutes, twice a day, using lavender, rosemary, and peppermint essential oils exerts more positive effects on hemiplegic shoulder pain, compared to acupressure alone, in women who have undergone stroke (Shin & Lee, 2007).

STROKE CASE STUDY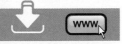

Mr. Andrews's father, uncle, and grandfather died of strokes. He wants to take any actions he can to prevent dying from a stroke himself.

HEALTH PROMOTION CHALLENGE

Develop a stroke prevention teaching/learning program for Mr. Andrews.

REFERENCES

Alper, B. S. (2008, April). Evidence-based medicine: Occupational therapy reduces post-stroke deterioration in ADLs. *The Clinical Advisor*, 129–130.

American Heart Association. (2008, February 22). Obesity linked to stroke increase among middle-aged women. *ScienceDaily*. Retrieved from http://www.sciencedaily.com/releases/2008/02/080221080606.htm

Atif, F., Yousuf, S., & Agrawal, S. K. (2009). S-allyl L-cysteine diminishes cerebral ischemia-induced mitochondrial dysfunctions in hippocampus. *Brain Research, 1265*, 128–137.

Cook, N. R., Cutler, J. A., Obarzanek, E., Buring, J. E., Rexrode, K. M., Kumanyika, S., . . . Whelton, P. K. (2007). Long term effects of dietary sodium reduction on cardiovascular disease outcomes: Observational follow-up of the trials of hypertension prevention. *British Medical Journal, 334*(7599), 855.

Doull, J., Boekelheide, K., Farishian, B. G., Isaacson, R. L., Klotz, J. B., & Limeback, H. (2006). *Committee on Fluoride in Drinking Water Board on Environmental Studies & Toxicology, Division of Earth & Life Sciences*, a scientific review of EPA's Standards. Washington, DC: The National Academies Press; 2006. Available for purchase online at: http://www.nap.edu

Edwards, R. L., Lyon, T., Litwin, S. E., Rabovsky, A., Symons, J. D., & Jalili, T. (2007). Quercetin reduces blood pressure in hypertensive subjects. *The Journal of Nutrition, 137*(11), 2405–2411.

Giaquinto, S., Spiridigliozzi, C., & Caracciolo, B. (2007). Can faith protect from emotional distress after stroke? *Stroke, 38*(3), 993–997.

Goldstein, L. B. (2010). Physical activity and the risk of stroke. *Expert Review of Neurotherapeutics, 10*(8), 1263–1265.

Hu, G., Sarti, C., Jousilahti, P., Silventoinen, K., Barengo, N. C., & Tuomilehto, J. (2005). Leisure time, occupational, and commuting physical activity and the risk of stroke. *Stroke, 36*(9), 1994–1999.

JAMA and Archives Journals. (2008, April 15). Blood pressure-lowering diet also may be associated with lower risk for heart disease, stroke. *ScienceDaily*. Retrieved from http://www.sciencedaily.com/releases/2008/04/080414161540.htm

Kuriyama, S., Shimazu, T., Ohmori, K., Kikuchi, N., Nakaya, N., Nishino, Y., & Tsuji, I. (2006). Green tea consumption and mortality due to cardiovascular disease, cancer, and all causes in Japan: The Ohsaki study. *Journal of the American Medical Association, 296*(10), 1255–1265.

Lui, M. H., Ross, F. M., & Thompson, D. R. (2005). Supporting family caregivers in stroke care: a review of the evidence for problem solving. *Stroke, 36*(11), 2514–2522.

Manz, F. (2007). Hydration and disease. *Journal of American College of Nutrition, 26*(5 Suppl), 535S–541S.

Mursu, J., Voutilainen, S., Tuomainen, T. P., Kurl, S., & Salonen, J. T. (2008). Flavonoid intake and the risk of ischaemic stroke and CVD mortality in middle-aged Finnish men: The Kuopio Ischaemic Heart Disease Risk Factor study. *British Journal of Nutrition, 1*, 1–6.

Myint, P. K., Luben, R. N., Welch, A. A., Bingham, S. A., Wareham, N. J., & Khaw, K. T. (2008). Plasma vitamin C concentrations predict risk of incident stroke over 10 years in 20 649 participants of the European Prospective Investigation in Cancer Norfolk prospective population study. *American Journal of Clinical Nutrition, 87*(1), 64–69.

Shi, F., Zhou, J., & Meng, D. (2001). Curative effect of soybean lecithin on cerebral infarction. *Zhonghua Yi Xue Za Zhi, 81*(21), 1301–1313.

Shin, B. C., & Lee, M. S. (2007). Effects of aromatherapy acupressure on hemiplegic shoulder pain and motor power in stroke patients: A pilot study. *Journal of Alternative and Complementary Medicine, 13*(2), 347–351.

University of California–Los Angeles. (2009, March 4). Green, black tea can reduce stroke risk, research suggests. *ScienceDaily.* Retrieved from http://www.sciencedaily.com/releases/2009/02/090223091806.htm

University of Helsinki. (2008, February 21). Listening to music improves stroke patients' recovery, study shows. *ScienceDaily.* Retrieved from http://www.sciencedaily.com/releases/2008/02/080219203554.htm

http://go.jblearning.com/healthpromotion (www)

For a full suite of assignments and learning activities, use the access code located in the front of your book to visit the exclusive website: http://go.jblearning.com/healthpromotion If you do not have an access code, you can obtain one at the site.

GLOSSARY

Acknowledging: an assertive response to criticism.

Active listening: paraphrasing back to the speaker what was heard.

Acupressure: a variant of an ancient art that uses the fingers to press key points on the surface of the skin to stimulate the body's natural self-curative abilities. When these points are pressed, they release muscular tension, promote the circulation of blood, and aid healing.

Acupuncture: complementary and alternative treatment in which a fine steel or copper needle is inserted into various points of the body that are selected in accordance to the *meridian*, or energy channel, most strongly associated with the patient's complaint or symptoms.

Acute disease: disease with a sudden onset; specific signs and symptoms that can be traced back to a disease process; lasts a short period of time and will end with recovery or death.

Adaptability: ability to change as situations change.

Adaptive dimension: one of Smith's dimensions of health the ability to adapt positively to social, mental, and physiological change, while illness demonstates, would mean a failure to adapt.

Affirmation: a positive thought one consciously chooses to immerse oneself in; a thought consciously chosen to produce a desired result.

Aggression: in communication, this can mean one of two things: (1) communicating in a manner that directs overt hostility, anger, or other negative feelings toward other parties; or (2) communicating in a manner intended to promote similar feelings in other parties.

Aggressiveness: interaction that has an element of control or manipulation. An aggressive interaction is one in which one party seeks to exert power or control over another.

Aromatherapy: the use of essential oils, via massage or inhalation, to improve health.

Assertiveness: the ability to clearly and willingly express thoughts, feelings, or desires in a respectful and cordial manner. Assertiveness means being able to define and stand up for reasonable rights, while being respectful of others' rights; setting goals for wellness; acting on these goals by following through consistently; and taking responsibility for the consequences of actions.

Avoidance: in the context of communication, taking steps to prevent a message from being delivered, either by impeding the messenger from transmitting it, or more commonly, simply refusing to receive it.

Awareness program: a health promotion program that typically uses newsletters, health fairs, posters, and screening to increase client interest. Awareness programs seek to educate a community about a health issue so that individuals will begin to consider their own behaviors or circumstances.

Ayurveda: a type of medicine developed in India thousands of years ago and continues to be practiced there today. The underlying goal of Ayurveda is to integrate body, mind, and spirit to promote wellness. It means "life science"; the name combines the Sanskrit words *ayur* (life) and *veda* (science).

Behavior change program: health promotion program that teaches skills, requires a supportive environment, and usually continues for 8–12 weeks to improve health.

Bio-psycho-social-spiritual model: disease, pain, wellness, and health may be the result of an interaction between biological, psychological, social, and spiritual dimensions.

Blamer: informal family role; a dictator who knows it all, thus finding fault.

Boundaries: invisible crossing points where one individual encounters another. In the physical sense, this is also sometimes referred to as "personal space," but boundaries are most commonly envisioned in nonphysical terms.

Bystander: informal family role; one who stands along the sideline with little involvement.

Caregiver: anyone who is providing help and treatment to someone who is in need of care.

Caretaker: informal family role; one who is called on the most for help and assistance; may also be called nurturer.

Centering: finding within oneself an inner reference of stability, a sense of self-relatedness that can be thought of as a place of inner being and a place of quietude within oneself where one can feel truly integrated, unified, and focused.

Chronic conditions: irreversible processes that require supportive care and self-care for continued function and prevention of further disability; continues indefinitely; becomes part of one's identity.

Chronic disease self-management model: a program developed by Dr. Kate Lorig for patients with chronic diseases; it incorporates modeling and social strategies that enhance self-efficacy, guided mastery of skills with action plans and feedback, modeling of self-management behaviors and problem-solving strategies, reinterpretation of symptoms, social persuasion through group support, and guidance. Program evaluation includes the areas of health status, health behaviors, perceived self-efficacy, and health services utilization.

Clark wellness model: this model examines nurse–client interactions from a wellness perspective and combines elements of systems theory. In this model, both nurse and client are complete systems that interact within themselves (that is, each has inputs, throughputs—activities within the system—and outputs), and interact with each other (intersystems) across interfaces to achieve jointly planned and achieved goals and feelings of well-being. The nurse's wellness is an important facet of this theory, and each nurse serves as a wellness role model for the client to emulate.

Client: implies an interactive consumer with free will and the ability to make choices about care.

Clinical dimension: one of Smith's dimensions of health; the absence of disease signs and symptoms indicates health, while illness is the extreme opposite, with obvious identifiable evidence of disease through specific signs and symptoms.

Clouding: a useful technique when one receives nonconstructive, manipulative criticism that one disagrees with. One states agreement with part of the statement but does not agree to change his or her position on the part with which one disagrees.

Community opinion survey: action that helps determine what are perceived to be the major community health problems. The procedure includes interviews with identified community leaders. The interviews are tools for analyzing the community and identifying community leaders and are among the first steps in the community organization process.

Concept: a general idea derived or inferred from specific instances or occurrences.

Conceptual model: includes a set of concepts, with propositions that describe them, expresses the relationship between them, or set forth the basic assumptions of the model.

Contracting: a written agreement between the nurse and client that sets down an agreed-upon way to achieve a health goal.

Coordinator: informal family role; one who is the planner and organizer of family activities.

Coping skills: actions taken to become healthy or well.

Correlation research: an investigation of the relationship between the study variables.

Cultural competence: identifying cultural differences between the nurse and the client, and maintaining an attitude of flexibility when dealing with a situation in which the client's norms differ from the nurse's.

Data analysis: the technique that organizes and gives meaning to data through the use of statistics.

Data collection: the gathering of information/data.

Dependent variable: the outcome or response that the researcher wants to explain.

Descriptive research: the exploration and description of a phenomenon in a real-life situation depicting accurate accounts of the characteristics of the participants, situations, or even the group as a whole.

Determinants of health: a range of factors, which include social, economic, and environmental categories.

Differentiation: the extent to which people intellectually distinguish themselves and their own needs from others in their emotional relationship system.

Disease: a condition that relates to a specific pathophysiologic process.

Disease prevention: the avoidance of illness and agents of illness, plus the identification of risks.

Dominator: informal family role; one who manipulates the family to be the primary authoritarian.

Dosha: one of three life forces in Ayurveda whose balance is unique in every person. The *doshas* are *vata*, *pitta*, and *kapha*, which have particular properties and relationships to specific bodily functions.

Double bind: receiving contradictory injunctions or emotional messages on different levels of communication.

Ecomap: a type of drawing useful in family health promotion; used to provide a visual overview of how the family interacts with different systems in the environment, such as work, church, school, etc.

Emotional cut-off: a concept developed by Murray Bowen that refers to the mechanisms people use to reduce anxiety from their unresolved emotional issues with parents, siblings, and other members of their family of origin. To avoid sensitive issues, they either move away from their families and rarely go home; if they remain in physical contact with their families, to avoid sensitive issues, they use silence or divert the conversation.

Though cutoff may diminish their immediate anxiety, these unresolved problems contaminate other relationships, especially when those relationships are stressed.

Emotional subtext: information about how a messenger is feeling.

Empathy: includes the ability to listen actively and to reflect back the essence of the client's communication that results in the client feeling understood and supported.

Encourager: informal family role; one who motivates others by making them feel important.

Ethnographic research: the collection and analysis of data specifically from a cultural behavior to develop theory.

Eudaimonistic dimension: one of Smith's dimensions of health; health is the positive interaction among the physical, social, psychological, and spiritual aspects of the environment, while illness is a lack of involvement or apathy/wasting away with life.

Evaluation: an integral part of the entire process of developing community-based health promotion programs. It is important to determine the extent to which proposed activities have been carried out (process evaluation) and the actual effectiveness of the program (i.e., what impact the program has had on the community's health risks).

Evidence-based research: provides valid results for effective strategies and stimulates decisions and actions.

Expanded health belief model: a later form of the health belief model that incorporates the assumptions that one has the desire to avoid illness or get well and that one believes a specific health action would prevent illness; the expanded model includes self-efficacy.

Experiment: highly controlled study; has the purpose of predicting and controlling a phenomenon between independent and dependent variables.

Family: two or more individuals who depend on one another for emotional, physical, and economic support (Hanson, 2001).

Family composition: sum of the individuals within a family.

Family health promotion model: developed from Pender's original health promotion model; in this versions, it is hypothesized that there are three broad influences on a family's behavioral outcome of health-promoting behaviors: general, health-related, and behavior-specific.

Family theory: extrapolated from systems theory; contains at least eight assumptions.

Follower: informal family role; one who passively accepts family decisions.

Functional limitations: any condition or situation that impedes activities of daily living.

Genetics Information Nondiscrimination Act (GINA): passed in 2008, this Act protects Americans from discrimination based on information found on genetic tests, forbids insurance companies from discriminating through such things as reduced coverage or pricing, and prohibits employers from making adverse employment decisions based on a person's genetic code.

Genogram: a visual diagram of family structure, with symbolic representation of family composition, health history, and relationships with other members.

Genome: the organism's complete set of DNA.

Goals: a broad, long-range aims that define a desired result associated with identified strategic issues.

Grand theories: explain a broad scope of happenings.

Grounded theory: inductive approach that has been developed from sociology, specifically the symbolic interaction theory; it involves formulation, testing, and redevelopment of propositions until a theory is developed.

Guided imagery: a process that involves the use of symbols to imagine the changes that the individual desires taking place. Clients are encouraged to relax and imagine a journey to relaxation and healing.

Harmonizer: informal family role; one who tries to keep peace within the family by acting as mediator.

Health: a condition of well-being, free of disease or infirmity, and a basic human right (World Health Organization [WHO], 2012). Health is the absence of disease plus physical, mental, and social well-being.

Health belief model: a value expectancy theory, incorporating the assumptions that one has the desire to avoid illness or get well (value) and a belief that a specific health action to that person would prevent illness (expectancy); originally developed in the 1950s to aid in explaining the widespread failure of people to participate in health promotion/prevention programs.

Health disparities: adverse effects on groups of people who have significantly greater obstacles to health than the general population.

Health education model: explains how educating clients can induce change in behavior.

Health policy: a decision made to direct the actions of individuals by health promotion.

Health promotion: a process of enabling people to increase control over their health and its determinants and thereby improve their health (WHO, 2012). Health promotion activities encourage well-being, quality of life, and the avoidance of illness for individuals, families, and communities; included under the concept of health promotion are health education, health protection, and disease prevention.

Health promotion model: developed by Nola Pender, the health promotion model contains 7 assumptions that reflect nursing and behavioral science perspectives, and 14 statements/propositions that provide a basis for investigative work on health behaviors.

Health-related quality of life: a life situation that includes health and physical function, emotional well-being, general health perceptions, and role and social function.

Healthy family: a family that has traits that are a combination of unity, flexibility, and communication.

Healthy People: an agenda of prevention for the United States; a tool that identifies what has been found to be the most significant preventable health threats.

Hidden agendas: goals that are not shared by a group but are still acted upon by individuals of the group.

High-level wellness: maximizing one's potential, having direction and purpose in life, meeting the challenges of the environment, looking beyond the needs of self to the needs of society, and doing it all with joy or a zest for life (Dunn, 1961).

Historical research: an analysis or narrative of specific events that have already occurred or are retrospective.

Hypnosis: a wakeful state of deep relaxation that includes an increase in the ability to focus on a particular situation. Under hypnosis, people are more open to suggestion.

Hypothesis: a testable prediction about the relationship between at least two events, characteristics, or variables.

Illness: the experience of symptoms and suffering and how an individual lives with and responds to these symptoms.

Independent variable: what the researcher is manipulating.

Interventions: planned efforts to produce change in a population.

Lifestyle change program: a health promotion program that changes not one, but multiple behaviors so that overall lifestyle is altered toward health.

Literature review: the process of compiling all known studies on a particular topic to become acquainted with the current extent of knowledge about said topic.

Mantra: a thought or word one focuses on in transcendental meditation until attention transcends its common meaning. As a result of this focus, subtler meanings of thought are perceived.

Martyr: an informal family role; one who sacrifices everything for the sake of the family.

Medicare Act: *see* Social Security Act Amendments.

Meditation: a self-directed practice that is used to relax the body and calm the mind; during that time, the body's internal mechanisms repair the body, providing physiological benefits.

Mental health: "a state of successful mental functioning, resulting in productive activities, fulfilling relationships, and the ability to adapt to change and cope with adversity" (WHO, 2020).

Mental health promotion: intervention to improve the coping skills of the individual, instead of eliminating symptoms and deficits as in the medical model.

Midrange theories: a set of related ideas focused on a limited dimension of reality.

Mindfulness meditation: an intentional and self-regulated focusing of attention, whose purpose is to relax and calm the mind and body.

Mirror practice: technique for enhancing assertiveness that gives feedback about facial expression, posture, and whether words fit with gestures and body position. It can also be helpful in rehearsing assertive statements prior to trying them with a real-life person. This kind of rehearsal can build confidence so that assertiveness in the real-life situation is more likely.

Model: a schematic description of a system, theory, or phenomenon that accounts for its known or inferred properties and may be used for further study of its characteristics.

Motivational interviewing: focuses on exploring and resolving ambivalence and centering on processes that facilitate change.

Music therapy: the use of music to stimulate, relax, and/or heal.

Nursing Workforce Development programs: part of the Patient Protection and Affordable Care Act, the goals of recruiting new nurses into the profession, promoting career advancement within nursing, and improving patient care delivery.

Objective evidence: an evaluation that includes such things as activity reports, surveys, changes in scores, and measurable changes in health (e.g., decreases in smoking rates or cholesterol levels).

Objectives: results of specific activities or outcomes to be achieved over a stated period of time and are specific, measurable, and realistic statements.

Opposer: informal family role; one who is negative to family ideas and suggestions.

Orem self-care model: describes the role of the nurse in helping a person experiencing inabilities in self-care, including universal care, which consists of self-care to meet physiologic and psychosocial needs; developmental care, the self-care required when one goes through developmental stages; and health deviation care, the self-care required when one has a deviation from a healthy status.

Outcome: the impact a health promotion program has had on the community's health risks.

Outcome evaluation: type of evaluation that measures consequences attributable to health promotion program activities and can show whether you are attaining your program objectives.

Passive aggression: expressing hostility or anger through passivity or silence—such as sullenly refusing to acknowledge a speaker or failing to do something one has agreed to do—as a way of annoying others.

Patient Protection and Affordable Care Act: healthcare reform passed in 2010, its major provisions include no insurance discrimination based on employee's wages; insurance rating variability on age, family composition, geographic location, and tobacco use, but not on health or gender; Medicaid to all individuals under age 65 at 133% of the federal poverty level; programs to support school-based health centers and nurse-managed health centers; benefits packages that provide a comprehensive set of basic services and mental health services; and support of training programs focusing on primary care models.

Phenomenological research: captures the lived experience of the participant; the research is inductive in nature.

Prana: the cosmic vibratory energy of the universe that is believed to connect an individual to a transcendental existence during which slow, rhythmic, nasal and abdominal breathing prevail.

PRECEDE-PROCEED framework: developed by Green and Kreuter in 2005, it is a systematic planning process with the primary goal of empowering individuals and communities to understand and engage in efforts to improve the quality of their lives. The two propositions of the model are that (1) health and health risks have multiple determinants, and (2) efforts to change the behavioral, physical, and social environment must be multidisciplinary and participatory.

Pretesting: the process of measuring the effectiveness of the tool. It will help identify problems with wording, interpretation, or information gaps.

Primary prevention: a set of actions that prevent a specific disease or condition.

Priorities: alternatives ranked according to feasibility, value, and/or importance.

Probing: an assertive response to criticism that is effective in determining whether the criticism is constructive or manipulative and clarifies unclear comments.

Problem: in research, a problem is the area of focus where there is a gap that will lead to the purpose or the goal or aim of the study.

Qigong: life-energy work. A powerful practice that cleanses and balances the body through a combination of movement, visualization, and specialized breathing.

Qualitative research: subjective research; examines the experience of the participants; describes the meaning related to an event.

Quality of life: general well-being as assessed by either the client or someone else various multidimensional tools and scales have been developed to assess socioeconomic, demographic, and life-style factors; personality characteristics; social and community environments; and well-being in physical and mental health.

Quantitative research: a formal and rigorous process for objectively generating information; or, to describe, explore, and/or examine new situations, events, or concepts.

Quasiexperimental research: not an experimental study as it lacks control by the researcher; there is no manipulation of treatment, setting management, or subject selection.

Reflexology: a physical stimulation therapy that is based on the premise that body organs have corresponding reflex points on other parts of the body. The reflex points are believed to be up to 20 times more sensitive than the corresponding organs. Reflex points also influence functional relationships to their corresponding organs.

Refuting irrational ideas: communication skill in which one identifies irrational ideas and associated emotions, selects one irrational idea to refute, and substitutes alternative self-talk.

Relaxation procedures: ways to relax the body, which leads to relaxation of the mind, and can reduce future cardiac events and enhance body processes.

Research design: the architectural blueprint for the study.

Resource inventory: an analysis that identifies what resources exist in the community to meet health needs. The procedure includes interviews with identified community leaders. These interviews are tools for analyzing the community and identifying community leaders and are among the first steps in the community organization process.

Rheumatoid arthritis: a chronic condition characterized by inflammation of the joint synovium.

Role ambiguity: a vague and insufficiently defined role causing the individual to have disharmony within.

Role conflict: inconsistent expectations in the role set, usually caused by incompatible interaction by two or more roles yielding unmet demands.

Role incongruity: similar to role conflict with incompatibility, but discrepancy is evident between the role and the person who holds it.

Role overload: inability to meet the role obligations or failing to meet them in a specified time.

Role-performance dimension: one of Smith's dimensions of health. In it, health is defined as the ability of the person to perform social roles, including work and family, based on societal expectations; illness is the inability to perform roles at this level of expectation.

Role strain: "the difficulty felt in fulfilling role obligations" (Goode, 1960, p. 483)

Role stress: the result of when environmental demands exceed an individual's natural regulatory capacity.

Sample: the part of the population being studied; those who become study participants.

Scapegoat: informal family role; the one who is blamed for problems.

Secondary prevention: the identification and treatment of asymptomatic persons who have developed risk factors or are at a preclinical state for an illness.

Self-determination theory: concerned with supporting our natural or intrinsic tendencies to behave in effective and healthy ways.

Self-efficacy: a concept proposed by Bandura in 1977; the conviction by an individual that he or she is able to successfully execute a behavior needed for producing a desired outcome.

Self-esteem: a confidence and satisfaction in oneself.

Self-evaluation: evaluating one's own performance.

Self-talk: the internal language we use to describe and interpret the world. When self-talk is accurate and realistic, health and wellness are enhanced. When self-talk is irrational and untrue, stress and emotional distress occur.

Shaping techniques: technique in which nurses act as sculptors, helping clients to approximate the behavior that will be successful for them.

Shiatsu: *see* Acupressure.

Social Security Act Amendments: a supplementary medical insurance program passed in 1965 that resulted in hospital and outpatient insurance for persons aged 65 and older. Also called the Medicare Act.

Socioecologic approach: provides a theoretical framework to analyze various contexts and focuses on the study of people in an environment and their influences on one another.

Spin-off effects: secondary benefits related to the principal benefits sought by participants in a program.

Supportive environment program: health promotion program that aims to alter aspects of community life to help maintain a long-term, sustained, healthy lifestyle.

Systems theory: originally described by Bertalanffy in 1950, assumptions of the model include: a system is composed of a set of elements that interact with each other; each system is a unique entity from the environment; an open system exchanges matter and energy with the environment, while a closed system does not and causes isolation from the environment; and systems depend on both positive and negative feedback to maintain homeostasis.

T'ai chi (pronounced "tye chee"): a mind–body movement therapy that draws from martial arts as well as qigong. It is sometimes called moving meditation because practitioners focus their attention and intention on the movements of the practice while breathing deeply. Also called t'ai chi chuan.

Tertiary prevention: the treatment and management of the client's clinical and chronic condition, restoring the person to optimum function for maintenance of life skills.

Theory: a coherent group of tested general propositions, commonly regarded as correct, that can be used as principles of explanation and prediction for a class of phenomena.

Theory of reasoned action: posits that individual behavior is driven by behavioral intentions that are a function of an individual's attitude toward the action and what other people important to the individual think of that action.

Thought stopping: used to control unwanted or useless thoughts by silently shouting STOP in one's head or using a negative reinforcer, such as snapping a rubber band on the wrist or finger, to end the thought.

Transcendental meditation: a technique of meditation derived from Hindu traditions that promotes deep relaxation through the use of a mantra or special word.

Triangulation: a situation in which two people who are involved in a relationship of emotional significance experience anxiety or stress building up between them, and to alleviate this stress, one or both of the individuals calls upon another person, issue, or object to intervene or disrupt the conflict and thereby decrease discomfort.

Value clarification: communication enhancement technique that can assist nurses and clients to develop larger portions of solid self and thus become more differentiated and open to health promotion actions.

Value expectancy theory: a theory that incorporates the assumptions that one has the desire to avoid illness or get well (value) and a belief that a specific health action to that person would prevent illness (expectancy).

Variables: include independent (the one the researcher manipulates), dependent (changes as a result of changing the independent variable), and controlled variables (kept constant).

Visualization: *see* guided imagery.

Wellness: *see* high level wellness.

Yoga: a mind/body movement modality that is not only a set of physical exercises, but an inner spiritual experience as well. Yoga incorporates specific postures and breathing techniques to strengthen the body and relax the mind. The practice of yoga is devoted to balance.

REFERENCES

Dunn, H. (1961). *High Level Wellness.* Arlington, VA: Beatty Press.

Goode, D. (1960). A theory of role strain. *American Sociological Review, 25*, 483–496.

Hanson, S. (2001). *Family health care nursing: Theory, practice, and research* (2nd ed.). Philadelphia, PA: FA Davis.

Healthy People 2020. Retrieved from http://www.healthypeople.gov/2020/default.aspx

NIH/NCCAM. (n.d.). *What is complementary and alternative medicine?* Bethesda, MD: National Institutes of Health. Retrieved from http://nccam.nih.gov/health/whatiscam/

World Health Organization [WHO]. (2012). Retrieved from http://www.who.int/en/

INDEX

Blamer role, 245

Blended families, 236, 237

Blocking body messages, 365

Blood disorders and safety, 158–159

Body image, 16

Body Mass Index (BMI), 461, 462

Body Message Theory, 363, 364–365, 366f, 367

Boryc, K., 337

Boundaries, 88–89

Bowen, Murray, 84, 85

Bow pose, 401

Brandt E., 423

Brazil, educational initiatives in, 312

Breast cancer
    environmental factors and, 167
    exercise and, 299
    genomics and, 278
    mammograms and, 272
    obesity and, 457
    physical health promotion for, 159
    substance abuse and, 455, 456

Breastfeeding, 319, 355, 458

Broken record approach, 110–111

Bullying, 212

Buy-in to health policies, 278

Bystander role, 245

C

Calgary family intervention model, 251

California health policies, 267–268

Canada, health promotion programs in, 427

Cancer. *See also specific types of cancer*
    aromatherapy and, 357, 358
    children and, 318
    exercise and, 299, 457
    food and nutrition and, 457–458
    genomics and, 278
    imagery and, 376
    locus of control and, 130
    mammograms and, 272

obesity and, 456, 457

oral health and, 179

physical health promotion for, 159–160

prevention of, 22, 159, 299, 456–458

risk factors, 277

substance abuse and, 455, 456

tobacco use and, 455, 456

treatment decision making (TDM), 318

Cardiovascular disease. *See* Heart conditions

Caretaker role, 245, 383

Car seats for children, 275–277

Cat stretch, 403

Center for Advanced Research in Phenomenology, 316

Centering/centering prayer, 104–105, 382

Centers for Disease Control and Prevention (CDC)
    on blood disorders and safety, 158–159
    on chronic conditions, 452, 454
    cover-your-cough campaign, 297f, 298
    goals and objectives, 290
    health policies, 270
    HIV/AIDS counseling, 54
    on mental health promotion, 220, 223
    obesity prevention, 434
    on quality of life, 463

Cervical cancer, 159, 455

Chi, 350

Children and adolescents
    aromatherapy and, 359
    bicycle helmets and, 279–281
    cancer and, 318
    car seats, 275–277
    diabetes and, 267–268, 278, 315
    exercise and, 47, 48, 158
    food and nutrition, 47, 157–158
    gynecologists' interactions with, 120

PHOTO CREDITS

Unless otherwise indicated, photographs and art are under copyright of Jones & Bartlett Learning.

Part and chapter openers © Myper/ShutterStock, Inc.

☐ Chapter 1

Page 15 © Monkey Business Images /ShutterStock, Inc.; **Page 18** © iStockphoto .com/kali9; **Page 19** © Phaitoon Sutunyawatchai/ShutterStock, Inc.

☐ Chapter 2

Page 47 © Cathy Yeulet/123RF; **Page 51** © oliveromg/ShutterStock, Inc.

☐ Chapter 3

Page 95 © iStockphoto.com/asiseeit; **Page 105** © iStockphoto.com/Bronwyn8; **Page 123** © Hasloo Group Production Studio /ShutterStock, Inc.

☐ Chapter 4

Page 163 © iStockphoto/Thinkstock; **Page 171** © Ryan McVay/Photodisc/Thinkstock; **Page 181** © Creatas/Thinkstock; **Page 194** © Reflekta/ShutterStock, Inc.

☐ Chapter 5

Page 207 © iStockphoto.com/Thomas_ EyeDesign; **Page 209** © Hemera/Thinkstock;

Page 210 © Monkey Business Images /ShutterStock, Inc.; **Page 211** © Blend Images /ShutterStock, Inc.; **Page 214** © Lisa F. Young /ShutterStock, Inc.

☐ Chapter 6

Page 240 © wavebreakmedia ltd/ShutterStock, Inc.; **Page 247** © iStockphoto.com/RichVintage

☐ Chapter 7

Page 276 © Ryan McVay/Photodisc /Thinkstock; **Page 296** © Purestock/Thinkstock

☐ Chapter 8

Page 317 © Jupiterimages/Comstock /Thinkstock

☐ Chapter 9

Page 384 © Robert Kneschke/ShutterStock, Inc.

☐ Chapter 10

Page 428 © Hemera/Thinkstock; **Page 432** © iStockphoto.com/dlewis33

☐ Chapter 11

Page 470 © Jupiterimages/Comstock /Thinkstock; **Page 471** © iStockphoto.com /vgajic